L. M. Portnoy

Radiologic Diagnosis of Gastric Cancer

A new Outlook

L. M. Portnoy

Radiologic Diagnosis of Gastric Cancer

A new Outlook

Springer

Dr. L. M. Portnoy
1st Aeroportovskaya, 6-196
125319 Moscow
Russia

Springer Medizin Verlag Heidelberg
ISBN-10 3-540-29120-2 1. Auflage Springer-Verlag Berlin Heidelberg New York
ISBN-13 978-3-540-29120-2

Bibliografische Information der Deutschen Bibliothek
Die Deutsche Bibliothek verzeichnet diese Publikation in der Deutschen Nationalbibliografie; detaillierte bibliografische Daten sind im Internet über http://dnb.ddb.de abrufbar.

Springer Medizin Verlag

SPIN 1156 0968
Umschlaggestaltung: deblik, Berlin
Satz: typographics GmbH, Darmstadt
Druck: Stürtz AG, Würzburg

Gedruckt auf säurefreiem Papier 18/5135/DK – 5 4 3 2 1 0

Author's Foreword

We chose the radiological diagnosis of gastric cancer as the subject of our monograph for the following reasons: First, the diagnosis of gastric cancer has not improved radically during the past 10 years despite the extensive use of endoscopy in practical medicine. Second, the potentials of radiological examination and traditional X-ray diagnosis of gastric cancer are greatly underestimated.

Our thorough and detailed analysis of the situation based on our experience, both scientific and practical, should serve to remind health-care authorities and most clinicians about the advantages of radiological methods in diagnosing gastric cancer. It is necessary to radically revise the diagnostic concept, which was formed in the 1960s–1970s and was based solely on endoscopic examinations.

This book emphasizes the objective necessity of returning to the radiological diagnosis of gastric cancer in close collaboration with endoscopy. The monograph will be helpful to both practical radiological diagnosticians and gastroenterologists, oncologists, surgeons, and health-care authorities. It presents entirely new methodological approaches to the X-ray examination of the stomach and corrected semiotics of the tumor. We also provide a list of clinical symptoms of the disease. A special section in the monograph deals with screening of populations for gastric cancer with special emphasis on radiology.

We present comparative data to show the relations between X-ray data and morphological evidence obtained by examination of resected stomach tissues.

We also describe in detail all currently used methods, such as single and double-contrast barium investigations, ultrasonography, computed tomography, and magnetic resonance imaging. We describe the methodology and semiotics of gastric cancer, which were verified by using these methods, and the results of comparative studies obtained using traditional X-ray examination and morphological studies.

In the section dedicated to ultrasonographic and tomographic methods of examination we explain our point of view regarding the possibilities of modern radiological diagnosis in staging gastric cancer, in determining its spread over the stomach walls and invasion of the neighboring organs and tissues.

In this monograph we also discuss the indications for radical surgery which, in our opinion, need correction as well, because only histological evidence is now regarded as an indication for the operative treatment of gastric cancer.

January, 2006

Dr. L. M. Portnoy

Preface

This book deals with problems which are sufficiently important to become the subject of studies. Cancer of the stomach remains one of the most pressing medical problems. Meanwhile, scientific and practical interest in this problem has markedly diminished during recent years. According to some experts, this can be explained first by the decreasing incidence of gastric cancer. But this concerns only some developed countries, where effective measures are taken for the prevention and early diagnosis of malignant tumors. It is noteworthy that everything concerning gastric cancer today requires objective and comprehensive analysis. Another important factor is the vast amount of scientific information which has been accumulated on this problem. According to popular opinion, all possible scientific research in the diagnosis of gastric cancer has already been completed. But this is not so. Factors that force us to reconsider the problem include the relatively high incidence and low percentage of cancer diagnosis at its early stages, the high occurrence of inoperable tumors and the low 5-year survival, certain changes in the concept of gastric cancer morphogenesis and, more particularly, the prevalence of diffuse forms, and »new« proportions regarding the primary locations of the tumor in various parts of the stomach, characterized by significantly increasing frequency of the primary lesion on the greater curvature and the anterior wall of the stomach.

The leading role of the traditional X-ray studies in the complex examination of gastroenterological patients was challenged by excessive indulgence in modern endoscopy, which became dominant in the diagnosis of gastroenterological pathologies. But close studies of this problem show that the diagnostic benefits of endoscopy are overestimated. The incorporation of new, highly informative technologies (quite unjustified in some cases) into the set of procedures used for primary diagnosis of gastrointestinal pathologies pushed back the traditional X-ray methods.

Needless to say, despite recent advancements in the treatment of gastric cancer, in surgery in particular, the efficacy of this treatment depends largely on timely diagnosis of the disease.

We believe that it is necessary to change the commonly held attitude regarding the relationship between endoscopy and X-ray methods of examination, with due consideration given to the changed views on the morphogenesis of gastric cancer. It should be remembered that in its essence, the traditional X-ray examination is now one of the branches of radiological diagnosis which has been supplemented with new possibilities owing to the appearance of up-dated technologies such as ultrasonography, computed tomography, and magnetic resonance tomography. They all, in combination with the traditional X-ray examination, have significantly improved the overall diagnostic potential of the X-ray in revealing gastric cancer.

The authors believe that the main objective of this book, i.e., to share the vast experience of the authors and our colleagues in the radiological diagnosis of gastric cancer with radiologists, gastroenterologists, oncologists, and surgeons, will justify the resolute manner in which our opinions are presented in some of the sections. This sort of confidence is also based on our firm belief that every error in clinical examination of the patient, and every incorrect interpretation of the findings, is detrimental to the effectiveness of treatment of patients with cancer of the stomach.

Introduction

Until the 1960s–1970s, X-ray examination was the leading method of diagnosing gastrointestinal diseases [1, 11]. A great army of experienced radiologists in Russia and other countries were able to effectively establish the diagnosis of gastrointestinal diseases. At that time, no one suspected that the X-ray examination might be ever displaced from the diagnostic algorithm.

Meanwhile, significant changes in the diagnosis of gastric cancer took place during the last decades of the twentieth century. This period (beginning with the 1960s–1970s) was characterized by the almost unrivalled prevalence of endoscopy [62, 79, 90]. In 1958, the appearance of fiber-optic endoscopic tools initiated a new diagnostic trend in gastroenterology and gastroentero-oncology. The physicians were given the chance to visualize the mucous membranes in vivo. Fiber-optic instruments were successfully used to diagnose diseases of the gastrointestinal viscera, including cancer of the stomach.

Beginning in 1964, fibergastroscopes became available, which could be used to take samples of new growth tissues. In 1978, instruments equipped with photo and cine cameras made it possible to record the endoscopic pictures.

On the whole, the increasing popularity of this trend could be described as an endoscopic boom. An avalanche of scientific papers, monographs, and other publications appeared. All were dedicated to the use of endoscopes in the diagnosis of practically all gastrointestinal pathologies, gastric cancer included. The number of physicians who started practicing endoscopic diagnosis increased accordingly. Meanwhile endoscopy is one of the main diagnostic tools, and each gastroenterologist must be able to use it in his or her examination of patients with gastroenterological diseases.

Once given the chance to visualize the surface of the mucous membrane (we do mean the surface of the mucous membrane, rather than the wall of the stomach), gastroenterology abruptly changed its diagnostic orientation: The proportion of X-ray examinations dramatically decreased, whereas endoscopy became practically the only instrumental method to reveal diseases of the gastrointestinal tract, gastric cancer included [32, 58].

The absolute domination of endoscopy did not, however, increase the percentage of diagnosed »minor« cancers of the stomach. Following the experience of Japanese physicians, who significantly improved the quality of diagnosis of gastric cancer, in its initial stages in particular, by population screening, physicians have also markedly improved the situation. Radiology and now radiological diagnosis and the traditional method of examination, is slowly but steadily regaining its position as one of the main diagnostic methods used for patients with gastroenterological pathologies. All this, after all, has markedly improved the effectiveness of uncovering gastric cancer and increased the 5-year survival of patients.

In 1962, an endoscopic classification of early gastric cancer was worked out. This classification was acknowledged not only by endoscopists but also by diagnosticians of other specialties, X-ray and morphology experts included. Endoscopy is undoubtedly a powerful tool for diagnosing various gastroenterological diseases. Many scientific and practical developments have been achieved using endoscopy, and many medical researchers and practitioners began to regard endoscopy as the gold standard for abdominal visualization. But during the last decades of the past century, the proportion of infiltrative gastric cancer increased significantly, and endoscopy often fails to answer many practical questions in such cases.

Practitioners often question which of the diagnostic tools is more informative, radiology or endoscopy. Their interest in this problem is easy to understand. They are often faced with a discrepancy between the results of diagnostic examinations and the final diagnosis. Thus, they cannot make a final decision about which primary examination method they should choose, and they tend to assume that endoscopy is the sole sufficient examination, simply because this was the traditional attitude to endoscopy in the second half of the twentieth century. Strange as it may appear, no one can give a definite answer to their question. This is a kind of medical paradox. Both methods are aimed at attaining the same goal. But they cannot be compared as regards their informative value, because the current roentgenosemiotics of gastric cancer is founded on a standpoint that is quite different from the former one. It is now based on the evaluation of the stomach wall rather than on characteristics of mucosal relief, including so-called microrelief. Neither can the two methods be regarded as being in contraposition to each other. In future, they can probably work together. Endoscopic ultrasonography and optical coherent tomography are a good example of how two examination methods can be combined. Informative value is a relative notion, and it depends largely on the particular diagnostic apparatus and materials used for examination of patients and, of course, on the professional skill of the examiner.

An oft-cited criticism of radiological diagnosis is the ionizing radiation, which is undoubtedly harmful for the patient. But modern X-ray units and digital technologies with high-quality contrast media can improve X-ray examinations and broaden the potentials of X-ray diagnosis with a substantially reduced radiation dose for the patient. Of course, updated digital X-ray units and MRI are expensive, but we cannot make a diagnosis without these new modalities in the twenty-first century.

The other reason for the inefficient organization of diagnostic examinations of gastroenterologic patients is related directly to radiological diagnosis, and more particularly to the almost complete dismissal of X-ray examinations as a way of uncovering gastric cancer. The opinion exists that tumors are exclusively the subject of oncology. But we believe that one of the main aims of the field of oncology is (in addition to treatment of patients) the organizational and methodological management of oncological services rendered to the population, with due consideration of medical and social aspects. The problem of early diagnosis of malignant tumors of the gastrointestinal tract, which constitute 25–30% of all tumors, will not be solved unless the thesis suggesting that the most common tumors, such as tumors of the lung, stomach, mammary gland, and rectum should be revealed at the stage of outpatient examination with active involvement of screening (selective screening in particular) is adopted as an axiom. Thus, X-ray diagnosticians must do their best to reveal tumoral diseases of the gastrointestinal tract.

Based on our long and vast experience in discovering gastric cancer, we must say that, since the introduction of endoscopy into gastro-oncology and the active dismissal of the X-ray method, there has been no improvement in the early diagnosis of gastric cancer. The 5-year survival, one of the major proofs of successful surgical treatment, remains at a very low level [6, 8, 16].

There are periodical discussions in the literature about the necessity of screening the so-called risk groups in the population for gastric cancer aimed at early revealing of carcinoma. On the whole, this problem has been solved only in Japan, where gastric cancer was extremely frequent in the 1960s, accounting for 40–45% of oncological morbidity. The Japanese used a modified X-ray examination with double-contrast X-ray investigation of the stomach to screen their population. Remote-control X-ray units were developed which reduced the radiation dose for the personnel and thus increased the number of examinations that could be conducted by one roentgenological team. It is worthy of note that Japan was the first country to employ modern endoscopy. Owing to economic considerations, this method did not become popular in countries where the incidence of gastric cancer was lower. A concept of examining risk groups was produced as an alternative, and programs for prevention of pre-cancer pathologies of the gastrointestinal tract were also adopted. These measures did, after all, substantially reduce the incidence of gastric cancer; they increased the number of early (minor) cancers diagnosed, and increased the 5-year survival in the USA, Great Britain, Canada, Belgium, and some other countries [125, 144, 165, 170, 186, 236].

The usefulness of the formation of such risk groups with the aim of increasing the effectiveness of gastric cancer diagnosis is indisputable. But now a new subject of special concern has appeared which is an important argument for improving the current disadvantageous situation in the diagnosis of this pathology, namely: the accents in the morphogenesis of gastric cancer have radically changed [102, 121, 244]. By using the double-contrast technique extensively in combination with elements of the traditional X-ray examination, we have acquired convincing evidence of the leading position of diffuse and mixed tumors among the anatomical forms of gastric cancer. Slowly developing and only manifesting clinically at later stages, intramural tumors are the most difficult to reveal, even using the most advanced technologies. Such tumors show themselves as minimal changes on the surface of the mucous membrane of the stomach and are a serious challenge to endoscopic diagnosis of the tumor. And finally, it is necessary to mention a significant increase in the incidence of cancer of the upper part of the stomach, the greater curvature, and the anterior wall of the stomach. This suggests that it is necessary to radically correct the existing viewpoints on the problem of gastric cancer diagnosis, based mostly on the endoscopic classification of 1962, and to emphasize the particular necessity of urgently resuming radiological diagnosis, such as the traditional X-ray technique. Working in close contact with endoscopists we became convinced that, in a significant proportion of cases, the current radiological and endoscopic semiotics of early cancer of the stomach, in its classical understanding, restricts the framework of diagnosis of carcinomas at their initial stages [28, 32].

In this connection we return to the problem of linitis plastica, the form of diffuse cancer, in which we see the origin of the difficulties that persist today and are connected with the diagnosis of gastric cancer on the whole. We appreciate the authors who, early in the twentieth century, interpreted linitis plastica as being the most common and fatal disease, but today we regard it from the standpoints of current possibilities of diagnosis of the disease at its early stage. Furthermore, guided by the pathogenetic mechanisms of propagation of blastomatous infiltration in linitis plastica patients, we have arrived at the conclusion that their major elements occur in most patients with gastric cancer.

We have formulated a special symptom complex characterizing the initial manifestations of gastric tumor [31, 32]. Thus it can be definitely stated that, if our aim is to improve the situation in gastroenterology and gastroentero-oncology, the traditional significance of radiology in the diagnosis of gastric cancer must be restored.

Radiological diagnosis methods have changed substantially, mainly because of developments in digital technologies. Modern digital X-ray units have greatly reduced the doses for patients and simultaneously increased diagnostic efficiency. Ultrasonography, CT and MRI have broadened the possibilities for radiological diagnosis of the gastrointestinal tract on the whole and of gastric cancer in particular [2, 20, 29, 49, 92, 230, 273].

Contents

Some Current Problems in the Epidemiology of Gastric Cancer

The epidemiology of gastric cancer changed substantially during the course of the past century. These changes were closely connected with social developments [23, 211]. We will discuss the current situation in detail in this chapter.

Tumors of the alimentary tract remain one of the main problems in gastroenterology. On the whole, cancer of the digestive organs is the leading pathology in the structure of oncological morbidity and mortality. The history of the genesis and development of oncology as a major and complex medical field shows that, for a long period of time, gastric cancer remained a kind of basic model for studies of numerous oncological problems. This was quite natural, because during the first decades of the past century it was generally belief that gastric cancer was the most common of all tumoral diseases. Many existing clinicomorphological and diagnostic oncological postulates were studied in detail in gastric cancer patients.

At the present time, the picture of the oncological morbidity and mortality of various cancers worldwide has changed somewhat. According to the International Agency for Research on Cancer (IARC), in 2000, 10.1 million new cases of cancer of all localizations were diagnosed; there were 6.2 million fatal outcomes of cancer and a total of 22 million patients with cancer in the 5-year survival period. Compared with the figures for 1990, cancer incidence in 2000 increased by 22%. The cancer profile varies within a wide range depending on the parameter studied (morbidity or mortality) [219, 220].

In 2000, 86 700 new cases of gastric cancer were diagnosed (8.4% of all cancer patients). Gastric cancer morbidity is fourth in line of frequency, after cancer of the lungs (1.2 million, or 12.3%), the mammary gland (1.05 million, or 10.4%), and colorectal cancer (94 500, or 9.4%). Nevertheless, gastric cancer mortality has remained consistently in second place for several decades, following only pulmonary carcinoma (10.4% vs 17.8%, respectively; ▸ Diagrams 1 and 2) [80, 220].

Diagram 1. Structure of global cancer morbidity

Pulmonary cancer	12.3%
Mammary cancer	10.4%
Colorectal cancer	9.4%
Gastric cancer	8.4%
Other cancers	59.2%

Diagram 2. Structure of global cancer mortality

Pulmonary cancer	17.8%
Gastric cancer	10.4%
Cancer of the liver	8.8%
Other cancers	63.0%

In recent years, the incidence of gastric cancer has decreased in some developed countries, and this decrease has been quite substantial in some of them, the mean reduction being 10–19% per decade. Thus, since 1930, the incidence of gastric cancer in the USA has decreased four times, dropping to as low as six to seven cases per 100,000 population. During the past 50 years, it has decreased from 33 to ten per 100,000 cases in male, and from 30 to five per 100,000 cases in female subjects. Nonetheless, gastric cancer remains 7th among malignant tumors in the USA [87, 200]. In 1996, gastric cancer was diagnosed in about 22,800 Americans, and it became the cause of death in 14,000. In Finland, the incidence of gastric carcinoma has decreased by 31% during the past two decades. In Great Britain, Belgium, and Canada, in the countries of Western Europe, North America, and Southern Asia, the situation is relatively positive [149, 237, 276].

The incidence of gastric cancer in the rest of the world is far more significant. Almost two thirds of the overall gastric cancer incidence is in the underdeveloped countries. But the morbidity is also high in some economically developed countries. These include the countries of Eastern Europe, Eastern Asia, South and Central America, some republics of the former Soviet Union, and most African countries.

In Russia, gastric cancer accounts for 12.7% of the overall oncological morbidity, which is much higher than the average world incidence. In men, it stands second (14.7%), in women, third (10.8%) in the list of malignant tumors. As regards cancer mortality, gastric tumors constitute 16.7% [8, 76]. Gastric cancer morbidity is the highest in Korea (70.02 per 100 000 men and 25.02 per 100 000 women) and in Japan (69.2 per 100 000 men and 28.6 per 100 000 women). Survival of gastric cancer patients is relatively high (52%) in Japan, where mass screening by gastrophotofluoroscopy has been performed since the 1960s, the time when the morbidity was dramatically high: 40–45% of overall tumor morbidity. Survival in the USA, Europe, and China varies from 20 to 25% [191, 267].

The relatively good survival rate in Japan is explained above all by early diagnosis of the disease, based on complex examination of the stomach, including primary X-ray with subsequent selective endoscopy. As a result, the disease in its first and second stages is diagnosed in 45.7% and 11.9%, respectively, whereas in the USA, where endoscopy dominates the diagnostic techniques, gastric cancer is diagnosed only at its third and fourth stages (35.% and 30.1%, respectively). As a result, the 5-year survival is twice as high in Japan as in the USA [112, 129, 130, 134, 221].

It is quite natural that specialists question why almost 50% of patients in Japan undergo surgery for minor cancer, whereas in the developed countries the percentage of such patients is below 10%, the diagnostic potential being practically similar in these countries. It is the opinion of pathological anatomists that one of the causes of this phenomenon is the different criteria for estimating malignant new growths. Meanwhile, these are decisive in the healthcare system. To be more explicit: Either the patients operated on in Japan had no cancer, or in the other developed countries they do not diagnose cancer early in order to avoid having to operate on the patients in the early stage of the disease. This dispute resulted in adoption of the Vienna classification of gastrointestinal neoplasia in 2000 [237]. According to this classification, morphological changes in the mucous membrane are divided into five groups:

1. Absence of neoplasia and dysplasia – normal mucous membrane, gastritis, intestinal metaplasia
2. Indefinite neoplasia or dysplasia, diagnosed in cases where it is not clear whether the changes are regenerative or neoplastic. Inflamma-tion and atrophic changes interfere with diagnosis.
3. Non-invasive neoplasia of low degree – low degree of dysplasia or adenoma
4. Non-invasive neoplasia of high degree:
   a. High-degree adenoma or dysplasia
   b. Non-invasive carcinoma (carcinoma in situ)
   c. Suspected invasive carcinoma
5. Invasive neoplasia
   a. Adenocarcinoma growing through proper mucous membrane
   b. Deeper carcinoma

Analysis of the international classification of neoplasia shows that pathomorphologists now agree with those concepts and terms

which they formerly rejected. First of all, dysplasia is now defined as neoplasia, i.e., tumor. It follows, therefore, that it shall be appropriately considered by clinicians.

However, the marked difference in percentage of patients operated on for minor cancer cannot be explained solely by the different approach to morphological characteristics of changes occurring in the mucous membrane. One of the causes is found in the different clinical approach to the problem of minor gastric cancer. The economically developed countries rely mostly on endoscopy, whereas in Japan the X-ray examination is used, followed by endoscopy. This explains the high percentage of early diagnoses of cancer in Japan: Based on X-ray findings, the endoscopist more accurately examines changes in the mucous membrane and takes tissue specimens for histological examination, and the results are estimated by the physician on the basis of the complex of findings rather than on the pathomorphological data alone.

In Russia, in more than 75% of patients with newly diagnosed primary gastric cancer the disease is already in the third and fourth stages of its development. At the same time, the number of X-ray examinations performed on the stomach is steadily decreasing, during the past decade from 6 to 3 million. It is worthy of note that early in the 1980s, the yearly number of X-ray examinations in Japan was 4 million.

Some Russian authors explain the observed reduction of gastric cancer incidence in the world as whole with the introduction of endoscopy into practical medicine, and they extrapolate this tendency onto Russia. Meanwhile, the situation in Russia is quite different. In the 1960s, the operability of tumors at the moment of establishing the diagnosis was only 20–35%. It remains at the same level today. According to medical statistics and the data of the information-analytical center of the Health Ministry of the Russian Federation, among 48,989 patients newly diagnosed with gastric cancer in 1998, a radical operation was performed in only 26% of cases. Only 17.6% of patients were diagnosed with tumors in the 1st and 2nd stage. The number of gastrointestinal cancer patients in whom test or explorative laparotomy is performed amounts to 13–28%; 58% of patients with a primarily established diagnosis die within the first year of observation.

One factor influencing the reduced global incidence of gastric cancer is connected with a thorough study of the effect of Helicobacter pylori on the onset of gastric cancer. H. pylori is one of the most common infections in the world. Epidemiological data supporting a connection between the genesis of malignant tumors of the stomach and chronic H. pylori infection appeared so convincing that the International Agency for Gastric Cancer Research classified H. pylori as a carcinogen of the first group. A marked reduction in the incidence of gastric cancer during the past decade is characteristic of those countries where H. pylori infection was eradicated in practically the entire population. If the H. pylori hypothesis is correct, then Belgium has carried out primary prophylaxis of the population for gastric cancer.

An analysis of epidemiological characteristics of gastric cancer in various regions of the world shows that there is a direct dependence of gastric cancer morbidity and mortality on the H. pylori infection level and on socioeconomic conditions. The following triad is characteristic of the underdeveloped countries: high occurrence of H. pylori infection, gastroduodenal ulcer, and gastric cancer. Gastric cancer mortality in such countries exceeds 30 per 100,000 population. Conversely, in economically developed countries with low infection indices, the gastric cancer death rate is less than 10 per 100,000 population.

Despite the high standard of living in Japan, gastric cancer morbidity in that country is among the highest. However, during the period from 1965 to 1995 mortality decreased by half. The H. pylori infection rate also decreased by half, whereas the incidence of atrophic gastritis decreased to one sixth of the previous value.

The incidence of gastric cancer associated with H. pylori is enormously high, especially in the developing countries. According to some authors, this neoplasia is four to six times higher in infected patients than in non-infected subjects. In a population of 100,000 aged over 30 with an infection level of 35%, gastric cancer occurs in about one per 100 infected subjects versus one per 750 non-infected persons. According to the data for prospective (cohort) studies, the relative risk associated with H. pylori infection is 2.5. The proportion of infected members of the population is higher in less developed countries (80–90%) than in developed countries (50%). In view of these data, H. pylori is regarded as a causative agent in 50% of gastric cancer cases worldwide, the proportion being 55% in less-developed countries (42% on the whole) [113, 138]. The results of epidemiological studies thus suggest that H. pylori is involved in the initiation of malignant transformation of the gastric mucous membrane [112]. Another possible infectious agent associated with gastric cancer is the Epstein-Barr virus [140].

In our opinion, this popular trend in explaining the problem is not fully justified and is due mostly to a certain boom in the research conducted in this particular field. We are firmly convinced that in the very near future, everything that is connected with the H. pylori problem will be verified, including the role that is attributed to these micro-organisms as the triggering factor of gastric cancer. However, a great many environmental factors also exist, for example, smoking tobacco and inadequate nutrition, namely, an imbalance between the excessive intake of salt, animal fats, nitrate-containing canned foods, and smoked foods, which may be involved in the onset of gastric cancer, and a deficient intake of vitamin C and antioxidants, which are contained in fruits and vegetables, etc.

Gastric cancer demonstrates a great variety of mutations in the genome of tumor cells and gene instability. These events may occur at the early stages of chronic gastritis, before detectable morphological, endoscopic, or clinical signs of neoplasia appear. Gastric cancer is characterized by a variety of genotypical forms. This accounts for the multifactorial pathogenesis and morphological variability of the pathology, whereas the clinical course is characterized by a large spectrum of syndromes and diseases which are associated with a high risk of cancer. Therefore, one specific carcinogen cannot be regarded as the sole cause of gastric cancer [135, 195, 233, 245, 246, 250, 256].

Studies on population migration showed that living conditions in early childhood are important for the genesis of gastric cancer. In migrants of the first generation, gastric cancer mortality is similar to that in the areas of their origin. This also holds for migration within one country. But among second-generation migrants, gastric cancer mortality nears that of the country where they were born and grew up [108, 171, 255].

Environmental effects and H. pylori infection are believed to be more important in the onset of the intestinal type of gastric cancer. The reduced incidence of gastric cancer in developed countries refers to this type. It occurs mainly in the distal part of the stomach and is characterized by expansive growth. Therefore, we would like to contradict some researchers who believe that the worldwide situation with gastric cancer incidence is gradually improving. As a matter of fact, the situation is somewhat different. Quite different again is the epidemiology of diffuse gastric cancer, and high priority problems of gastro-oncology are associated with this type.

At the dawn of endoscopy, exophytic cancer (a morphologically intestinal type) prevailed. Endoscopy unambiguously diagnosed this type of cancer, and most physicians hurriedly (without sufficient substantiation) concluded that endoscopy was an absolutely suitable method of examining patients with gastrointestinal pathologies. They therefore excluded the X-ray from the diagnostic algorithm.

At the present time, despite the controversial estimates of the role of H. pylori in the onset of gastric cancer of the intestinal and diffuse types, it has been proved that both of these cancers are associated to a certain degree with H. pylori infection. However, the higher incidence of H. pylori infection occurs in patients with intestinal type cancer.

The incidence of H. pylori infection is the same in male and female patients, but in the age group under 60, gastric cancer in men occurs 2.2 times more frequently than in women, whereas in men over 60 it occurs 1.4 times more frequently. This suggests the existence of risk factors other than H. pylori in young men and certain defense factors in young women. It can thus be concluded that the global reduction of morbidity refers only to the intestinal type of gastric cancer with predominantly distal location, and only to those countries where the economic potential is sufficiently high to allow prevention of pre-cancer pathologies [21, 25, 32].

The onset of diffuse gastric cancer is believed to depend largely on genetic factors. This type of cancer occurs at about the same frequency in men and women, and is associated with the blood group II(A); it occurs more frequently in the young [99, 108]. Cases of familial gastric cancer have been known for a long time. In recent years, marked progress has been attained in studies on the genetic causes of infiltrative forms. In familial forms of pathology, genetic defects are inherited and may be found by statistic, cytogenetic, and molecular-biological analysis. Thus, the 21st chromosome is found in three of four members of a family with a high risk of gastric cancer [21].

The incidence of diffuse cancer has never decreased, but since 1976 it has been slowly but steadily increasing. Moreover, this tendency is observed worldwide. In all regions of the globe where the incidence of intestinal-type cancer has shown a tendency to decrease, the incidence of diffuse cancer has remained the same or even increased despite various preventive measures. High mortality and low 5-year survival are also associated with this type, because diffuse cancer is characterized by infiltrative propagation and relatively rapid metastasis and (especially important) is very difficult to diagnose by endoscopy. According to some authors, it occurs in 52–88% of all gastric cancer cases [30, 152, 179, 269].

During three recent decades, in contrast to the general tendency of the incidence of gastric cancer to decrease, the incidence of proximal cancer of the stomach has increased [175, 270]. Studies conducted from 1985 to 1996 at two hospitals in Little Rock (Arkansas, USA) showed an increasing incidence of gastric cardia cancer. The researchers divided their patients into three cohorts by age to establish that the frequency of gastric cardia cancer in cohorts 1, 2, and 3 was 31%, 36%, and 42%, respectively; the survival was 5, 8, and 8 months, respectively [137].

According to some authors, cancer of the proximal stomach occurs in about 16% cases, and according to others, in 30%, compared with the classical 10% as reported by R. Borrman (1926). It should be noted that the incidence increases by 4% a year [52, 96, 134, 186, 233, 259, 267]. During the past 38 years, the incidence of cardioesophageal cancer in the southeastern regions of the United Kingdom tripled [171]. Studies conducted at the Moscow Region Research Institute MONIKI during the past decades also demonstrate the increasing incidence of cancer of the upper part of the stomach, the diagnosis of which is especially difficult [27, 39]. According to our statistical data, the overall incidence of this cancer in the period of the past 34 years was 20.28% (293 cases). But during the 5-year period of 1971–1975, the number of cases was 24 (11.3%), and during the period from 1996 to 2000 this number increased to 55 (27.9%).

The causes of these changes in topography remain so far unknown. True, it was found that this situation agrees with the increasing incidence of Barrett's esophagus and adenocarcinoma of the lower third of the esophagus.

A relationship between H. pylori infection and cancer of the gastric cardia has not been proved. But there exists an opinion that the eradication of H. pylori may increase the incidence of cancer of gastric cardia and the esophagus. It is believed that this happens because of increasing acidity, which provokes the onset of reflux esophagitis, which in turn promotes the onset of Barrett's esophagus. In 1997–1998, publications appeared with paradoxical (at first sight) titles, such as »H. pylori prevents esophageal cancer«. Based on these data, M. Blaser formulated a hypothesis according to which H. pylori may have not only a pathogenic but also a protective effect on the human body. But it would be dangerous to eradicate H. pylori, a micro-organism which has cohabited with the human race for millennia [94]. This ambiguity in estimating H. pylori suggests the necessity of further studies on the protective potentials of this micro-organism.

The phenomenon of a protective effect of one disease against another has been known. But it would be hasty to use it in practical medicine at the present time. On the whole, H. pylori are not now regarded as useful bacteria but rather as micro-organisms causing chronic inflammation, which impairs the function of the parietal cells and possibly causes atrophic gastritis. Evolution of gastritis of this type and the markedly increasing longevity will eventually restore gastric cancer to the position it formerly occupied in the statistics of morbidity and mortality.

Based on cancer morbidity and mortality data of the past, one can predict the future of cancer (of course, with numerous limitations). It is possible to estimate demographic effects (growth of population and its aging) on the incidence of cancer in forthcoming decades, because we know that cancer attacks mostly the aged, and the proportion of the aged in the near future is predictable. The rapidly increasing absolute and relative number of aged people, owing to a longer life span, was the main characteristic of the human race in the twentieth century. According to current prognosis, if the existing rate of population growth persists, the number of people with cancer of all localizations will be 15 million in 2020 and about 24 million in 2050. The mortality will be 10 million in 2020 and 156 million in 2050 [220]. Aging of the human population indicates that the proportion of the aged patients with cancer will steadily increase in both less and more developed countries. This is only a tentative prognosis, but it definitely illustrates the increasing morbidity and mortality owing to aging. This illustration, however, suggests the imperative necessity of searching for new tools to control the pathology.

It is quite evident that the diagnostics of gastric cancer by no means influences its morbidity. We therefore suggest that this problem be solved by gastroenterologists. But mortality and the 5-year survival depend entirely on diagnosis. As far back as the first half of the past century, it became clear that only timely radical surgery can help cancer patients. Therefore, timely diagnosis of early forms of cancer, especially its endophytic forms, which are difficult to visualize endoscopically, is the pressing problem today. It follows that, in view of the overall situation, it is urgently necessary to revive radiological diagnosis, and especially the traditional X-ray, and to put it back into gastroenterology, where it must occupy its rightful position alongside of endoscopy. Only reasonable combination of the two methods (endoscopy and X-ray) can radically change the discouraging situation in the diagnosis of gastric cancer.

Morphology of Gastric Cancer

(with I. A. Kazantseva and L. E. Gaganov)

Introduction

Intensive studies carried out during the past several decades have made important corrections in our understanding of gastric cancer. According to modern concepts, gastric cancer is subdivided into three major histological types: intestinal, diffuse, and mixed. This classification was proposed by P. Laurent, who grouped cancer by its etiology, morphogenesis, macro- and microcharacteristics, the specific features of the course, and prognosis of the disease [178].

Intestinal carcinoma is represented by adenocarcinomas of various natures. This tumor is often called expansive, after the specific character of its growth. Its other name is epidemic cancer, which reflects the relative prevalence of this tumor in the structure of cancer morbidity and mortality in the first half of the twentieth century. It should be noted, however, that this epidemiological characteristic of intestinal cancer no longer corresponds to modern statistics, because there is much evidence for the appreciable reduction of its incidence. Our own findings also confirm this thesis. Morphogenesis of intestinal cancer is associated with chronic atrophic gastritis, dysplasia, and intestinal metaplasia [61, 110, 163]. The tumor would normally occur in the distal part of the stomach of aged male patients [246]. Macroscopically, the intestinal type of gastric cancer would more frequently be formed by the exophytic component of the tumor, although our research at MONIKI does not suggest that this phenomenon can be regarded as an absolute rule [36, 37, 48].

Diffuse carcinoma is represented by the signet-ring cell and non-differentiated forms. The tumor is characterized mostly by infiltrative growth, which accounts for its name of *infiltrating* cancer. It contrasts with intestinal carcinoma and has a different name: endemic cancer. The incidence of such cancer increases slowly but steadily. This is confirmed by the results of our observations over many years.

The prognosis of the tumor is much worse, and as a rule the tumor develops without visible endoscopic signs of the preceding mucosal affections [146, 228, 234].

Incidence

A mixed tumor combines the elements of the intestinal and diffuse carcinomas; in other words, it is an adenocarcinoma of various differentiation with the signet-ring cell component. The incidence of such forms of cancer tends to increase, which is confirmed by studies conducted at MONIKI during recent decades [31, 33].

Application of the epidemiological method to gastric cancer studies helped to establish climate-geographic, socioeconomic, genetic, and other factors influencing morbidity, and to estimate their importance in the etiology and pathogenesis of each particular form of cancer [109, 154, 245, 254, 270]. Statistical findings indicate that the incidence of gastric cancer in many economically developed countries has decreased during the past three or four decades. But these changes in the epidemiology of cancer are due to the decreasing incidence of carcinomas of the intestinal type (► see Diagram 3). Unfortunately, gastric cancer morbidity and mortality remain high in the countries of Latin America, China, Serbia, Montenegro, Finland, and Russia [218].

Dynamic observations of the past decades show that reduced incidence of intestinal carcinoma is not the only novelty in epidemiology of cancer. Researchers report a steady growth of diffuse and mixed cancer morbidity. Note that both diffuse and mixed cancers are diagnosed at their early stage only in rare cases; they are characterized by a rapid course and early metastasis, which markedly aggravate the prognosis. Thus, the increased number of cases of carcinoma of diffuse and mixed type suggests the necessity of revising the current approach to the diagnosis of gastric cancer.

Histogenesis

The current theory of the histogenesis of gastric cancer explains development of this malignancy by successive gene mutations in epithelial cells of the glandular generative zone (which later turn into tumor cells), which can stimulate the onset of the intestinal forms of gastric cancer with its subsequent transformation into diffuse cancer; or they can stimulate directly the onset of purely diffuse cancer [101, 122, 199, 212].

In normal mucous membrane, proliferating cells move upwards from the gland neck (for renewal of the superficial epithelium) and downwards (to form the gland) (► see Scheme 1). Glandular fragments containing mutated epithelial cells may, in some cases, be obliterated and incorporated into the proper mucous membrane. Entrapped malignant cells may remain inside such glands for a long time and later initiate the onset of gastric cancer of the intestinal type (► Scheme 2b) [127, 128, 200].

In diffuse type gastric carcinoma, malignant cells of the generative zone of the glands (due to mutation of genes that are responsible for maintenance of intercellular contacts and protein synthesis by the basal membrane) can migrate into the depth of the proper mucous membrane, thus initiating diffuse type cancer (► see Scheme 2a) [22, 239, 258].

These processes are closely connected with the functioning of the system, which is controlled mainly by intracellular genes such as p53 and bcl-2 [103, 194]. Gene p53 controls cell proliferation, differentiation, DNA synthesis and reparation, and also programmed cell death, called apoptosis [104, 166, 173, 177]; bcl-2 protein controls apoptosis [198]. Malignancy is possible in cases of reduced apoptosis activity and at intensive proliferation [142, 199, 215, 253, 256]. Apoptosis decreases in case of a mutation of p53, as a result of which it skips gene damage [152, 275].

Localization

As a rule, gastric cancer originates at junctions of the anatomical parts of the stomach, e.g., the prepyloric and antral parts, the lesser curvature, or the gastroesophageal junction [120]. According to the majority of reports, in 50% of cases cancer occurs in the pyloric part of the stomach (so-called distal cancer) (◘ Fig. 1). In 15% of cases, the carcinoma originates on the lesser curvature (◘ Fig. 2). In 16% of cas-

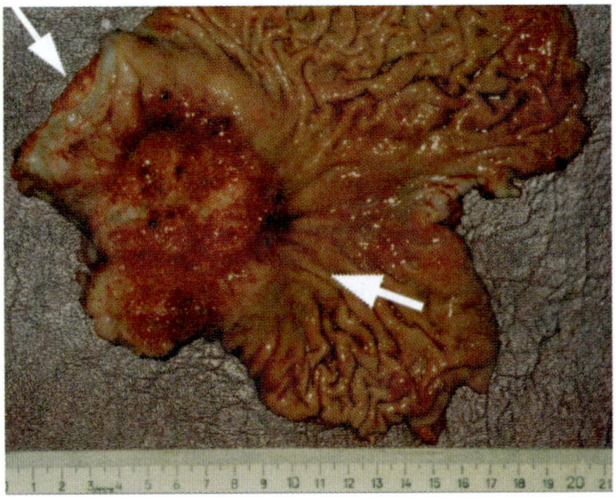

Fig. 1. Macrospecimen of a resected stomach. A 9×9-cm ulcer is seen in the pyloric part on the lesser curvature with a ridge of infiltration (arrows); the ulcer spreads over onto the anterior and posterior walls (distal cancer). Histologically, a moderately differentiated adenocarcinoma of the stomach with invasion of the serosa

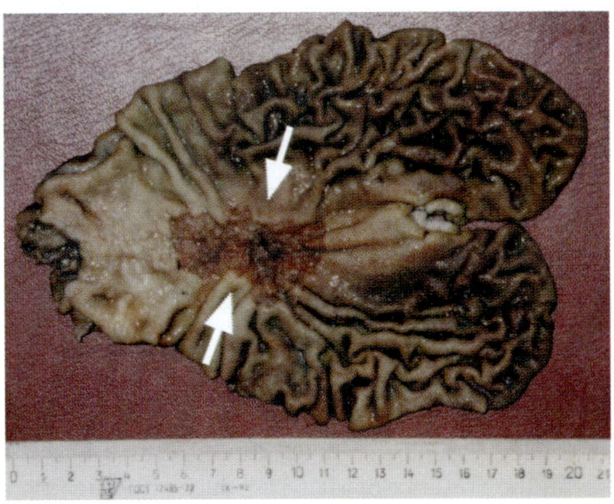

Fig. 2. Macrospecimen of a resected stomach. A 5×3-cm infiltrative-ulcerous cancer (arrows) on the lesser curvature, 5 cm from the distal and proximal edges of resection. Histologically, a signet-ring cell carcinoma of the stomach with invasion of the muscular coat

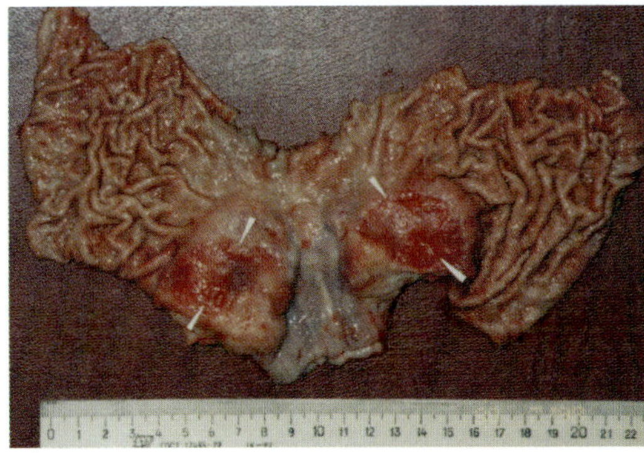

Fig. 3. Macrospecimen of a resected stomach. Ulcerated 9×4.5-cm endophytic tumor (dissected in two parts) in the vicinity of the esophagus (arrows). Histologically, a poorly differentiated adenocarcinoma with the signet-ring cell component and invasion of the muscular coat

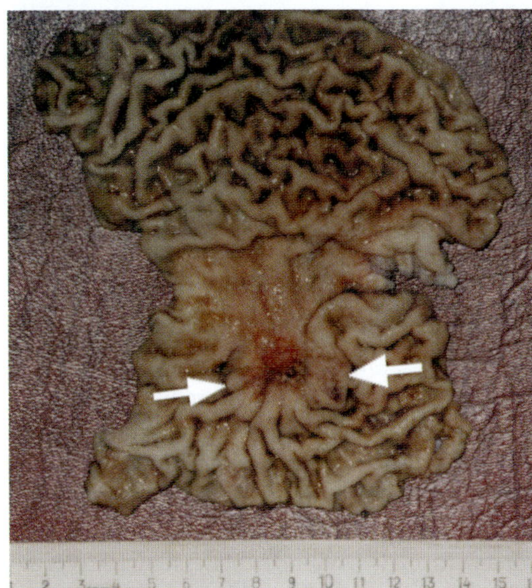

Fig. 4. Macrospecimen of a resected stomach. Infiltrative-ulcerous cancer (1 cm diameter) with eroded edges (arrows). Histologically, a moderately differentiated adenocarcinoma of the stomach

es cancer develops in the cardiac part, the upper third of the body, and the fundus – so-called proximal cancer (Fig. 3) [196, 271]. The greater curvature is attacked by the tumor in 8–9% of cases. Tumor activity on the anterior wall of the stomach is relatively rare (Fig. 4).

However, screening data suggest that tumors in the greater curvature and the anterior wall occur far more frequently than might be expected [33, 58, 129, 224]. In most cases, the newly revealed cancers extend over a significant length, and at the time of discovery the tumor cannot be regarded as located at the site of its origination.

During the past 30 years, the incidence of distal cancer has decreased, whereas the number of cases of proximal carcinoma has increased [86, 271], which agrees with the results of studies conducted at MONIKI (▶ see Diagram 4). Diagnosis of proximal gastric cancer is a difficult problem. Such tumors are normally accompanied by invasion of the esophageal wall, which makes endoscopic diagnosis much more difficult and sometimes even infeasible (Fig. 5). Moreover, the tumor often metastasizes into the para-esophageal lymph nodes. This worsens the prognosis and makes it difficult to treat the patient surgically. »Displacement« of the traditional site of cancer from the distal part of the stomach to its proximal part must stimulate a revision of the current approach to diagnosis.

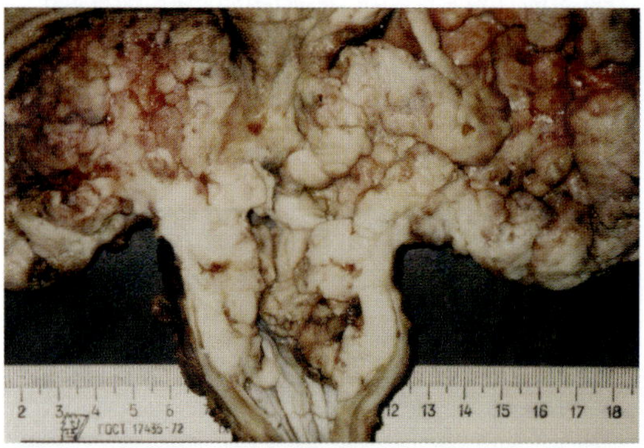

Fig. 5. Macrospecimen of a resected stomach. Large tumor in the area of the gastroesophageal junction invading the esophageal wall. Histologically, a moderately differentiated adenocarcinoma invading the serosa and the esophageal wall

According to some authors, the prognosis of the disease depends on the localization of the tumor, but in our opinion, such a dependence is quite disputable. As a rule, the prognosis would be best with tumors in the pyloric part and on the lesser curvature, and worst with total involvement of the stomach. It is evident that the prognosis would normally depend on the tumor's histological type and its stage. Intestinal carcinomas would have a better prognosis (they are easier to diagnose), while with diffuse carcinomas the latent course is longer and hence the prognosis is worse.

Multiple Gastric Cancers

The data on multiple gastric cancers are quite controversial. Their incidence varies from 2% to 38% [202]. According to Japanese researchers, they constitute 5–10% of all intestinal carcinomas [119, 259]. Studies conducted at MONIKI revealed this variant of carcinoma origination in 45% cases of primary cancer; the majority are mixed signet-ring cell carcinomas. Multiple gastric cancers, which originate in two to eight sites, dominate among the multiple cancers of the stomach [39]. In former times, many authors associated multiple gastric cancer with polyps of the stomach, but according to current concepts, the malignant transformation of polyps is very rare [219, 255].

Staging

Staging of gastric cancer was proposed by the American Joint Committee on Cancer. To that end, they used the TNM system [84, 266], which is based on the following three criteria: T (tumor) – the primary tumor, N (nodulus) – regional lymph nodes, and M – metastasis. The stage of the disease is thus identified according to the degree of each of the three components:

- Stage 0 (in situ): Tins, N0, M0
- Stage I:
  - A: T1, N0 M0
  - B: T1, N1, M0 or T2, N0, M0
- Stage II: T1, N2, M0; T2, N1, M0; T3, N0, M0
- Stage III:
  - A: T2, N2, M0; T3, N1, M0; T4, N0, M0
  - B: T3, N2, M0; T4, N1, M0
- Stage IV: T4, N2, M0, or any degree of T and N in the presence of M1

The T criterion is evaluated as follows (Scheme 3):

- Tx – primary tumor cannot be estimated
- T0 – no signs of primary tumor
- Tins – intraepithelial carcinoma without invasion of the mucous membrane proper
- T1 – invasion of the proper mucous or submucous membrane
- T2 – tumor invades the muscular and serous membranes
- T3 – tumor penetrates the serosa without invasion of the adjacent structures
- T4 – tumor invades adjacent tissues and organs (spleen, transverse colon, liver, diaphragm, pancreas, abdominal wall, adrenal glands, small intestine, and retroperitoneal space)

Involvement of regional lymph nodes (N) is estimated according to the scheme which follows below. Regional lymph nodes include pericardial, left ventricular, common liver, splenic, and those of the celiac artery. Involvement of the other intra-abdominal lymph nodes (hepatoduodenal, retropancreatic, mesenteric, and para-aortic) are regarded as distal metastases.

- Nx – regional lymph nodes cannot be evaluated
- N0 – no metastases to the regional lymph nodes
- N1 – metastases to the regional lymph nodes within a distance of 3 cm from the margin of the primary tumor
- N2 – metastases to the regional lymph nodes located farther than 3 cm from the margin of the primary tumor, or metastases to the lymph nodes along the entire left border of the stomach, common hepatic, splenic, and iliac artery
- Remote metastases:
  - Mx – presence of remote metastases cannot be estimated
  - M0 – no remote metastases
  - M1 – remote metastases

The proposed scheme is recommended only for carcinomas and should not be used to evaluate sarcomas, carcinoids, or lymphomas.

Gastric cancer is characterized by high variability, multiple forms, and combinations of various macroscopic forms. A great number of factors influence tumor growth: its histological structure, location, stage of the process, degree of hyperplastic (background) changes in the stomach wall, involvement of the stromal component, immune response of the body, age of the patient. However, it is possible to identify the major variants. The macroscopic concepts of gastric cancer are based on the first classification proposed by R. Borrmann in 1926 [96]. However, classifications which were proposed later proved more popular. They were produced by P. Laurent [78, 179], S. Ming [197], the WHO (1990) [272], and the American Joint Committee on Cancer (1992) [248]. The classification proposed by the Japanese Gastric Cancer Association [153] is now widely used. It identifies the following macroscopic types of gastric cancer:

- Type 0 – superficially spreading carcinoma, subdivided into five subtypes, presented in the section dedicated to early cancer
- Type 1 – polypiform
- Type 2 – ulcerating cancer with distinct borders and elevated edges
- Type 3 – ulcerating cancer infiltrating the surrounding tissues
- Type 4 – unclassifiable tumor; as a rule, this is diffusely propagating cancer without ulceration

Superficially Spreading Gastric Cancer

Superficially spreading gastric cancer (Fig. 6) is the earliest macroscopically visible form of gastric cancer [249]. The tumor growing in the surface of the mucous and submucous membrane is characterized by an elevated or sinking surface, sometimes affected with small ulcers; the area of carcinoma does not exceed 25 mm2. The tumor tends to stretch mucosal folds, making them rigid, and to fix them to the muscular coat. In about 80% of cases the stomach wall is thickened to 0.8–1.0 m (versus normal 0.6–0.7 m in the pyloric part and 0.4–0.7 m in the body) due to sclerosis and edema of the submucous membrane of varying degrees. The depth of invasion corresponds mostly to Tins–T1, less frequently T2. All forms of gastric cancer which will be described below develop later. Histologically, superficially spreading gastric cancer has, in most cases, the structure of poorly differentiated adenocarcinoma or signet-ring cell carcinoma.

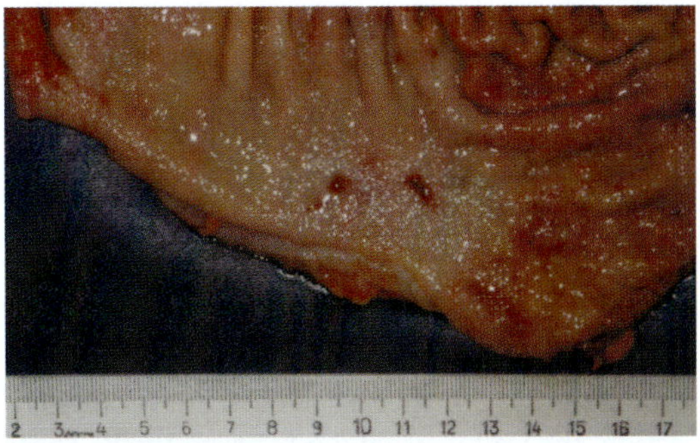

Fig. 6. a Fragment of a macrospecimen of a resected stomach. A 6x4-cm specimen of the mucous membrane with an elevated surface in the region of the greater curvature affected with 0.2- to 0.6-cm ulcers.

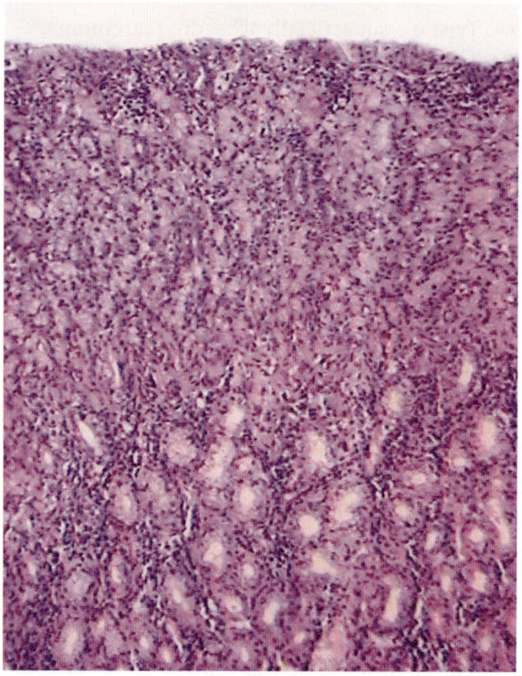

Fig. 6. b Fragment of a microspecimen of gastric mucosa with growing complexes of poorly differentiated adenocarcinoma on the proper mucous membrane surface. Hematoxylin and eosin, x100

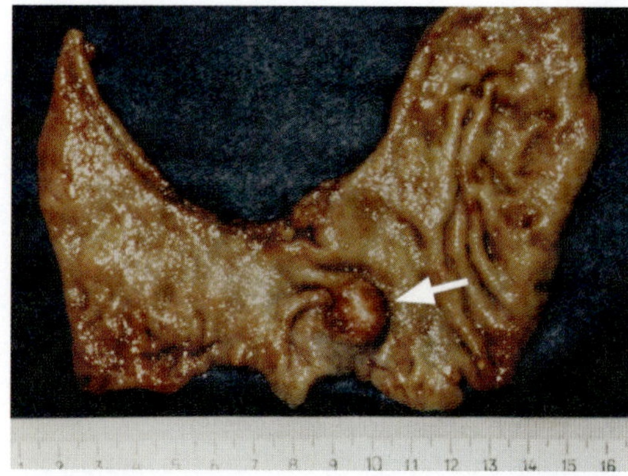

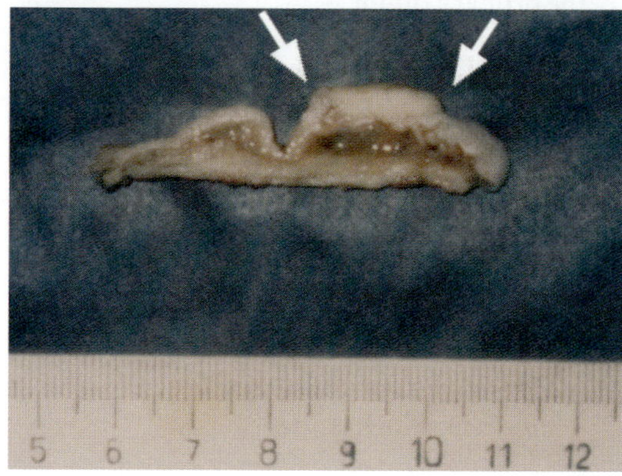

Fig. 7. a Fragment of a macrospecimen of a resected stomach. A 1.5x1.5x0.7-cm polypiform tumor (arrow) is seen in the immediate vicinity of the gastroesophageal junction. Histologically, an adenocarcinoma invading the submucous membrane. **b** The same preparation (section). Exophytic growth appears as a whitish firm tissue (arrows)

Polypiform Cancer of the Stomach

Polypiform cancer of the stomach (Fig. 7) occurs in 17% of cases. The tumor grows into the stomach cavity and varies in shape and size. As a rule, this is the late stage of endophytic carcinoma. Histologically, it has the structure of tubular or papillary well-differentiated adenocarcinoma, possibly with formation of mucus, and sometimes developing against the background of preceding adenoma.

Ulcerated Cancer of the Stomach

Ulcerated cancer of the stomach (Figs. 1, 2, 4) occurs in 25% of cases. This is an endophytic tumor of variable size, with rigid elevated or eroded edges, surrounded by a ridge of infiltrated tissue and converging flattened folds of the mucous membrane. The floor of the ulcer formed by cell detritus is rough. In section, the wall is usually 0.8–1.5 cm thick. These changes are due to sclerosis of the submucous membrane and specific cancer infiltration spreading between muscular strands and attended by desmoplastic response of varying degree. Firm, whitish cancer tissue underlies the ulcer over a length of 2–3 cm on each side. This tissue normally grows into the serous membrane (Fig. 8); the depth of invasion corresponds to T1–T3. Ulcerated carcinomas have the structure of both intestinal and diffuse cancer.

Diffusely Spreading Cancer of the Stomach

Diffusely spreading cancer of the stomach (linitis plastica) (Fig. 9) occurs in 16% of cases. Massive cancer infiltration combines with a pronounced desmoplasia. Invasion depth corresponds to T2–T3.

Histological Classification

Practical experience shows that the importance of the above differentiation of types of gastric cancer growth

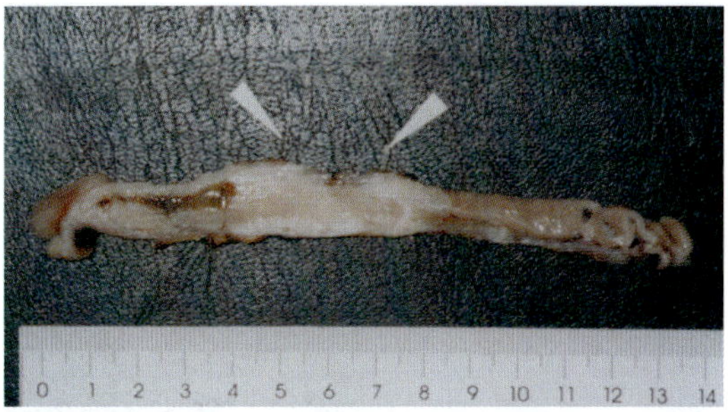

Fig. 8. Fragment of a preparation of a resected stomach (section). Whitish, firm cancerous tissue, growing to invade the serosa, underlies a flat ulcer (arrows), 4 cm on each side. Histologically, a poorly differentiated adenocarcinoma of the stomach invading the serous membrane

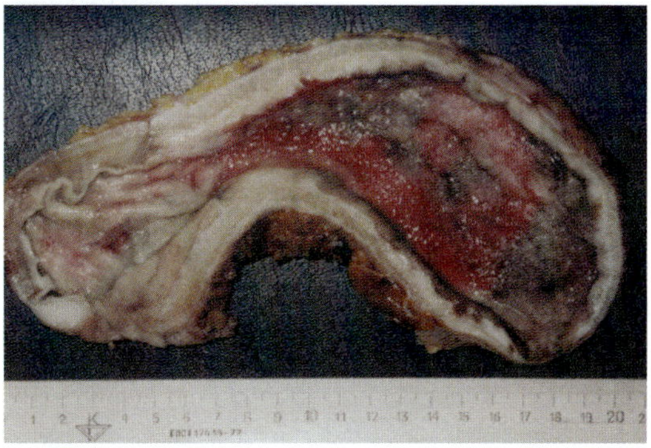

Fig. 9. Macrospecimen of a resected stomach. A 1- to 1.5-cm thick (versus normal 0.4–0.7 cm) rigid wall is distinctly seen in the section. Histologically, a signet-ring cell gastric cancer with the pronounced stromal component invading the serous membrane

is only relative, because it should be remembered that they are only specific stages of development of gastric carcinoma [22], whereas polypiform tumor is, as a rule, an exophytic component of carcinoma characterized by predominantly endophytic growth.

Many histological classifications of gastric cancer have been proposed, the most popular being those proposed by P. Laurent, S. Ming, and the American Joint Committee on Cancer (1992). The histological classification proposed by the WHO in 1990 differentiates between the following groups of gastric carcinomas:

1. Adenocarcinoma:
   a. papillary
   b. tubular
   c. mucous
   d. signet-ring cell carcinoma
2. Adenosquamous
3. Squamous
4. Small-cell
5. Non-differentiated
6. Other carcinomas (choriocarcinoma, embryonic carcinoma)

The histological variants of carcinomas listed above are subdivided into the following five grades, depending on their differentiation:

1. GX: grade cannot be estimated
2. G1: well-differentiated carcinomas
3. G2: moderately differentiated carcinomas
4. G4: poorly differentiated carcinomas
5. G4: non-differentiated carcinomas

Adenocarcinoma

Well-, moderately, and poorly differentiated adenocarcinomas (Fig. 10) are classified according to their degree of differentiation. Well-differentiated carcinomas grow at a faster rate than poorly differentiated ones [127].

Papillary adenocarcinoma. This is adenocarcinoma of tumor complexes in the form of fingerlike projections. The tumors are characterized by various degrees of cell and nucleus polymorphism; they can contain well-differentiated tubular structures, and in this case they are called papillotubular. Macroscopically, papillary adenocarcinoma is characterized mostly by exophytic growth.

Tubular adenocarcinoma. This is adenocarcinoma consisting of branching tubules. Their diame-

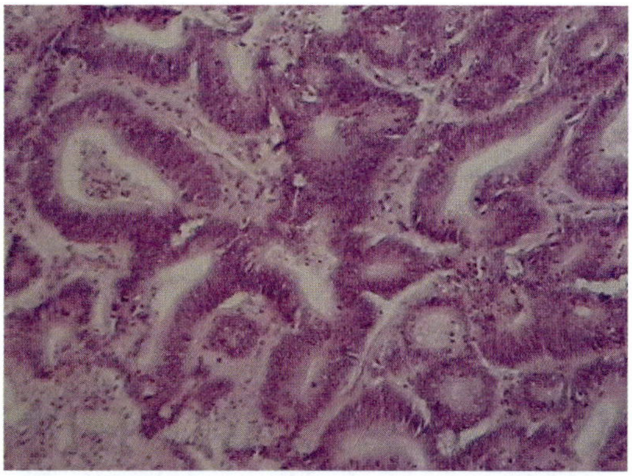

Fig. 10. Papillo-tubular adenocarcinoma: adenocarcinoma of tumor complexes in the form of tubules and fingerlike projections with a fibrovascular base. Hematoxylin and eosin, x400

ters vary within a wide range, e.g., owing to the accumulation of mucus in their lumen.

Mucous adenocarcinoma. The term mucous adenocarcinoma is synonymous with colloid, mucinous, and muconodular (use of the latter should be avoided). This adenocarcinoma involves the glands actively producing extracellular mucus. Two types of this adenocarcinoma are distinguished: one involving glands secreting mucus into the stomach lumen or stroma, and the other involving scattered or grouping signet-ring cells floating in the »lakes« of mucus.

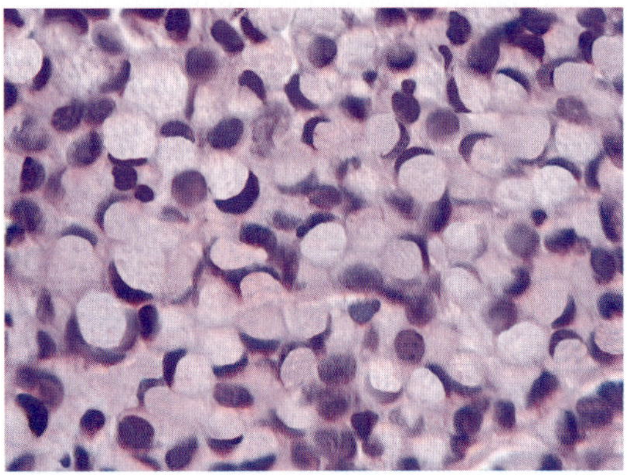

Fig. 11. a The first type of signet-ring cell carcinoma presents as scattered tumor cells of classical fingerlike shapes with optically light cytoplasm, containing intracytoplasmic mucus. Hematoxylin and eosin, x200.

Signet-ring cell carcinoma. This is adenocarcinoma, the dominant component of which is single or grouped tumor cells containing intracytoplasmic mucus. Characteristic of the latter cells are (a) the displacement of their nucleus towards the periphery and (b) the formation of fingerlike shapes. Four types of signet-ring cells are differentiated. The first type have the classical fingerlike shapes with optically light cytoplasm (Fig. 11a) containing acid intracytoplasmic mucin (pH 2.5) which is stained violet with alcian blue. The second type is characterized by a less eccentrically located nucleus with eosinophilic granular cytoplasm (Fig. 11b), presented by cytoplasmic granules containing neutral PAS-positive diastase-resistant mucin, which is stained pink. The third type is goblet-like cells, with cytoplasm containing granules of acid or neutral mucin. The nucleus of these cells is displaced towards the periphery, and in most cases it is rounded (Fig. 11c).

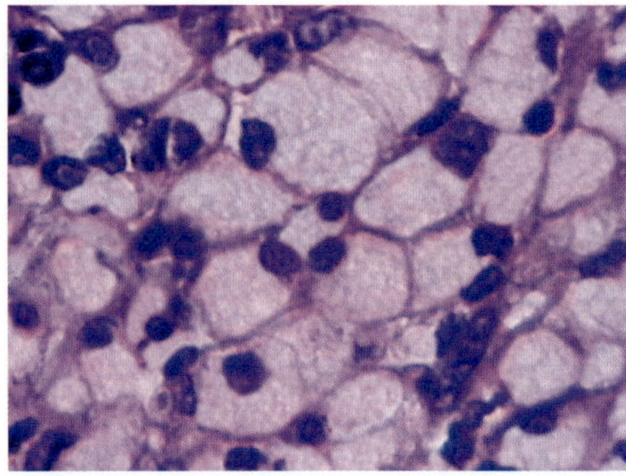

Fig. 11. b The second type is characterized by a less eccentrically located nucleus with eosinophilic granular cytoplasm. Hematoxylin and eosin, x400.

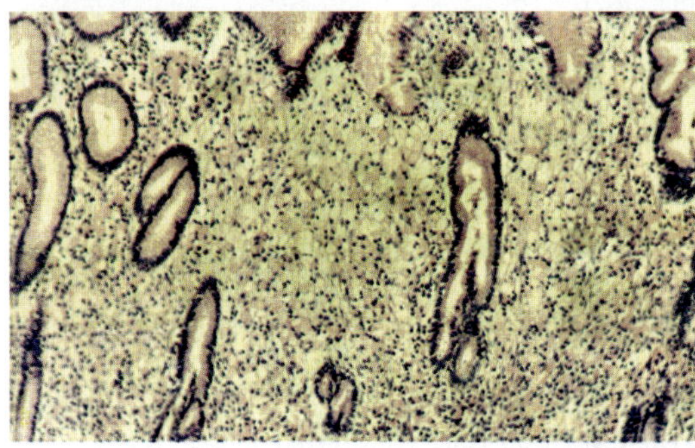

Fig. 11. c The third type presents as goblet-like cells, in which the rounded nucleus is displaced towards the periphery. Hematoxylin and eosin, x100; d The fourth type presents as mucus-free cells. Hematoxylin and eosin, x400

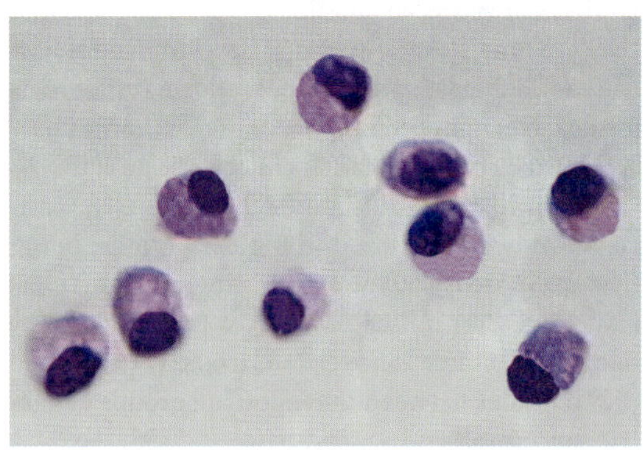

Fig. 11. d The fourth type presents as mucus-free cells. Hematoxylin and eosin, x400

The fourth type of cell contains no mucus (Fig. 11d). These four types of cells can occur in various combinations within one tumor.

Signet-ring cell carcinomas show the tendency to diffusely infiltrate the stomach wall, and they can be attended by a marked stromal component. In this case, this carcinoma is called scirrhous carcinoma, characterized by the presence of single neoplastic cells scattered in the cancer stroma, which are often undetectable without special staining. The entire stomach may be involved, in which case the condition is termed linitis plastica. PAS, mucicarmine, or alcian blue are normally used for their detection. The immunohistochemical method using antibodies to cytokeratine is also effective.

Studies on signet-ring cell carcinoma showed its tendency to preferably horizontal, rather than declining growth [140]. During the past two or three decades, the frequency of signet-ring cell carcinoma has tended to increase slowly but steadily. The terms »signet-ring cell carcinoma« and »mucocellular carcinoma« are synonymous, but the former is preferable. Adenocarcinoma with the signet-ring cell component is called mixed cancer (Fig. 12).

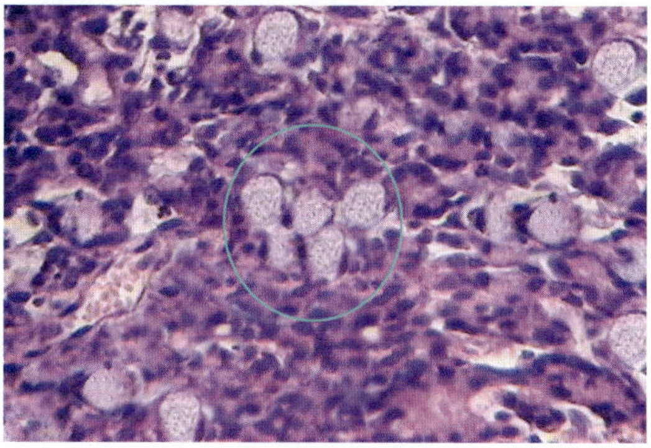

Fig. 12. Adenocarcinoma with the signet-ring cell component. A group of fingerlike cancer cells is encircled in the center of the microphotograph. Hematoxylin and eosin, x200

Adenosquamous Carcinoma

Adenosquamous carcinoma develops from the foci of squamous cell metaplasia. The prognosis is worse than for adenocarcinoma, probably because of the high degree of invasion [203].

Squamous Cell Carcinoma

One case of squamous cell carcinoma (Fig. 13) was described as developing in the middle third of the stomach, affected with polyps on the lesser curvature [83]. It was noted that squamous cell carcinoma aggravates the course of tertiary syphilis of the stomach, with acid burns; it also occurs in the stomach stump and can develop from foci of ectopic, multilayered squamous epithelium [116, 229].

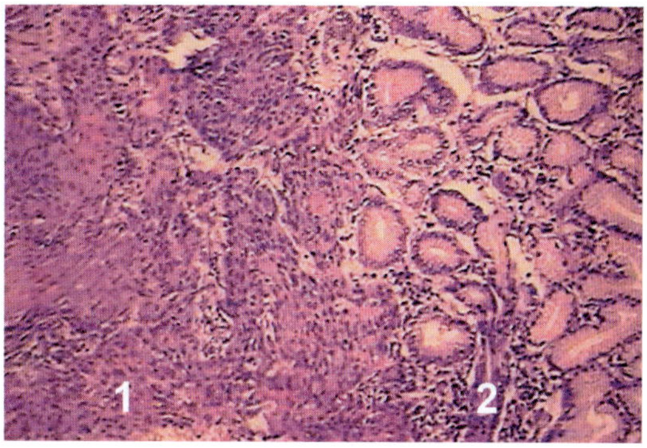

Fig. 13. Fragment of a microspecimen of gastric mucosa. Complexes with moderately differentiated squamous cell cancer (1) and glands of the stomach (2) can be seen in the mucosa. Hematoxylin and eosin, x100

Small-cell Carcinoma

Small-cell carcinoma occurs in 0.6% of all gastric carcinoma cases and can be regarded as an endocrine or neuroendocrine tumor. The tumor often includes adenocarcinoma complexes, especially inside the mucous membrane at the early stage of growth. This tumor is often mistaken for carcinoid.

Non-differentiated Carcinoma

A non-differentiated carconoma is a malignant epithelial tumor with no signs of differentiation. The carcinoma is characterized by a solid arrangement of atypical polygonal cells [197]. The terms »simplex carcinoma«, »solid carcinoma«, »medullar« and »trabecular« cancer were formerly used to designate this type of tumor.

Others

Primary choriocarcinoma and embryonic carcinoma are very rare tumors of the stomach. Not more than 60 cases of choriocarcinoma have been reported. The tumor occurs in subjects aged between 25 and 80 and produces human chorionic gonadotropin (hCG) [204, 274].

Embryonic carcinoma is also a very rare tumor of the stomach, containing elements comparable to those of the tumor of gonadal endodermal sinus and embryonic carcinoma. Many tumor cells express AFP [207].

Early Gastric Cancer

Early gastric cancer is the concept covering carcinomas confined between the mucous and submucous membranes, regardless of tumor size or metastases to the lymph nodes (◘ Fig. 14), as distinct from so-called advanced cancer growing into the underlying layers of the wall [208]. Marked macroscopic changes in the mucosa are normally absent, except for decreased motility and smoothed-down surface ulcers [104, 106]. This differentiation is explained by substantial deviations in the prognosis of these two groups of carcinomas. The term »early« gastric cancer is not synonymous with »intramucosal cancer«, in situ carcinoma, or superficial spreading carcinoma.

The clinical importance of this form of cancer depends on the longer postoperative survival (about 90%) compared with other cancers of the stomach. Early gastric carcinoma can exist inside the mucous membrane without appreciable growth for about a year, but at its later stages it grows rapidly. There is evidence that early cancer progresses into advanced cancer during 37 months on average. Resection of the stomach at the early stage of the tumor therefore

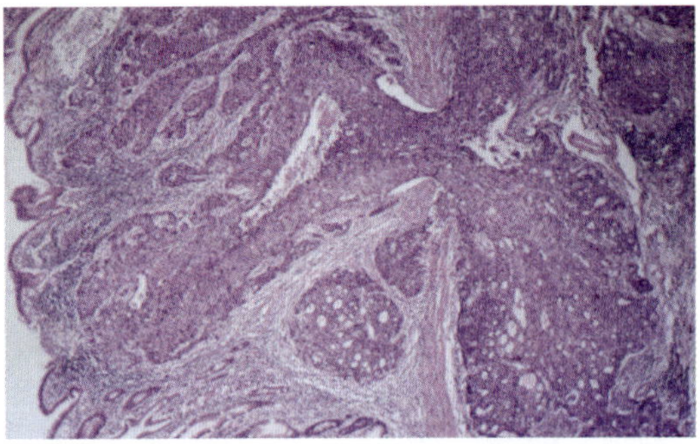

◘ **Fig. 14.** Fragment of a microspecimen of gastric mucosa. Complexes of poorly differentiated adenocarcinoma invading proper muscular coat of the mucous membrane and growing into the submucous layer. Hematoxylin and eosin, x50

guarantees a good prognosis in most cases. Prognosis of early gastric cancer remains good even if the patient is operated on later than in 6 months after the diagnosis was established. In a 10-year period, gastric cancer evolved into the advanced form in only 51% of patients operated on for early cancer [206, 252, 264, 265].

The macroscopic classification of early gastric cancer that is currently used worldwide was proposed in 1962 by the Japanese Gastroenterological Endoscopic Society [153]. In this classification, gastric cancer is divided into the following three major types (► see Scheme 4):

- Type I protruded cancer, characterized by 0.025–0.15 cm thick mucosa (twice as thick as the surrounding normal mucosa)
- Type II superficial cancer, further subdivided into three subtypes:
  - Type IIa slightly elevated tumor
  - Type IIb flat, the rarest tumor, especially characteristic of poorly differentiated adenocarcinoma and often preceding depression or ulceration of the mucous membrane
  - Type IIc slightly depressed tumor, which may have signs of scarred (uls) or existing superficial ulcer (ul) with folds converging toward it (conv); these details are parenthesized
- Type III distinctly excavated tumor; the lesion is characterized by penetration to the submucous membrane, the tumor tissues being detectable only at the ulcer edges

Combined types include several versions, such as IIa +IIc, IIc + IIa, I + IIc, and IIc + III. With IIa + IIc the changes are characterized by protruding, circular, slightly elevated edges around the central depression, at the level of the normal surrounding mucous membrane. With IIc + IIa – a macroscopic version of early carcinoma – the depression corresponding to IIc is often surrounded by slightly elevated mucosa, represented at the histological level by the glands lined with reactive and hyperplastic epithelium. In those cases where the surrounding mucosa is elevated only slightly, type IIa is often disregarded.

Minute (under 5 mm) and small (6–10 mm) cancers are distinguished. Minor cancers have some specific morphological features: They are classed as squamous cancer (lib), and histologically they are well-differentiated adenocarcinomas [204].

It should be noted that depth of lesion in early cancer does not correlate with tumor size. Despite the minimal invasion, the tumor metastasizes into lymph nodes in 10–20% of patients. It is important to note that the presence of metastases depends on the depth of cancer invasion [167]. According to P. Laurent, most early cancers are the intestinal type [205].

Diagnosis

Originating in the depth of the gastric mucosa, the diffuse form of early cancer attacks mostly the deep parts of the mucous and submucous membranes with only minimal changes to the surface structures. This adds difficulties to establishing the primary diagnosis. Guided by the results of X-ray examination, the problem may be made less difficult by taking many tissue samples during endoscopy. Based on X-ray data, and more particularly on the traditional X-ray examination, we suggest that the symptom of intramural blastomatous infiltration be used as the specific sign of early diffuse and mixed gastric cancers [31, 32, 58, 223]. The symptom will be described in detail in the chapter dedicated to the evaluation of signs of gastric cancer using various methods of X-ray examination (▼ Chap. 5).

Our point of view is that the possibilities of endoscopy for revealing endophytic tumors are limited. Our experience in the study of gastric cancer at MONIKI demonstrates convincingly the benefits of the traditional X-ray examination. The symptom of rough contours of the stomach filled with barium suspension, along with the symptom of a thick wall revealed by double contrast, helps to diagnose gastric cancer in its early stages.

Establishing the diagnosis of early cancer, as we understand this pathology today, is possible only with an adequate histological examination of resected stomach tissues. Therefore, the concept of »minor« cancer should be preferred in the radiological diagnosis.

Prognosis

The 5-year survival of patients operated on for early gastric cancer is 95–100% [169, 252, 269]; with an invasion depth corresponding to T2, T3, or T4 this drops to 60–80%, 50%, or 10–20%, respectively [136, 144]. The prognosis of multifocal carcinoma is slightly worse. Repeated analyses of macro- and microscopic factors has established that the depth of invasion of the stomach wall is decisive for the postoperative prognosis [213]. Less important are macroscopic form, size of the tumor, the character of its growth, the degree of differentiation, the presence of metastases, and some other factors [114, 150, 188].

Important features of diffuse and mixed cancers include their endophytic (intramural) growth (mostly without distinct borders), spreading via the intravisceral lymph ducts. This is associated with the high proliferative activity of cancer cells owing to a p53 gene mutation, and to acquisition of the second mutation in genes responsible for maintenance of intercellular contacts. Thus, the tumor borders are not always easy to locate with sufficient accuracy at the preoperative or the intraoperative stage of diagnosis. Early diagnosis of the disease, and hence less depth and area of invasion, are therefore the main factors for successful treatment and postoperative survival of 5 and more years. In this connection, the necessity of objective estimation of the size and type of tumor infiltration of the stomach wall is indisputable. But these factors can be estimated only by radiological examination.

Staging

Postoperative management of patients requires accurate determination of the stage and grade of gastric cancer. Sometimes, early carcinoma recurs in the stump of the operated stomach, either as a second primary tumor or as a result of the operation which was performed without removal of the adjacent healthy tissue [191]. According to some authors, relapses are more common in patients with the elevated type of early carcinoma and with the exophytic form of tumor growth [139, 171].

The DNA content of tumor cells evaluated by flow cytometry has certain prognostic importance.

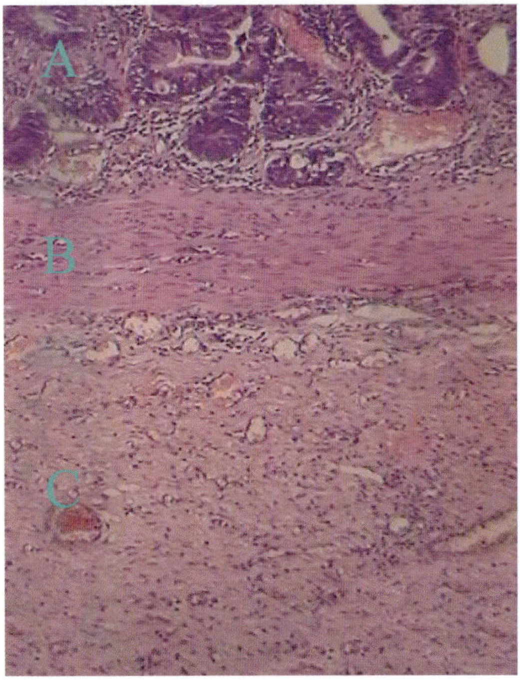

Fig. 15. Fragment of a microspecimen of gastric mucosa. Glands affected by severe dysplasia and foci of cancer in situ can be seen in the upper part of the microphotograph (A). Tunica muscularis propria of the mucous membrane (B). Marked sclerosis of the submucous membrane (C). Hematoxylin and eosin, x50

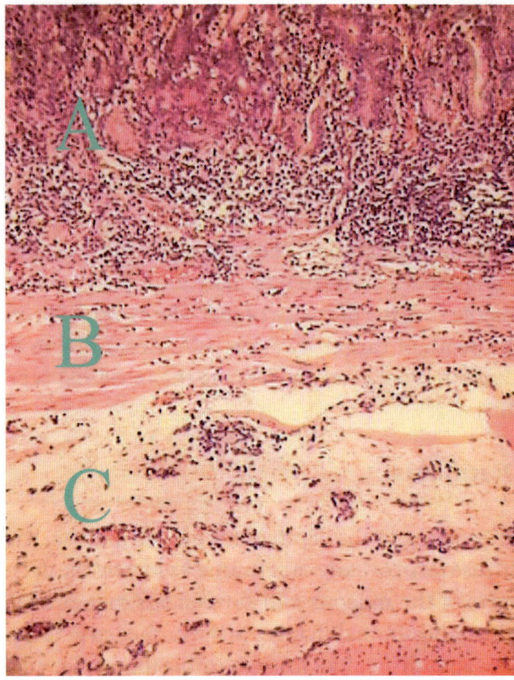

Fig. 16. Fragment of a microspecimen of gastric mucosa. Glands affected by severe dysplasia and foci of cancer in situ can be seen in the upper part of the microphotograph (A). Tunica muscularis propria of the mucous membrane (B). Marked edema of the submucous membrane (C). Hematoxylin and eosin, x50

Gastric carcinoma may be diploid (68.4%), aneuploid (14.8%), or mixed (12.9%), or it may contain complex aneuploid cell populations (3.7%). All cancers contain polypoid populations, but early cancer normally has fewer polypoid cells compared with advanced cancer. Statistics suggest that a correlation exists between metastases and high DNA content [161].

Examination of a great number of tissue specimens of the stomach resected for early cancer shows that in 60% of cases, sclerosed submucous membrane displaces the muscular coat, or grows over it, in the area of growing carcinoma (under the tumor or in its immediate vicinity; Fig. 15) [111]. In 15% of cases these changes occur at some distance from the tumor, where atrophy of the mucous membrane of varying degree and also dysplasia of the integumentary epithelium may develop. The structure of newly formed connective tissue is dissimilar in such cases, probably dependent on the different mechanisms and duration of its formation. Fibrous and, less frequently, cellular connective tissues are formed. This process is usually associated with chronic inflammation or is interpreted as a response to metabolites of anaplastic cells and products of their decay [157]. But other mechanisms are also possible. It is quite probable that such tissue can be formed in the presence of persistent edema followed by hyalinosis (Fig. 16).

In addition to the described changes in the submucous membrane of the stomach, in 17% of early cancer cases, the walls of the intramural vessels (mostly in the submucous membrane) thicken at the expense of the muscular coat and sclerosed inner coat, to narrow the vessel lumen (Fig. 17). Such changes do not depend on the stage of carcinoma, histological type, or localization of the tumor in the stomach, or on the age and gender of the patient. In addition, the intravisceral veins remain without visible pathological changes.

The described hyperplastic changes associated with early gastric carcinoma inevitably cause mac-

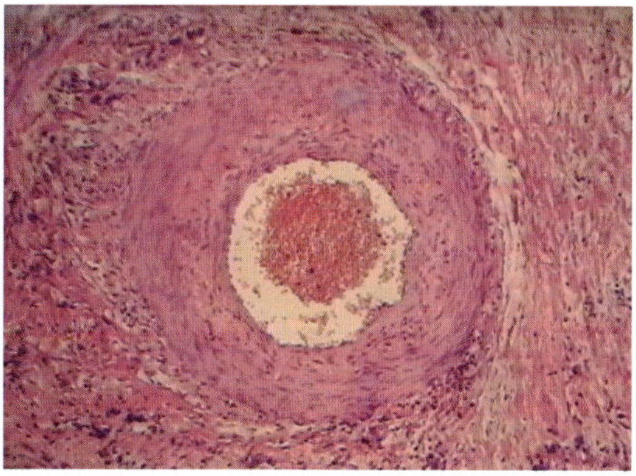

Fig. 17. Fragment of a microspecimen of the stomach wall. Sclerosed submucous membrane. Arterial type vessel with the wall thickened at the expense of the muscular coat and sclerosed inner coat. Hematoxylin and eosin, x200

roscopically visible thickening of the stomach walls. This feature of early cancer was taken into consideration while studying the stomach by the radiological diagnostic methods. It is evident that these changes require further thorough studies [34, 36, 37].

Diagram 3. Incidence of the three major histological types of gastric carcinomas during the period 1970–2003 (histological studies of 1440 resected stomachs of patients operated on at MONIKI). This 34-year period is characterized by reduced incidence of the intestinal type of gastric cancer and simultaneously increasing incidence of carcinomas of the diffuse and mixed types

Scheme 1. Gastric glands of the pyloric zone, which are subdivided into three parts – villiform, cervical, and glandular. The generative zone of the glands is located in the cervical part

Scheme 2 a,b. Histogenesis of diffuse (**a**) and intestinal (**b**) forms of gastric cancer. a Malignant cells of the glandular generative zone (as a result of mutation of genes that are responsible for maintenance of intercellular contacts and protein synthesis by the basal membrane) can migrate into the depth of the proper mucous membrane (bold black) thus initiating diffuse cancer. Figures 1 and 3 represent cancer originating in the fundic glands, Figs. 2 and 4 cancer in the antral glands. b Intestinal type cancer develops in cases where gland fragments containing mutated epithelial cells are obliterated and incorporated into the proper mucous membrane (bold black in 2, 3, and 4). Figure 1 shows mutated cell separation in normal mucosa

Diagram 3

Number of cases N Number of cases	------x------ diffuse type ------x------ intestinal type ------x------ mixed type
Five-year periods	

Scheme 1

	generative zone	
glandular part	cervical part	villiform part

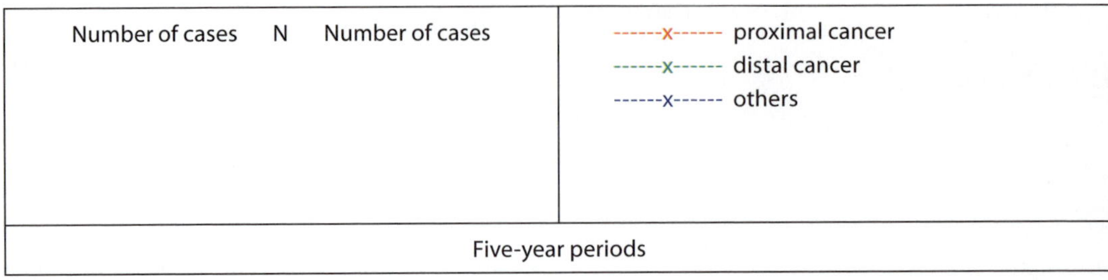

◘ Diagram 4

Diagram 4. Location of cancer in different anatomical parts of the stomach in 1440 patients operated on 1970–2003. This 34-year period is characterized by reduced incidence of cancer of the distal part of the stomach and simultaneously increasing incidence of carcinomas of its proximal part. The incidence of tumors of other locations remained at about the same level

Scheme 3. Tumor invasion of the stomach wall consisting of five layers:
1 (Tins) – proper mucous membrane;
2 (T1) – proper muscular coat of the mucous membrane;
3 (T2) – submucous membrane;
4 (T3) – muscular coat;
5 (T4) – serous membrane

Invasion of adjacent structures

Scheme 4. Macroscopic classification of early gastric cancer

Clinical Symptoms of Gastric Cancer

Introduction

The clinical symptoms of gastric cancer were established on the basis of the concept dominant in the 1960s, according to which the intestinal forms of gastric cancer are representative of the entire diagnostic aspects of this problem, the clinical symptoms included. We have already stated that this concept should be corrected.

We plan to discuss two main questions:

1. What new can be added to the known clinical symptoms of gastric cancer? (This chapter deals with this problem.)
2. What signs of gastric cancer can currently be detected using X-ray methods? (This problem will be covered in more detail in ▼ Chap. 5.)

If we describe the currently accepted clinical symptoms of gastric cancer, based on the analysis of a great number of monographs, manuals, papers, etc., we must conclude that they need serious revision and correction. This is connected with the rapidly changing morphological signs of gastric cancer. No one today doubts that the intestinal forms of gastric cancer have switched with its diffuse and mixed forms; the latter two have become prevalent, whereas the intestinal forms have decreased in incidence accordingly. Beginning in the 1960s in connection with the development of endoscopy, which is recognized as an indispensable tool for diagnosing gastric diseases, the use of X-ray examination of the stomach has decreased substantially [31]. This has not improved the diagnosis of gastric cancer. The reason is that endoscopy is useful mainly in cases of intestinal-type gastric cancer, which is known to show actively on the surface of the gastric mucosa (◘ Fig. 18). It is also useful in advanced cases of mixed gastric cancer, when changes in the mucous membrane are accessible for endoscopic visualization. Tissue specimens taken from such patients are suitable for histological verification of gastric cancer. Meanwhile, the diffuse forms of gastric cancer that originate in the deep parts of the mucosa develop inside the stomach wall and remain inaccessible for endoscopic visualization for a long period of time [24, 38, 98, 185].

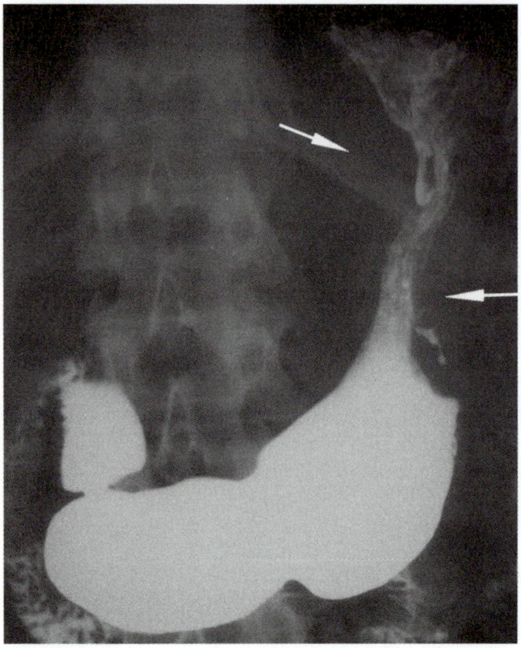

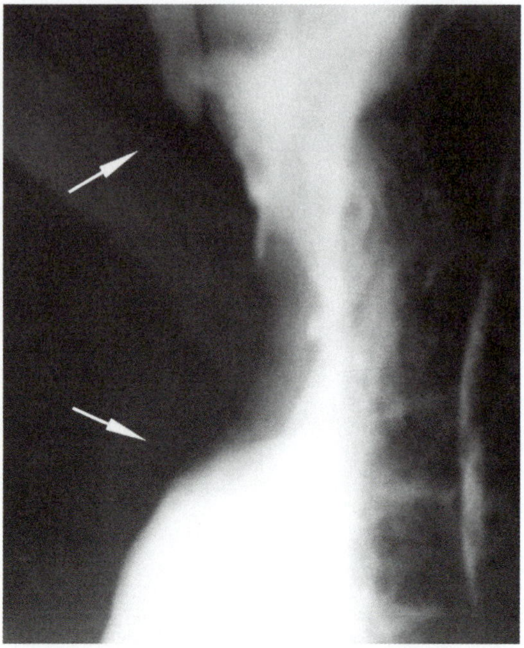

▲ **Fig. 18 a.** ▼ **Fig. 18 b.** ▲ **Fig. 18 c.** ▼ **Fig. 18 d.**

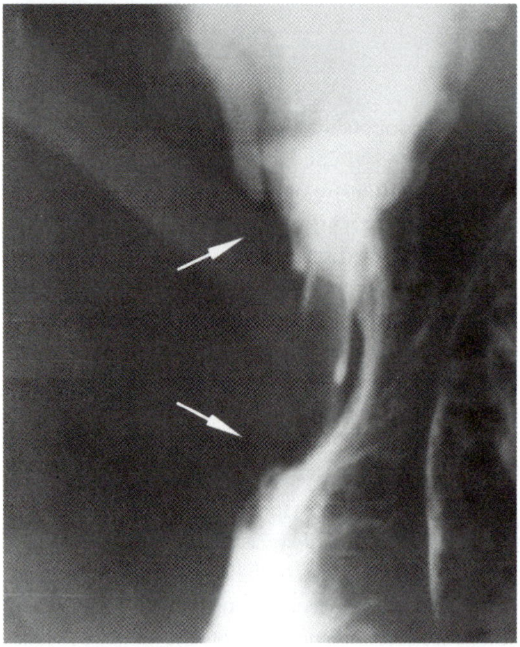

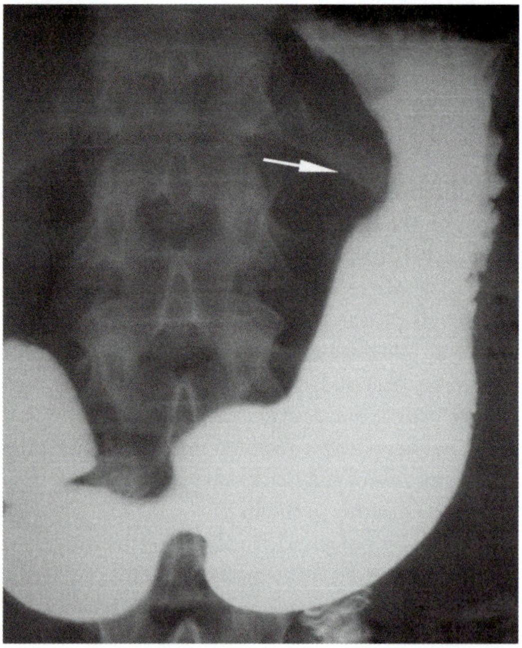

Fig. 18a–o. Female patient A., age 58. Diagnosis: gastric cancer. **a** Stomach X-ray (tight filling, vertical position, anterior projection): contours of the lesser and greater curvatures of the stomach body are uneven (arrows). **b, c** Series of X-rays (tight filling, vertical position, anterior projection): the contour of the lesser curvature is uneven and eroded (arrows). **d** Stomach X-ray (tight filling, vertical position, anterior projection) taken after additional portion of barium meal. The contour of the greater curvature is not changed; uneven contour of the lesser curvature (considerable depression) remains stable (arrow). **e** Stomach X-ray (tight filling, vertical position, left oblique projection): so-called filling defect with a small niche which does not extend beyond the stomach contour (arrow). **f** Stomach X-ray (double contrast, horizontal position, anterior projection): significant thickening of

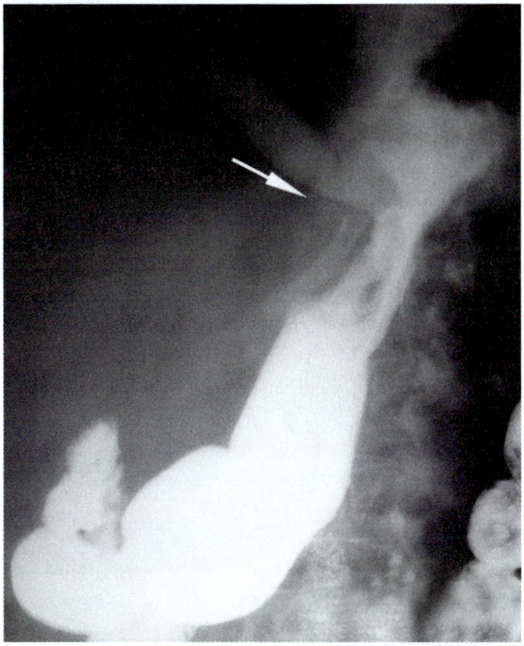

▲ Fig. 18 e. ▼ Fig. 18 f.

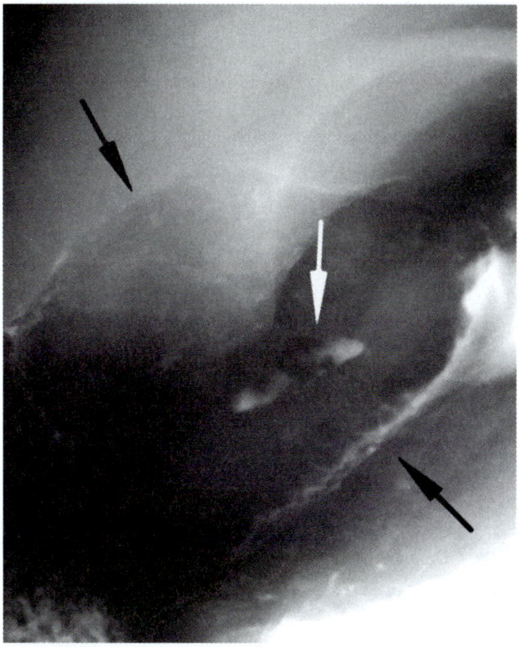

▲ Fig. 18 g

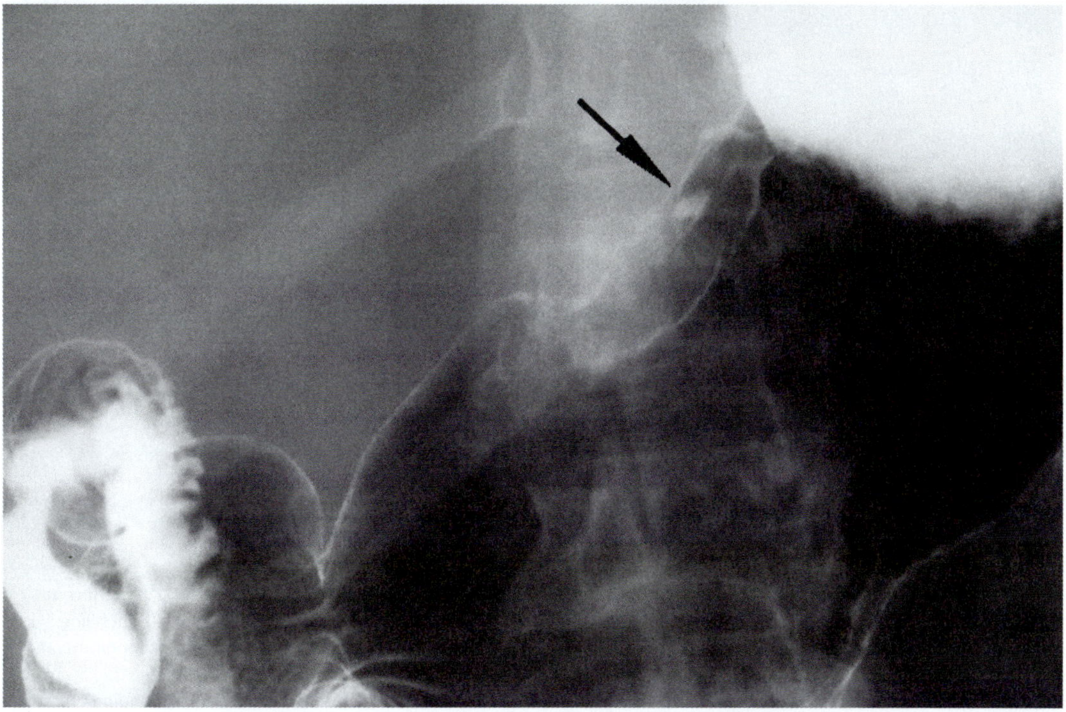

the lesser curvature wall depressed into the cavity, with a small depot of contrast medium (arrow). **g** Stomach X-ray (double contrast, horizontal position, left oblique projection): large tumor of the upper third of the stomach body, bypassed by the contrast medium (black arrows), with insignificant ulceration (white arrow). Conclusion: Cancer of the stomach body with mixed growth. The patient was examined by computed tomography to verify tumor spread.

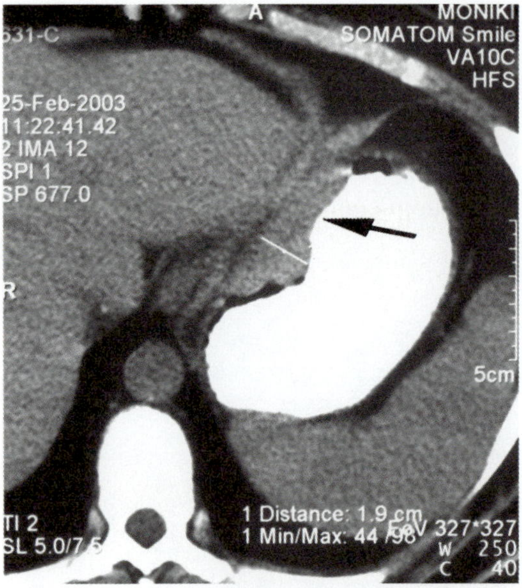

▲ **Fig. 18 h.**

▼ **Fig. 18 i.**

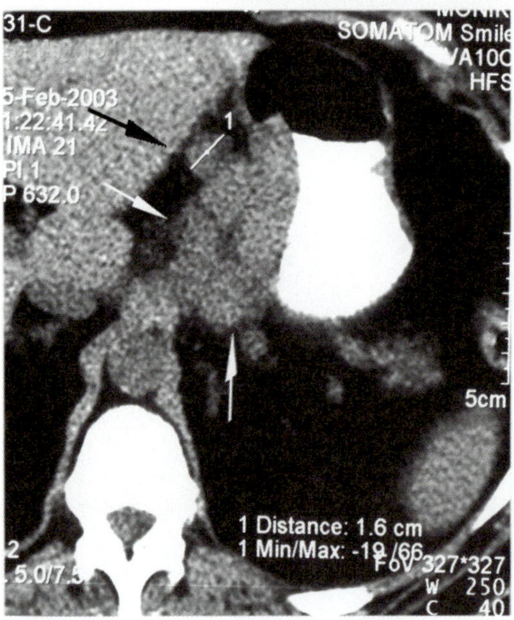

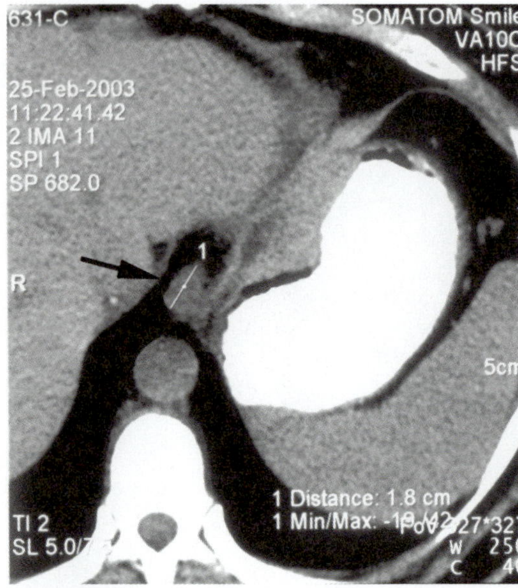

▲ **Fig. 18 j.**

▼ **Fig. 18 k.**

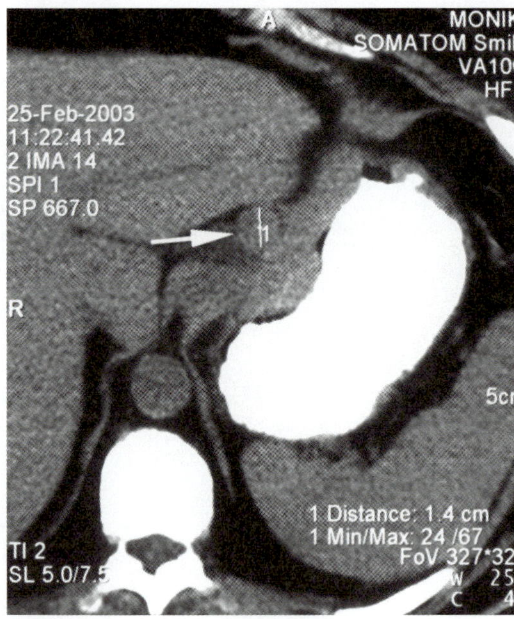

h Computed tomogram of the stomach (tight filling with E-Z-CAT DRY, supine position): distinctly visualized is thickened wall of the upper third of the stomach body; uneven inner contour (arrow). **i** Computed tomogram of the stomach (tight filling with E-Z-CAT DRY, supine position): The infiltrative component spreads to the lesser omentum to form a tumor conglomerate together with the regional and para-aortic lymph nodes (white arrows); an enlarged lymph node is differentiated (black arrow). **j, k, l** Series of CT images: distinct visualization of enlarged lymph nodes (arrow). Conclusion: gastric cancer extending onto the lesser omentum with metastases into the lymph nodes of the abdominal cavity and the retroperitoneal space. **m** Macrospecimen of a resected stomach: exophytic component of the tumor with insignificant ulceration. **n** Fragment of a macrospecimen (strip): thick gastric wall, tumor infiltration extends onto all layers; area of necrosis in center of tumor (arrows). **o** Macrospecimen of a resected stomach wall: moderately differentiated adenocarcinoma

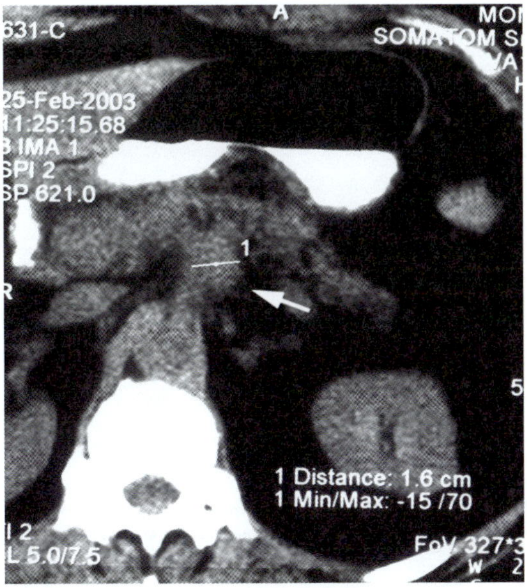

▲ Fig. 18 l. ▼ Fig. 18 m.

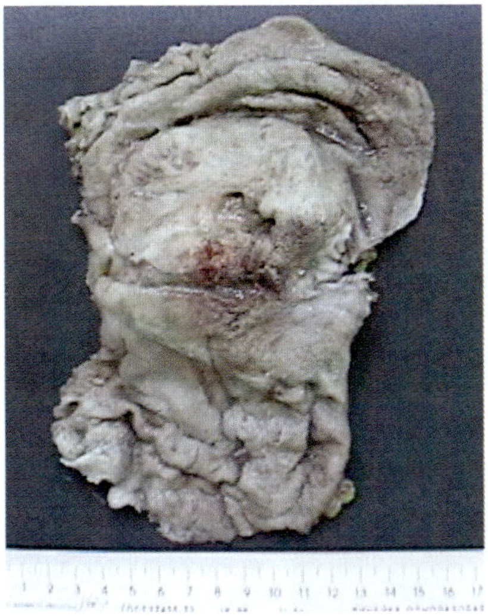

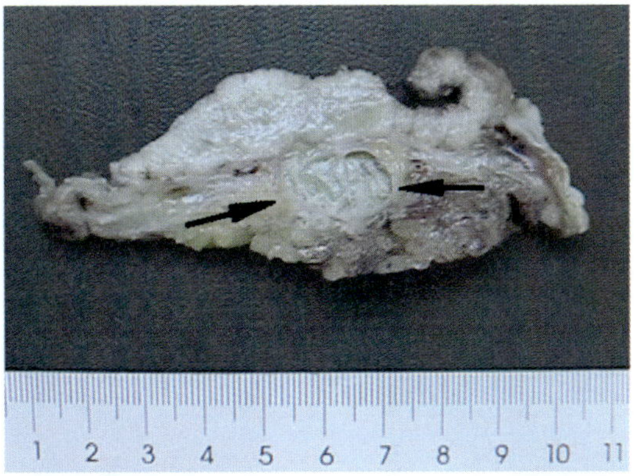

▲ Fig. 18 m. ▼ Fig. 18 o.

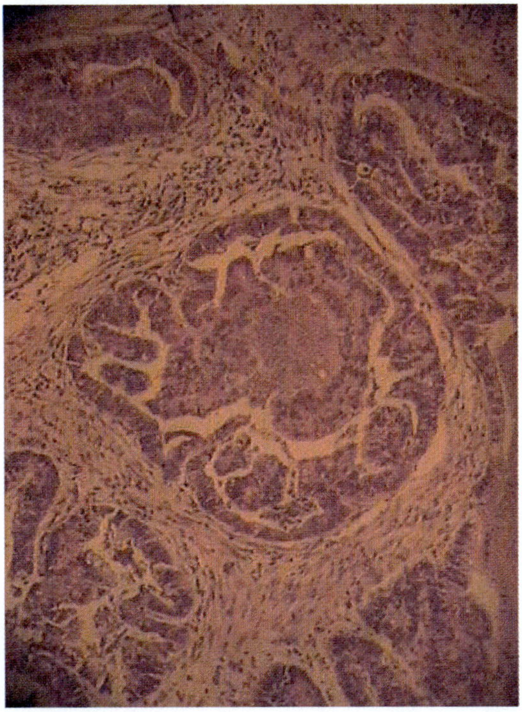

During about the same period, diffuse and mixed forms of gastric cancer started their ascending march, to slowly but steadily displace the intestinal forms of cancer. For this reason, in this and subsequent chapters we place special emphasis on the clinical symptoms of the diffuse (◘ Fig. 19) and mixed morphological forms of gastric cancer (◘ Fig. 20).

If we evaluate the symptoms based on modern ideas, we note that the discussion concerns mainly the clinical symptoms, characterizing a whole group of diseases of the so-called gastroenterological profile. These symptoms are almost unsuitable for the differential diagnosis of gastric cancer and non-cancerous diseases of the stomach. We have already noted that during the last decades of the past century, diffuse and mixed forms of gastric cancer became the dominant morphological forms. Accordingly, the »old« set of clinical symptoms of gastric cancer became even more useless for diagnostic purposes (◘ Fig. 21).

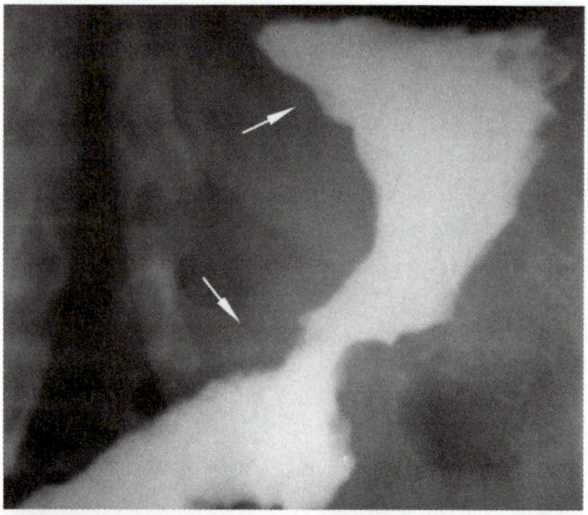

▲ Fig. 19 a.

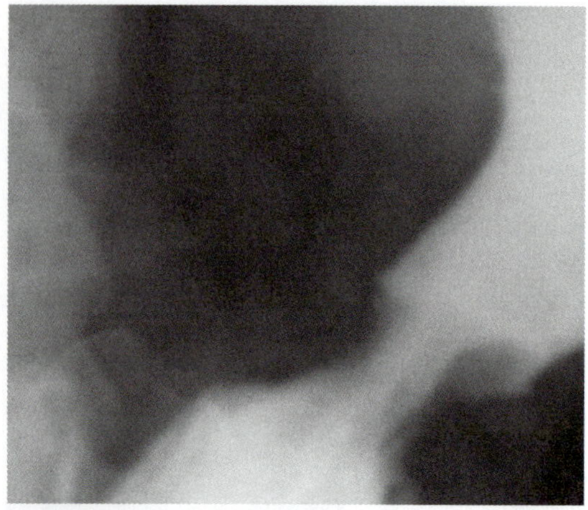

▲ Fig. 19 b.

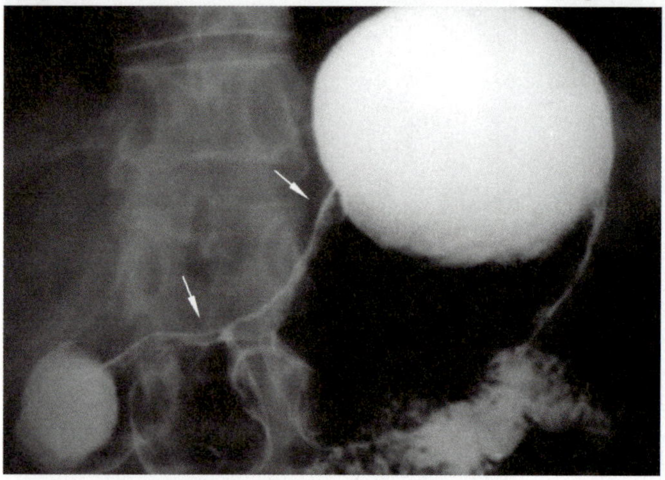

▲ Fig. 19 c. ▼ Fig. 19 d.

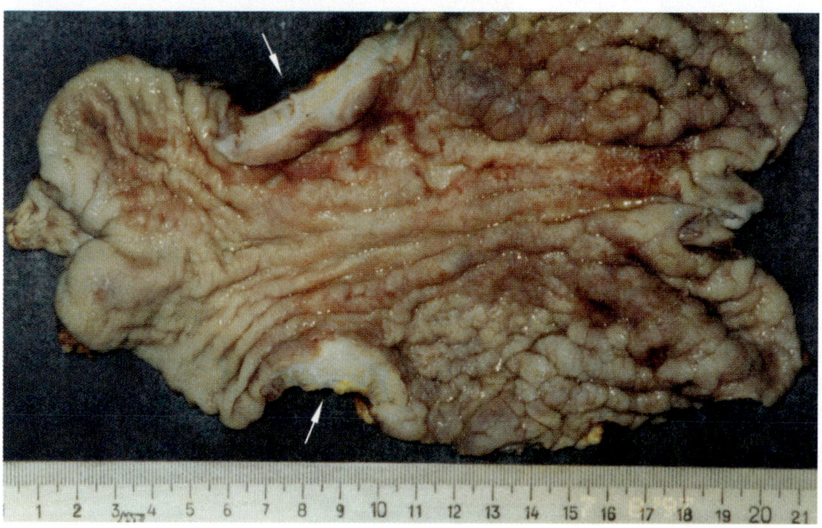

Fig. 19a–e. Female patient T., aged 60. Diagnosis: gastric cancer. **a** Stomach X-ray (tight filling, vertical position, anterior projection): lower third of stomach body irregularly narrowed by circles; the walls are rigid, the angular notch is straightened, the lesser curvature is depressed over a significant length (arrow). **b** Target X-ray of the stomach (tight filling, vertical position, anterior projection): stable narrowing, uneven and eroded contours. **c** Stomach X-ray (double contrast, horizontal position, anterior projection): circular infiltration of lower third of the stomach body; the wall of the lesser curvature at the notch and the proximal antral part is thickened due to expansion of intramural infiltration in the distal direction; the wall of the lesser curvature is thickened over a long distance because of predominant spread of the tumor in the proximal direction (arrows). Conclusion: infiltrative cancer of the antral part and the body of the stomach. **d** Macrospecimen of a resected stomach: part of the intramural infiltration of 3–4 cm on the greater curvature (arrows); relief of the lesser curvature with no visible changes (longitudinal folds persist). **e** Fragments of a macrospecimen (strips): gastric wall is thick over a long distance due to intramural infiltration (arrows). Histologically, a signet-ring cell carcinoma

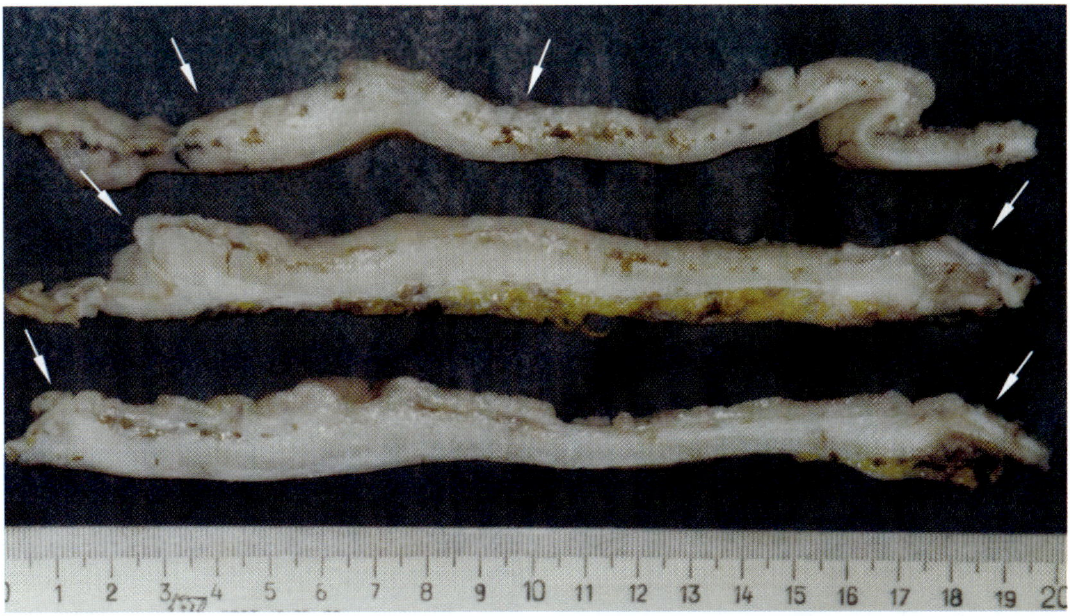

▲ **Fig. 19 e.**

▼ **Fig. 20 a.**

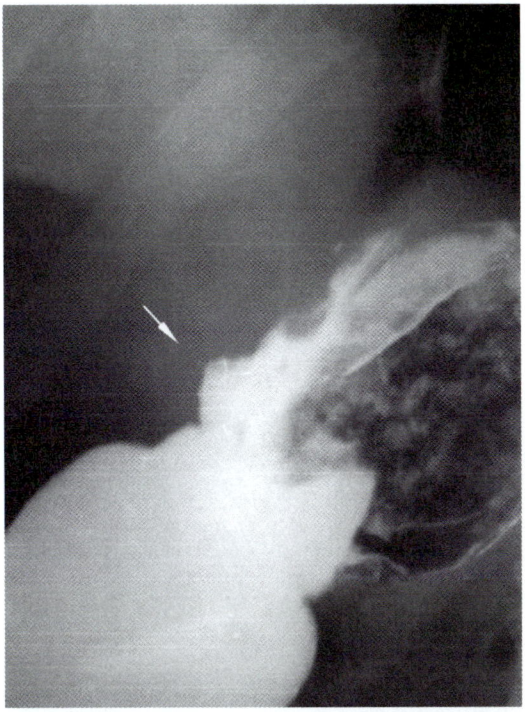

▼ **Fig. 20 b.**

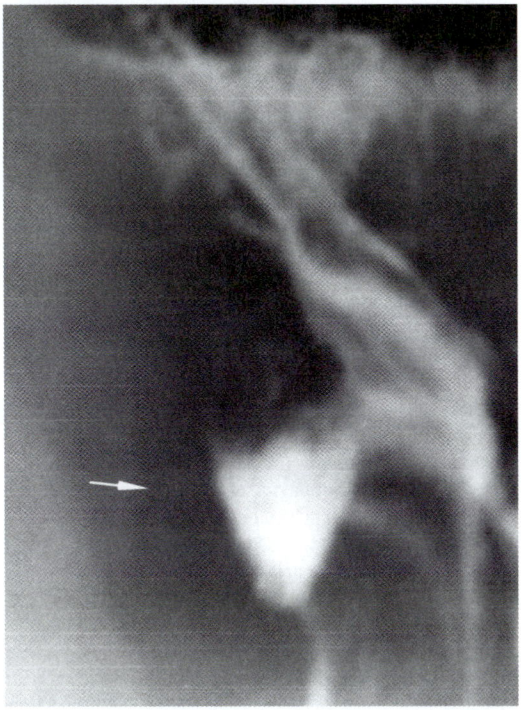

Fig. 20a–g. Female patient K., age 72. Diagnosis: gastric cancer. **a** Stomach X-ray (tight filling, horizontal position, left oblique projection): markedly uneven contour of the anterior wall of upper third of the stomach body with an ulcer niche not extending beyond the stomach contour (arrow). **b** Target X-ray of the stomach (tight filling, vertical position, anterior projection): in projection of the lesser curvature of the anterior wall in the upper third of the stomach body, there is a depot of contrast medium surrounded by areas with changed relief (arrow).

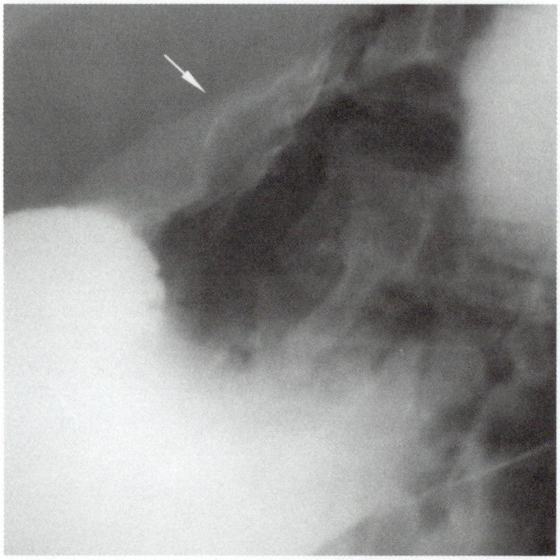

▲ Fig. 20 c. ▼ Fig. 20 d.

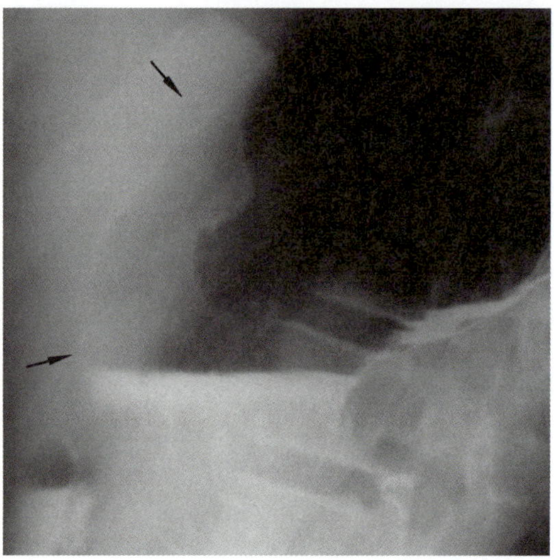

c Stomach X-ray (double contrast, horizontal position, left oblique projection): the anterior wall of the upper third of the stomach body is thickened due to intramural infiltration (arrow). **d** Stomach X-ray (double contrast, vertical position, left oblique projection): infiltrative component of the tumor with ulceration (arrows). **e** Stomach X-ray (double contrast, vertical position, left oblique projection): pronounced thickening of the anterior wall of the body and the upper part due to intramural infiltration (arrow). Conclusion: infiltrative-ulcerative cancer of the anterior wall in the upper third of the stomach body and the upper part of the stomach. **f** Macrospecimen of a resected stomach: a portion showing infiltration of the anterior wall and the upper part with ulcerated surface coated occasionally with fibrin. Peripheral convergence of the folds toward smooth parts of the relief near the infiltration ridge slightly elevated over the surface of the mucous membrane (arrows).

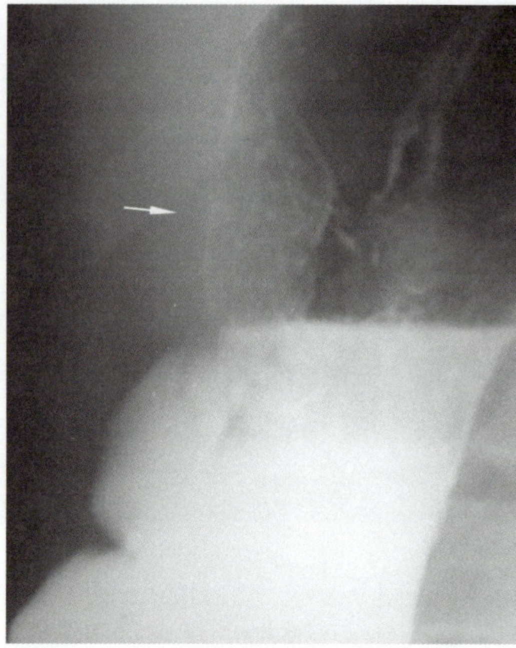

▲ Fig. 20 e. ▼ Fig. 20 f.

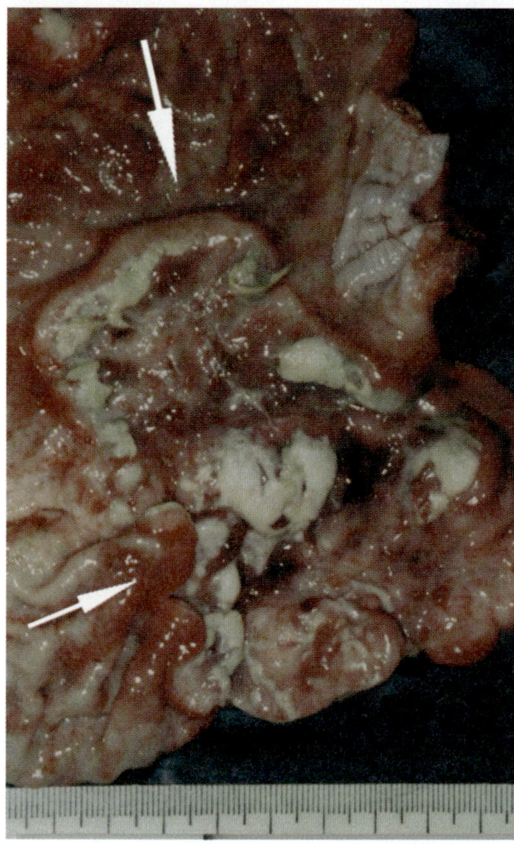

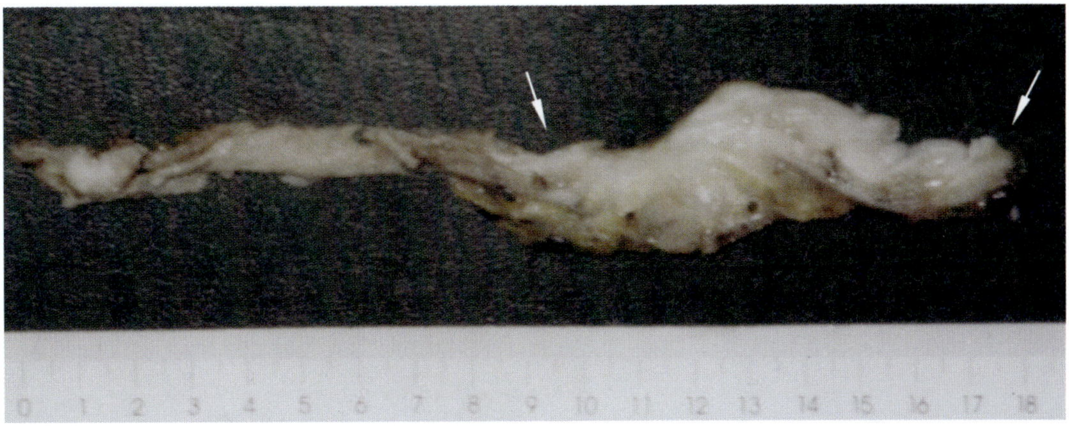

▲ **Fig. 20 g** Fragment of a macrospecimen (strip): stomach wall is thickened due to intramural infiltration over a length of 9 cm (arrows). Histologically, an adenocarcinoma with the signet-ring cell component

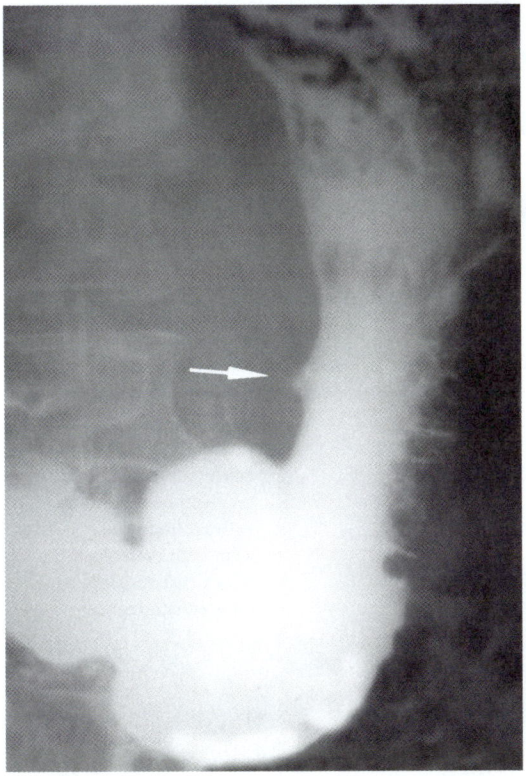

▲ **Fig. 21 a.**

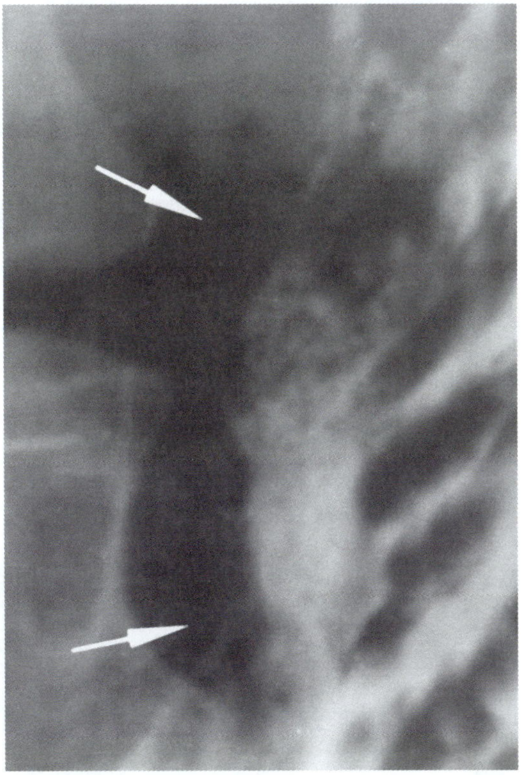

▲ **Fig. 21 b.**

Fig. 21a–d. Female patient B, age 46. Diagnosis: gastric cancer. Complained of weakness and epigastric pain unassociated with meals. Endoscopy: ulcerous defect in middle third of the stomach body. Histolological studies failed to reveal tumor cells. Pain persisted for about 6 months and intensified despite active outpatient treatment. In the absence of improvement, X-ray examination was done. **a** Stomach X-ray (tight filling, vertical position, anterior projection): ulcer niche in the lower third of the stomach body (arrow) and uneven contour of the lesser curvature in the form of a small depression in the middle third of the stomach body. **b** Target stomach X-ray (tight filling, vertical position, anterior projection), dosed compression: a flat niche with converging folds in the lower third of the stomach body (arrows).

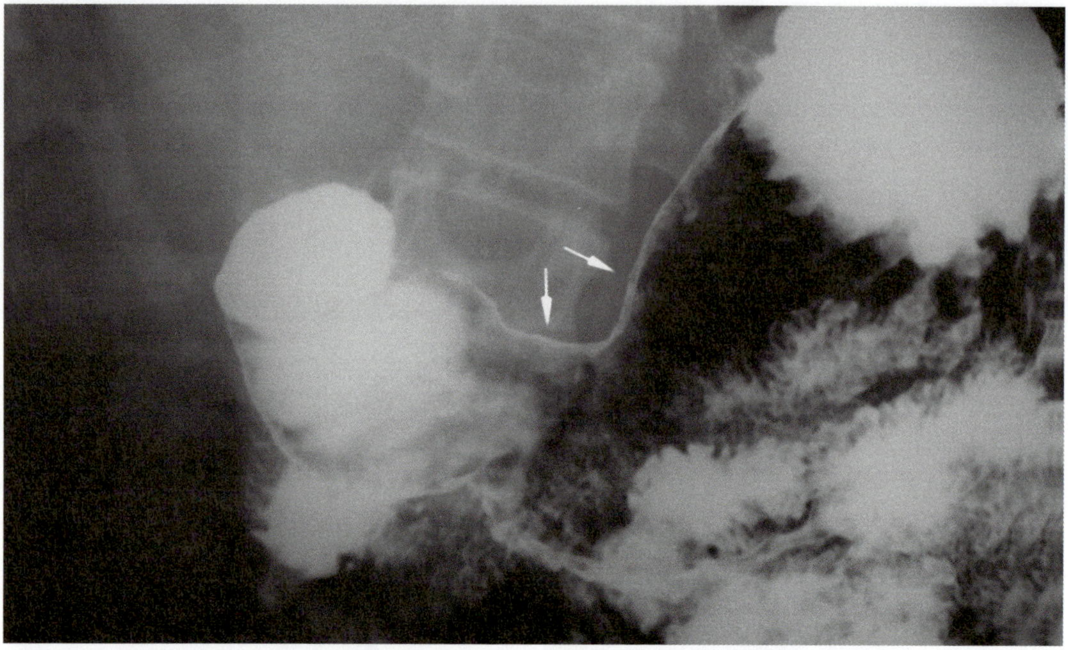

▲ **Fig. 21 c.**

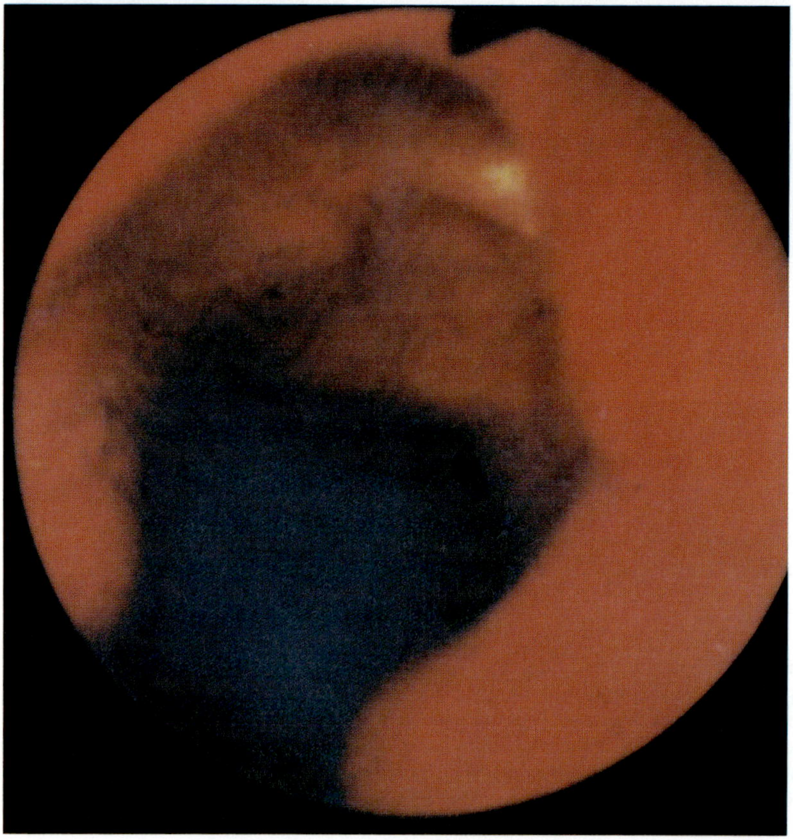

c Stomach X-ray (double contrast, horizontal position, anterior projection): wall of the lesser curvature is thick and rigid, with converging folds, due to intramural infiltration (arrows). Conclusion: infiltrative-ulcerous cancer of the stomach body. **d** Endophotograph: disfigured stomach lumen; the lesser curvature is straightened and rigid, with a rounded ulcer sized at 1 cm, with even, sloping edges. Histologically, a non-differentiated cancer

◄ **Fig. 21 d.**

Symptomatology

What are the main clinical manifestations of gastric cancer nowadays? In other words, what should be changed and what should be added to the known clinical symptoms? In the clinical diagnosis of early gastric cancer it is necessary to consider the patient's age and the presence of the symptom of rapid satiability while taking food. It should be noted that this symptom, which is more characteristic of advanced gastric cancers, can also occur in the early stages. True, this symptom may be discovered only by very thorough observation of the patient by a gastroenterologist or general clinician, or else by the family doctor. A further symptom is transient epigastric pain which rapidly subsides in response to the treatment of endoscopically diagnosed gastritis or peptic ulcer.

It should be noted that the clinical picture of gastric cancer, which is far from being conspicuous, is now blurred by medications which suppress gastric secretion. Drugs such as Omez, Losec, Ortanol, Promezol (omeprazole) Nexium (esomeprazole, S-isomer of omeprazole), Pariet (rabeprazole), omeprazole and its analogues inhibit the H+, K+-ATPase in the parietal cells of the stomach to block the final stage of gastric juice secretion.

In addition, the following important aspect should be mentioned. During recent years, the primary focus of cancer has changed its location in the stomach; the incidence of affections of the upper part have increased significantly. The situation is the same with the primary site of cancer on the greater curvature and the anterior wall. It therefore follows that in characterizing the clinical symptoms of gastric cancer these factors will be taken into consideration [38, 125].

Generally speaking, the problem of gastric cancer inevitably requires a revision of the screening strategy. Radical improvement in the early diagnosis of gastric cancer is infeasible without mass screening [144]. It is also important to note that, despite the existing opinion that the incidence of gastric cancer is decreasing, epidemiological data convincingly show that gastric cancer remains one of the leading oncological pathologies, and that in most regions of the world it constitutes 12–13% of all oncological diseases.

In our concise review of the clinical symptoms of gastric cancer, it is necessary to note that the centuries-old concept of a malignant tumor as a rapidly progressing pathology is unacceptable today. The concept was based on the fact that in earlier times the tumor was diagnosed at the advanced stage when its size was quite significant and the progress appeared to be »rapid«.

As a matter of fact, up to a certain moment a tumor grows slowly, sometimes for 3 or 4 years, and does not extend beyond the limits of the mucous and submucous membranes, nor does it manifest itself clinically [206]. For this reason, any clinical symptom may be regarded as the late manifestation of the tumor. In order to avoid misunderstanding, it is necessary to be more accurate: The presence of clinical symptoms of gastric cancer should not be interpreted as a sign of advanced cancer. It was established that anorexia (the absence of appetite) and decreasing body weight (and some other symptoms), which were formerly regarded as symptoms specific for advanced and neglected cancer and, according to some authors, occur in 19–25% and 20–88% of patients, respectively, may appear in patients with relatively early forms of the disease [99, 131, 189, 201, 217].

The rate of tumor growth can be estimated beginning only from the moment of its discovery on; and it is impossible to tell the age of a particular tumor before this moment. There have been times when, during the clinical examination of a patient who had no complaints or any clinical symptoms that might suggest pathologies of the gastrointestinal tract, the X-ray examination discovered minor gastric cancer which had been resolutely precluded by preceding endoscopy and histological studies. A year or more later, repeated endoscopic and histological examinations confirmed the radiological diagnosis.

At its earliest stages, gastric cancer does not show itself clinically for a long time. This time varies depending on the primary location of the tumor, and no one can say (even approximately) how long it may last. But it is precisely during this period that surgical treatment may result in complete cure [66].

The first clinical signs of the disease appear only when the tumor growth is so significant that it interferes with normal function of the stomach by decreasing its capacity, narrowing the gastroesophageal junction, and evacuating its contents. As the tumor starts to disintegrate, the destroyed vessels begin to bleed. This, in turn, evokes gradually increasing hypochromic anemia. Absorbed products of tumor decay cause toxicity. Infection develops in the tumor and the surrounding tissues, and the bacterial toxins are also absorbed, causing specific symptoms. Nerve trunks become involved in the process and the tumor invades the adjacent organs to result in the development of an unbearable and persistent pain syndrome. Remote metastatic tumor nodes discovered accidentally in persons who are regarded as being »in full health« are sometimes the first symptoms of the disease. These nodes may be revealed on the X-ray images of thoracic organs (PA chest, for example). Sometimes, an ultrasonographic follow-up examination for some pathology which by no means is connected with the stomach reveals free fluid in the abdominal cavity, which is also an indirect sign of carcinomatosis. The search for the primary focus then reveals gastric cancer. Even when the presence of distant metastases suggests infeasibility of radical intervention, the patient's complaints might not give grounds to suspect gastric disease. In some cases, even in the presence of specific complaints the physician does not think it reasonable to suspect a blastomatous process in the stomach, and only steadily intensifying clinical symptoms force the physician to continue the diagnostic search.

The first clinical symptoms of gastric cancer are quite varied and depend on many factors, the main ones being location of the tumor in a particular part of the stomach, the nature of tumor growth, its morphological structure, involvement of the adjacent organs, and bodily dysfunctions.

The common clinical symptoms are connected with the intoxication syndrome (non-motivated weakness, flaccidity, decreased working capacity, fatigue, impaired appetite, gastric discomfort, loss of body weight in the absence of visible reason, depression). These symptoms may be so insignificant that it is only their persistent character that makes the patient seek medical aid. It is easy to understand that many diseases are connected with intoxication, but the diagnostic investigation should always be conducted with the awareness of possible oncological involvement [6, 189]. While physicians should be alert, they should not exaggerate the danger of tumor and prescribe X-ray or endoscopic examination to all their patients during influenza epidemics, because influenza is manifested by marked intoxication.

Epigastric Pain

The most typical symptom of gastric cancer is disturbed patency of the gastrointestinal canal, which is narrowed by the growing tumor. It is evident that such disorders will be the relatively early and more pronounced signs of tumor in the cardiac and prepyloric parts, the pylorus included, because these are the most narrow portions of the stomach cavity. And these symptoms may be absent if the tumor is located in the stomach body or the fundus, especially on the greater curvature or the anterior wall of the stomach.

The feeling of an overfilled epigastrium is believed to be the sign of the initial process of obstruction of the pylorus, the antral, and the prepyloric parts. In other words, this feeling is characteristic of cancer. At the same time, development of the obstructive symptoms in the presence of invasive carcinoma in the pyloric part, which causes its steno-

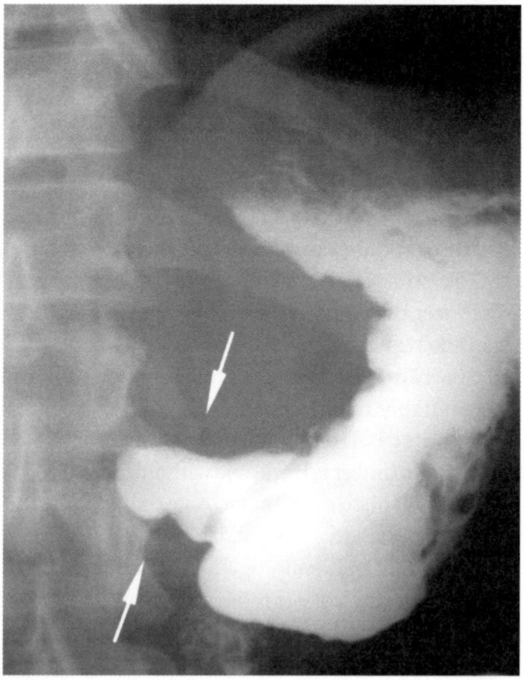

Fig. 22 a.

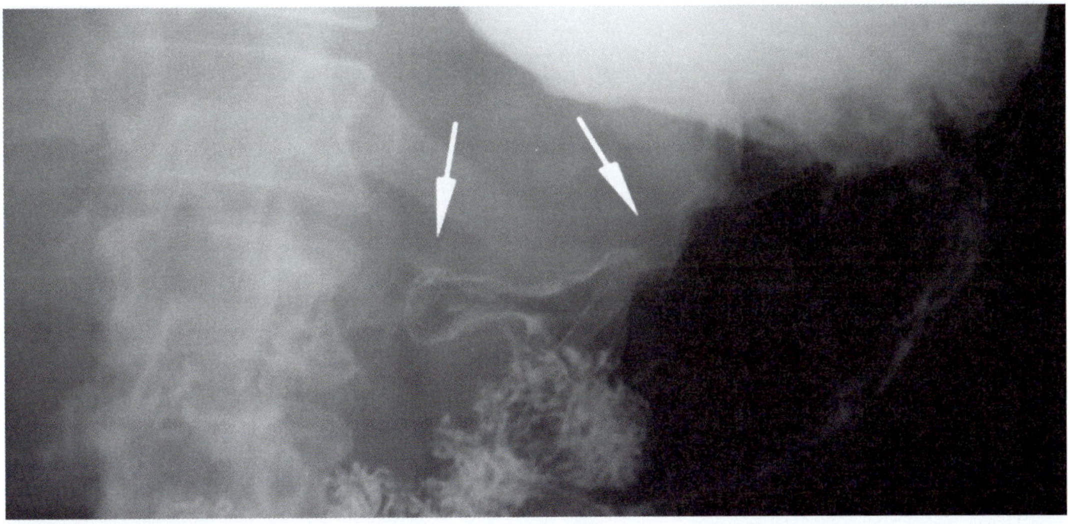

Fig. 22 b.

sis, may be associated with a relatively insignificant invasion of the submucous membrane of the stomach. In addition, even in the presence of cancer infiltration over a short length, marked clinical symptoms may appear. But this relates only to tumors, the primary location of which is the pylorus proper [31, 222]. In patients with exophytic carcinoma, evacuation disorders develop mostly in cases where the tumor passes from the expansive growth stage to mixed-type cancer, which is associated with a strongly advanced process.

First, the evacuation disorders may occur only occasionally, especially in severe abuse of foods, especially bitter dishes or alcohol. The disorders are especially marked in patients who suddenly stop drinking strong alcoholic drinks to replace them with soft ones. Such patients may develop obstruction all of a sudden, while they are »totally healthy«. Epigastric pain and vomiting may develop. All these symptoms may persist for several days or weeks, and then subside as a result of dietary restrictions. The patient may feel healthy for several weeks or months, until another attack of obstruction occurs. In some patients, obstruction fails to be removed, but rather progresses steadily. Gradually increasing symptoms are more common. Even small meals cause an unsurpassable feeling of gravity in the stomach, and sometimes eructation. Voiding of gas through the mouth is explained by congestion of food in the stomach. The wind is first odorless, but later, as the congestion is characterized by putrefactive decomposition of the stomach contents, eructation becomes fetid, and the patient complains of »rotten-egg eructation«. Pyrosis (heartburn) is also not infrequent. This is due to irritation of the esophageal mucosa with regurgitated acid stomach contents. This may occur as well in the case of normal gastric secretion and also when organic acids are formed during decomposition of gastric contents. Therefore, hypoacidity patients with this complaint should undergo both an X-ray and endoscopic examination immediately, regardless of how recent their previous examination was (Fig. 22).

Fig. 22a–d. Patient D, age 54. Diagnosis: gastric cancer. Complained of overfilled stomach after eating very small meals, and of heartburn which persisted for 8 months. Slow but steady intensification of the symptoms led the patient to seek medical aid. **a** Stomach X-ray (tight filling, vertical position, anterior projection): the stomach contains much liquid, the antral part is disfigured, narrow, uneven walls are rigid (arrows), markedly disordered evacuation. **b** Stomach X-ray (double contract, horizontal position, right oblique projection): the pyloric and antral parts are disfigured and narrow, the walls are thick and rigid due to intramural circular infiltration (arrows). Conclusion: infiltrative cancer of the pyloric and antral parts of the stomach. **c** Macrospecimen of a resected stomach: the distal part is narrow, the walls are thick and firm (arrows). **d** Fragment of the macrospecimen (strip): the stomach wall is thick due to intramural infiltration (arrows). Histologically, an adenocarcinoma with the signet-ring cell component

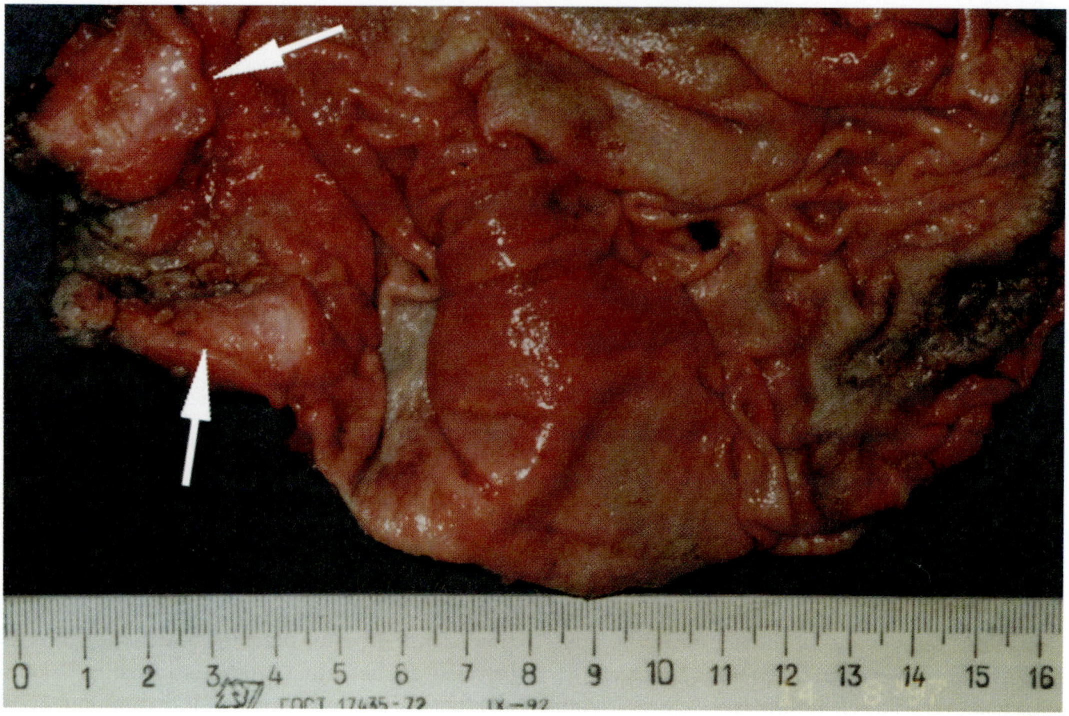

▲ **Fig. 22 c.**

▼ **Fig. 22 d.**

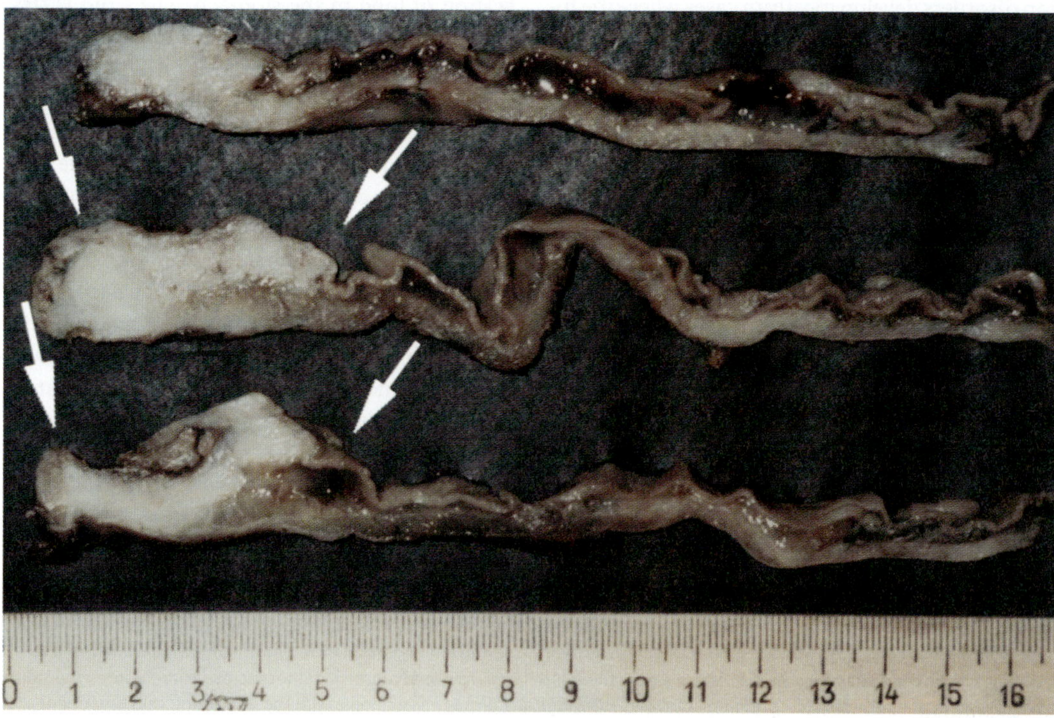

If the evacuation dysfunction is severe and the stomach is not emptied, the patient starts vomiting. A typical picture of the so-called stenosed pyloric part of the stomach develops [28]. It is characterized by the patient's relatively good condition with a fasting stomach (in the morning). But after the first meal, the patient feels epigastric discomfort and dull pain. After the next meal the discomfort and pain increases. By the evening, these symptoms intensify, becoming unbearable after supper. The patient vomits all food taken during the day, and sometimes the erupted gastric contents include residues of »old« food ingested the day before. The odor is fetid. The patient feels better. Improvement is so significant that if vomiting does not occur spontaneously, the patient tries to provoke it artificially.

Despite an increasing feeling of hunger, the patient refuses much food in fear of the painful consequences, and an aversion to food may develop. Daily lavage of the stomach is indicated for such patients. After this procedure the patient feels much better, but the amounts of water and nutrients in the body remain deficient, which leads to loss of weight and dehydration.

Some patients with an involved pyloric part do not develop obstruction; rather, the pylorus loses the ability to contract, and all food leaves the stomach through an open passage. The same situation can develop when a part of the pylorus wall remains uninvolved, but the pylorus does not contract and fails to close the outlet from the stomach, owing to affection of the relevant nerve endings or because of the lost reflex in the presence of disordered secretion of gastric juice and the absence of hydrochloric acid in it. The rapid passage of non-digested food into the intestine results in a permanent feeling of hunger. The patient begins to eat a large amount of food but continues to lose weight rapidly because the food is inadequately absorbed in the intestine. Stools become frequent and liquid, containing much undigested food. Involvement of the pancreas is of great importance: Digestion becomes upset not only in the stomach but also in the intestine.

If the tumor affects the middle third of the stomach, especially on its anterior and posterior walls, and also on the greater curvature, the patient does not have any complaints associated with gastric dysfunction for a long time. Epigastric pain may develop against the background of general symptoms. Pain develops after meals and abates after defecation. In contrast, the patient may experience pain which develops only in the fasting stomach and abates after food is ingested (just like fasting pain in duodenal ulcer). If the tumor does not grow beyond the limits of the stomach, fasting fain is either mild or completely absent. Strong permanent pain not connected with meals and radiating to the back, at times dull or acute, almost incurable by medication, is often the result of tumor propagation to the retroperitoneal organs and anatomical structures, e.g., the pancreas, solar plexus, nerve trunks. Appetite is often absent; the patient frequently develops an aversion to food in general, and sometimes to a particular food, most often to meat.

Stomach capacity may decrease significantly in patients with endophytic tumors which are difficult to diagnose endoscopically, especially the linitis plastica type tumor. The rapid satiability symptom develops in such patients (35–45%). The patient feels epigastric discomfort and an overfilled stomach, with the symptoms developing following a small meal. According to patients' complaints, they can eat only half, one fourth, or even less of the normal amount of food. If the tumor grows circularly, the stomach can be narrowed to the extent where it resembles an hourglass in scirrhous carcinoma, or it may occupy considerable space in fibrous carcinoma, to form a rigid tube, which is usually characterized by expansive infiltration along the lesser curvature reaching the esophagus. The stomach capacity decreases, evacuation of its contents from the upper part, and sometimes from the esophagus, becomes difficult. This condition develops not only if the tumor encircles the stomach to diminish its lumen, but much earlier, because the infiltrated muscular coat becomes unable to contract and interferes with the peristaltic movement of the gastric wall (▫ Fig. 23).

Symptoms of gastric involvement with tumors of this localization usually develop at late stages of the disease when the tumor becomes very large and begins to disintegrate and bleed. The symptoms of tumor bleeding (melena, hypochromic anemia) may thus become the first clinical symptoms of gastric disease.

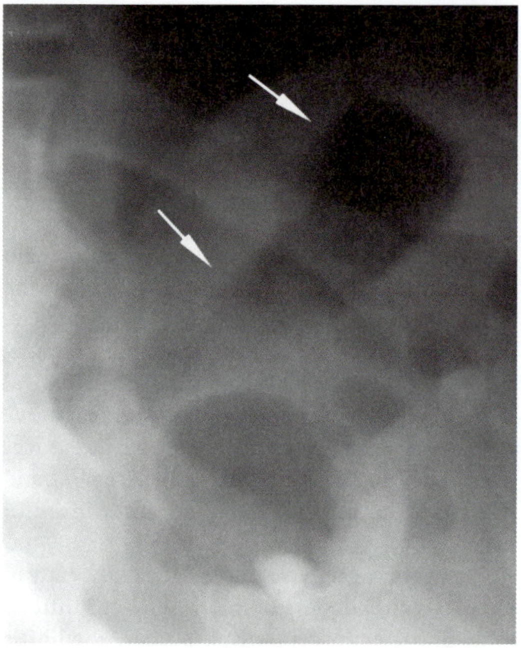

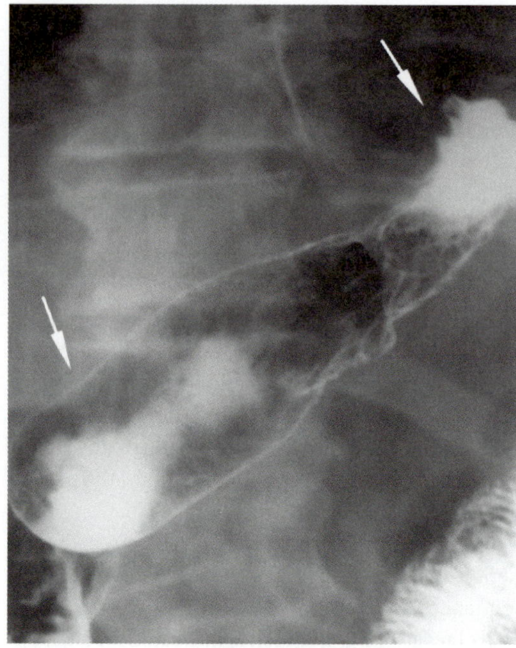

▲ Fig. 23 a. ▼ Fig. 23 b.

▲ Fig. 23 c. ▼ Fig. 23 d.

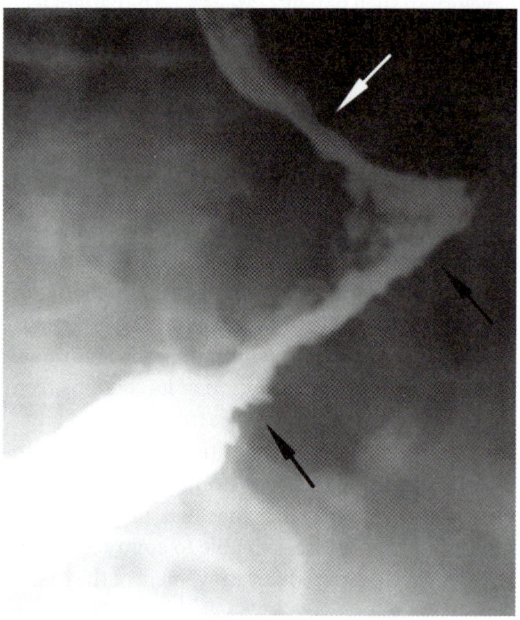

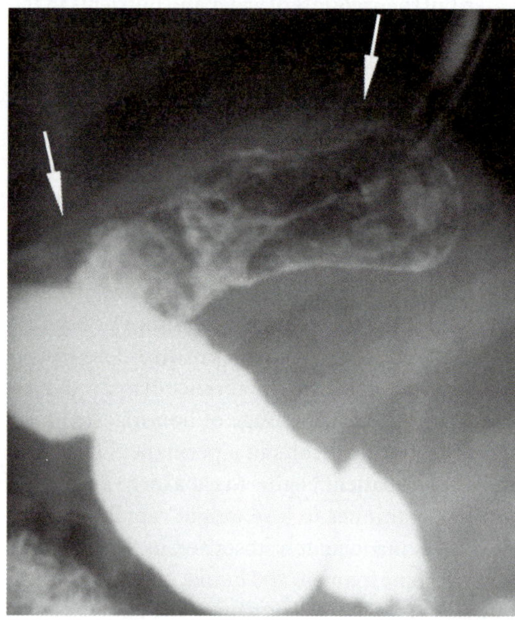

Fig. 23a–h. Patient A., age 58. Diagnosis: gastric cancer. Complained of rapid fatigue, rapid satiability after eating small meals, moderate dysphagia. Diseased for 2 years (from the time when he first felt epigastric discomfort after meals). Received outpatient treatment with no positive results. Anamnesis: the first X-ray examination revealed infiltrative cancer of the stomach. Multiple endoscopy, including the taking of 6–8 tissue specimens, failed to reveal organic involvement. Histological studies did not reveal tumor cells either. The first symptom of dysphagia had occurred about a month earlier. The patient was given another X-ray examination. **a** Stomach X-ray (vertical position, anterior projection): symptom of gas redistribution in the stomach, the gastric air bubble is extended (arrows); **b** Stomach X-ray (tight filling, vertical position, anterior projection) at the moment of contrast medium passage through the gastroesophageal junction; the abdominal segment of the esophagus is irregularly narrow,

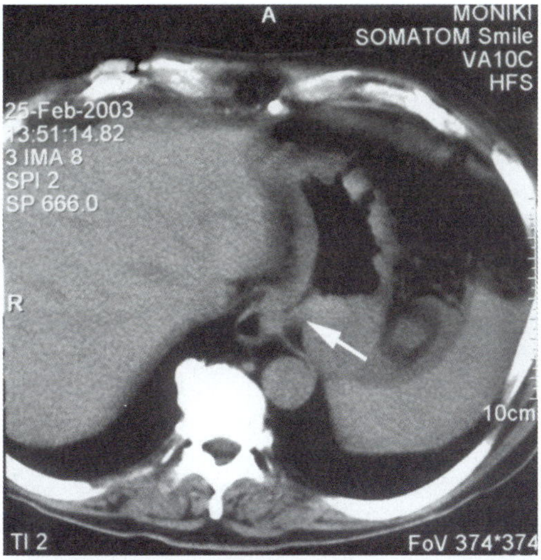

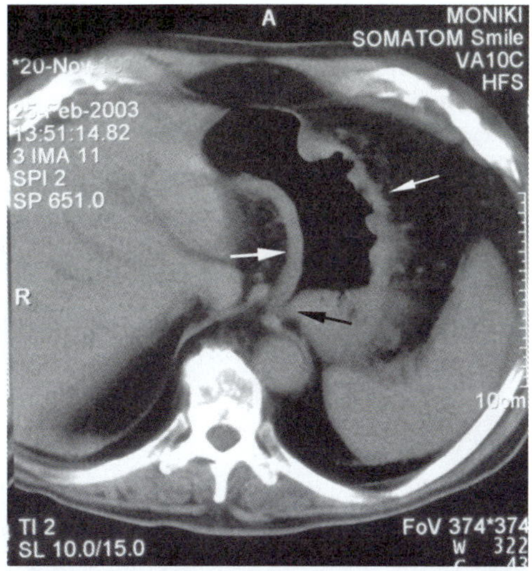

▲ **Fig. 23 e.** ▼ **Fig. 23 g.** ▲ **Fig. 23 f.**

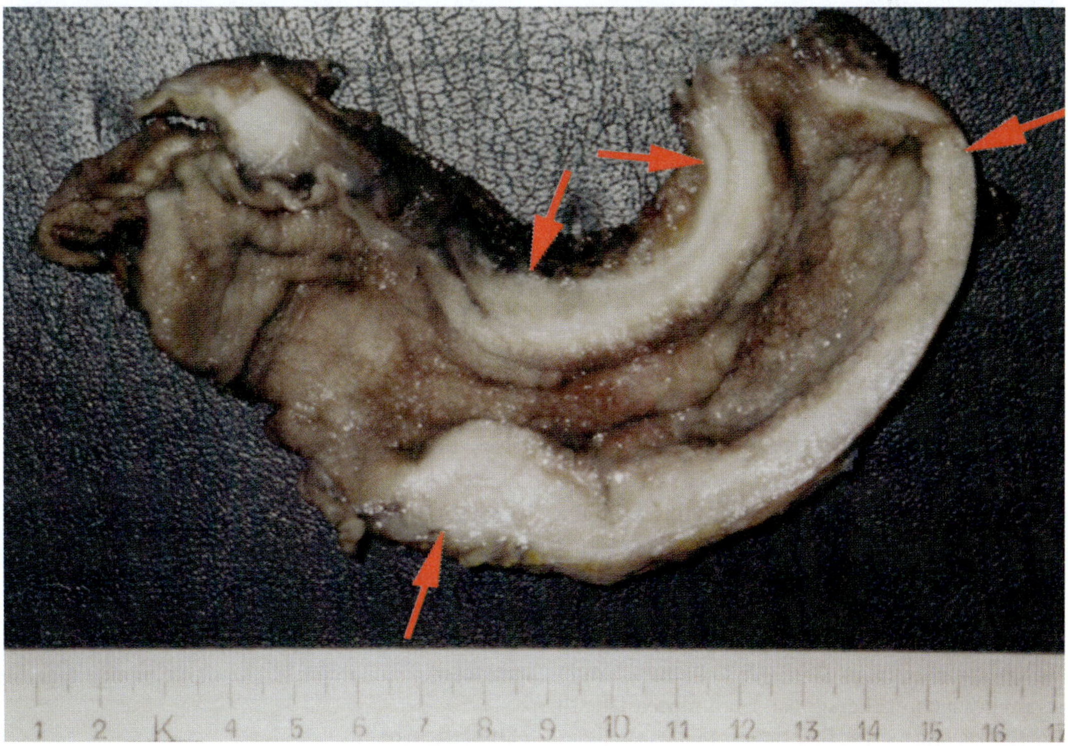

with uneven contours (white arrow), stomach capacity is decreased considerably, uneven contours (black arrows). **c** Stomach X-ray (double contrast, horizontal position, anterior projection): the walls are rigid, the capacity decreased significantly (arrows), markedly accelerated evacuation, contrast medium drops straight to the duodenum; **d** Stomach X-ray (double contrast, horizontal position, left oblique projection) after additional intake of gas-producing mixture and barium meal: thick walls of the stomach body and the upper part; rigid due to circular infiltration (arrows). Conclusion: infiltrative cancer of the stomach spreading to the abdominal segment of the esophagus. Control endoscopy and histological examination of tumor samples failed to reveal tumor cells. **e** Computed tomogram of the stomach (native study in supine position) at the level of the abdominal segment of the esophagus: walls of the abdominal esophagus are thick due to intramural infiltration (arrow). **f** Computed tomogram of the stomach (native study, supine position) at the level of the upper third of the stomach body: the walls of the upper part are thick due to circular intramural infiltration (white arrow); infiltration extends to the esophagus (black arrow). Conclusion: infiltrative cancer of the stomach with spread to the abdominal segment of the esophagus. **g** Macrospecimen of a resected stomach: inner cavity is diminished, walls are thick and firm due to circular intramural infiltration which extends onto the esophagus (arrows). **h** Fragment of a macrospecimen (strip): stomach wall is thick due to intramural infiltration (arrows). Histologically, a signet-ring cell carcinoma

▼ **Fig. 23 h.**

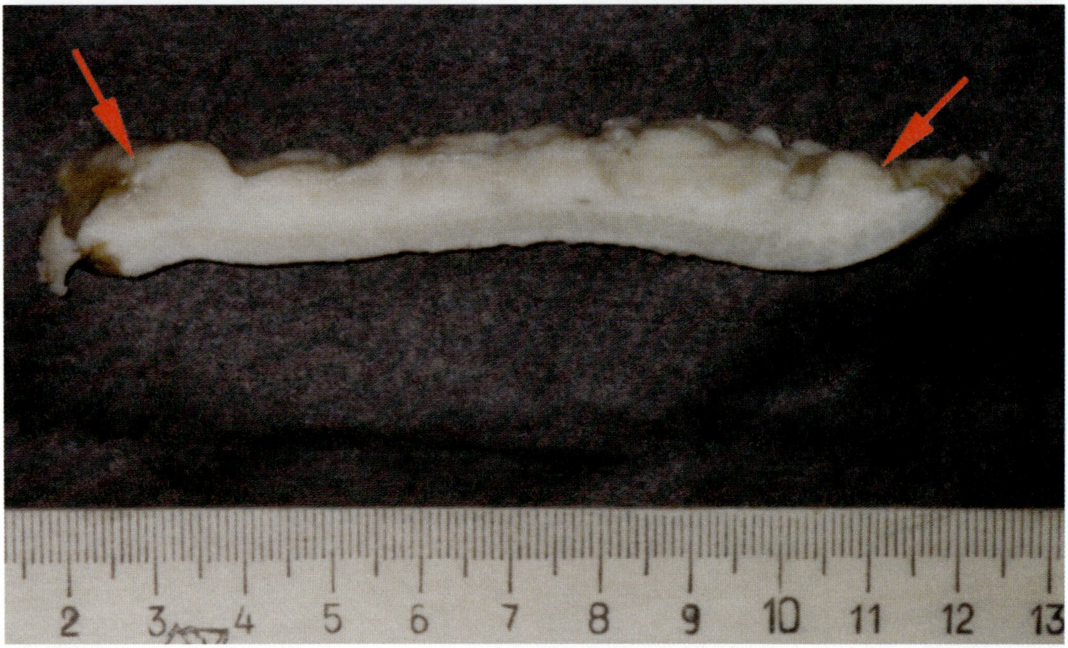

Ulceration

Clinical symptoms become more pronounced in the presence of ulceration. This helps in the differentiation of non-differentiated and signet-ring cell carcinoma from the great variety of other forms, among which infiltrative cancers dominate. The clinical picture of the disease depends mainly on infiltrative-ulcerous carcinomas, which now prevail. This, in turn, interferes with the differential diagnosis of malignant and benign ulcers. Ulcer in the anamnesis makes a clinical diagnosis even more difficult. Correct diagnostic and therapeutic tactics are therefore decisive for the prognosis. According to some authors, symptoms specific for peptic ulcer are absent [117, 177]. This means that if epigastric discomfort and pain intensify after meals, and the feeling of full stomach, nausea, and vomiting develop, this suggests a very high probability of malignancy (◘ Fig. 24).

At the same time, the clinical picture of malignant ulcers, which often attack the lesser curvature, is not specific either, as distinct from scirrhous affections of the greater curvature and the anterior and posterior walls of the stomach. Meals intensify pain in such patients, but the feeling of a full stomach is the main symptom. The symptoms intensify at a comparatively rapid pace and, if therapy is not given in due time, the pronounced clinical picture of gastric cancer develops with prevalence of the obstructive signs [37].

Dysphagia

Dysphagia is another symptom connected with difficult patency. Since dysphagia is a symptom of blastomatous affection of the cardia, which according to the topographic classification refers to the proximal part of the stomach (the most complicated part from the anatomical standpoint), it should be regard-

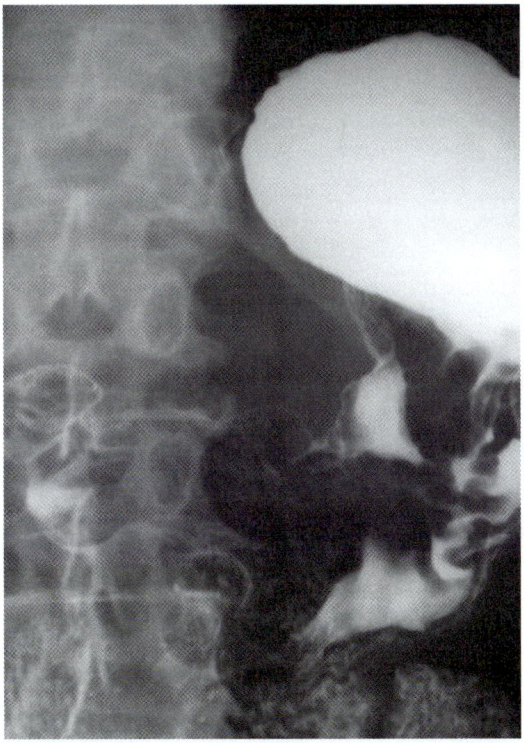

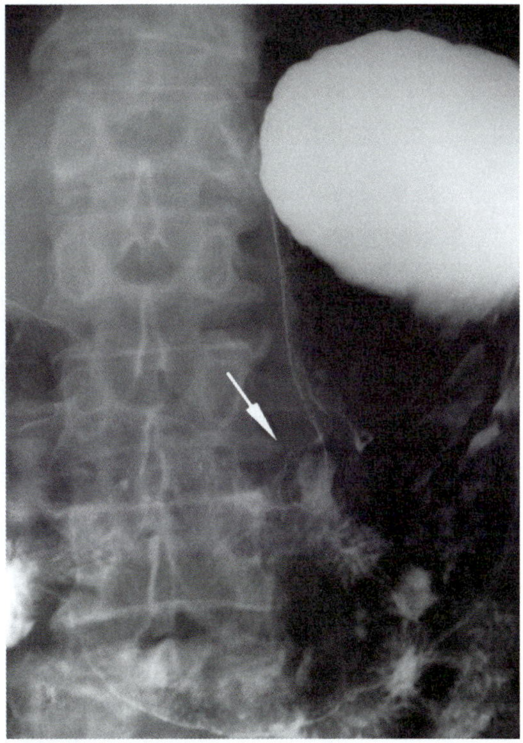

▲ Fig. 24 a. ▼ Fig. 24 c. ▲ Fig. 24 b.

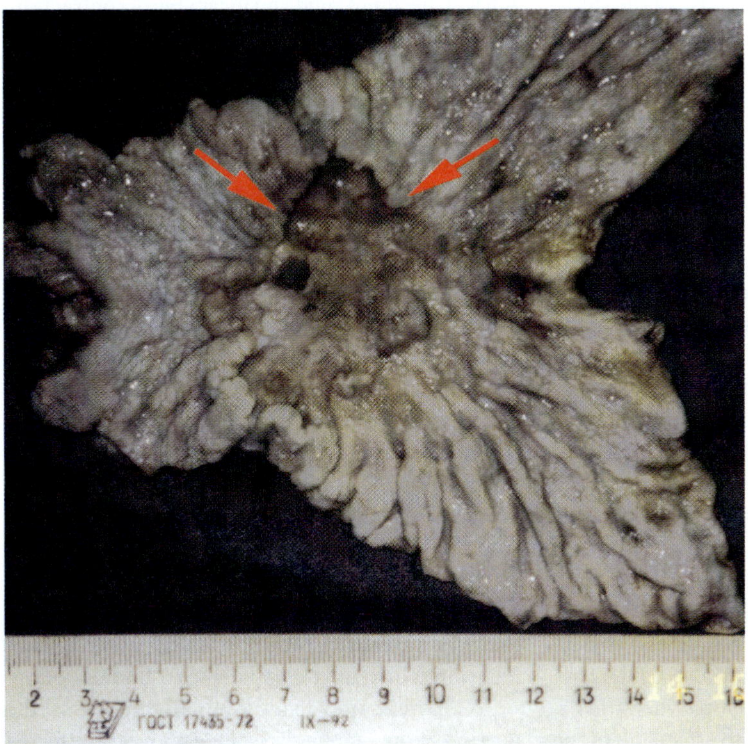

Fig. 24a–d. Patient B., age 64. Diagnosis: gastric cancer. Complained of epigastric discomfort which intensified after meals. The symptom had increased steadily during the preceding month. Nausea occurred periodically. **a** Stomach X-ray (double contrast, horizontal position, right oblique projection): depot of irregular shapes with converging folds on the lesser curvature. **b** Stomach X-ray (double contrast, horizontal position, anterior projection): after the ulcer crater is emptied of the contrast medium, thick wall of the lesser curvature with converging folds is visualized (arrow). Conclusion: infiltrative ulcerous cancer of the stomach body. **c** Macrospecimen of a resected stomach: firm walls, flat ulcer on the lesser curvature (arrow). **d** Fragments of the macrospecimen (strips): white tumor tissue underlying the ulcer crater and infiltrating the stomach wall (arrows). Histologically, an adenocarcinoma with the signet-ring cell component

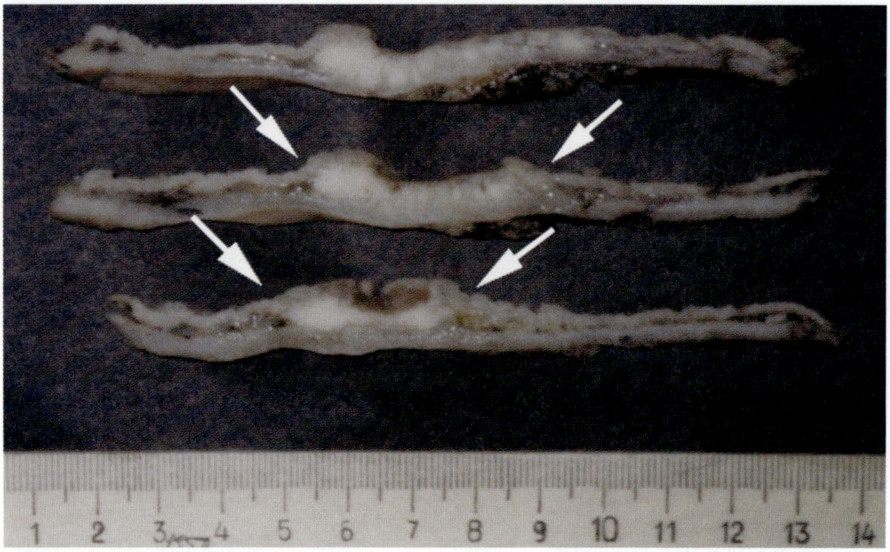

◂ Fig. 24 d.

ed together with all clinical symptoms of cancer of the upper part of the stomach.

Clinical symptoms of proximal gastric cancer and the time of their development depend even more on the primary (initial) site of tumor location within the limits of this anatomical part, as compared with tumors developing in other parts of the stomach. Note that, in addition to the general clinical symptoms, an important symptom such as dysphagia develops in some patients with cancer of the upper part of the stomach only at late stages of the disease, and in some patients not at all. The idea that dysphagia is an obligatory companion of cancer of the upper part of the stomach is therefore incorrect. A tumor originating in the immediate vicinity of the cardiac sphincter very soon spreads to the abdominal part of the esophagus to cause dysphagia. At the same time, a tumor of the upper part of the stomach located at a distance from the cardiac rosette (cardioesophageal junction), e.g., on the posterior wall, the greater curvature, or the fundus, produces these symptoms either much later or not at all.

Dysphagia occurs in about 89.4% of cases of proximal gastric cancer. First the patient may feel only scratching, burning, or pain when swallowing food. Passage of food through a narrowed canal becomes more difficult with time. A sudden complete obstruction of the esophagus may also be the first sign, but dysphagia usually develops when the tumor size is considerable enough to affect half of the canal circumference or even greater. Marked dysphagia can also develop in the presence of very small tumors, owing to spasm of the stomach wall at the moment of food passage. However, sometimes dysphagia does not develop in patients with extensive disease. This may happen when the involved stomach wall becomes rigid and incapable of contraction. Food drops freely through the open tube of the esophagus in such patients (◘ Fig. 25).

Cardiac impatency develops more often in patients with tumors infiltrating the wall of the stomach. Blastomatous infiltration spreads onto the muscular coat to involve nerve endings. First this increases the sensitivity of the muscular membrane and induces mild spasms, but later, the contractility of the muscles becomes impaired. Exophytic tumors, which rarely occur now, interfere with food passage to the stomach less frequently and at later stages of the disease. Ingested food in most cases passes freely over a mushroom-like tumor, provided the latter does not affect the rosette proper, where the mucous membrane is immobile relative to the muscular coat and the tumor can obstruct the entrance to the stomach.

Most often, dysphagia first manifests as a difficulty in swallowing solid food, and the patient has to drink water after each portion is ingested. Later it becomes difficult to swallow semi-liquid food.

As cardiac impatency gradually increases, the portion of the esophagus located above the affected

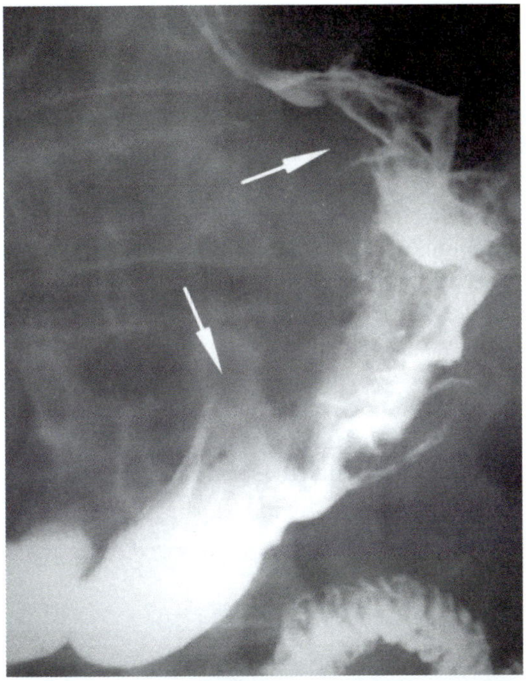

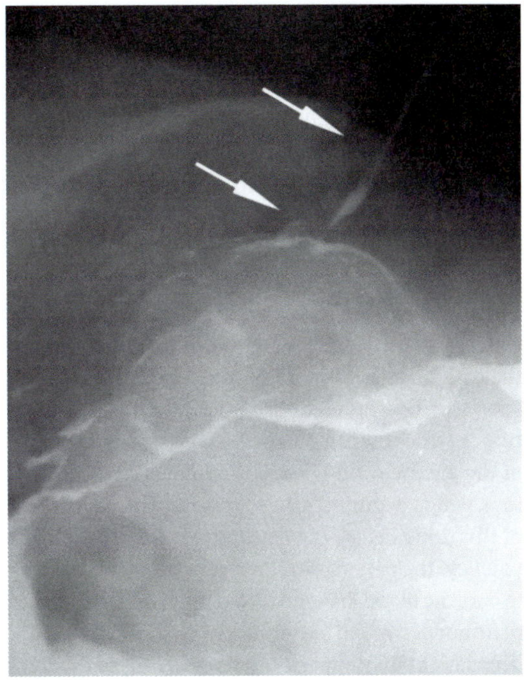

▲ **Fig. 25 a.** ▼ **Fig. 25 b.**

▲ **Fig. 25 c.** ▼ **Fig. 25 d.**

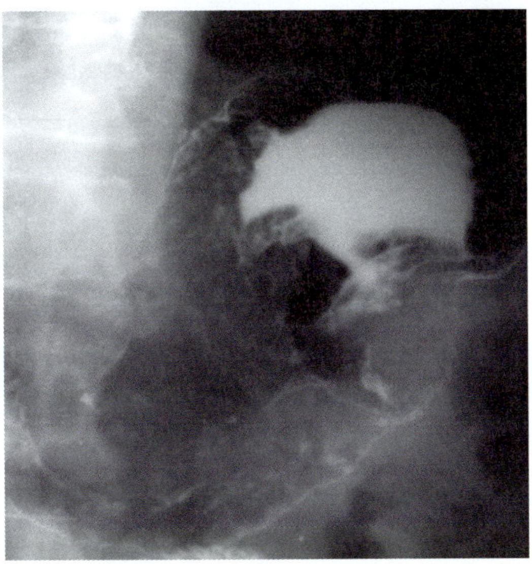

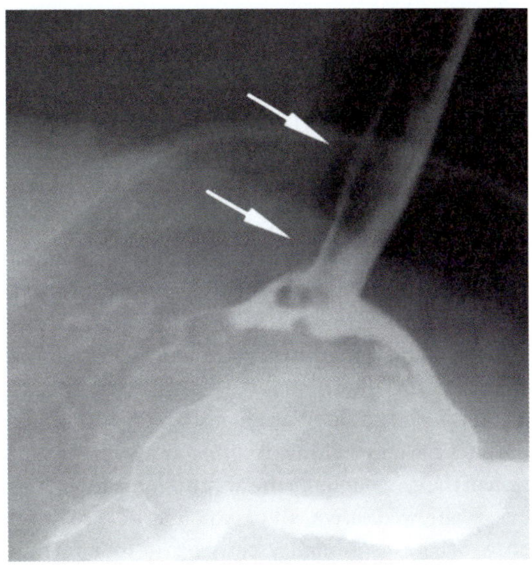

Fig. 25a–d. Patient Z., age 68. Diagnosis: gastric cancer. **a** Stomach x-ray (tight filling, vertical position, anterior projection): the stomach body is disfigured to a rigid tube with uneven contours (arrows). **b** Stomach X-ray (double contrast, horizontal position, anterior projection): walls of the body and the upper part are thick and rigid; the inner surface is tuberous. **c** Stomach X-ray (double contrast, vertical position, left oblique projection): posterior wall of the body and the upper part is thick due to infiltration extending to the cardia; the walls of the esophagus are rigid, the lumen is wide open (arrows). **d** X-ray of the stomach and abdominal segment of the esophagus (double contrast, vertical position, left oblique projection): relief of the cardiac rosette (cardioesophageal junction) is changed, cardia is wide open, the abdominal esophagus is a rigid tube owing to spreading of the intramural infiltration (arrows). Conclusion: infiltrative cancer of the stomach body and its upper part, with extension of the tumor onto the esophagus

site distends to accumulate food masses, which are partly propelled to the stomach by esophageal contractions and partly evacuated by vomiting.

The patient rapidly loses weight and water. The skin becomes dry and flaccid, tissue turgor decreases markedly. When tested, skin folds do not straighten for a long time. This condition may develop very soon if the tumor is found in the cardia proper. As the tumor grows, it soon obstructs the entrance to the stomach to account for the typical symptoms of cancer before development of general disorders in the patient. If the tumor is at a distance from the rosette (cardioesophageal junction), then, before the tumor closes the lumen, it affects considerable areas of the gastric wall. Ulcers often develop on the tumor, which begins to disintegrate and bleed. In view of this, long before the development of cardiac impatency, the patient develops general disorders due to chronic blood loss and intoxication with products of tumor decay and bacterial toxins. The ESR is high. The patient may experience pain owing to involvement of the nerve elements of the stomach wall or the adjacent organs.

If the tumor resides in the upper part of the stomach, the patient feels retrosternal pain or pain between the shoulder blades. Very often this is interpreted as heart pain. This pain may be the result of intensified contractions of the esophagus in patients with disordered cardiac patency. As a rule, pain develops at the moment of swallowing when the esophagus must contract. These contractions may be very painful and the patient has to drink water, to take a deep breath, assume a special position, etc. If the esophagus is strongly distended above the point of obstruction, pain may be absent immediately after small portions of food are ingested. Pain develops only after a lapse of time in connection with distension of the esophagus by the accumulated food, mucus, swallowed saliva, all of which irritate the mucosa of the esophagus, causing it to contract vigorously. In such cases the patient does not associate pain with meals but relates its development to disorders of his/her cardiovascular system.

Tumors with their primary location in the region of the fundus, on the posterior or anterior wall, or on the greater curvature may manifest for a long time only as general disorders. Gastric disorders may be either absent or so mild that the patient disregards them. The disease is often identified correctly only when the tumor attacks the stomach wall close to the entrance, which manifests as dysphagia, or when pain of specific localization develops. Hiccup is the most common clinical symptom of cancer in the zone of the fundus and the supracardiac part; it is due to involvement of the diaphragm. Among other symptoms may be pain irradiating by the diaphragmatic nerve; diaphragmatic pleurisy is not infrequent either. Left-sided pleurisy occurs in tumors not only of the stomach fundus but of its body as well, which spread onto the cardiac part. This is sometimes the first sign of the disease.

When located on the greater curvature, a tumor more often grows into the splenic portal. In patients with affections of the posterior wall, the tumor

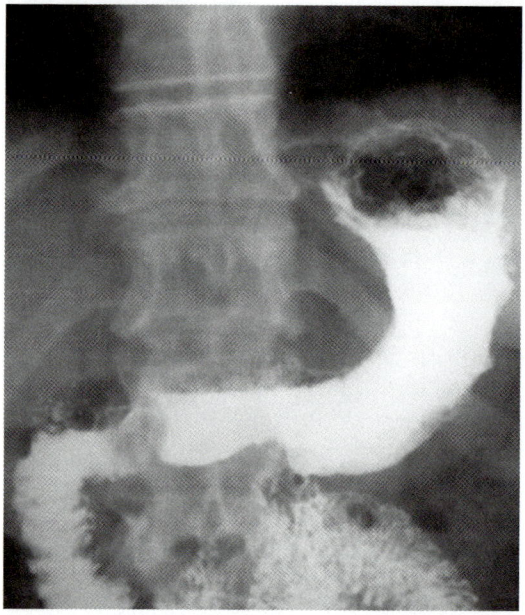

▲ **Fig. 26 a.** ◘ **Fig. 26a–e.** Patient S., age 59. Diagnosis: gastric cancer. **a** Stomach X-ray (tight filling, vertical position, anterior projection): stomach inner volume is diminished, the stomach is disfigured (rigid tube type); the contours are uneven. **b** Target stomach X-ray (tight filling, vertical position, anterior projection): the angular notch is straightened, the lesser curvature is depressed, the walls are rigid. **c** Stomach X-ray (double contrast, horizontal position, anterior projection): walls of the distal part and the body are thick and rigid due to circular infiltration. Conclusion: infiltrative cancer of the stomach. **d** Macrospecimen of a resected stomach: walls are thick due to intramural infiltration (arrow). **e** Fragments of the macrospecimen (strips): the wall is thickened due to the white tumor tissue (arrows)

spreads to the retroperitoneal space and first of all into the pancreas, sometimes also into the left kidney [158]. Of course, it should be understood that we are speaking here about neglected or advanced cancers, and that involvement of the diaphragm and the adjacent organs is more frequent in diffuse cancers than in the intestinal form.

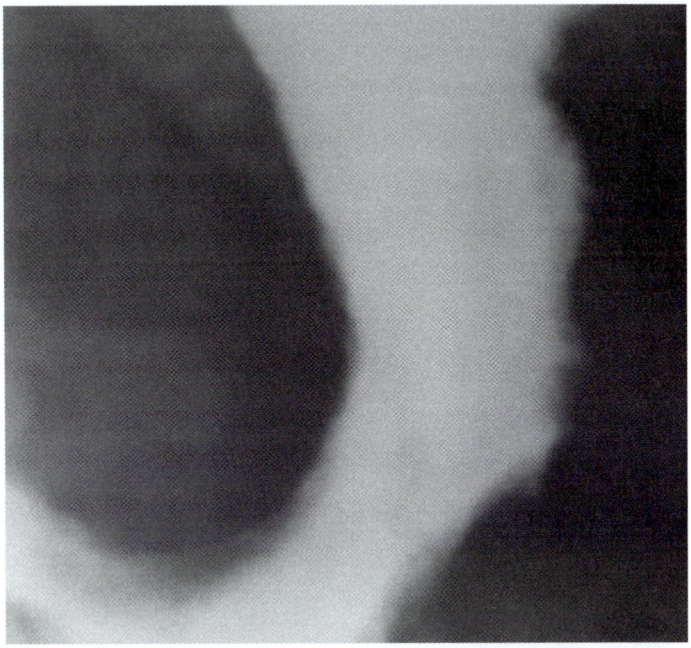

▲ Fig. 26 b.

▼ Fig. 26 c.

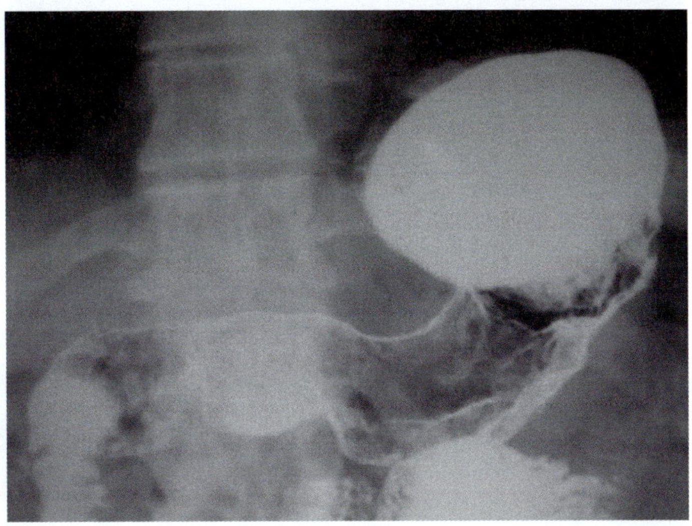

Conclusion

To conclude our survey of the symptoms which are currently acknowledged as characteristic of gastric cancer, it should be noted that the markedly high frequency of latent cancer (which is diagnosed only at its advanced stages) is due to the prevalence of the diffuse forms. In other words, the absence of clinical symptoms is more typical of endophytic cancer of the stomach (disregarding the terminal stage of the disease).

The special features of clinical symptoms of infiltrative tumors (which often develop in the absence of specific symptoms of malignancy due to tumor development in the submucous membrane and often with only microscopic signs on the mucosal surface) have been known for several centuries. The changes in the stomach wall in such cases were interpreted as the result of inflammation.

Lilientaud was the first to describe this pathology (1779). Andral (1829) interpreted the discovered thickening of the stomach wall as a result of hypertrophy. This standpoint was supported by W. Brinton (1864), who gave the name of linitis plastica to the discovered pathological changes. The name was deemed quite appropriate, and it has persisted up to the present to designate new growth inside the submucous membrane, which markedly thickens the stomach wall (◘ Fig. 26) [88]. If this disease runs an asymptomatic course, the tumor may spread over a significant area and become manifest only when the entire stomach has already been involved.

Early diagnosis of gastric cancer in the young is especially difficult. The time from appearance of the first complaints till the moment of establishing the diagnosis in aged patients is 6 months on average, whereas for persons aged 40–45 this period extends

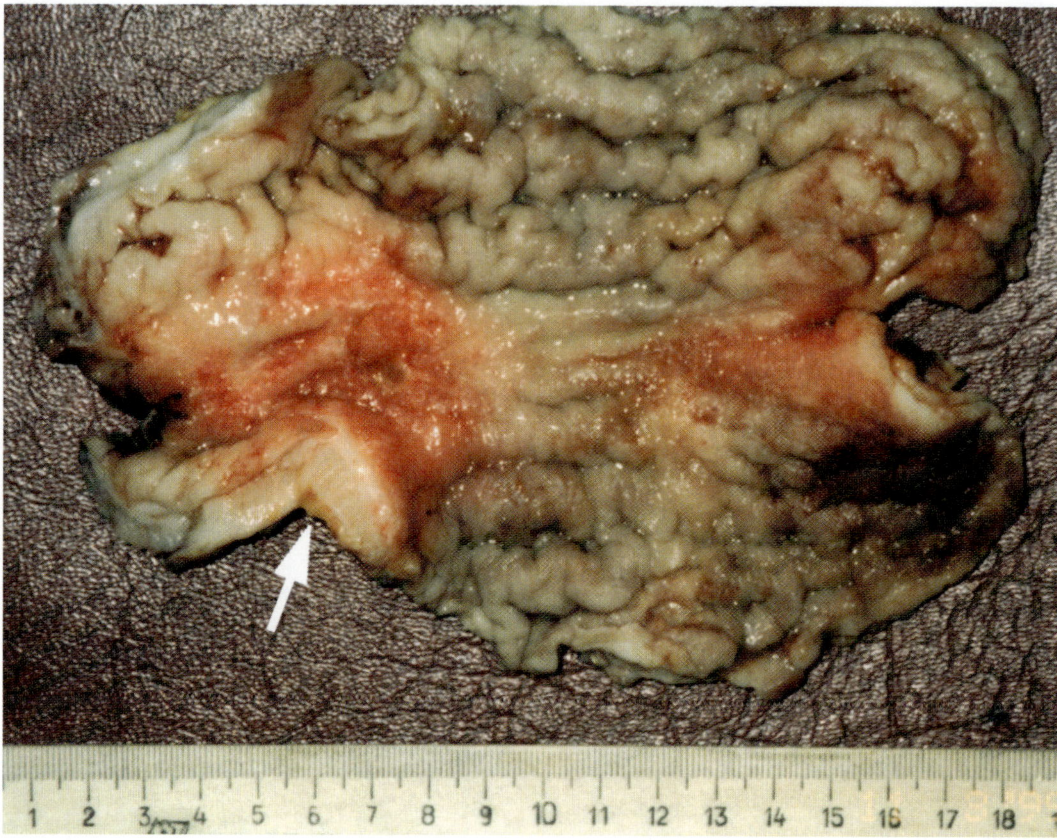

▲ Fig. 26 d.

▼ Fig. 26 e.

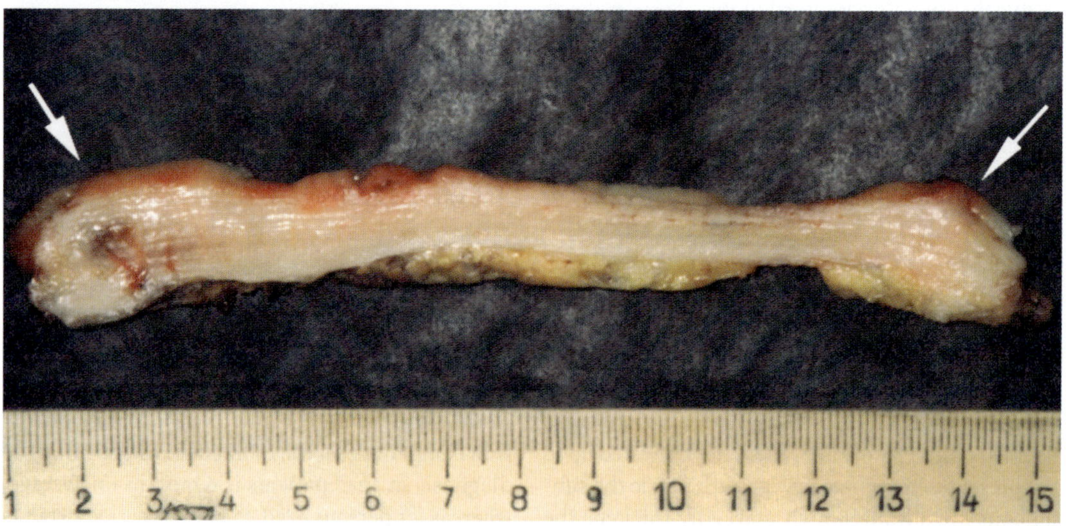

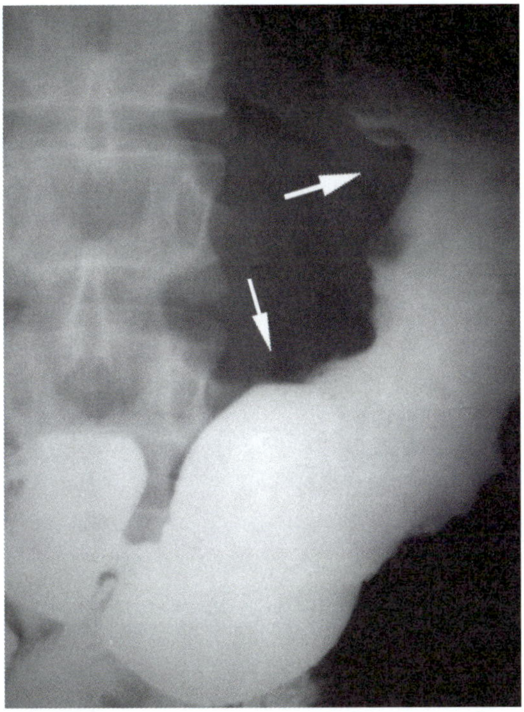

▲ Fig. 27 a. ▼ Fig. 27 b.

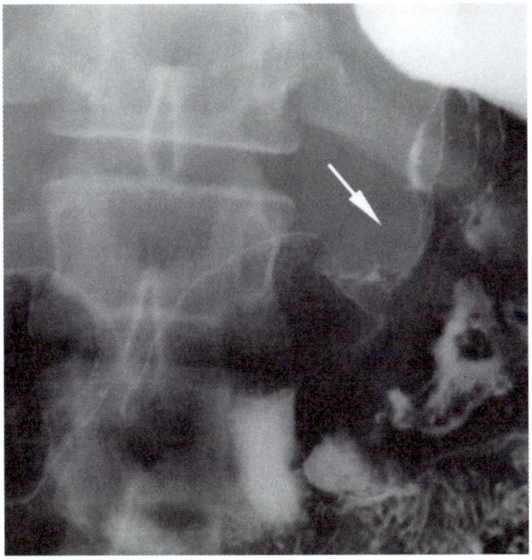

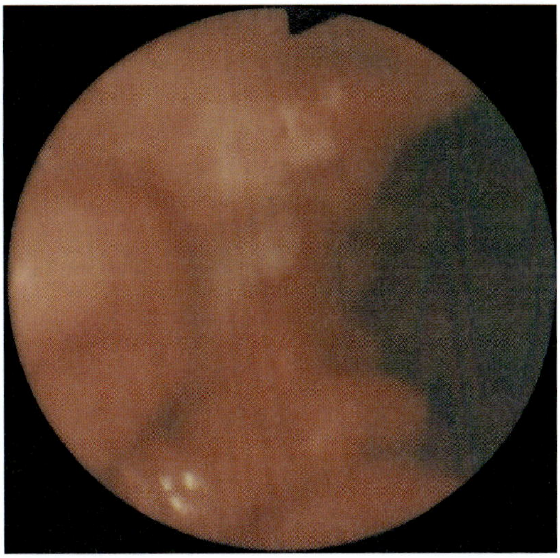

▲ Fig. 27 c.

Fig. 27a–c. Patient T., age 19. Diagnosis: gastric cancer. Anamnesis: the patient complained of epigastric pain for about 6 months. Primary endoscopy revealed ulcerous defect on the anterior wall of the stomach. Examination of bioptates did not reveal signs of inflammation or tumor cells. The absence of improvement suggested X-ray examination. **a** Stomach X-ray (tight filling, vertical position, anterior projection): markedly disfigured stomach body, uneven contours, eroded at some points (arrows). **b** Stomach X-ray (double contrast, horizontal position, anterior projection): stomach walls are thick and rigid due to circular intramural infiltration (arrows), with some irregular rounded spots with contrast medium at the periphery (ulcers). Conclusion: infiltrative-ulcerous cancer of the stomach. **c** Endophotograph (following X-ray examination): 2.5-cm ulcer with rough floor covered with necrotic tissues, with thick converging folds. Infiltration into adjacent mucous membranes. Histologically, non-differentiated cancer

to 10 months, even if the patient visits the doctor within the first 5–10 weeks. These patients are usually subjected to an endoscopic examination which establishes the diagnosis of gastritis, and the patient is given relevant treatment, whereas the true character of their complaints is not established [45].

This situation can be explained as follows: First, the physician is not on the alert while examining the young; cancer occurs far less frequently in young patients than in the aged. But physicians should never underestimate the danger of cancer even in persons under 20 (Fig. 27). Second, most carcinomas of the young are characterized by intramural growth (in 70–75% of cases). Therefore, any patient presenting with gastrointestinal complaints must be examined by both X-ray and endoscopy [45, 53].

To complete our discussion of the clinical symptoms of gastric cancer we should return to the problem of its early diagnosis. When the diagnostic search begins only after the appearance of clinical symptoms, radical change is necessary. In most cases gastric cancer need not be diagnosed only at the clinical stage of its development; indeed, this must be done earlier, because gastric cancer belongs to the group of diseases that are diagnosed mainly by instrumental methods. The situation with early diagnosis of gastric cancer may be improved only if a complex of diagnostic tools, including a primary X-ray survey of the entire stomach and subsequent endoscopy, is used. In other words, risk group patients should be examined. It must also be noted that in view of recent advances in technology, the diagnostic algorithm of patient examination for gastric cancer must include ultrasonography, computed tomography, and magnetic resonance tomography. These should be regarded as methods additional to the traditional X-ray investigation and endoscopy.

4

Radiological Diagnosis of Gastric Cancer

(with O.V. Vyatchanin and G.A. Stashuk)

Introduction

This chapter deals with one of the most important problems in the radiological diagnosis of gastric cancer, namely, the characteristics of various methods and their practical use. The change of emphasis in the morphogenesis of gastric cancer and in the »favored« location of cancer's appearance in the stomach make it necessary to radically revise the methodological approach to radiological diagnosis of gastric cancer.

The method of X-ray examination of the stomach which was worked out in the first half of the past century is now outdated and requires radical correction. In addition, if we consider the fact that a group of new technologies such as ultrasonography, computed tomography, and magnetic resonance imaging (MRI) has appeared, it becomes quite obvious that the outdated method of radiological examination in gastroenterology on the whole, and in gastric cancer in particular, needs to be thoroughly revised. Based on this postulate, we will discuss the methodological aspects of using radiology to diagnose gastric cancer in this chapter.

Traditional X-ray Investigations

With the introduction of contrast media, which help to visualize the alimentary tract without inflicting any damage on the patient, the classical X-ray examination became the leading method for diagnosing gastric cancer. Gastroenterology was qualified as a relatively independent branch in medicine, and by the 1960s–1970s it had accumulated vast experience in the diagnosis of gastric cancer. A group of experienced radiologists emerged who mastered the X-ray examination of the stomach. A roentgenosemiotics of gastric cancer was then compiled; some of the signs remain valid today, but some require re-evaluation.

Unfortunately, the indisputable successes of X-ray methods achieved in gastroenterology led to the erroneous belief that these methods had reached their climax. Some researchers in the 1960s declared that the effectiveness of the X-ray investigation in diagnosing gastric cancer was 95–98%. This statement was not valid, because the statistical data were based on experience at specialized hospitals, to which patients were admitted long after the appearance of their first complaints; in other words, these patients had far advanced forms of cancer.

It is easy to understand why endoscopic study of the gastric mucosa was regarded by physicians as the gold standard for the diagnosis of gastric cancer. The visualization of ulcers and the possibility of taking tissue specimens for morphological examination proved to be advantageous in the diagnosis of gastrointestinal pathologies [90, 232]. All these factors accounted for the endoscopic boom. But as time passed, many things became clearer. While it provides objective information on changes in the mucosal surface, endoscopy has limitations in estimating organic changes of the stomach wall on the whole (◘ Fig. 28).

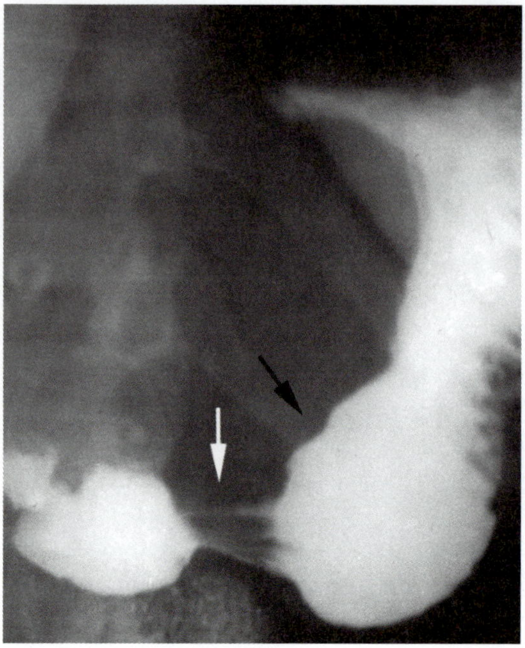

▲ Fig. 28 a.

About 40 years have passed since endoscopy was introduced into practical gastroenterology, but the diagnosis of gastric cancer has not improved. On the contrary, it has worsened somewhat. Diagnosis of minor cancers has remained at the same low level. The majority of patients who are admitted to specialized hospitals have cancer in far advanced forms. Physicians seem to underestimate endophytic cancer of the stomach, which is characterized by intramural growth, and to overestimate the diagnostic potentials of endoscopy. The extent of intramural infiltration in diffuse cancer proved to be more significant than it was possible to estimate by means of endoscopy [24]. Methods were then proposed for taking tissue specimens from deep layers of the stomach wall. First, however, one must know where exactly a tissue specimen should be taken and, second, endoscopic biopsy carries the danger of stomach perforation. It then became clear that X-ray methods must be restored to their important position in gastroenterology.

Like any science, radiology continues to develop. Its potentials have been strengthened by such advanced technologies as ultrasonography, CT, MRI, and digital X-ray methods. As information on the advanced working method was accumulated, it turned out that gastroenterology, despite its vast and long experience, entails a contradiction. On the one hand, there is a huge amount of knowledge in gastroenterology, which was accumulated over a period of almost 100 years and is used now in daily practice. On the other hand, the old methodological approaches to the diagnosis of pathologies and the original roentgenosemiotics continue to be employed mechanically and without reflection under changed conditions. True, there have been some positive shifts in organizational and methodological aspects, such as the examination of risk groups using X-ray fluoroscopy and digital X-ray spot imaging with subsequent target endoscopy. But interpretation of the findings (roentgenosemiotics) should be revised and corrected in the light of current concepts in morphology of gastric cancer [40, 67].

A comparative analysis of morphological estimates of infiltrative cancer conducted early in the twentieth century and today shows significant differences in how the essence of the problem is understood. Thus, at the present time, we observe a tendency toward compartmentalization of the pathological process, consisting in the artificial differentiation of tumors depending on the prevalence of particular signs, which sometimes are far from being equivalent. Meanwhile, according to some re-

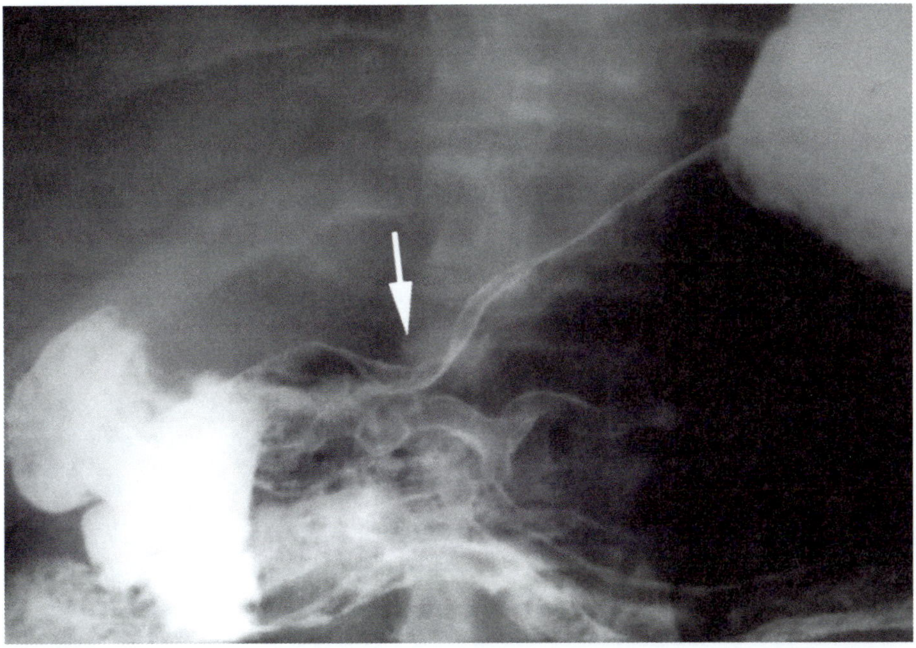

◂ **Fig. 28 b.**

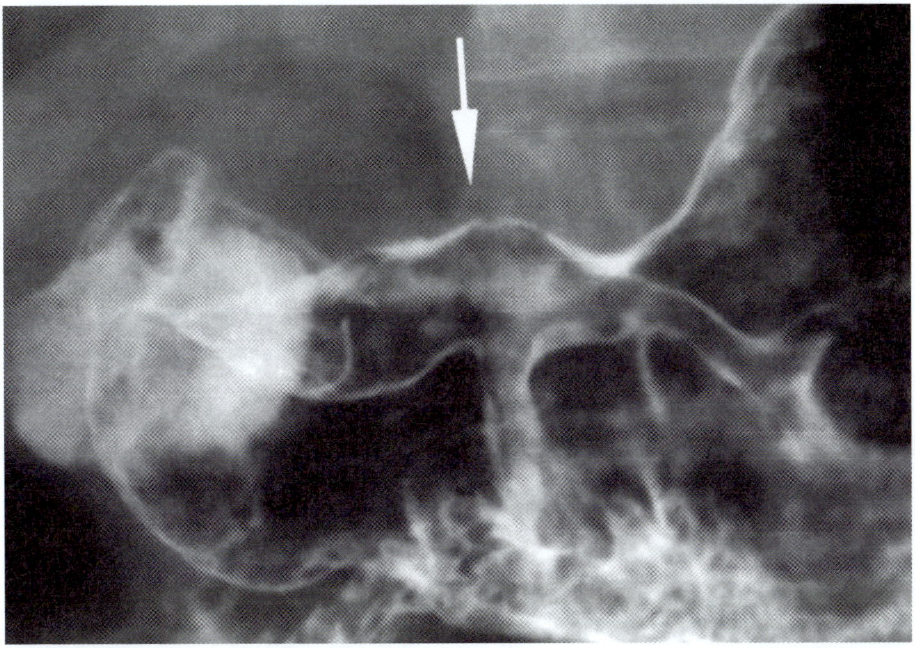

◂ **Fig. 28 c.**

Fig. 28a–f. Patient K., age 55. Diagnosis: gastric cancer. **a** Stomach roentgenogram (tight filling, vertical position, anterior projection): the angular notch contour is uneven, slightly depressed (black arrow); rigid platform on the lesser curvature of the antral part of the stomach (white arrow). **b** Stomach roentgenogram (double contrast, horizontal position, anterior projection): broad infiltrated folds of the mucous membrane converge toward the thick wall of the antral part and the notch (arrow). **c** Target stomach roentgenogram (double contrast, horizontal position, anterior projection): more distinctly visualized are thick walls of the antral part of the stomach and the notch with the infiltrated folds converging toward the lesser curvature (arrow). Conclusion: Infiltrative cancer of the lesser curvature and the angular notch.

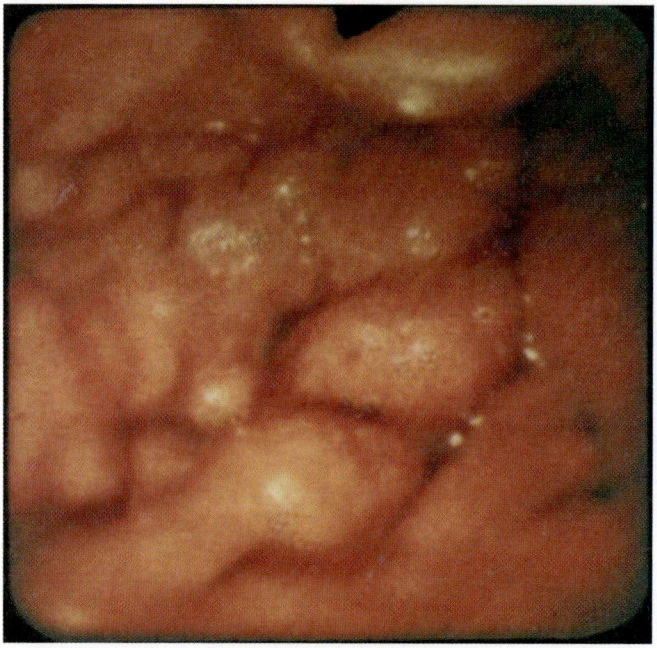

d Endophotograph: very thick folds of the gastric mucosa. The mucosa is pale pink and glassy. Deep biopsy. Histologically, a signet-ring cell carcinoma. **e** Macrospecimen of a resected stomach: portion of the wall of the lesser curvature is firm due to intramural infiltration (white arrow), in the direction of which thick folds converge (black arrows). **f** Fragment of a macrospecimen (strip): white tumor tissue infiltrating the stomach wall to the serosa, covered on top with visually intact mucous membrane (arrows)

◂ **Fig. 28 d.**

▾ **Fig. 28 e.**

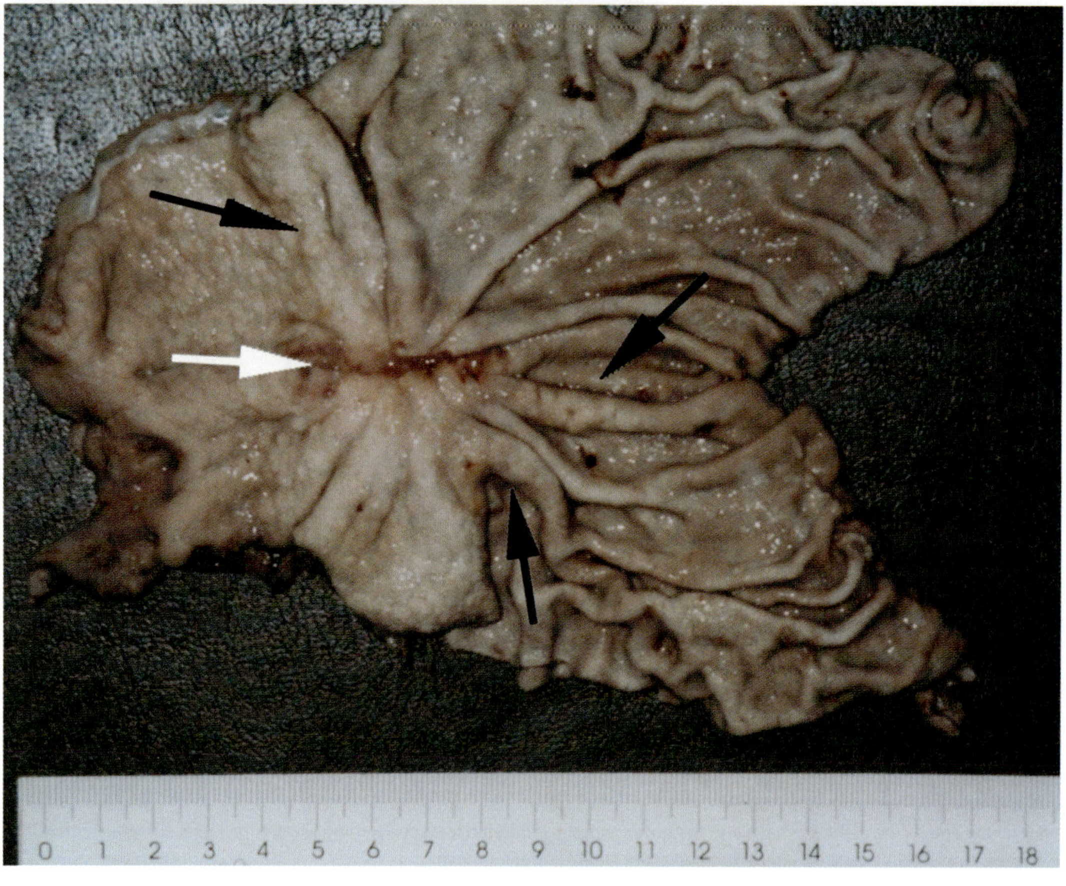

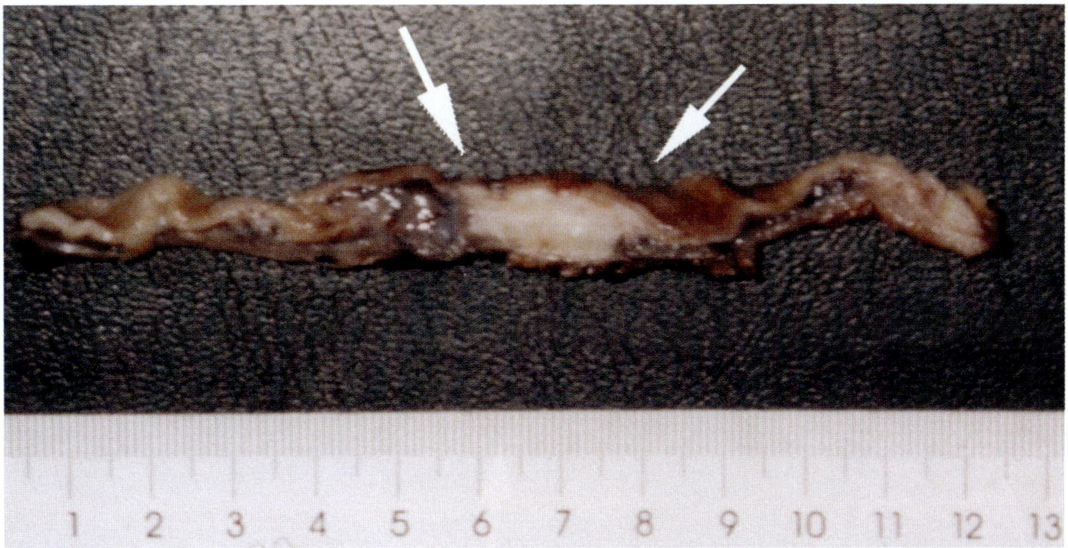

▲ **Fig. 28 f.**

searchers of the first half and the middle of the past century, the definition of intramural infiltration as the basis for tumor changes demonstrated the closest connection between separate forms of infiltrative cancer. Their estimation of the morphological substrate of the tumor was thus outside the framework of various classifications or schemes (◘ Fig. 29) [122, 123].

Some authors now use the terms »ulcerous cancer«, »cancer ulcer«, and others to characterize a

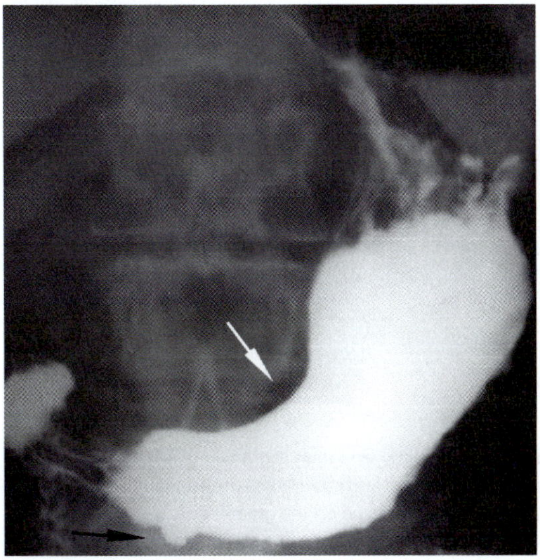

▲ **Fig. 29 a.**

definite stage of the tumor. But early in the past century, authors indicated only the tendency of infiltrative cancer to ulceration, which emphasized the importance of its endophytic growth. Data on the so-called cycles of malignant ulcer »healing« (when the ulcer epithelializes and then appears again) can be used only as confirmation of the classical works. The following question is justified in such a situation: If a malignant tumor »heals«, does it mean that the disease is cured? Nothing of the kind. Therefore, those authors who define an exophytic tumor resting on a large base with ulceration as the infiltrative form of gastric cancer are more correct than modern authors who define such new growth as the ulcerous form with submucous spread.

While characterizing X-ray examination of the stomach with reference to practical health care problems, we would like to emphasize some methodological aspects in order to better explain the role of radiological diagnosis in gastro-oncology. What is understood today to be traditional radiology differs considerably from what was practiced in the first half of the past century. The double-contrast method developed by Japanese physicians in the mid 1950s made it possible not only to visualize the mucous membrane impregnated with a barium suspension, but also to estimate the elasticity of the stomach wall by inflating it with air. The extent of affection could

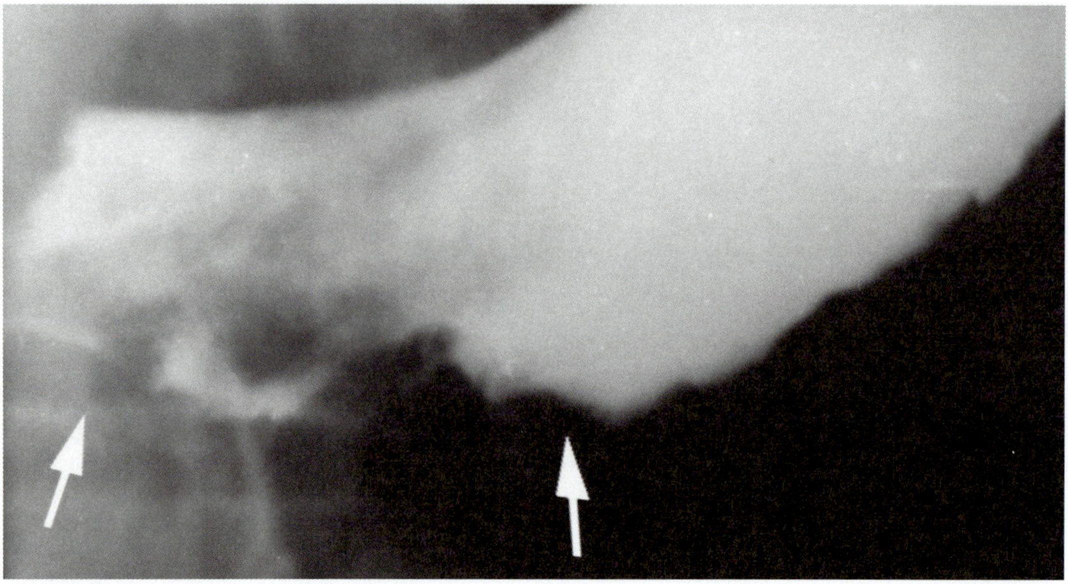

▲ Fig. 29 b.

▼ Fig. 29 c.

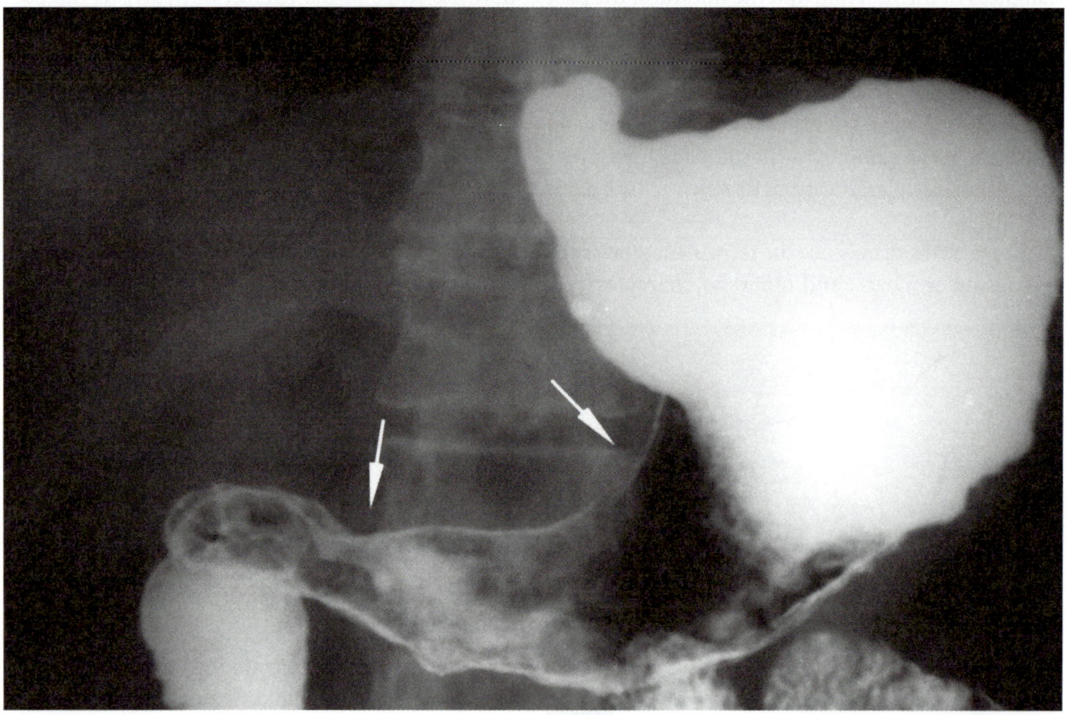

Fig. 29a–e. Female patient U., age 63. Diagnosis: gastric cancer. **a** Stomach roentgenogram (tight filling, vertical position, anterior projection): the lesser curvature of the distal part of the stomach is depressed and straightens the angular notch (white arrow); the prepyloric part is irregularly narrowed over its entire length; planar ulcer niche on the greater curvature (black arrow). **b** Target stomach roentgenogram (tight filling, vertical position, anterior projection), dosed compression: the lesser curvature is depressed, the angular notch straightened; the greater curvature contour is uneven and eroded owing to the ridge of infiltration encircling a flat niche (arrows). **c** Stomach roentgenogram (double contrast, horizontal position, anterior projection): rigid walls

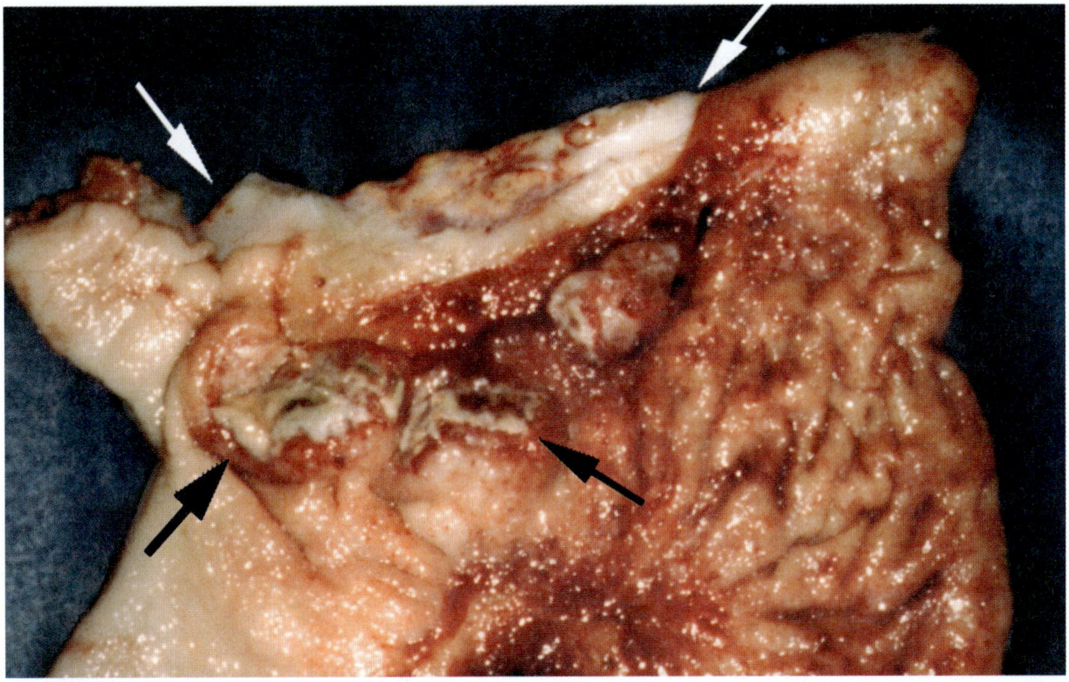

▲ **Fig. 29 d.**

▼ **Fig. 29 e.**

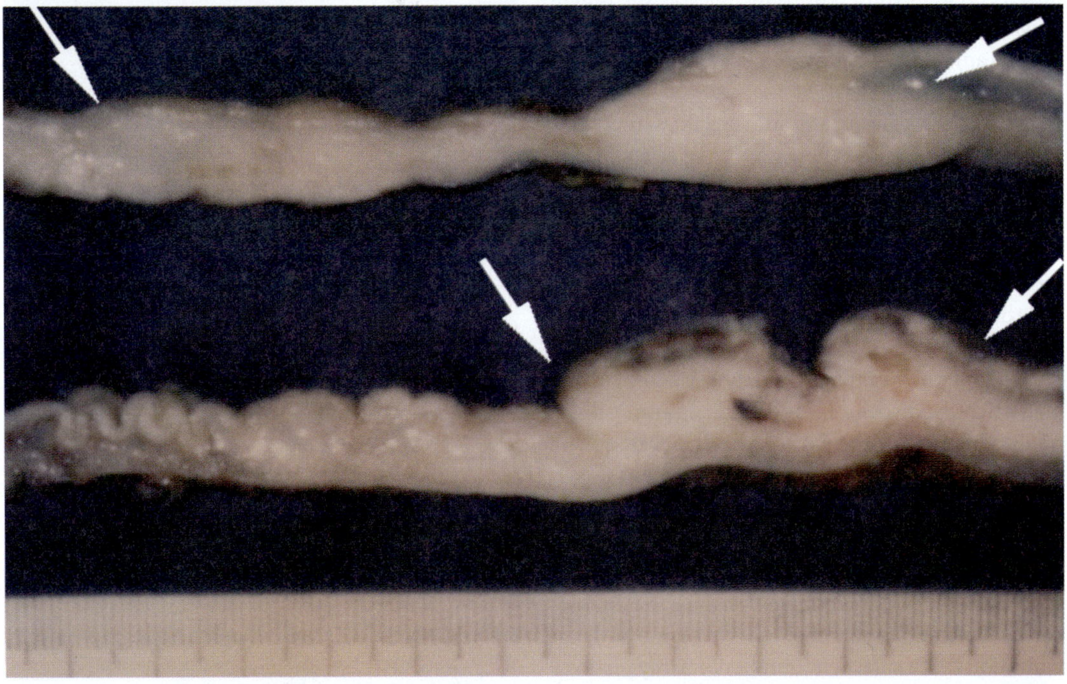

of distal part due to circular infiltration spreading over the entire body of the stomach (arrows). Conclusion: Infiltrative-ulcerous cancer of the distal part of the stomach with spread to the stomach body. **d** Macrospecimen of a resected stomach: firm wall; ulcers on the inner surface, occasional sites coated with fibrin (black arrows); intramural infiltration (white arrows). **e** Fragments of a macrospecimen (strips): white tumor tissue infiltrating the stomach wall (arrows) with ulceration thus be evaluated with sufficient accuracy. Combined with the classical method, double-contrast radiology significantly broadened the diagnostic potentials of roentgenogastroenterology [31, 58, 185]. This combined examination with tight filling, dosed compression, double contrast, and other technical features, turned into a study that differs substantially from the relatively simple procedure that was practiced 50 years ago.

Like the numerous currently used diagnostic methods on the whole, the traditional multi-component X-ray study of the stomach should be used reasonably and effectively with proper consideration of all its component parts. Standardization is one of them. This is an approach which joins the economic and diagnostic aspects of radiology and which allows another specialist to comment, whenever necessary, on the results of the examination.

At the present time, traditional radiology has several standard methods for examining the stomach which do not differ in principle except in minor and unimportant details. These methods are based on several important requirements, the fulfillment of which allows the most effective use of the traditional radiology, which is now a component of radiological diagnosis.

First, X-rays pictures should be taken in various projections, because if new growths are small and the morphological signs of their early forms are insignificant, organic changes may be masked by various elements of the stomach X-ray picture. The radiologist has to take pictures in optimal projections in order to correctly evaluate the stomach condition.

Second, the radiologist must be aided by X-ray TV, which is indispensable today for obtaining high-quality pictures of the pathology. The prerequisite for an adequate X-ray examination of the stomach is an X-ray unit that enables computerized analysis of the X-ray picture.

Another important requisite is obligatory recording of the obtained image, because the double-contrast technique can give reliable results only on condition that a sufficient number of X-ray pictures of various parts of the organ are taken. This requirement also holds for tight filling – one of the main elements of the traditional X-ray examination of the stomach (Fig. 30).

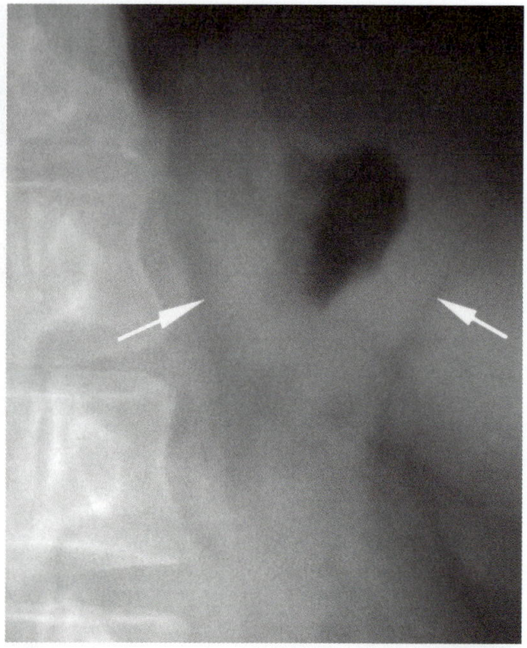

▲ **Fig. 30 a.** ▼ **Fig. 30 b.**

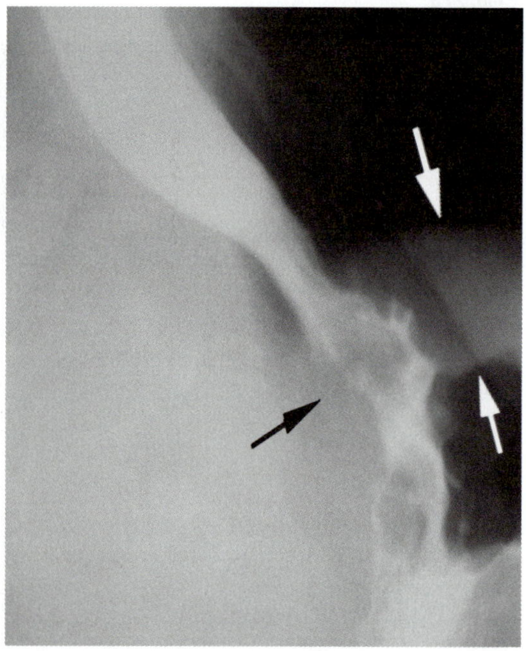

Fig. 30a–h. Female patient S., age 67. Diagnosis: gastric cancer. **a** Stomach roentgenogram (vertical position, anterior projection): air bubble redistribution in the stomach, which is elongated; the walls are thick (arrows). **b, c** Series of pictures of the upper part of the stomach and the lower third of the esophagus (tight filling, vertical position, anterior projection) at the moment of contrast medium passage through the gas-

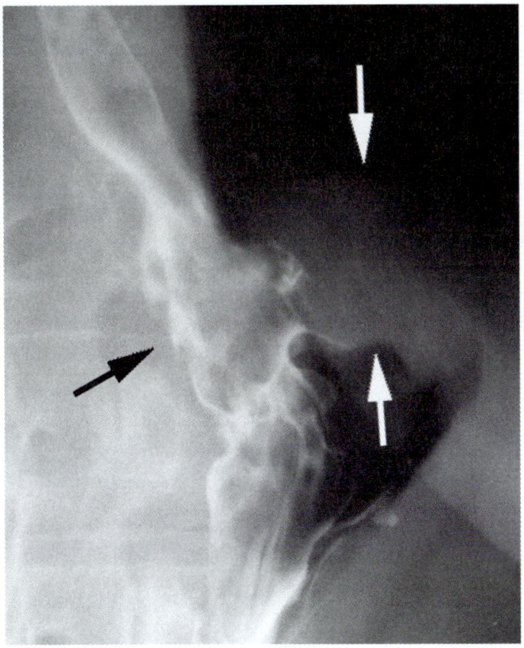

▲ **Fig. 30 c.**

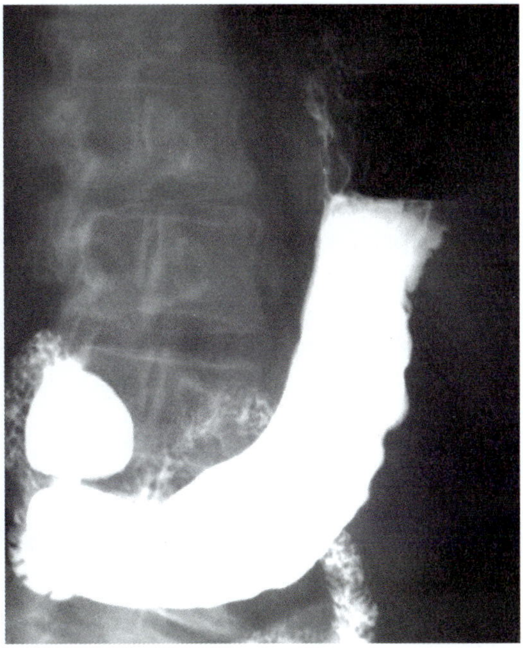

▲ **Fig. 30 d.**

▼ **Fig. 30 e.**

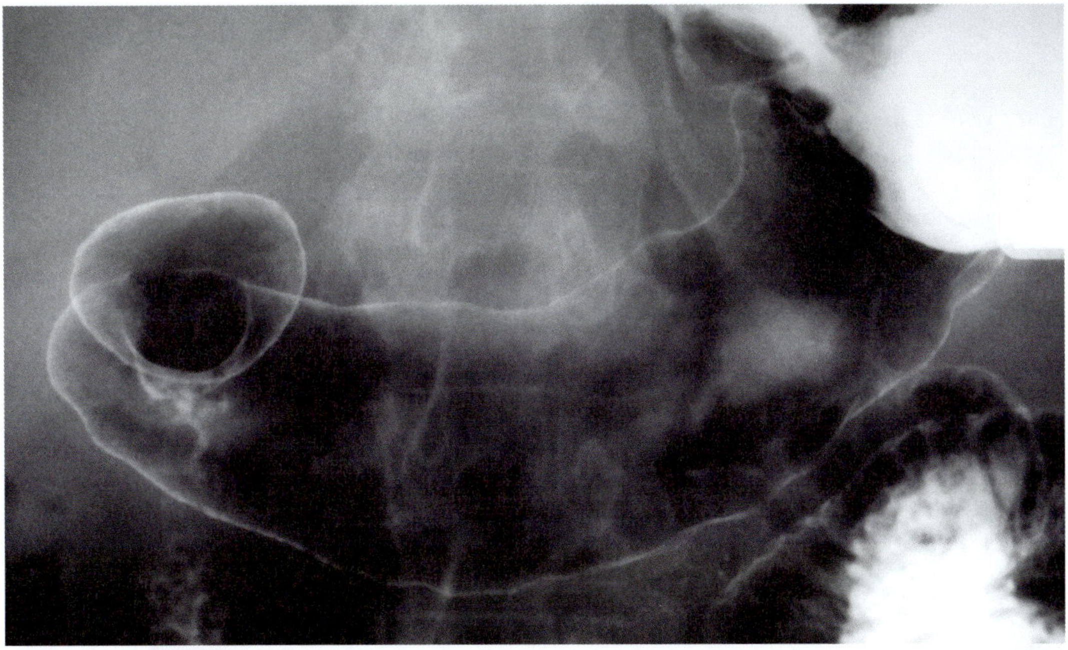

troesophageal junction: the abdominal segment of the esophagus is disfigured, its walls are rigid, the relief of the inner surface is changed (black arrow), the stomach–diaphragm distance is increased (white arrows). **d** Stomach roentgenogram (tight filling, vertical position, anterior projection): the cavity volume is decreased, the angular notch is straightened, the lesser curvature is short and depressed. **e** Stomach roentgenogram (double contrast, horizontal position, anterior projection): the stomach is disfigured into a rigid tube over almost its entire length except for the pyloric part and the pylorus proper due to circular intramural infiltration. Depot on the posterior wall of the middle third of the esophagus. The disfigured upper part of the stomach is tightly filled. Contrast medium regurgitated to the esophagus due to dysfunction of the gastroesophageal junction as a result of

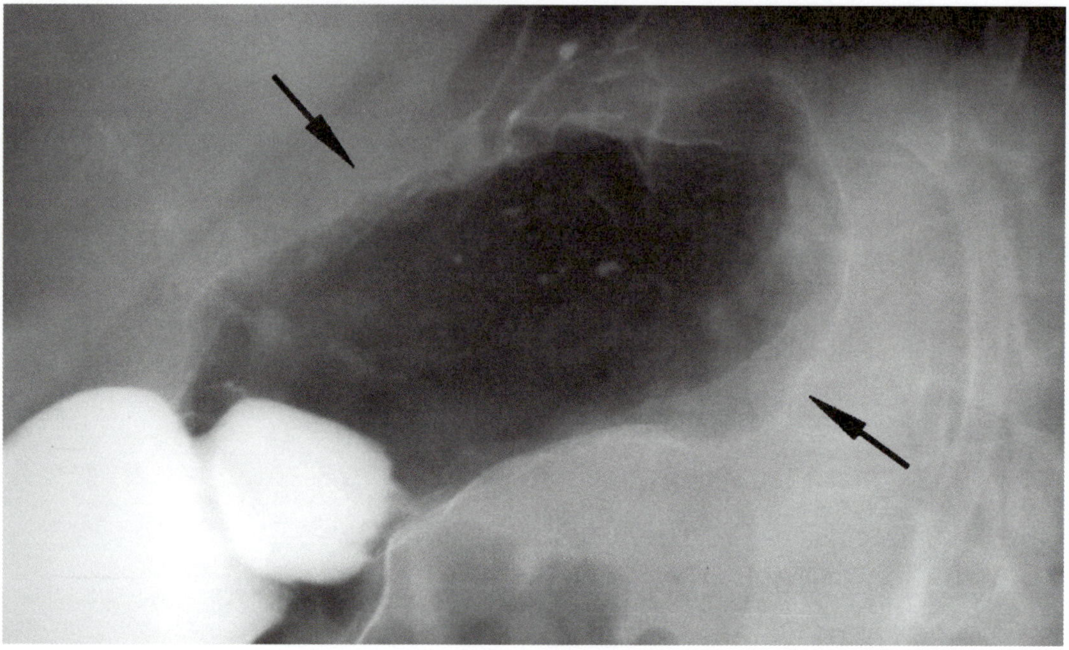

▲ Fig. 30 f. ▼ Fig. 30 g.

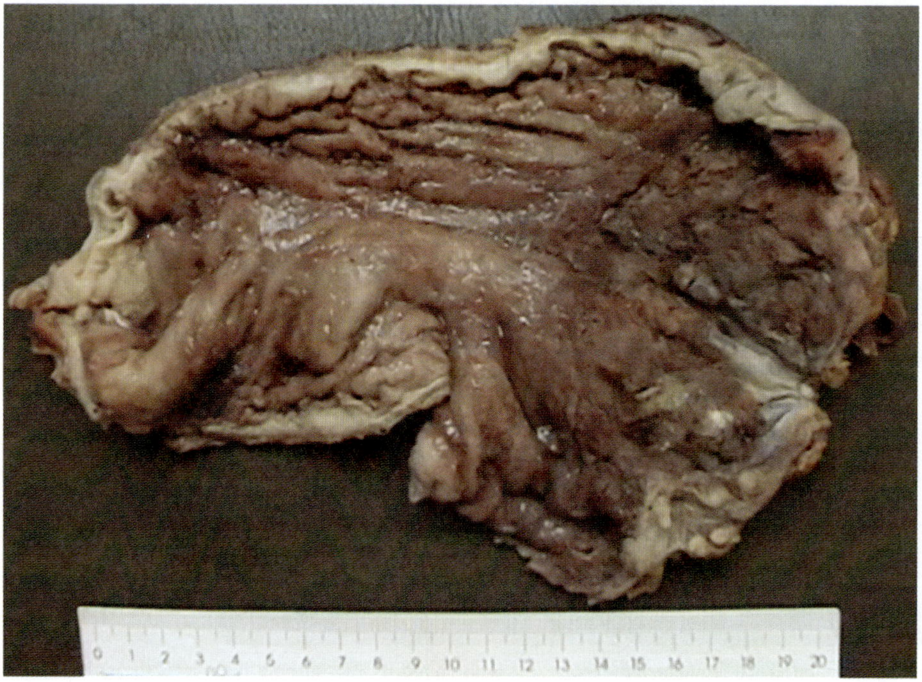

infiltration expansion onto the abdominal segment of the esophagus. **f** Stomach roentgenogram (double contrast, horizontal position, left oblique projection): thick walls of the upper part due to expansion of intramural infiltration (arrows). Conclusion: Infiltrative cancer of the stomach with involvement of the esophagus. **g** Macrospecimen of a resected stomach: firm wall over its entire length due to tumor infiltration expanding to the esophagus. **h** Fragment of a macrospecimen (strip): the wall is thick; white tumor tissue infiltrating the stomach wall is seen (arrows). Histologically, a signet-ring cell carcinoma

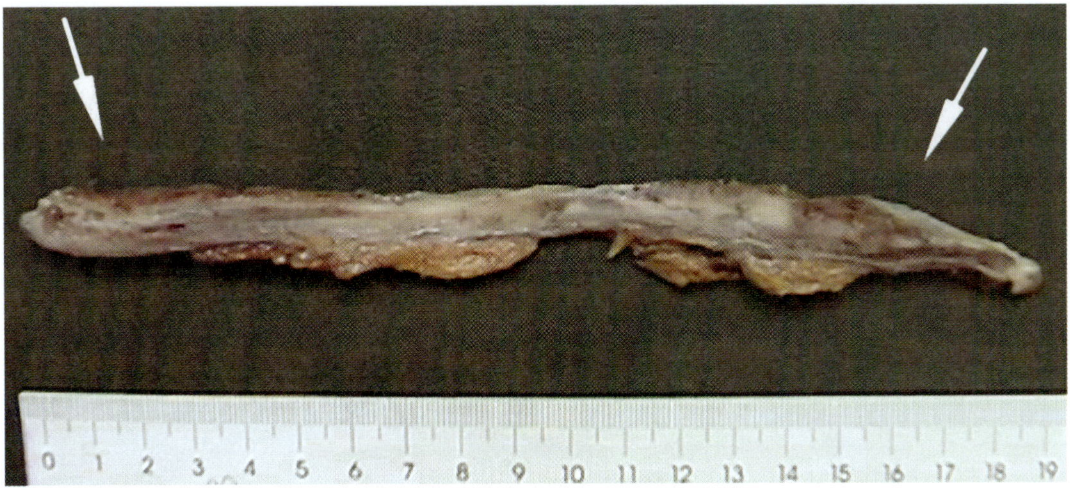

▲ **Fig. 30 h.**

Fulfillment of said requirements increases the cost of the X-ray examination and the patient's dose. Therefore, it is necessary to reasonably limit the number of pictures taken in various projections. Digital X-ray imaging is also used now on an ever-increasing scale. It is more informative owing to computerized processing of the obtained image of the stomach.

In order to optimize the X-ray examination we have standardized the procedure. We take a limited number of pictures in certain projections in a defined sequence, the projections being so selected that all parts of the stomach are imaged. Strict adherence to the methodology of stomach examination gives a full review of the stomach and accounts for its quality. However, standardization does not imply obligatory filming with the patient in strictly fixed positions, because an individual approach to each particular patient is necessary depending on his or her constitutional features, different shapes of the stomach (the form of a horn or a hook), the position of the duodenum, etc. The optimal position of the patient can be chosen only under visual control.

The X-ray imaging is a point of special importance. Fluoroscopy should be used as the primary method. In addition to selection of the optimal projection, X-ray fluoroscopy guidance must ensure flexibility of the investigation program. Thus, if, during the examination, the radiologist discovers changes requiring verification, he or she may alter the course of the examination by taking additional pictures in non-standard projections with detailed imaging of the affected site. The importance of correct primary estimation of the character of the pathology based on the results of X-ray fluoroscopy will be given special emphasis. But in revealing gastric cancer, especially its minor forms, this stage is important only for the tentative location of the lesion (e.g., the pyloric, cardiac part, etc.). A detailed study is done by analyzing stored images or X-ray films (◘ Fig. 31).

▼ **Fig. 31 a.**

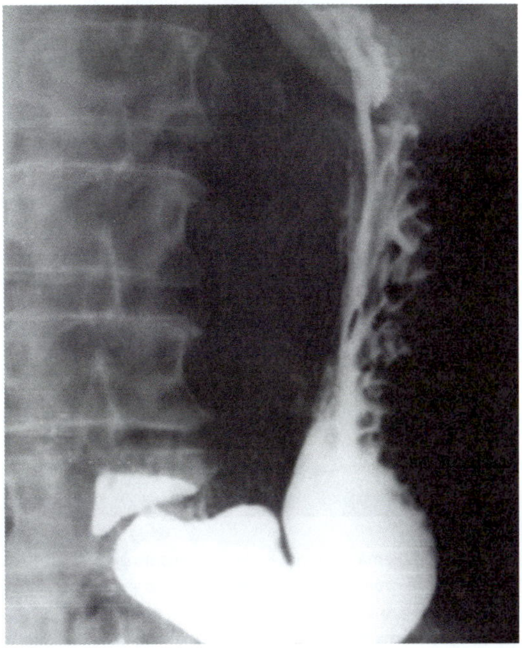

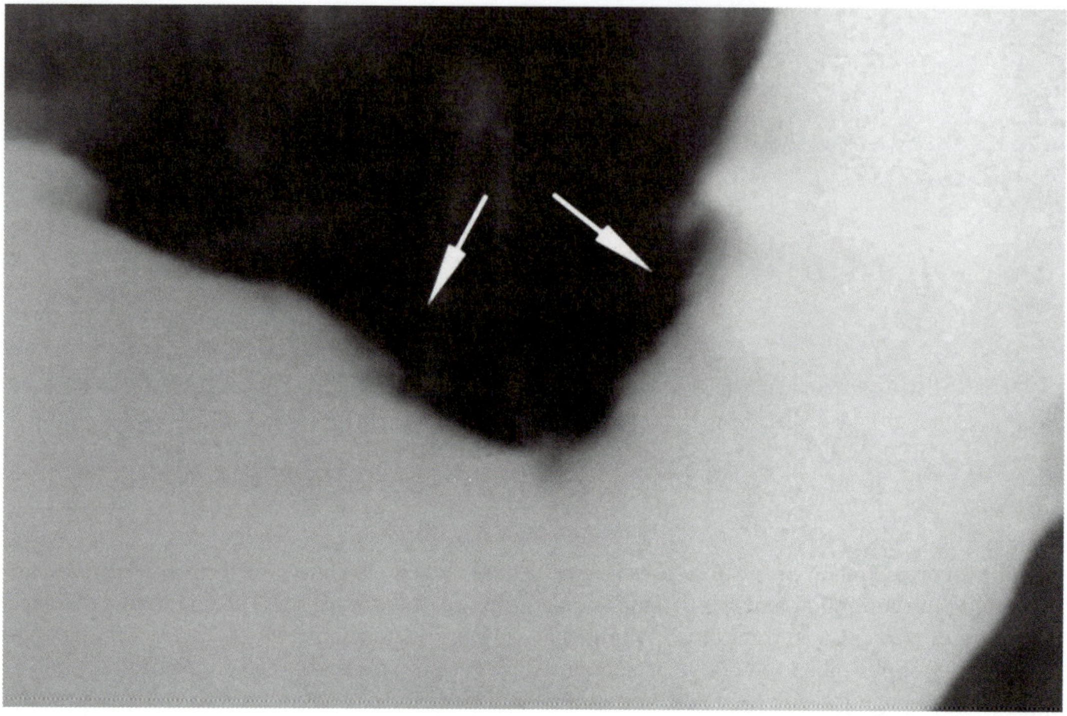

▲ Fig. 31 b.

▼ Fig. 31 c.

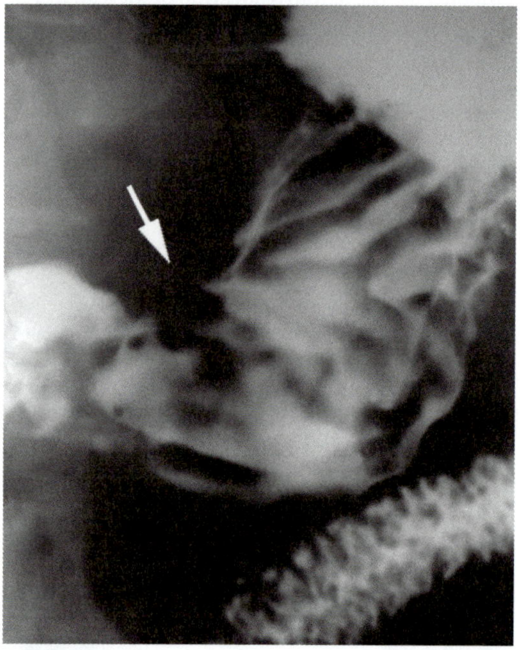

▼ Fig. 31 d.

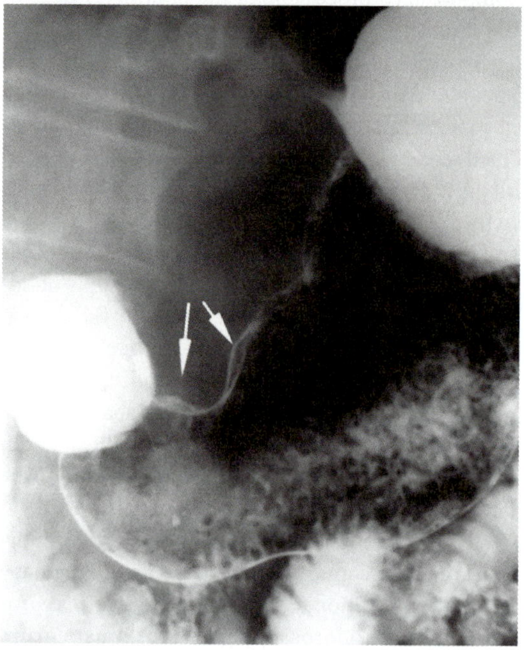

Fig. 31a–f. Female patient K., age 60. Diagnosis: gastric cancer. **a** Stomach roentgenogram (tight filling, vertical position, right semi-oblique projection) at the moment of peristaltic wave passage over the involved zone: no organic changes, stomach contours are even. **b** Stomach roentgenogram (tight filling, vertical position, anterior projection): uneven and eroded notch contour (arrows). **c** Stomach roentgenogram (pneumo-relief, horizontal position, right oblique projection): marked convergence of the

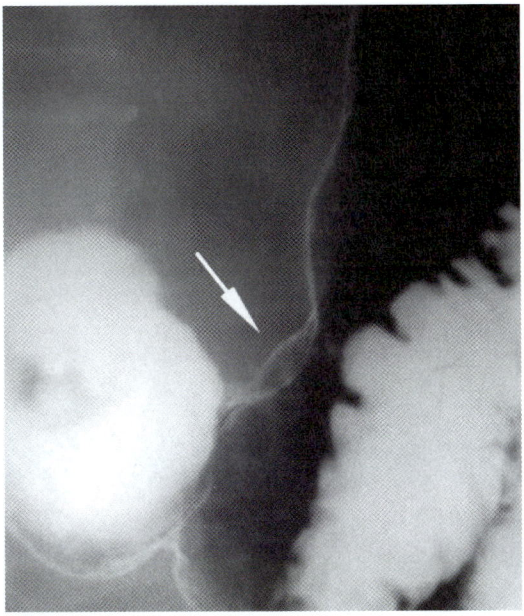

▲ **Fig. 31 e.** ▼ **Fig. 31 f.**

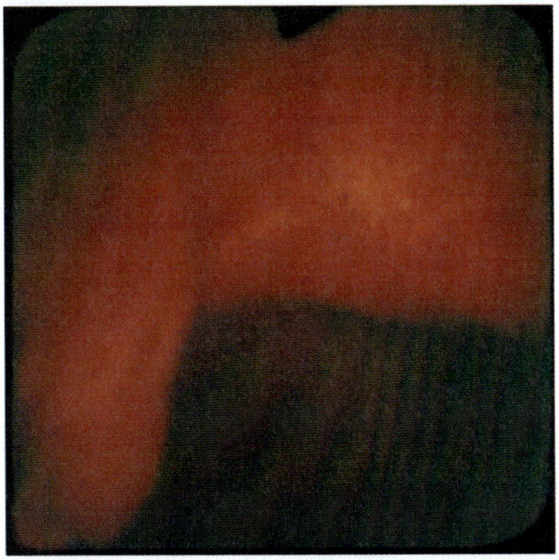

folds toward the angular notch (arrow). **d** Stomach roentgenogram (double contrast, horizontal position, right semi-oblique projection): thick wall in the notch projection (arrows); peristalsis can be seen over the entire length. **e** Stomach roentgenogram (double contrast, horizontal position, right oblique projection): thick wall appears more distinct with the optimal projection due to intramural infiltration (arrow). Conclusion: Early infiltrative cancer of the angular notch. **f** Endophotograph: gray-yellow portion of mucosa, to 1 cm in diameter, with indistinct borders and irregular surface on the lesser curvature of the lower third of the stomach. Histologically, a signet-ring cell carcinoma

The standardization problems have been under discussion for several decades in Japan, the mother country of gastrofluorographic examinations. The protocol for a standard X-ray examination of the stomach suggests taking six to eight pictures. According to our own experience and that of our colleagues, pictures taken in five standard projections are quite sufficient for the diagnostic procedure [28, 31, 54, 58].

We suggest that the study begin with a short surveillance of the abdominal cavity as a whole. As the first portions of the barium meal are ingested (at the phase of tight filling, pneumo-relief, and wall collapse), the condition of the esophagus is evaluated in the anterior and right oblique projections. At the tight-filling phase, the configuration and contours of the esophagus are estimated, and an attempt is made to detect possible protrusion, narrowing, curvature, disfigured contours, or obturation. As the esophagus empties itself of the barium suspension, the character of wall collapse and the mucosal condition are estimated based on the relief and the pattern of the folds. Analysis of the esophagus picture at various degrees of filling gives information on the functional parameters of the esophagus and the condition of its sphincter zones: wall elasticity, sphincter competence, rate of barium meal passage through the esophagus, and the contractile function of the esophagus.

The stomach is then examined in the vertical position. As its cavity is filled with barium suspension, the shape, size, position, and contours of the stomach are estimated. Two projections should be preferred to visualize the stomach contours: anterior projection with a 10°–15° tilt and left lateral projection.

Two pictures are taken in the vertical position:

1. Anterior or right oblique, half-oblique, quarter-oblique, depending on the particular topography of the patient's stomach (for estimation at tight filling of the body, sinus, antral and pyloric parts, and also duodenal bulb). This projection helps to visualize the contours of the lesser and greater curvatures of the afore-mentioned stomach parts with tight filling and also the state of the air bubble.
2. Left lateral projection for estimation at tight filling of the anterior and posterior walls of the stomach body, and also the anterior and poste-

rior walls of its upper part against the background of a natural amount of air.

Then the patient ingests a gas-producing mixture or granules, and drinks a barium suspension in small portions. The patient keeps the last gulp in his mouth and assumes the horizontal position for the posterior left-oblique projection. As the last portion of the barium meal is swallowed, the condition of the esophagus is estimated in the left-oblique projection; the function of the gastroesophageal junction is also evaluated. Next the patient is asked to turn slowly about his or her long axis in a counterclockwise direction for better permeation of the entire gastric mucosa and to reduce the volume of foam that has formed.

Then pictures are taken in the horizontal position of the patient in the following projections:

1. Left posterior oblique projection to visualize the distal third of the esophagus, the gastroesophageal junction, the upper part of the stomach (double contrast), the distal third of the stomach, and the duodenal bulb (tight filling).
2. Anterior projection (double contrast) to study the stomach body wall and the contour of the upper part with tight filling.
3. Right anterior oblique projection – double contrast of the distal half of the stomach, duodenal bulb, and visualization of the fundus contour at tight filling.

Examination according to this program visualizes every part of the stomach tightly filled with barium suspension using the double-contrast technique. As has been noted, an effective examination depends on high quality of the barium meal and the gas-producing mixture. Owing to the simplicity of the standardized method using digital technology, it is possible to increase the number of examinations by several orders of magnitude, whereas its low cost can considerably increase the profitability of the service. In our opinion, its high efficiency in detecting affections of various localizations meets current requirements for the traditional X-ray examination of the stomach (Fig. 32).

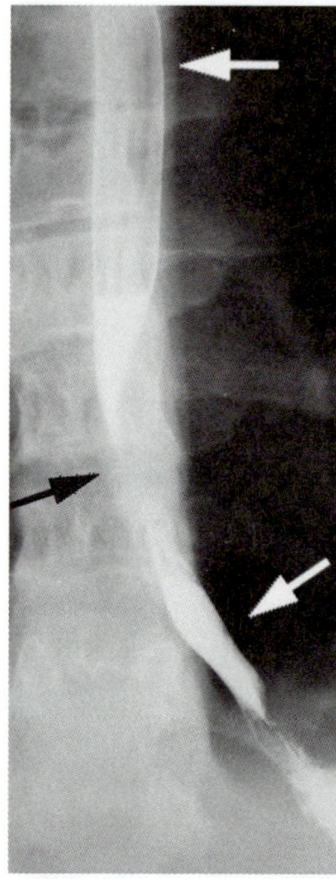

▲ **Fig. 32 a.**

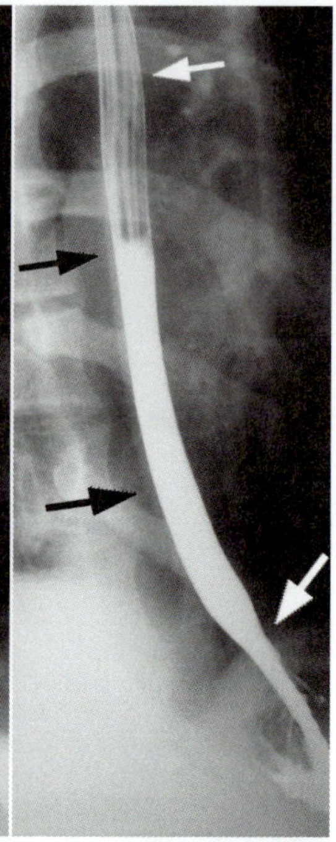

▲ **Fig. 32 b.**

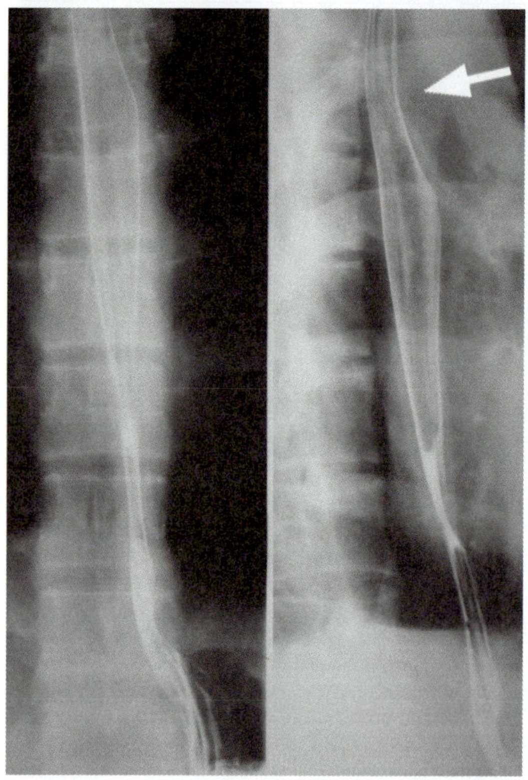

▲ **Fig. 32 c.**

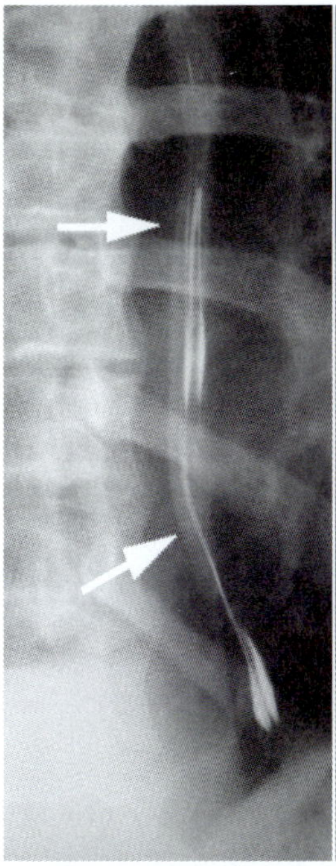

▲ **Fig. 32 d.**

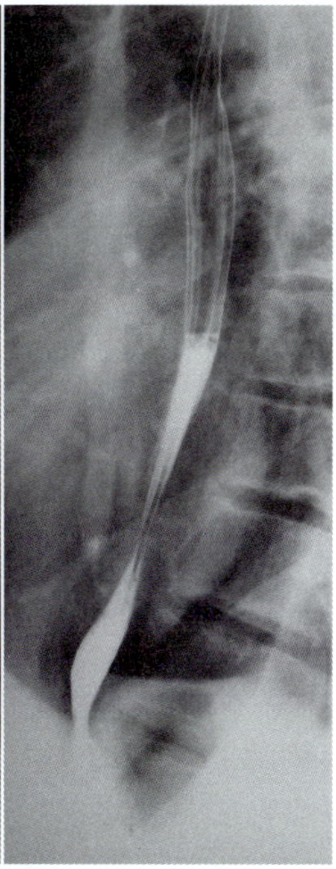

▲ **Fig. 32 e.**

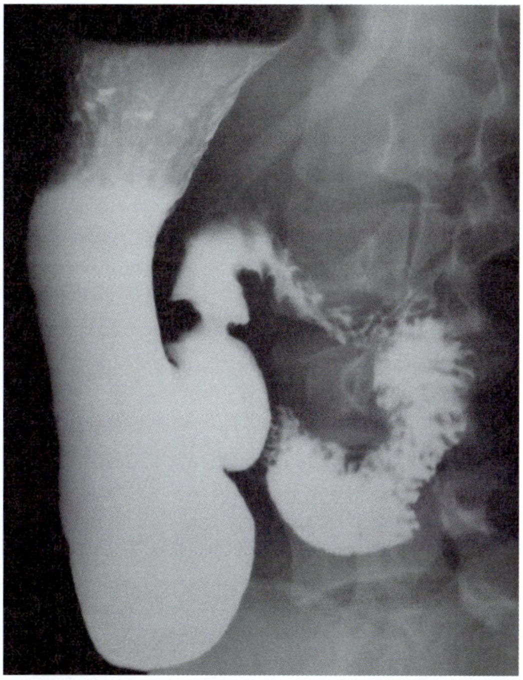

▲ **Fig. 32 g.**

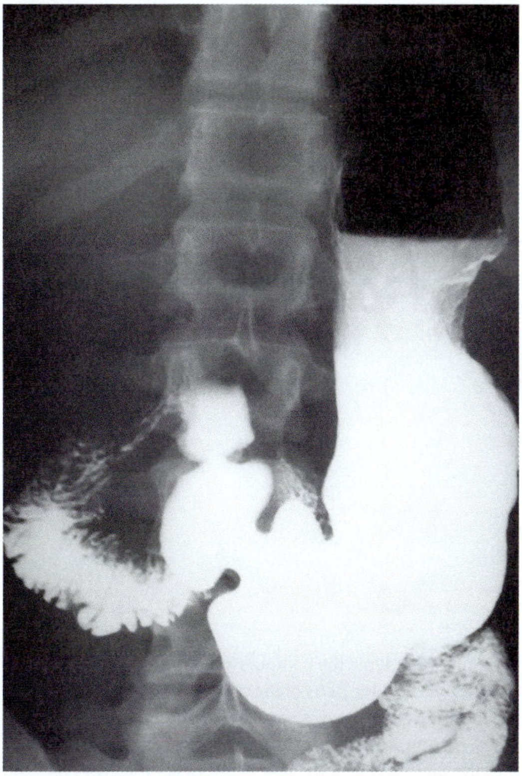

▲ **Fig. 32 f.**

Fig. 32a–n. Individual version of X-ray imaging of the esophagus, stomach, and duodenum. **a** Esophagus roentgenogram (tight filling, vertical position, right quarter-oblique projection): even contours, distinct over the entire length (white arrows), smooth transition to the narrow portion resulting from peristaltic contraction of the muscular coat of its wall (black arrow). **b** Esophagus roentgenogram (tight filling, vertical position, right oblique projection): even contours, distinct over the entire length (white arrows). About 2- to 3-mm-thick »paraesophageal« strip, repeating the esophagus course to mark its right posterior wall and the periesophageal fat tissue (black arrows). **c** Esophagus roentgenograms (double contrast, vertical position, straight and right oblique projections): the walls of normal thickness are elastic. Smooth impression of the aortal arch by the left anterior contour (arrow). **d** Esophagus roentgenogram (reflection phase of mucosal relief, vertical position, right oblique projection): rectilinear parallel mucosal folds. More distinct visualization of the »paraesophageal« strip (arrows). **e** Esophageal roentgenogram (pneumo-relief, vertical position, left oblique projection): distinct visualization of specifically rectilinear parallel folds of the mucosal relief. **f** Stomach roentgenogram (tight filling, vertical position, anterior projection): distinct visualization of the stomach body, sinus, antral and pyloric parts of the stomach, the bulb, and the proximal half of the duodenum. Even contours of the lesser and great curvature over their entire lengths. Symmetric peristalsis. Air bubbles of regular shape. The medial and lateral walls of the upper part and the wall of the stomach fundus are elastic, of normal thickness. The duodenal bulb of normal configuration. The duodenal lumen is not changed, the folds are of normal caliber. The narrowed upper horizontal part is due to peristaltic contraction of the muscular coat of the duodenal wall. **g, h** Roentgenograms of asthenic and hypersthenic stomachs (tight filling, vertical position, left oblique projection): distinct visualization of the body and the distal third of the stomach, duodenal bulb, and loop. Even contours over the entire length of the anterior and posterior walls of the stomach body; normal shapes of the air bubbles. The anterior and posterior walls of the upper part are elastic and of normal thickness. The duodenal loop lumen is not changed; the folds are of normal caliber. **i, j** Roentgenograms of asthenic and hypersthenic stomachs (double contrast, horizontal position, anterior projection): the upper part is distinctly visualized by barium suspension. The body of the stomach, its distal part, and the duodenum at the double-contrast phase. The contours of the upper part are slightly uneven due to the specific anatomy of the folds and the mucosa; the stomach–diaphragm distance is normal. The walls of the lesser and greater curvatures of the stomach and of the duodenal bulb are elastic and of normal thickness. Unaltered folds of the duodenal loop can be seen. **k, l** Roentgenograms of asthenic and hypersthenic stomachs (double contrast, horizontal position, right oblique projection): the upper part is distinctly visualized by barium suspension. The stomach body, its distal part, and the duodenum are in the double-contrast phase. The projection makes it possible to study in every detail the contours of the upper part, which are even and distinct. The walls of the lesser and greater curvature of the antral and pyloric parts of the stomach, and of the duodenal bulb, are elastic and of normal thickness. Unaltered folds of the duodenal loop are more distinct. **m, n** Stomach roentgenograms (double contrast, horizontal position, left posterior oblique projection): barium suspension distinctly visualizes the lower half of the stomach body, its distal part and the duodenum, the upper part in the double-contrast phase. Contours of the lower half and the distal part of the stomach are even, the duodenal bulb is of normal configuration, location of the duodenal loop and its lumen

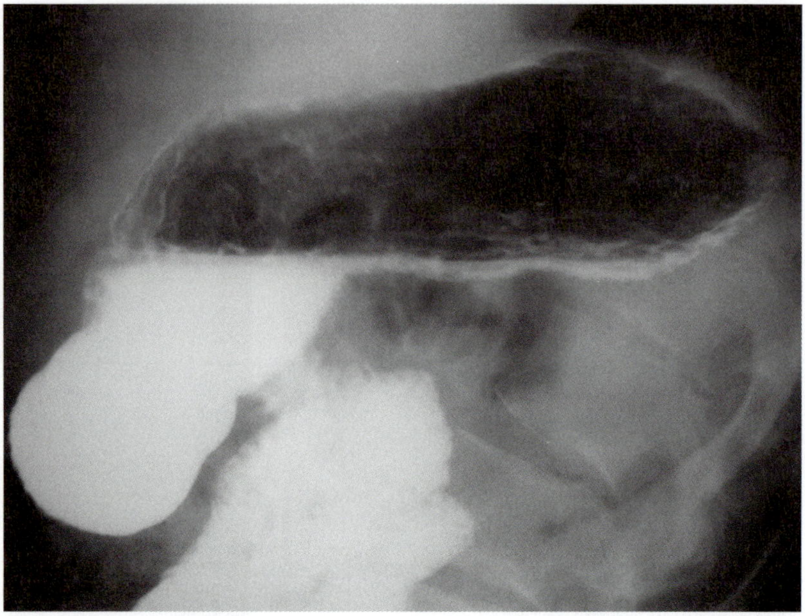

▲ **Fig. 32 h.**

▼ **Fig. 32 i.**

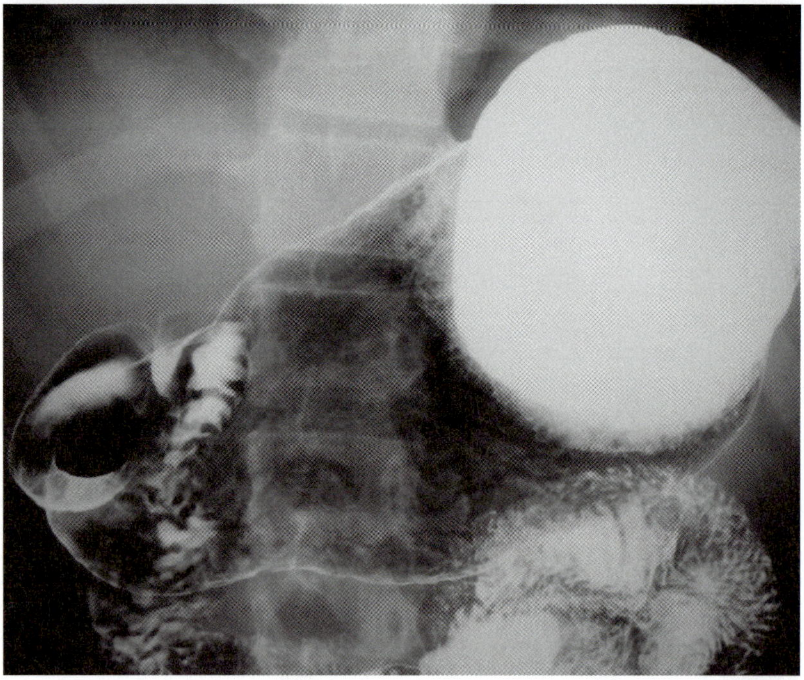

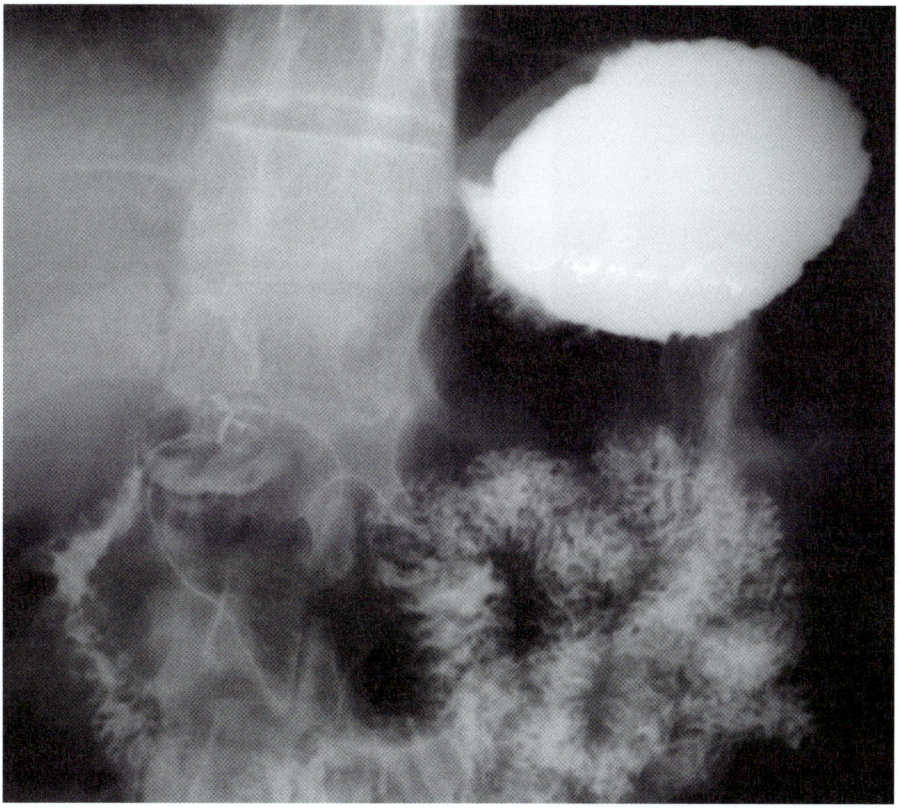

◀ **Fig. 32 j.**

▼ **Fig. 32 k.**

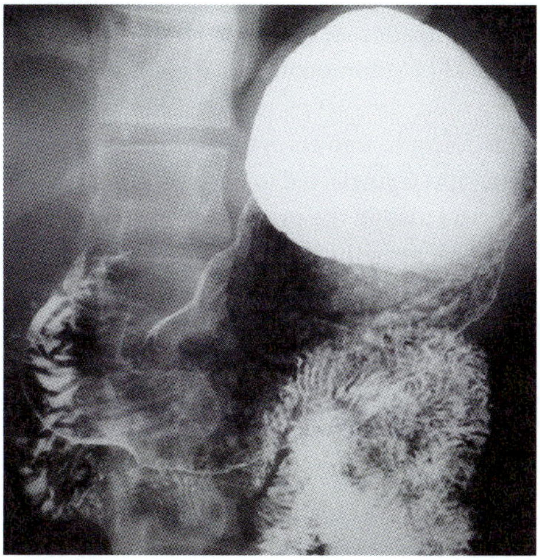

are normal. The walls of the upper part are of normal thickness, the relief of the cardiac rosette (cardioesophageal junction) has the specific radiating pattern (arrow)

▼ **Fig. 32 l.**

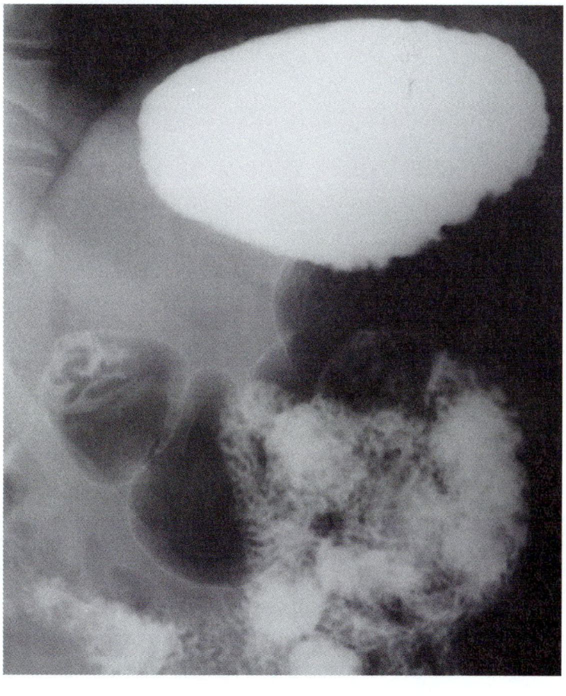

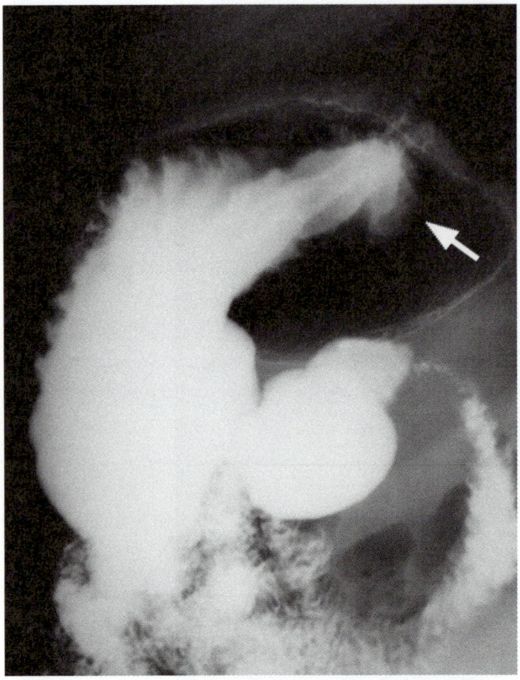

▲ Fig. 32 m. ▼ Fig. 32 n.

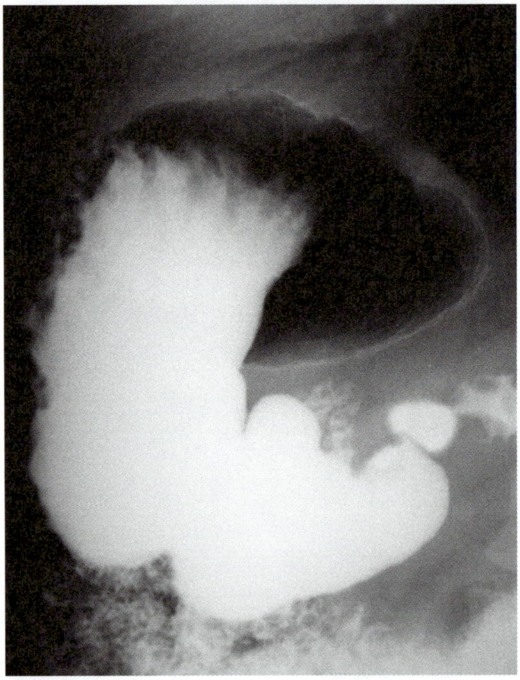

While describing in general current methods for the traditional X-ray examination of the stomach, it is necessary to mention some provisions that can be regarded as the fundamental principles. At present, standardization is the main prerequisite for any radiological study of the stomach. But the methodology should not be turned into a standard scheme restricted to taking five pictures. It should be applied to screen the population for gastric cancer. In case of any deviation from the »radiology norm,« however, it is necessary to take pictures in additional projections which enable a more objective estimation of the findings [28, 31, 33, 58, 144, 224].

Our experience with X-ray examination of gastric cancer, accumulated over many years, indicates that the specific anatomy of separate parts of the stomach (greater curvature, anterior wall, cardiac part, etc.) should also guide the radiologist in selecting an additional technique. We have already mentioned that minor errors, which inevitably occur in standardization, are especially numerous with primary localization of cancer in these parts of the stomach. In this connection, the necessary additional techniques and methodological approaches will be discussed in the relevant sections of the monograph dealing with cancer in these parts of the stomach.

To continue our discussion of the fundamentals of X-ray examination of the stomach, it is necessary to note some important problems connected with the use of additional techniques aimed at improving the visualization of changes. First, there is the possible use of compression. It is usually employed to obtain a more distinct picture of abnormalities of mucosa relief and contours of the stomach, especially if the patient is suspected to have early endophytic cancer, and also in the presence of minor benign exophytic new growths (small polyps, leiomyomas, etc.). Sometimes, organic intramural infiltrations become visible only as slightly detectable irregularities of the contour with tight filling of the stomach. Additional compression helps to reveal a specific picture of infiltrative-ulcerous (saucer- or cup-shaped, according to the formerly used nomenclature) cancers, both minor and advanced (Fig. 33).

By compression we mean the classical techniques, which remain an important tool. But with the introduction of double contrast, these techniques have acquired quite new forms, especially in situations where it is necessary to examine in more detail the anterior and posterior walls of the stomach. The double-contrast technique is especially effective in

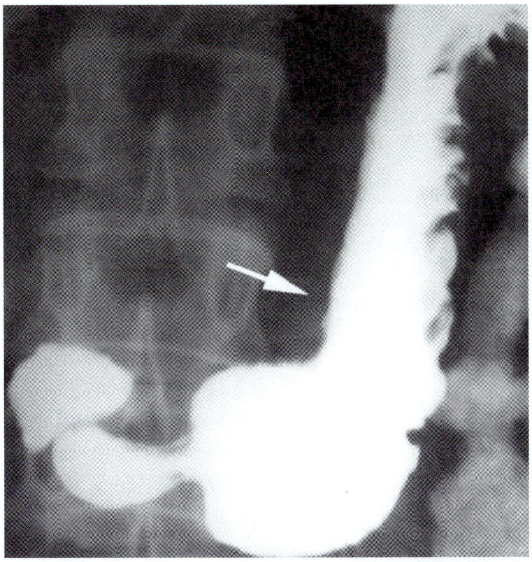

▲ **Fig. 33 a.**

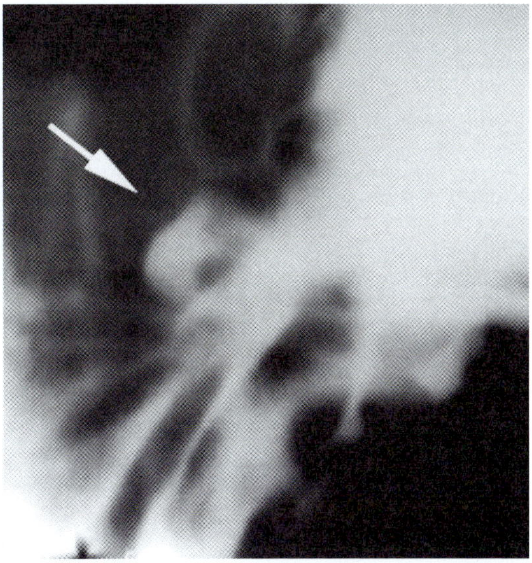

▲ **Fig. 33 c.**

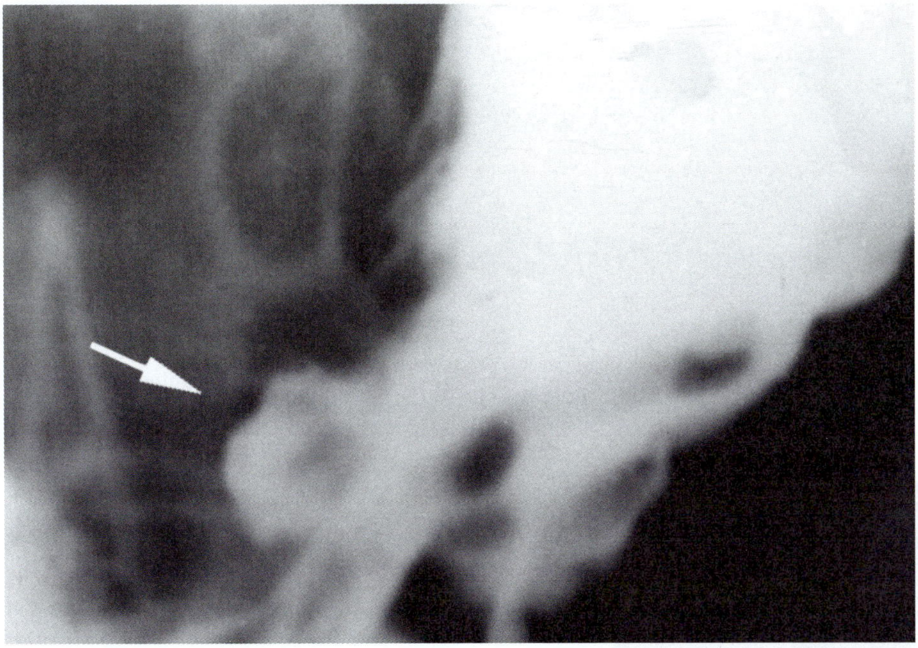

◄ **Fig. 33 b.**

Fig. 33a–f. Female patient L., age 68. Diagnosis: gastric cancer. **a** Stomach roentgenogram (tight filling, vertical position, anterior projection): uneven contour of the lesser curvature in the lower third of the stomach body, closer to the angular notch (arrow); no visible changes in the contour of the greater curvature. **b, c** Series of target stomach roentgenograms (tight filling, vertical position, anterior projection), dosed compression: depot of contrast medium on the posterior wall of the stomach body with converging folds (arrow) imitating an ulcer niche owing to depressed wall of the lesser curvature. **d, e** Series of target stomach roentgenograms (double contrast, horizontal position, anterior projection): circular infiltration in the lower third of the stomach body (black arrows); a rounded light spot corresponding to the ulcer crater with a ridge of infiltrated tissue and converging folds (white arrow) on the posterior wall, closer to the greater curvature. Conclusion: Infiltrative-ulcerous cancer of the lower third of the stomach body. **f** Endophotograph: ulceration with eroded edges on the greater curvature, in the center of infiltration, elevated over the surrounding mucous membrane. Histologically, a non-differentiated cancer

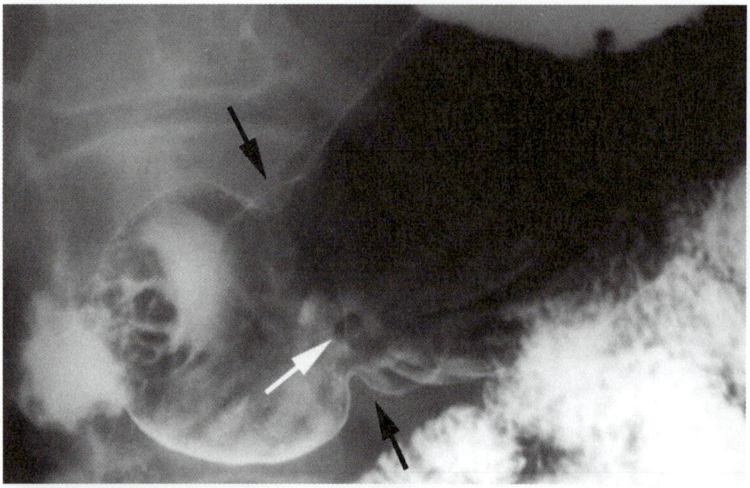

▲ Fig. 33 d.

▼ Fig. 33 e.

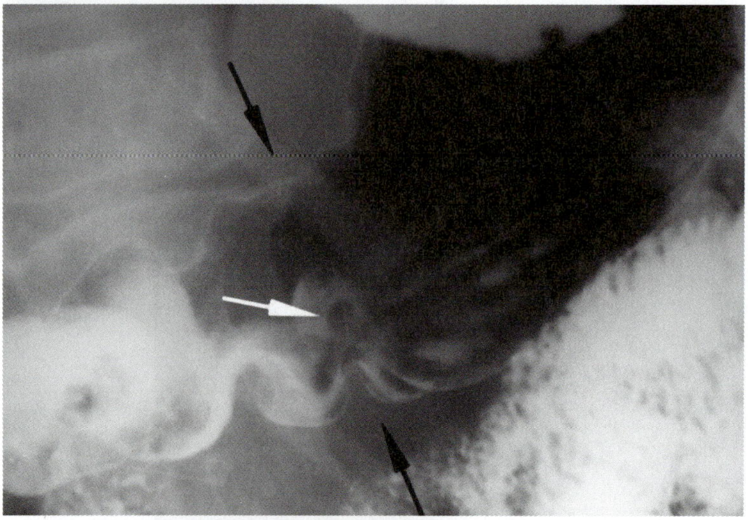

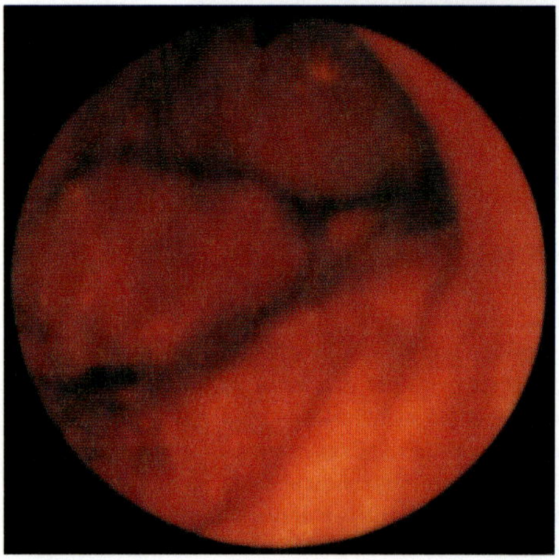

◀ Fig. 33 f.

studying the upper parts of the stomach, in verification of causes of cascade stomach, etc. (Fig. 34).

It should be noted that in cases suspected to have any deviation from the »radiology standard«, it is not sufficient to take pictures only in the five standard projections. In each particular case, the radiologist must use all his talent and experience and take as many pictures in various projections as necessary to arrive at a correct conclusion on the presence or absence of changes in the stomach.

Thus, while stating the necessity of qualitative changes in the methodology of the traditional X-ray examination, it must be said that a correct diagnosis can be established only with due consideration of the morphogenetic changes that have recently occurred and the initial site of the primary tumor in the stomach, especially when the patient has diffuse forms of cancer. Today, not only clinicians but also well-known radiological experts openly denounce the role of current radiological diagnosis of gastric cancer and the role of the X-ray examination in gastroenterology and gastro-oncology on the whole. This is nothing but professional error and populism. Diffuse cancer of the stomach now accounts for 88% of all gastric cancers. Regretfully, this tendency is becoming more evident in Russia, while in all other countries opin-

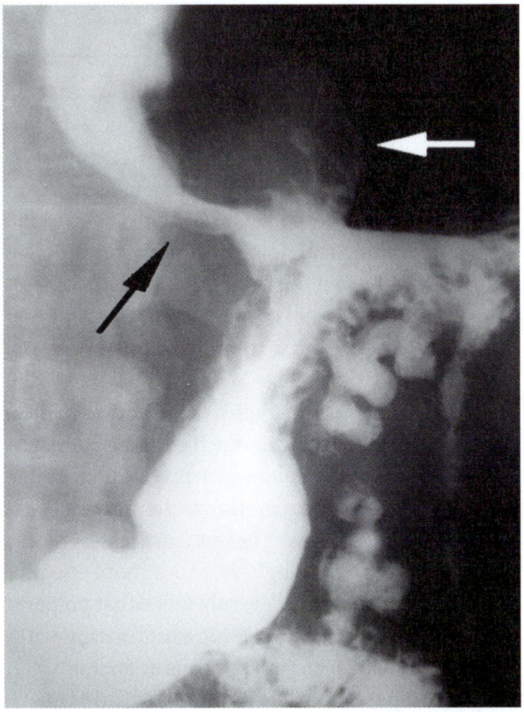

▲ **Fig. 34 a.**

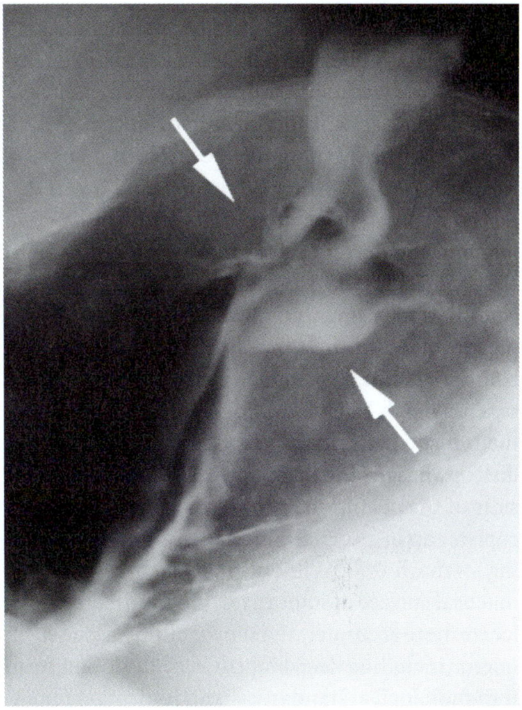

▲ **Fig. 34 c.**

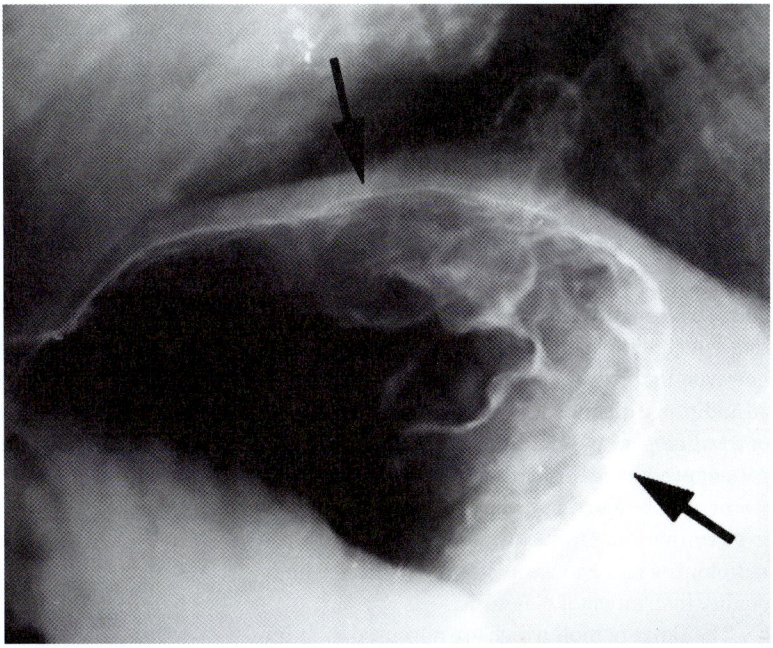

▼ **Fig. 34 b.**

Fig. 34a–c. Patient B., age 72. Diagnosis: gastric cancer. **a** Stomach roentgenogram (tight filling, vertical position, anterior projection) at the moment of contrast medium passage through the gastroesophageal junction: unevenly narrowed abdominal segment of the esophagus, uneven and eroded contours, rigid walls (black arrow); the air bubble of the stomach is disfigured due to intramural infiltration of the medial wall (white arrow). **b** Roentgenogram of the upper part of the stomach (double contrast, horizontal position, left posterior oblique projection): walls of the upper part are thickened due to the circular infiltration (arrows); altered relief. **c** Roentgenogram of the upper part of the stomach (double contrast, horizontal position, left lateral projection) at the moment of contrast medium passage through the gastroesophageal junction: abnormal relief of the cardiac rosette (arrows), infiltration spreads over onto the abdominal segment of the esophagus. Conclusion: Infiltrative cancer of the upper part of the stomach with invasion of the esophagus. Histologically, an adenocarcinoma with the signet-ring cell component.

ions about the role and possibilities of radiological diagnosis in gastroenterology, and especially of traditional roentgenology, are radically changing. As a result of underestimating the importance of radiology in Russia, most gastric cancers are diagnosed at late stages.

Meanwhile, significant advances made in X-ray technology in recent years guarantee an even higher efficiency of radiological diagnosis of gastric cancer. The main additional technique for examining patients following their primary examination according to the complex X-ray program is fibergastroscopy with biopsy. Supported by the findings of the traditional X-ray studies, the usefulness of endoscopy has increased several-fold. Based on the results of the primary X-ray examination, the endoscopists can inspect more closely the involved part of the stomach wall. Without finding changes on the mucosal surface in some cases, the endoscopists can locate more accurately the site for taking tissue specimens (including deep biopsy). Any deviation from the »radiological standards« is an indication for endoscopy. These may include malignant and benign tumors, polyps, ulcers, marked hyperplasia of the mucosal folds (Ménétrier's disease, excessive folding), various deformities of the stomach (Haudek's sign, cascade stomach, incomplete turn of the intestinal tube, etc.). Patients who need this examination must be directed to the endoscopist. According to our own data and findings of our colleagues, X-ray screening uncovers 6–7% of those subjects who require endoscopy; those among outpatients who present with no specific complaints do not exceed 3–4%, and 8–9% of patients with pronounced gastric symptoms need endoscopy. It should be remembered, however, that we are speaking about endoscopy as an additional diagnostic examination on the request of a radiologist. We emphasize once again that any patient producing this or that gastrointestinal complaint must be given a primary X-ray and endoscopic examination. Only close cooperation between radiologists and endoscopists can guarantee high-quality instrumental diagnosis.

The range of tools which are now used in radiological diagnosis has been enriched with ultrasonography, CT, and MRI. Therefore, radiological diagnosis is equipped with everything it needs to solve diagnostic problems.

Ultrasonography

Sonographic studies are included in the set of techniques now used in the radiological diagnosis of gastric cancer. During recent years, ultrasonography has been used extensively in diagnosing diseases of the abdominal organs [5]. Rapid advancements in ultrasonographic technologies, their high efficiency, safety, and possibility of simultaneously examining many abdominal organs make ultrasonography the best primary tool for examining the abdomen.

Standard ultrasonography of the abdominal organs is done on a fasting stomach with the patient lying in the horizontal position, after preliminary measures have been taken to minimize the amount of gas in the intestinal loops. These measures include a cleansing enema, although there is a more effective method, using Fortrans, the substance that prepares the patient for ultrasonographic examination without preliminary dietary restrictions or enema.

We compared various methodological versions of ultrasonographic studies of the stomach to conclude that the method proposed by H. Worlicek in 1989, and modified by us and our colleagues, is the most suitable for the purpose. It includes filling the stomach with normal boiled water (500–1000 ml). The stomach is then examined in the five standard projections [42, 273]:

1. On the left side in Trendelenburg's position (head end of the bed is tilted upwards 20°). This projection is used to study the fundus and the body of the stomach.
2. On the left side with the head end of the bed tilted upwards 30°–40°
3. Supine patient on the bed in the same position. Both projections are used to study the body and the proximal part of the antral part of the stomach.
4. On the right side in the same position
5. In the vertical position. Both projections are suitable for the study of the pylorus, the antral part of the stomach, and the duodenal bulb.

Ultrasonographic study of the stomach begins with the search for the pylorus, which is found to the right of the median line, dorsal or caudal of the liver border. When scanned in the sagittal plane, it appears

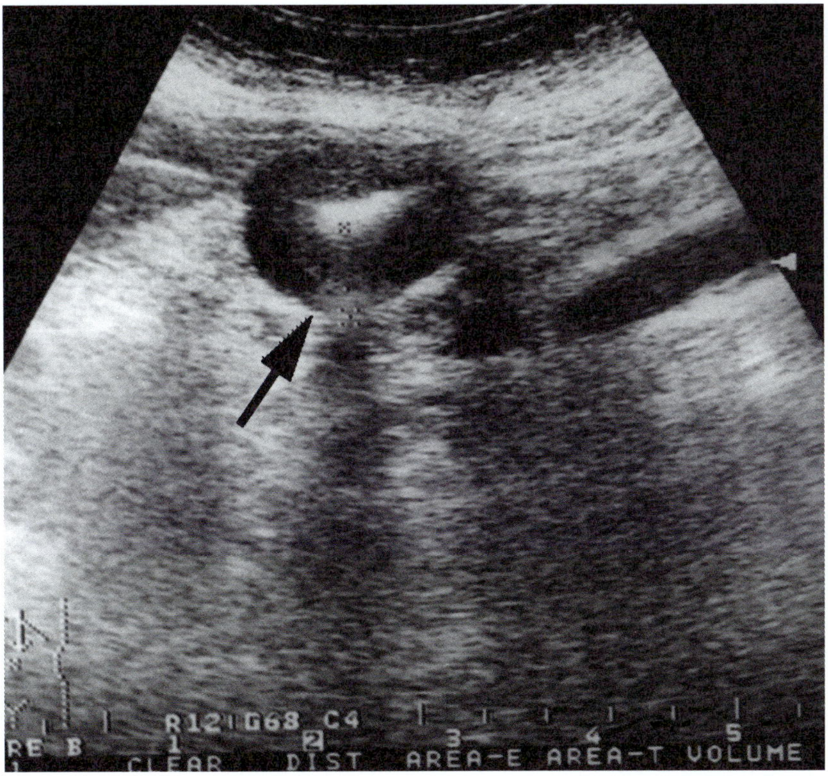

Fig. 35.
Patient V., age 62. Diagnosis: infiltrative gastric cancer. Transverse echotomogram of the lower third of the stomach body: natural hyper-pneumatization sign (hyperechogenicity) of the stomach lumen with thickening of its wall (arrow)

as a ring with poor echogenic properties, encircling a hyperechogenic center. The ring, which is normally 6–7 mm thick, is the reflection of the walls in the pyloric part of the stomach. The hyperechogenic center corresponds to the interfold spaces. On completion of examination of the pylorus, the scanner is moved to the left in the same horizontal direction. Now the prepyloric and the antral parts of the stomach are examined, up to the angular notch. Scanning of these parts ends by gradually or rapidly (depending on the stomach shape) changing the sensor's position to the horizontal plane for subsequent examination of the stomach body. In some cases, where the angular notch is not pronounced, it is possible to scan by consecutive oblique sections.

Ultrasonography is especially effective with the sensor perpendicular to the long axis of each part of the stomach: their normal ultrasonographic image is then similar to the image of the pylorus. In the transverse section, this is a ring with a hypoechogenic periphery and a hyperechogenic center. The walls of the stomach body and the antral part are normally thicker than those of the pyloric part (4–7 mm). Asymmetry of the stomach walls can be observed in a fasting stomach, which is probably due to the presence of pronounced folds and higher tone of the smooth transverse muscles of the greater curvature. It should be noted that the dynamic scan of the stomach reveals inconstancy of its ultrasonographic image. Peristaltic movements steadily propel air of the stomach toward the duodenum, each portion interfering with visualization of the posterior wall. An acoustic shadow that appears behind the air changes the ring into a semi-ring.

While ultrasonography on the whole is a useful tool, it should be noted that its effectiveness is maximum only when the antral part and the lower half of the stomach body are studied, whereas visualization of the upper half of the body, and especially of the upper part of the stomach is difficult (Fig. 35).

In order to increase the potential of ultrasonography, we and our colleagues proposed an additional projection: scanning of the stomach in a supine patient with the leg end of the bed elevated to facilitate filling of contrast medium into the upper part of the stomach (Fig. 36) [42]. Filling the stomach

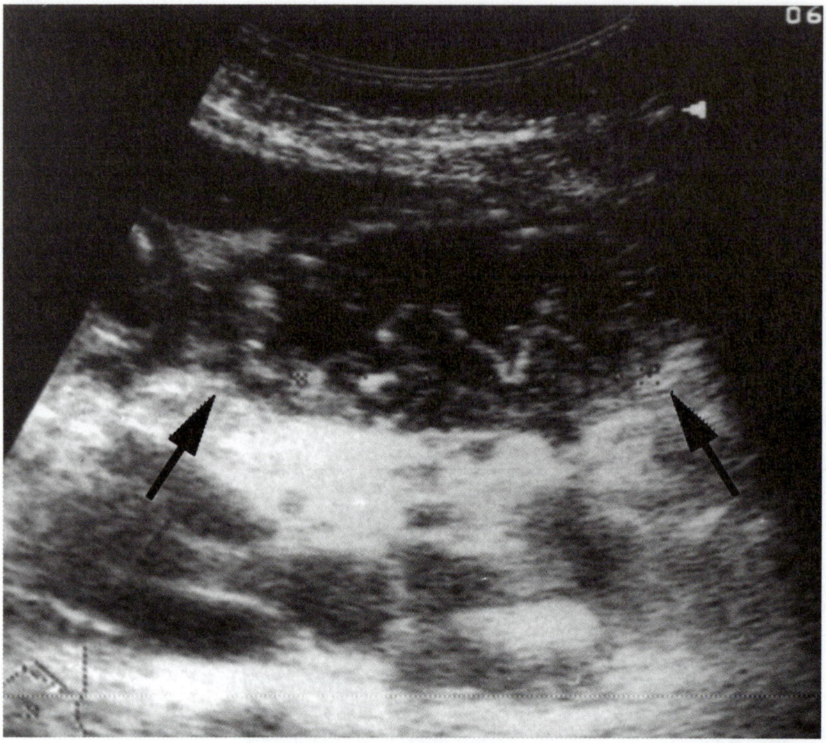

Fig. 36. Female patient R., age 75. Diagnosis: infiltrative cancer of the upper third of the stomach body. Echotomogram of the stomach filled with water. Oblique section at the level of the upper third of the stomach body (additional projection). Uneven thickening of the stomach wall to 7–22 mm over a length of 8–9 cm due to tumor infiltration. The inner contour of the changed wall is uneven and tuberous. Normal five-layer structure is absent (arrows)

with water maintains it in the field of scanning and also helps with orientation of the anatomical parts. In addition, the use of hypotonic preparations becomes unnecessary, which substantially reduces the time for the procedure without having an adverse effect on the final results.

Using the protocol we devised as a component of the common standard ultrasonographic examination of the abdominal organs can help to reveal metastases and to evaluate the possible primary location of a tumor prior to the use of special methods of tumor localization (traditional X-ray examination and endoscopy).

Computed Tomography

The development of computed tomography was an important contribution of science and technology. In 1979, A. Cormack and G. Hounsfield were awarded the Nobel Prize for this invention, which revolutionized the diagnosis of pathologies. Today, CT is widely used in the diagnosis of many diseases of various organs [273, 277].

CT technology is important in the following cases: staging of malignant tumor, diagnosis of tumor relapses, dynamic observation to evaluate the efficacy of therapy, verification of causes of displacement of the stomach and the duodenum, verification of the character of palpable formations in the abdominal cavity in situations where the traditional X-ray examination is of low effectiveness, detection of metastases, and determination of lymphatic system involvement (Fig. 37) [3, 18, 20, 85, 92, 196, 261, 262].

Publications which have appeared in recent years propose an even broader use of CT of the stomach. Some offer various methods for CT examinations of the stomach and describe the normal CT anatomy of the stomach and CT signs of blastomatous affection. Some deal with the differential diagnosis of epithelial and non-epithelial tumors of the stomach using CT, as well as to the staging of gastric cancer [47, 126, 267].

There is no consensus regarding the best method of conducting a CT examination of the stomach, and some authors continue to search for alternative methodological approaches. In order to obtain the necessary contrast, they use oral contrast media, wa-

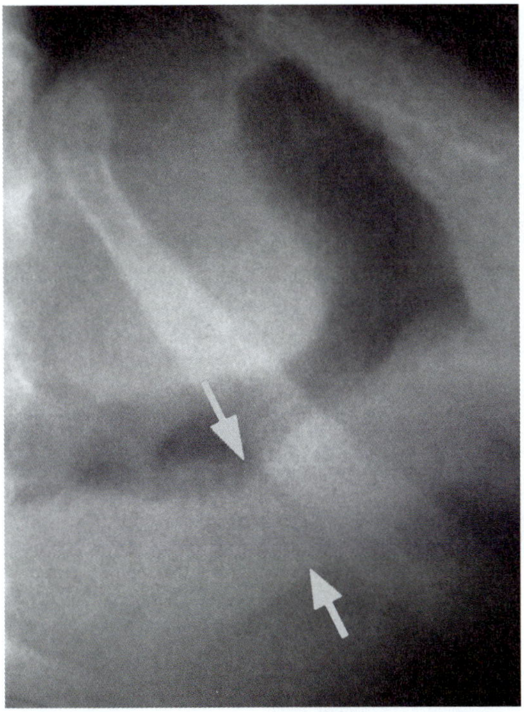

▲ **Fig. 37 a.**

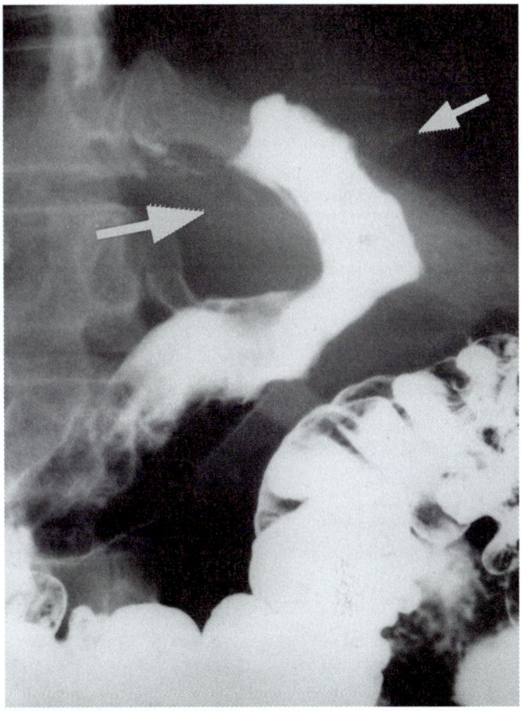

▼ **Fig. 37 b.**

▲ **Fig. 37 c.**

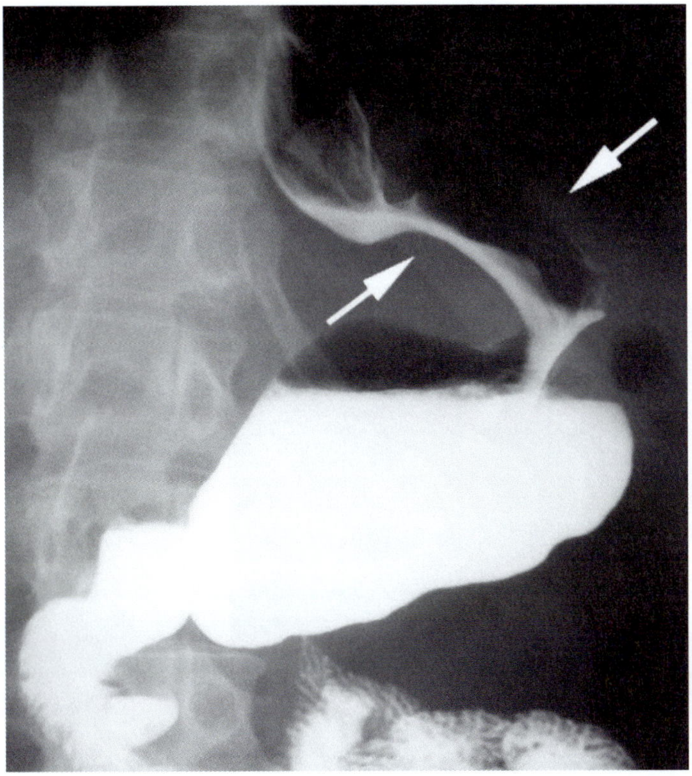

Fig. 37a–f. Female patient S., age 52. Diagnosis: gastric cancer. Complained of epigastric pain and discomfort after small meals. According to her estimate, she had been ill for 9 months. The patient was repeatedly examined by endoscopy which did not reveal organic changes. Ultrasonography detected much fluid in the abdominal cavity. The patient underwent an X-ray examination. **a** Stomach roentgenogram (vertical position, anterior projection): symptom of air redistribution in the stomach; the air bubble is elongated in the form of a comma; the stomach walls are thick (arrows). **b** Stomach roentgenogram (tight filling, vertical position, anterior projection): the cavity of the stomach upper half is reduced significantly; contours are uneven (arrows). **c** Stomach roentgenogram (double contrast, horizontal position, anterior projection): the stomach body and its upper part are tightly filled with barium meal; stomach cavity is significantly decreased (arrows); stomach walls are rigid, evacuation is rapid. **d** Stomach roentgenogram (double contrast, horizontal position, left oblique projection) after additional intake of a gas-producing mixture and barium meal:

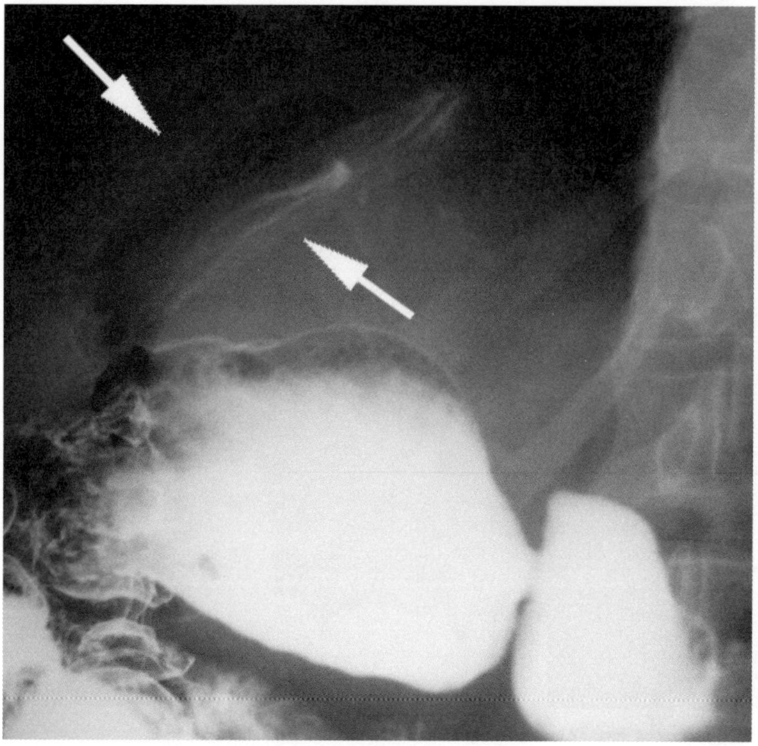

walls of the stomach body and its upper part are rigid due to circular infiltration (arrows). Conclusion: Infiltrative cancer of the body and the upper part of the stomach. In the absence of histological verification, the patient underwent CT examination of the stomach. **e** Computed tomography of the stomach (tight filling with E-Z-CAT DRY): stomach cavity decreased (white arrows), walls are thick due to intramural infiltration (black arrows), much fluid in the abdominal cavity. **f** Computed tomography of the stomach (under dosed inflation with air): the walls of the stomach body and its upper part are thick and rigid due to a circular intramural infiltration (arrows); much fluid in the abdominal cavity. Conclusion: Infiltrative cancer of the body and the upper part of the stomach. Ascites (indirect sign of carcinomatosis)

◄ **Fig. 37 d.**

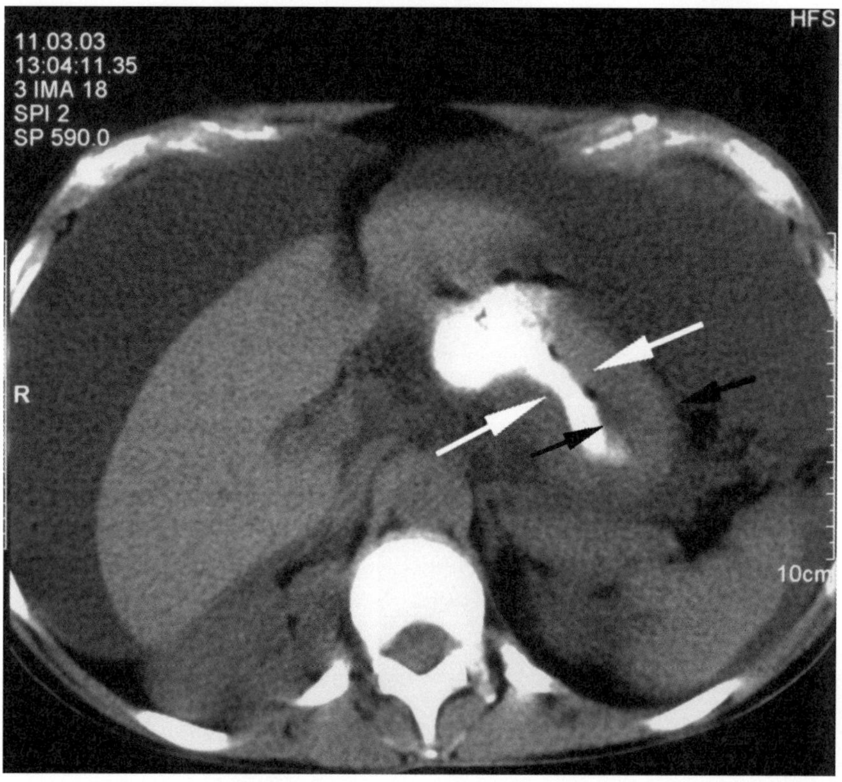

◄ **Fig. 37 e.**

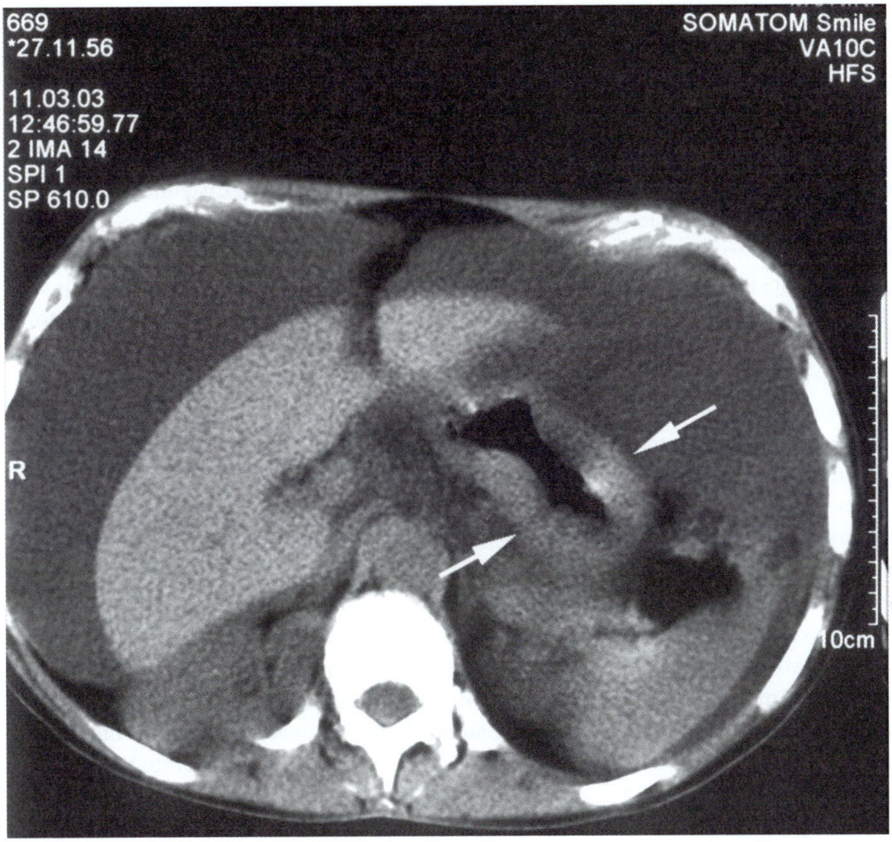

◂ **Fig. 37 f.**

ter, air, oral contrast in combination with intravenous injections of iodine preparations aimed at layered imaging of the stomach wall, as well as spasmolytics in conditions of hypotension; the principle of polypositional scanning is also proposed [47, 80, 180].

Owing to the high contrast of imaging, most researchers prefer using water to fill the stomach for its adequate distension and they explain their choice by good tolerability of water and good miscibility of water with gastric contents (as distinct from positive contrast media). M. Minami et al. recommend that the patient drink 400 ml of water for dynamic CT [196]. In order to intensify stomach wall imaging, M.S. Chen et al. suggest the following method: after receiving an intramuscular injection of Buscopan and 600–1000 ml water orally, the patient is given intravenous iodine contrast medium using an automatic injector which is synchronized with the computed tomograph [105]. J.S. Cho et al. used two-phase dynamic CT with intravenous injection of 150 ml contrast medium at a rate of 5 ml/s for 30 s and subsequent tomography at 30 s and at 2 min after the start of the injection [107]. All these different methods have one common feature: They all are used either to reveal or to confirm the presence of an infiltrative tumor. It is not obligatory to use multislice tomographs in order to scan the entire stomach within a short period of time. Not all medical institutions can afford to acquire the apparatus. Therefore, we propose two simple methods for conducting CT of the stomach.

One method is based on dosed inflation of the stomach with air as the only contrast medium. The method consists in the following:

1. Air is used as contrast medium.
2. A thin elastic tube is passed into the stomach for insufflation of air, which is kept in the stomach cavity for the length of the study.
3. The stomach is repeatedly inflated with air during scanning, with detailed assessment of the zone of interest.

In the other method, E-Z-CAT DRY barium suspension (EZEM company) is used as the contrast medium. This substance is especially intended for CT of the stomach. Both methods are equally suitable, but each has its particular advantages and disadvantages. It is not always possible to introduce the tube into the stomach, especially in patients with cancer of the upper part of the stomach with involvement of the esophagus. It is true that the tube may remain in the esophagus and then air alone may be used as contrast medium, but only small tumors of the wall can be detected with inflation of the stomach. The method including administration of barium sulfate suspension as the contrast medium is noninvasive, but the absence of considerable stomach distension decreases reliability of the CT signs of early blastomatous infiltration. Therefore, the choice of method for CT of the stomach should be decided separately for each individual patient in consideration of the findings of the traditional X-ray examination (Fig. 38).

Computed tomography is done in a fasting stomach and conducted in two phases – before and after administration of a contrast medium. The stomach is first studied in its native state with the patient in a supine position; axial scans are obtained localize the tumor in the stomach. The second phase is following the administration of either barium sulfate suspension or air into the stomach cavity. This phase is used to reveal and verify the character of changes in the zone of interest (tumor infiltration of the stomach wall). The multi-positional principle is fundamental to CT of the stomach. Whenever necessary, the patient is examined in additional positions (prone, lateral). If the tumor is in the cardiac and pyloric parts, the most optimal position is with the patient lying on his right side. T. Shiravaca et al. studied the value of the right lateral position while determining the spread of gastric cancer to the adjacent organs [242]. According to M. Rossi et al., the patient lying in a prone position after having drunk 500 ml of water and received glucagons administered intravenously (drug-induced hypotonia) improves distension of the stomach with tumors of the lesser curvature and the pyloric part of the stomach [231].

Analysis of the signs of tumor infiltration of the stomach wall is based on the study of CT images of its intact wall, which, being distended by contrast medium, appears as a distinct 1.5- to 2.5-mm line with distinct inner and outer contours. It is only in the prepyloric and cardiac parts that the wall is 5–6 mm thick (after adequate distension of the stomach cavity), which can be explained by the anatomical thickening of the muscular coat in these parts, as well as by the specific anatomical position (transverse) of the stomach in some patients, hypersthenics in particular. Therefore, if the walls of the upper and lower parts of the stomach are thick, it would be reasonable to conduct repeated CT (following additional inflation) with thinner sections (2–5 mm). It should be remembered that if the stomach wall is not affected by a tumor its thickness never exceeds 5–6 mm. Despite the difficulties of topical localization of the pathological process in the upper parts of the stomach, the proposed method has one advantage: As the gastric tube is passed into the lumen of the gastroesophageal junction, its imaging on computed tomograms is more distinct, which helps in staging the tumor of the upper part of the stomach and in determining tumor infiltration into the esophagus. The specificity of CT data on tumor infiltration to the esophagus is 95% [16, 28, 123, 196].

Various contrast media have been used to diagnose tumor infiltration of the stomach wall with CT. E.J. Balthazar et al. show that with CT it is possible to diagnose scirrhous carcinoma by a thickening of the stomach wall [92]. K. Tsuda et al. indicate that this method can be used not only to show intramural tumor infiltration, but also to reveal early gastric cancer in 49% cases; moreover, the specificity of the method is as high as 93–100% [262]. Assuming that CT reveals affections of the stomach wall in patients with epithelial tumors, G. Potente et al. regard this as only an adjunct method in view of its limitations in determining tumors at the first and second stages; furthermore, the method sometimes fails to diagnose pronounced tumor infiltration sufficiently [226]. According to some authors, thickening of the stomach wall cannot be regarded as a specific sign of tumor. Meanwhile, others indicate that in pa-

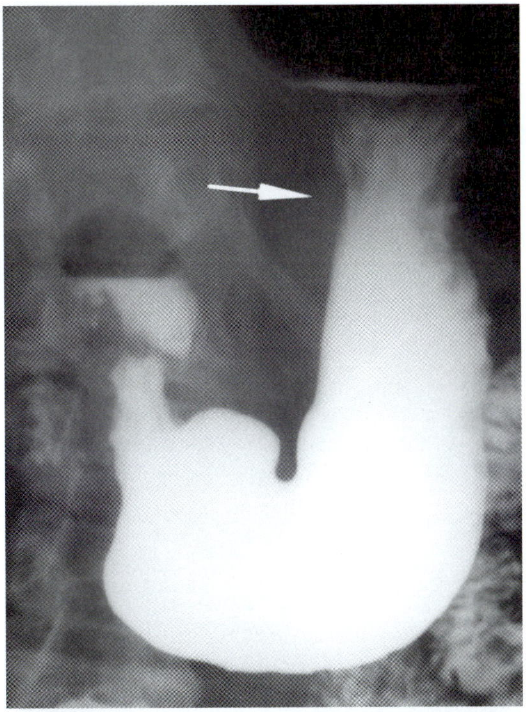

▲ Fig. 38 a.

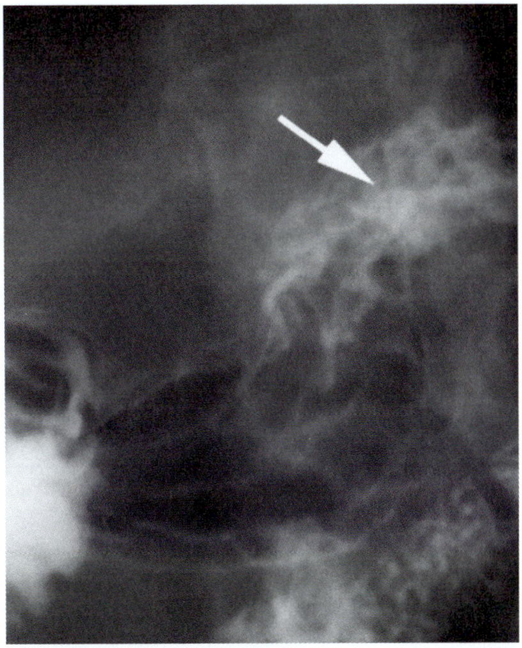

▲ Fig. 38 c.

▼ Fig. 38 b.

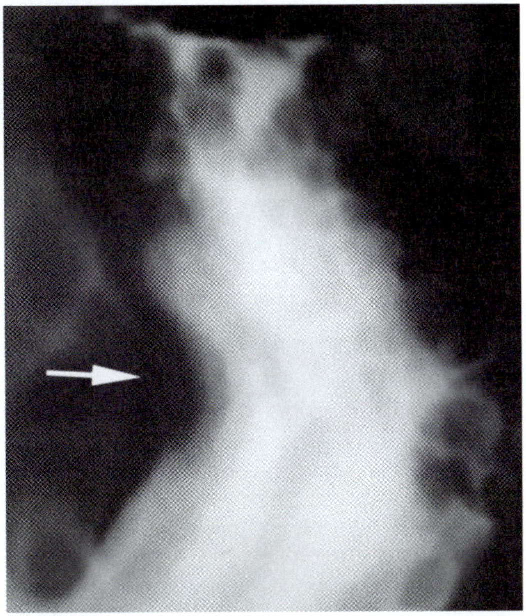

▼ Fig. 38 d.

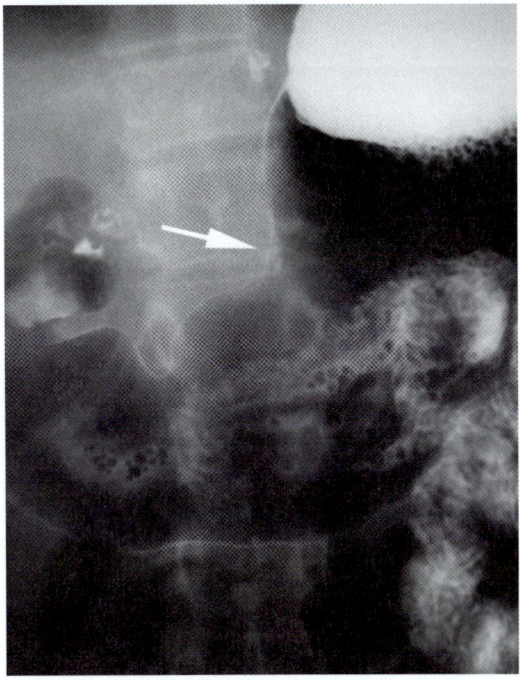

Fig. 38a–o. Female patient P., age 57. Diagnosis: gastric cancer. **a** Stomach roentgenogram (tight filling, vertical position, anterior projection): uneven contour of the lesser curvature of the upper third of the stomach (arrow). **b** Target stomach roentgenogram (tight filling, vertical position, left quarter-oblique projection): optimal projection in roentgenotelescopy distinctly visualizes uneven contour of the upper third of the stomach body (arrow). **c** Stomach roentgenogram (pneumo-relief, horizontal position, anterior projection): a depot of contrast medium on the anterior wall with folds converging towards the depot (arrow). **d, e** Series

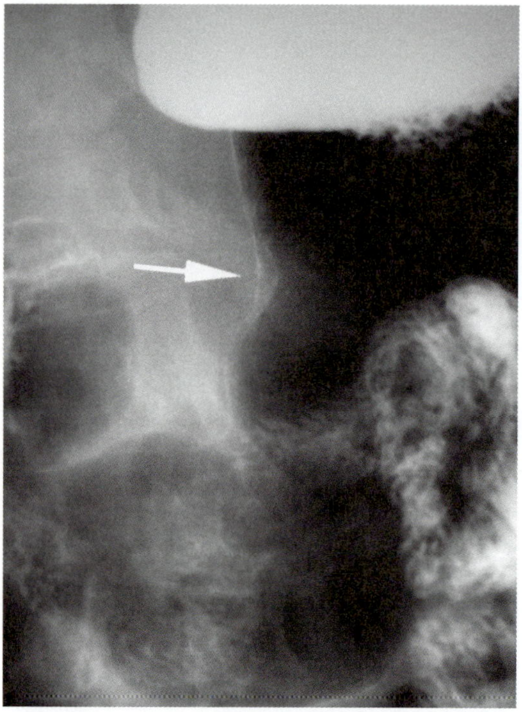

▲ **Fig. 38 e.** ▼ **Fig. 38 f.**

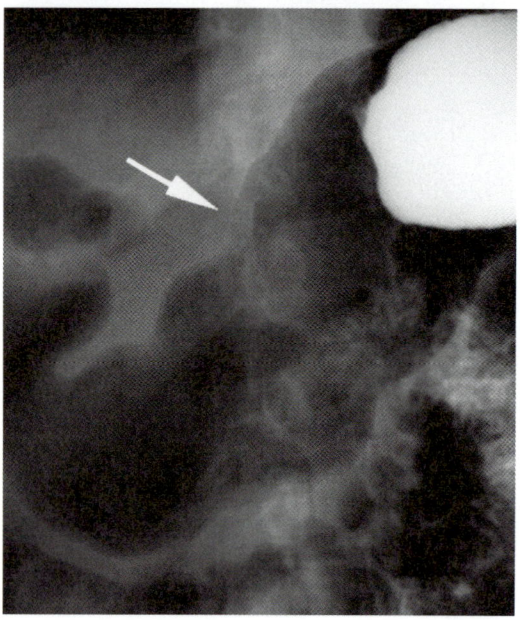

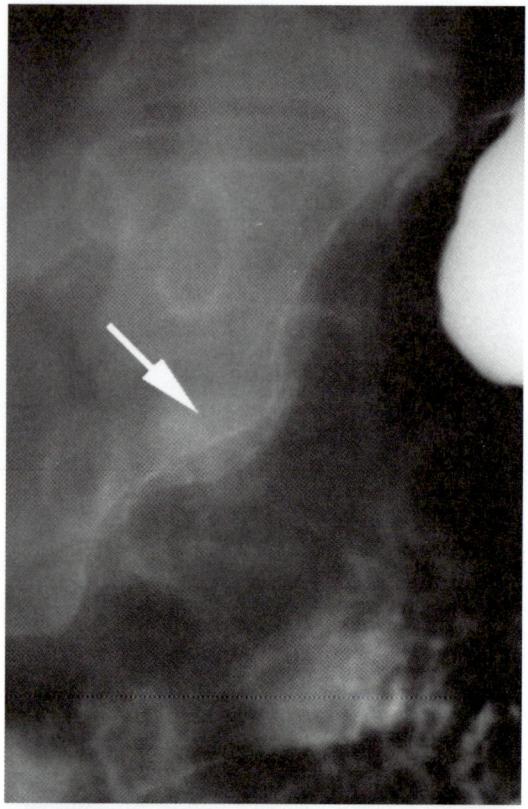

▲ **Fig. 38 g.** ▼ **Fig. 38 h.**

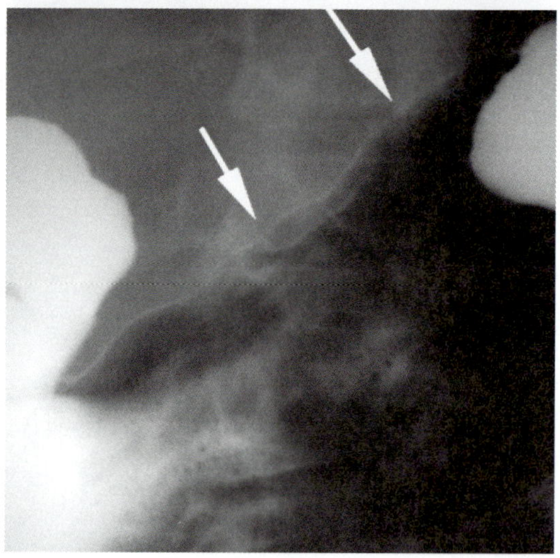

of stomach roentgenograms (double contrast, horizontal position, anterior projection): the wall of the lesser curvature in the upper third of the stomach body is thickened over a short length (arrow). **f, g** Series of stomach roentgenograms (double contrast, horizontal position, left half-oblique projection): walls thickened due to intramural infiltration (arrow) are visualized more distinctly; **h** Stomach roentgenogram (double contrast, horizontal position, left oblique projection): optimal projection in roentgenotelescopy distinctly visualizes infiltration of the anterior wall in the upper third of the stomach body over a significantly greater length

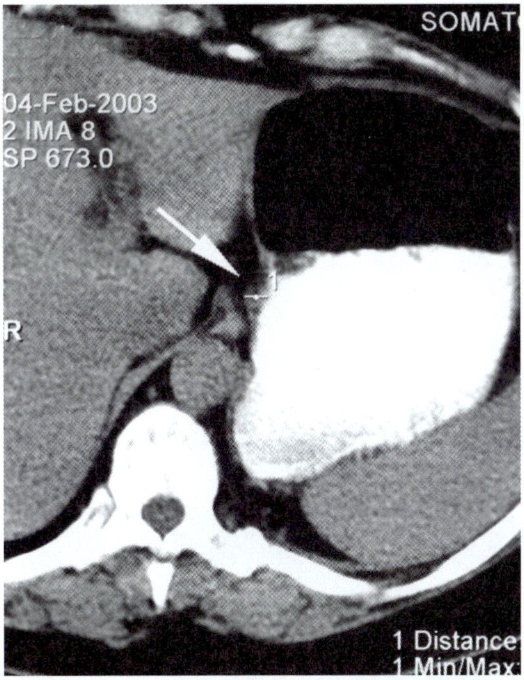

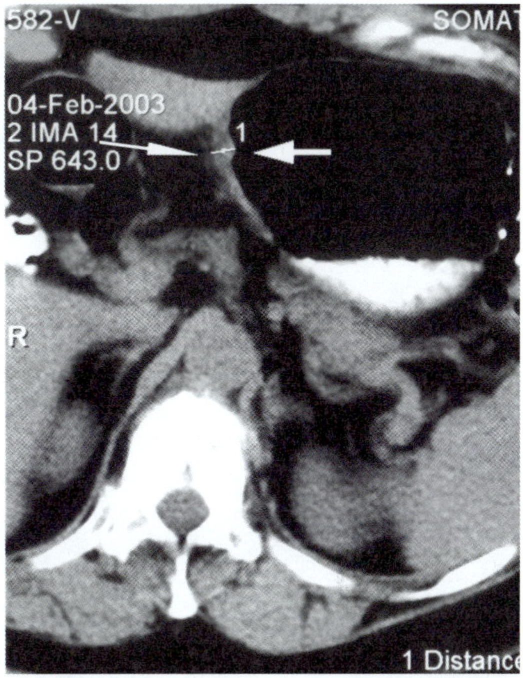

▲ **Fig. 38 i.** ▼ **Fig. 38 j.** ▲ **Fig. 38 k.** ▼ **Fig. 38 l.**

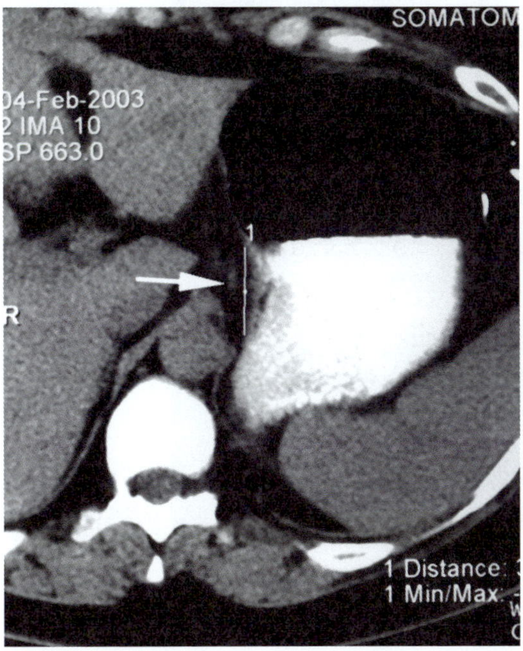

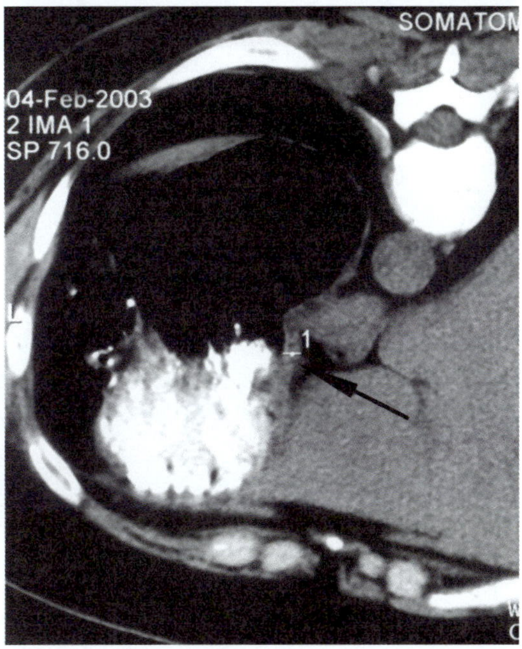

compared with other projections (arrows). Conclusion: Minor infiltrative cancer of the anterior wall of the upper third of the stomach body. Histological study of tissue specimens taken during endoscopy failed to find tumor cells. The patient was examined using computed tomography. **i, j**Series of CT images of the stomach (tight filling with E-Z-CAT DRY, supine patient): insignificant thickening of the stomach wall to 8 mm over a length of 3.2 cm (arrow). **k** CT image of the stomach (after additional inflation with air; supine patient): after inflation of the stomach, wall thickness does not change (arrows). **l** CT image of the stomach (after addi-

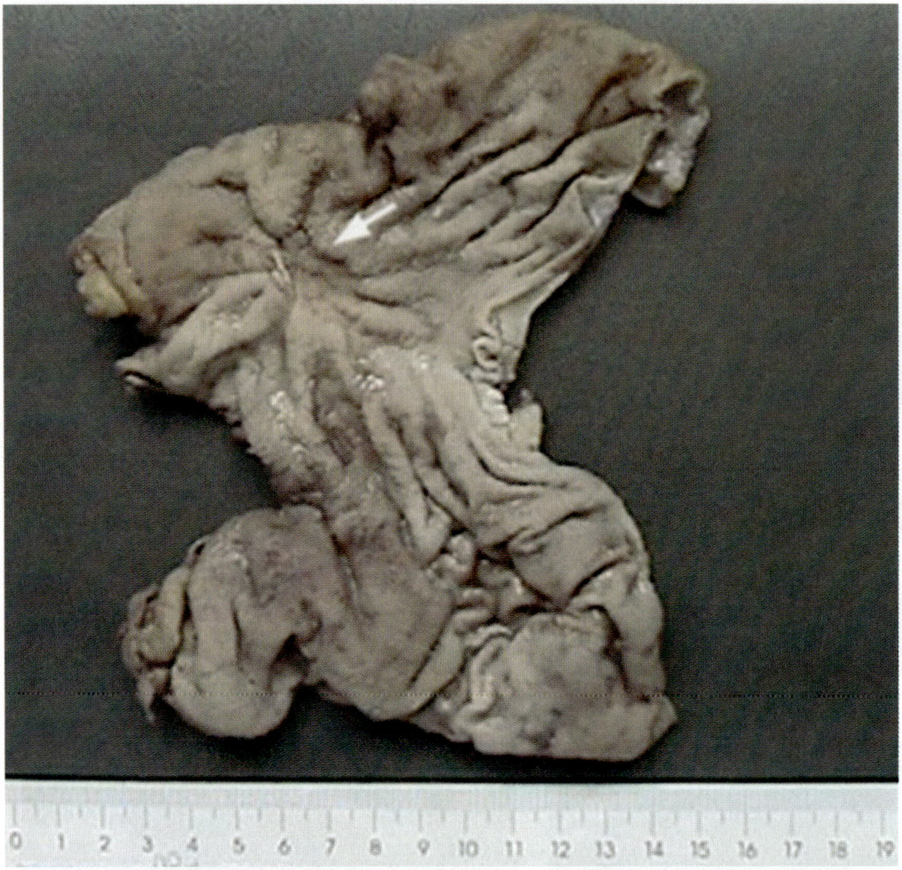

◂ **Fig. 38 m.**

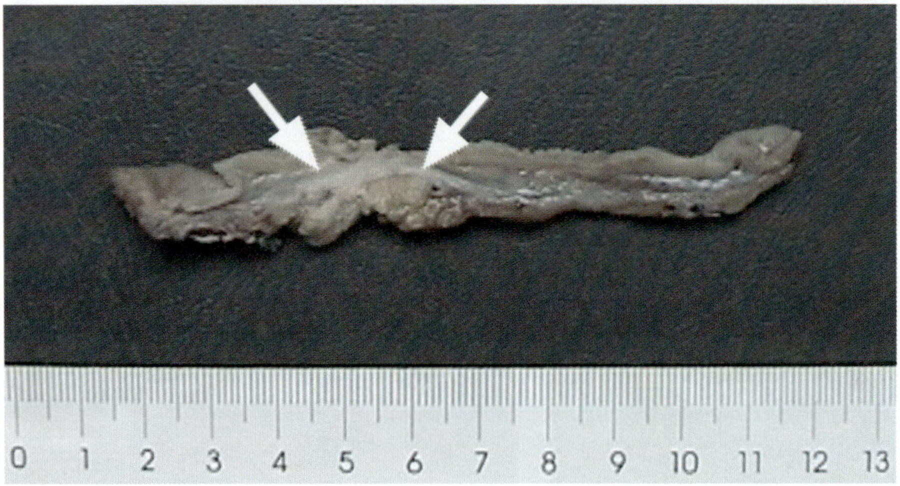

◂ **Fig. 38 n.**

tional inflation of the stomach; prone position): as the patient changes position, thickness of the stomach wall remains stable (arrows). Conclusion: Minor infiltrative cancer of the upper third of the stomach body. **m** Macrospecimen of a resected stomach: folds converging towards the firm part of the wall (arrow). **n** Fragment of the macrospecimen (strip): arrows indicate white intramural infiltration extending over a distance of 3 cm, mostly in the submucous layer. **o** Microspecimen of the wall fragment: signet-ring cell carcinoma. Tumor cells have the classical fingerlike shapes floating in »lakes« of mucus

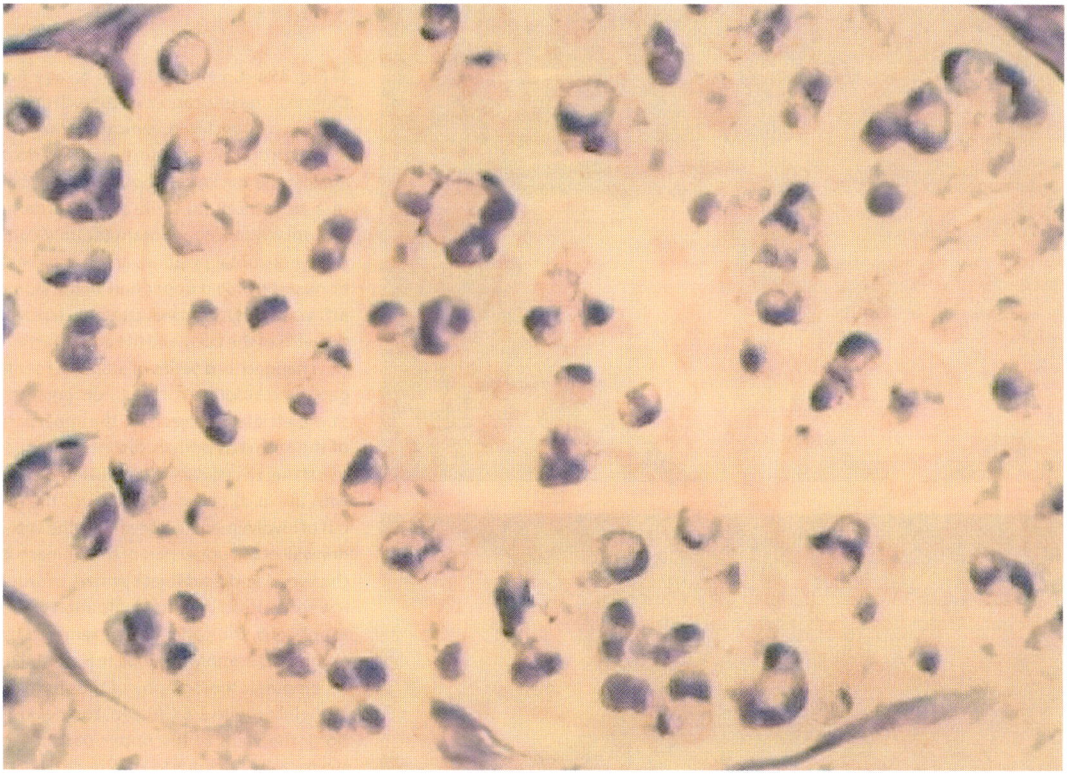

▲ Fig. 38 o.

tients with endophytic cancer, in whom the tumor grows intramurally, this sign gives a specific CT image of a limited or diffuse thickening of the stomach wall (◘ Fig. 39) [33, 35, 53, 180].

Analysis of data in the literature, presenting quite controversial current concepts of the potentials of CT in the diagnosis of gastric cancer, shows that this problem is still pressing, and that further studies are needed. At the same time, based on our own experience and that of our colleagues with the use of CT to diagnose stomach affections in more than 300 studies, most of which were done in suspected cases of cancer and other diseases requiring differential diagnosis [31, 33, 36, 38, 47], we can state that the role of computed tomography in the examination of patients with gastric tumors is quite well defined. This will be described in detail in Chap. 5, which is dedicated to the radiological signs of gastric cancer.

Magnetic Resonance Imaging

The physical phenomenon of nuclear magnetic resonance has been known for quite some time. F. Bloch and E. Purcell were awarded the Nobel Prize for this invention in 1946, but it was introduced into practical medicine only in recent decades.

In a comparatively short time, from the early 1980s until today, MRI has become one of the most informative methods of noninvasive diagnosis. This is explained by the fact that MRI has great advantages over the other radiological diagnostic methods. Most important are its noninvasive character, the complete absence of ionizing radiation, the ability to produce multiplanar images, the unsurpassable contrast of imaging soft tissues, the natural contrast of the circulating blood, and the absence of artifacts of bone tissues and gas-containing structures [15].

Owing to continuous improvement of the method, its field of use has broadened as well. MRI is known to physicians of various profiles as a meth-

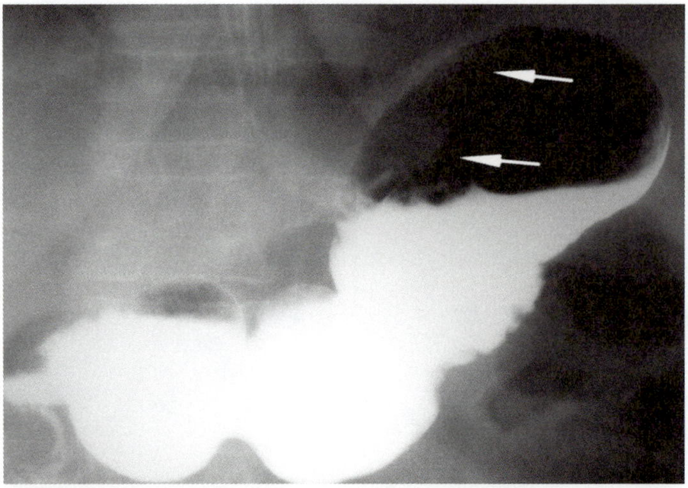

◂ **Fig. 39 a.**

Fig. 39a–l. Female patient S., age 68. Diagnosis; gastric cancer. **a** Stomach roentgenogram (tight filling, vertical position, anterior projection): additional shadow against the background of the air bubble due to intramural infiltration (arrows). **b** Stomach roentgenogram (double contrast, horizontal position, anterior projection): tightly filled upper part of the stomach visualizes its uneven contours (arrow); the walls of the body and the antral part are not changed. **c, d** Series of stomach roentgenograms (double contrast, horizontal position, left lateral projection): the upper part of the stomach body is disfigured (hourglass) due to circular intramural infiltration with the folds converging towards the focus of involvement (white arrow); the anterior wall of the upper part of the stomach is thickened and rigid (black arrow). In order to verify spread of tumor infiltration to the esophagus, the patient was examined by computed tomography of the stomach. **e** Computed tomography of the stomach (tight filling with E-Z-CAT DRY, supine position): the walls of the upper part of the stomach are thick due to intramural infiltration (white arrow) which spreads over onto the abdominal segment of the esophagus and the left crus of the diaphragm (black arrow). **f, g, h** Series of CT images (tight filling E-Z-CAT DRY, supine position): the walls are thick due to intramural infiltration. **i** Computed tomography of the stomach (pneumo-CT, prone position): stable thickening of the stomach wall is visualized over a significantly greater length. Conclusion: Infiltrative cancer of the stomach body and its upper part with invasion of the abdominal segment of the esophagus and the left crus of the diaphragm. **j** Macrospecimen of a resected stomach: white tumor tissue (white arrows) infiltrating the wall; changed relief of the cardiac rosette relief can be seen (black arrow). **k** Fragment of a macrospecimen (strip): the stomach wall is thick due to white tumor infiltration. **l** Microspecimen of a fragment of the stomach wall: moderately differentiated adenocarcinoma (white arrows) with the signet-ring cell component (black arrow)

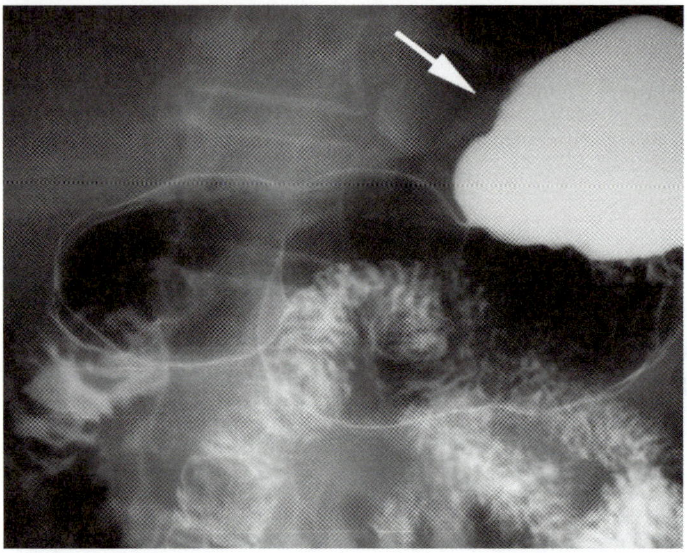

◂ **Fig. 39 b.**

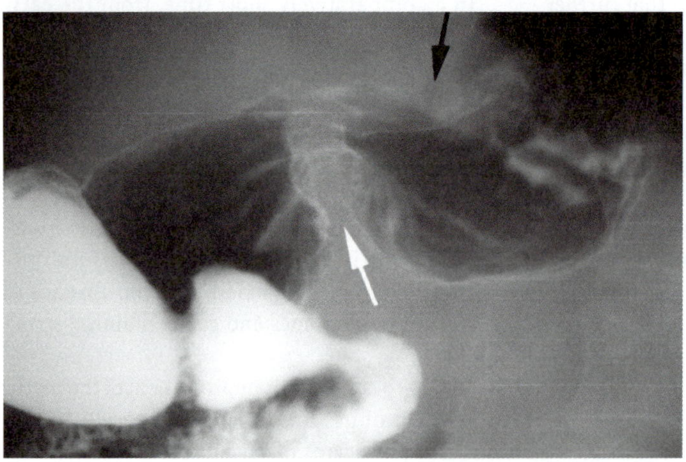

◂ **Fig. 39 c.**

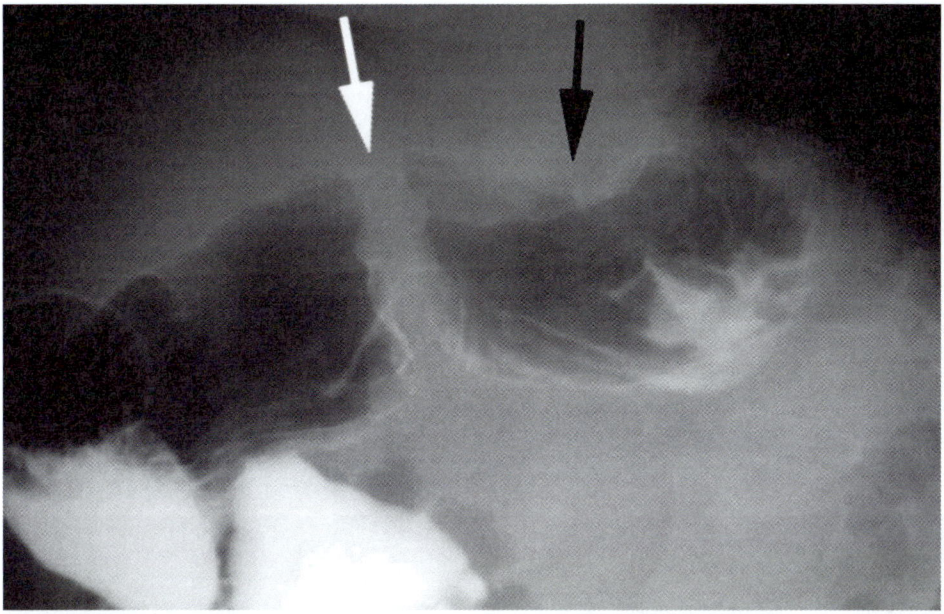

◄ **Fig. 39 d.**

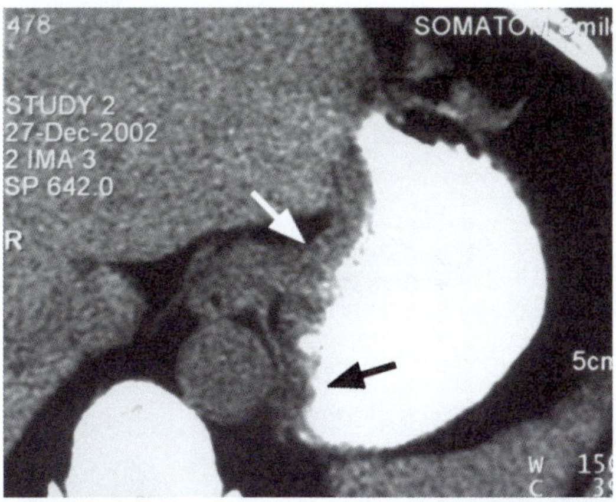

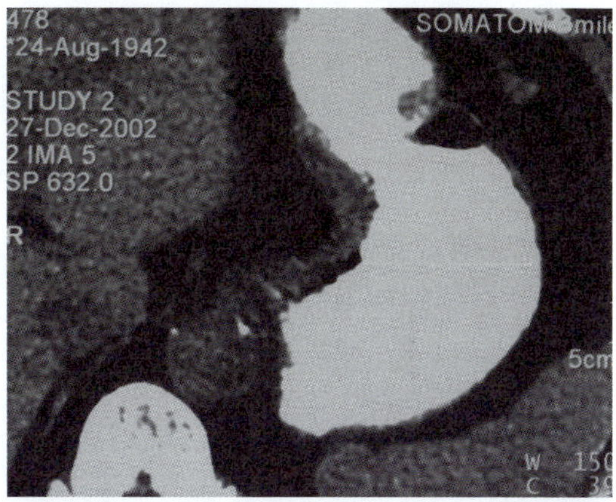

▲ **Fig. 39 e.** ▼ **Fig. 39 f.** ▲ **Fig. 39 g.** ▼ **Fig. 39 h.**

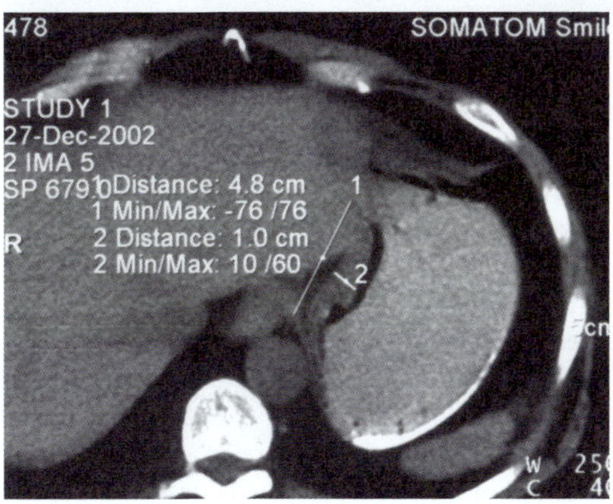

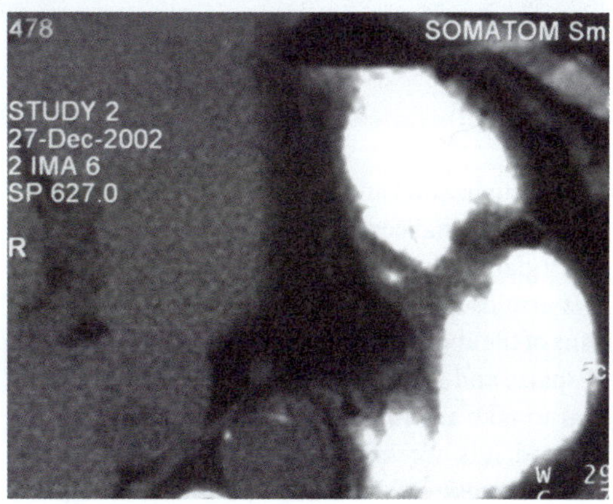

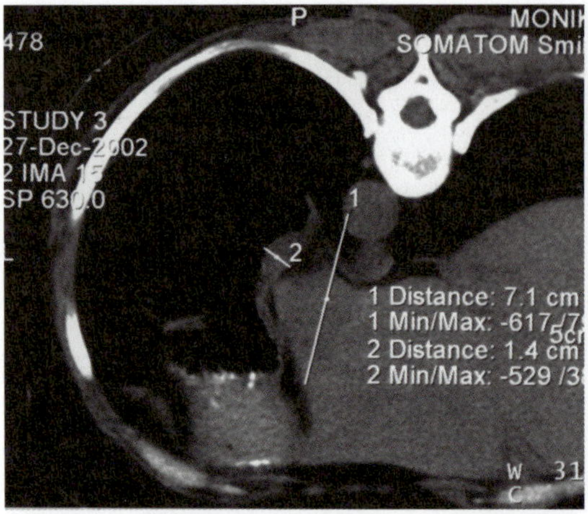

▲ **Fig. 39 i.**

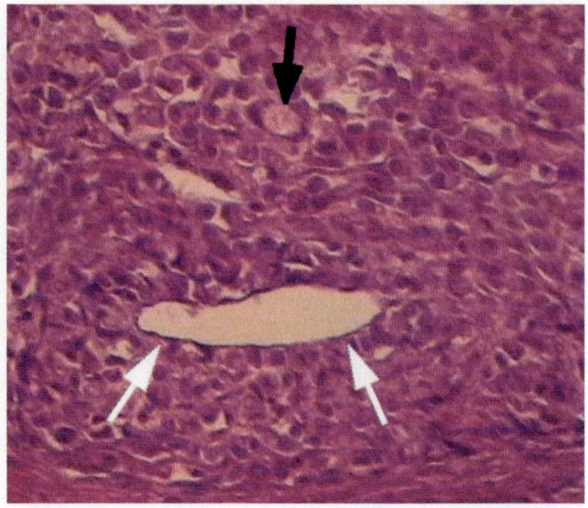

▲ **Fig. 39 l.**

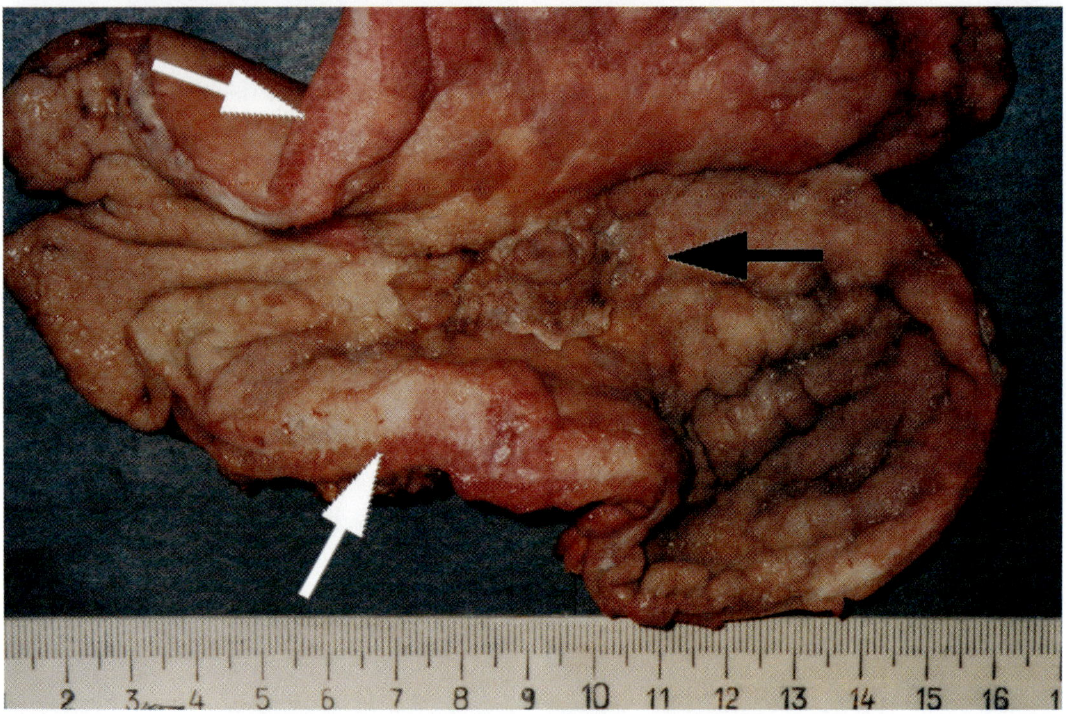

▼ **Fig. 39 j.**

od of visualization and diagnosis of affections of the brain and spinal cord, spinal column, joints, mammary glands, thyroid gland, heart and large vessels. It is also used in the study of parenchymatous organs of the abdominal cavity and the retroperitoneal space, and the pelvic organs. It should be noted that to take advantage of all the potentials of this method, it is necessary to acquire MR tomographs with magnetic induction of a permanent magnetic field of not less than 0.35–0.5 T (Tesla). From an economic standpoint, it is more advantageous to acquire tomographs with a moderate field (0.5 T < B < 1.0 T), although »open« tomographs of 0.35 T can also be used. This is of decisive importance when conducting MRI of the abdominal organs, the stomach in particular.

The few publications by foreign authors concerning MRI of the stomach actually deal with experi-

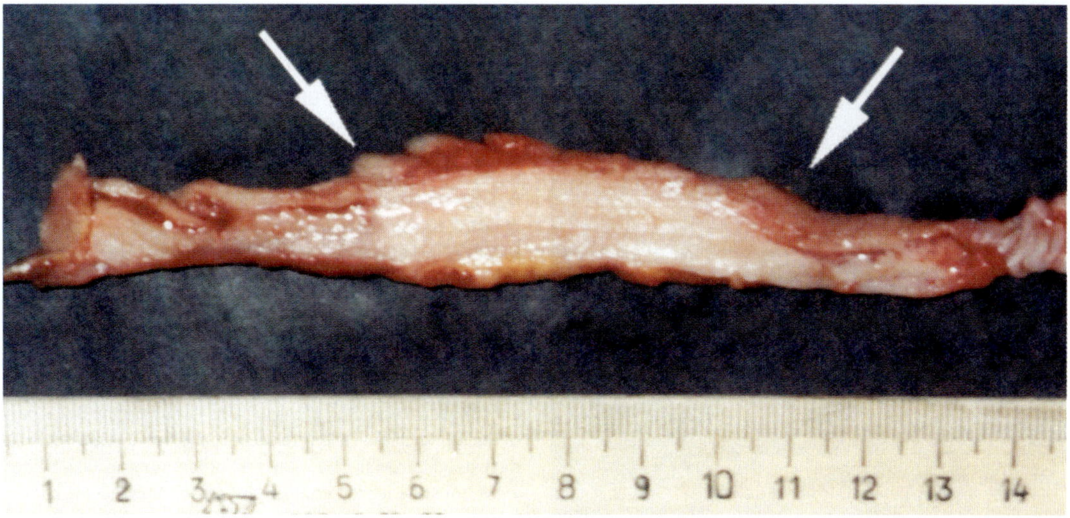

▲ **Fig. 39 k.**

mental studies of macrospecimens of resected stomachs, or far-advanced tumors. However, these publications offer no comparative analysis of the results. Our position is different. We used findings not only of endoscopy but also of traditional X-ray investigations to characterize the role of ultrasonography, CT, and MRI in the diagnosis of gastric cancer (▣ Figs. 40, 41) [79, 115, 137]. While evaluating them, we laid special emphasis on comparison of the results obtained by new methods with those of the traditional X-ray.

One of the things that impedes the use of MRI in the diagnosis of gastric tumors is the fact that endoscopy, ultrasonography, and CT are generally as-

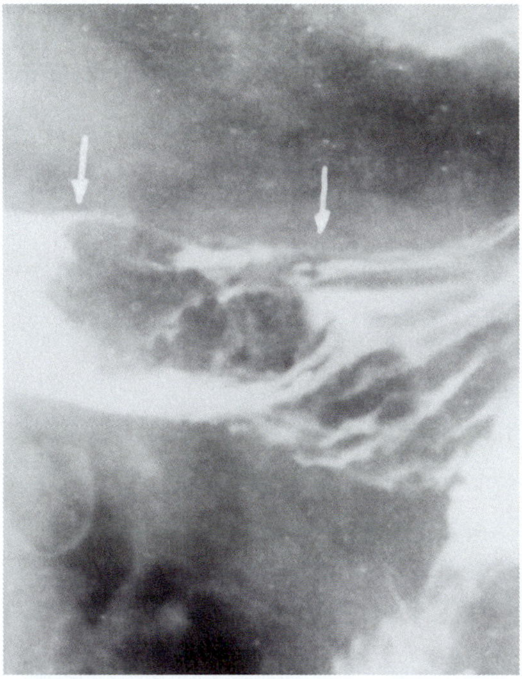

▲ **Fig. 40 a.**

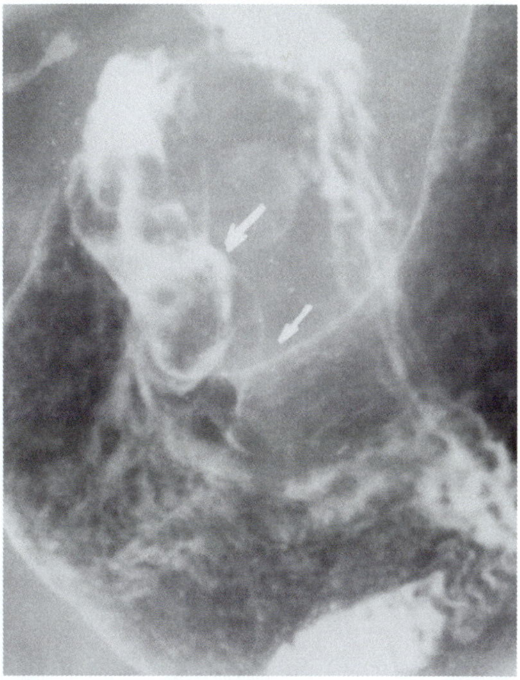

▲ **Fig. 40 b.**

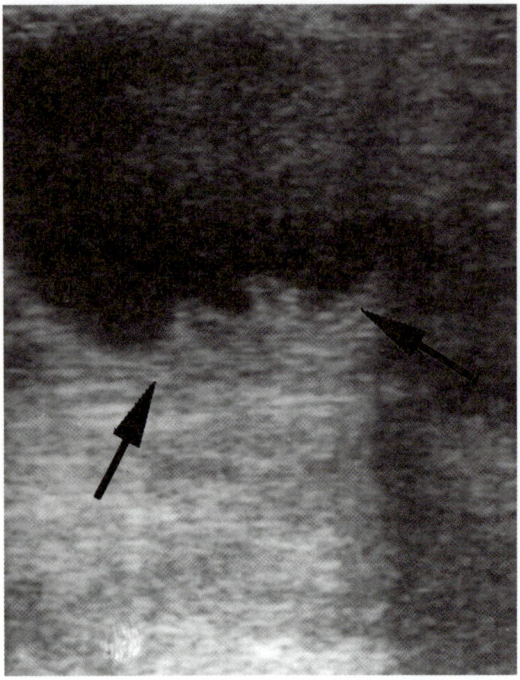

▲ Fig. 40 c.

Fig. 40a–c. Female patient V., age 64. Diagnosis: gastric cancer. Endoscopy revealed a polyp in the antral part of the stomach. Histological studies of tissue specimens taken during endoscopy discovered fragments of a hyperplastic polyp with focal dysplasia of the epithelium. **a** Stomach roentgenogram (tight filling, vertical position, right half-oblique projection), dosed compression: the distal portion of the antral part is disfigured, the lesser curvature contour is uneven, with a flat niche (arrows). **b** Stomach roentgenogram (double contrast, horizontal position, left quarter-oblique projection): walls of the lesser curvature of the antral part are thick and rigid due to intramural infiltration (arrows). Conclusion: Infiltrative-ulcerous cancer of the antral part of the stomach. In the absence of histological confirmation, the patient underwent ultrasonographic examination of the stomach. **c** Ultrasonographic picture of the stomach: uneven thickening of the wall (to 12 mm) in the distal part of the stomach over a length of 3 cm; the five-coat structure is destroyed (arrows). The X-ray and ultrasonographic findings were not sufficient to confirm the presence of gastric cancer without histological verification (no tumor cells were discovered). Radical treatment was not given. A repeated examination was done 2 months later with MR

▼ Fig. 41 a.

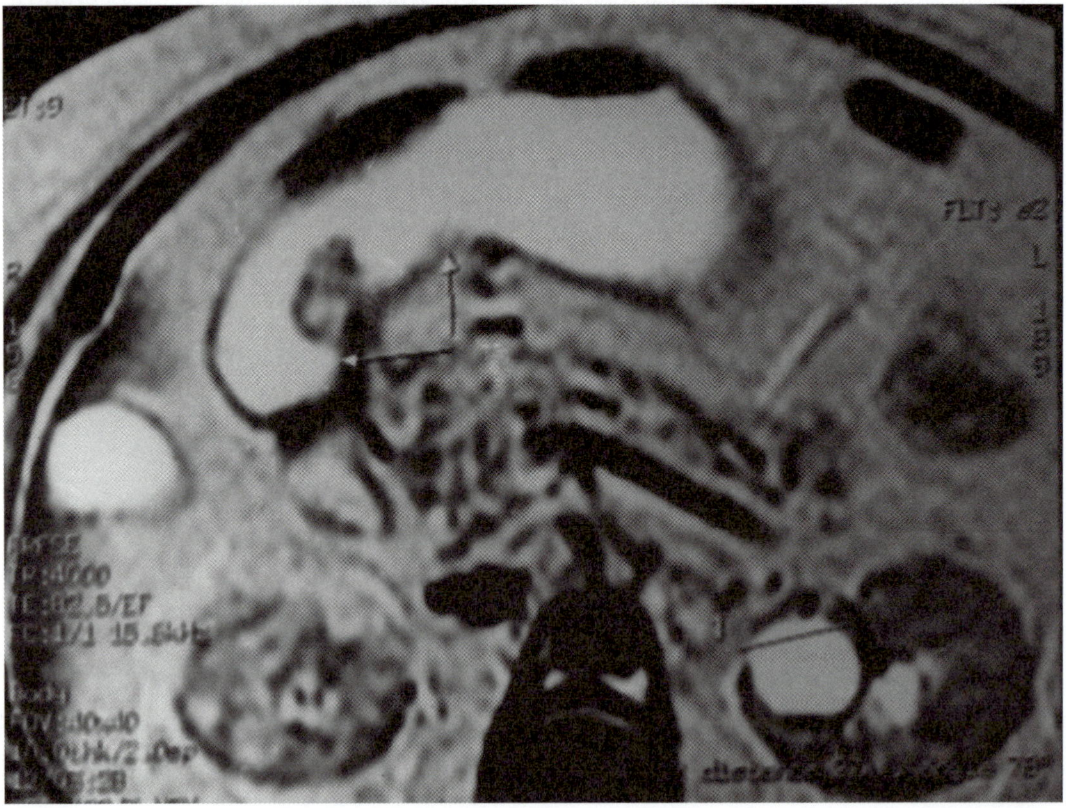

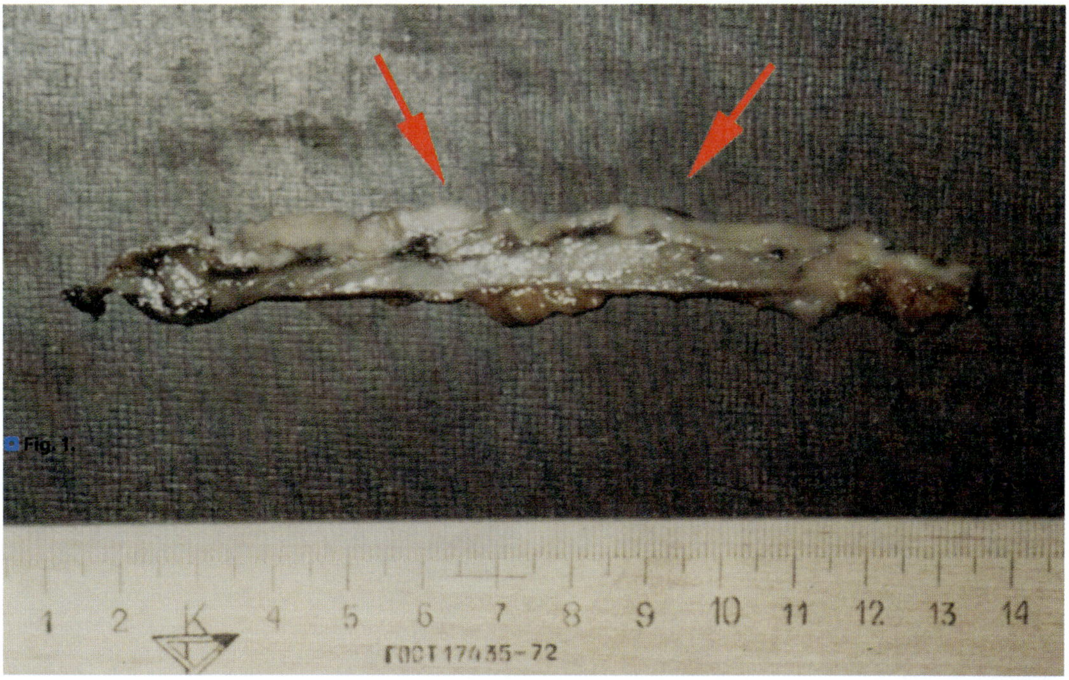

▲ **Fig. 41 b.**

▼ **Fig. 42 a.**

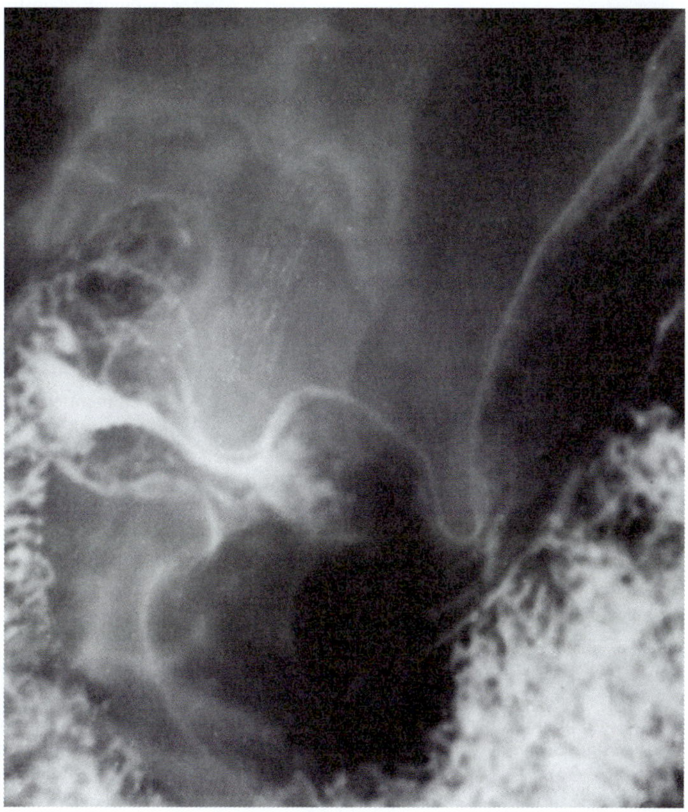

Fig. 41a, b. The same patient 3 months later. **a** MRI of the stomach (axial projection, T2 image): superfluous growth (3.5 x 2 cm) originating from a broad base on the stomach wall and extending into the stomach lumen can be seen at the lesser curvature and the adjacent parts of the posterior wall. Uneven contours of the exophytic component with a slightly eccentrically located hyperintensive fragment corresponding to fluid in the crater of the ulcer. In addition, the posterior wall of the stomach is thickened at the base of the new growth in the proximal direction, over a length of 2 cm. The absence of a hypodense strip by the posterior contour of the new growth suggests involvement of gastric serosa (arrows). MRI confirmed sufficiently distinct symptoms of blastomatous infiltration of the stomach wall. It also revealed involvement of the serous membrane of the stomach. Endoscopy with taking of eight tissue specimens did not reveal tumor cells either, but only 1 month later a control study of a bioptate revealed single cells of signet-ring cell carcinoma. **b** Fragment of a macrospecimen (strip): the arrows indicate a white intramural infiltration extending over 2.5 cm

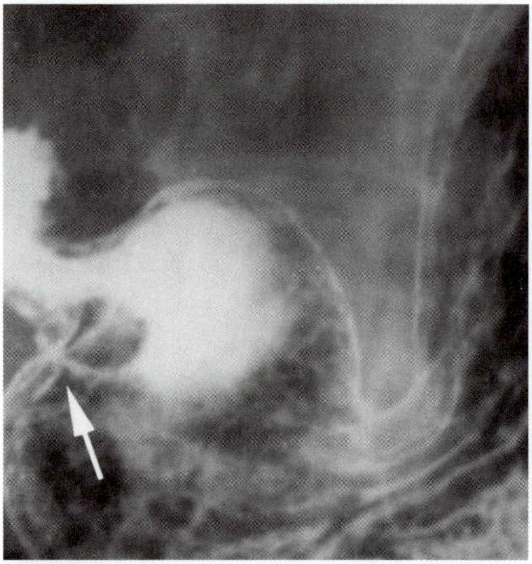

▲ **Fig. 42 b.**

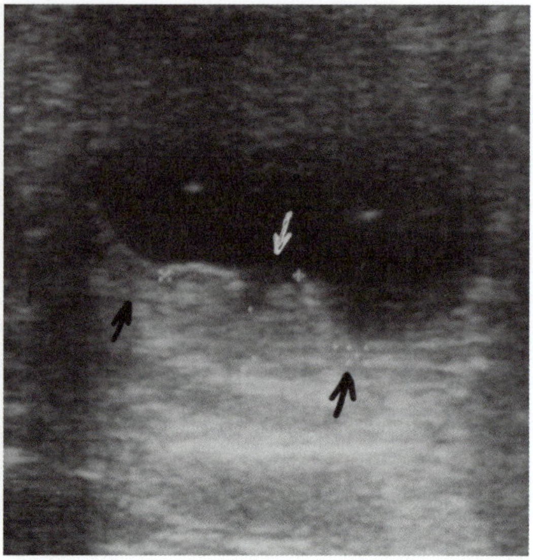

▲ **Fig. 42 d.**

▼ **Fig. 42 c.**

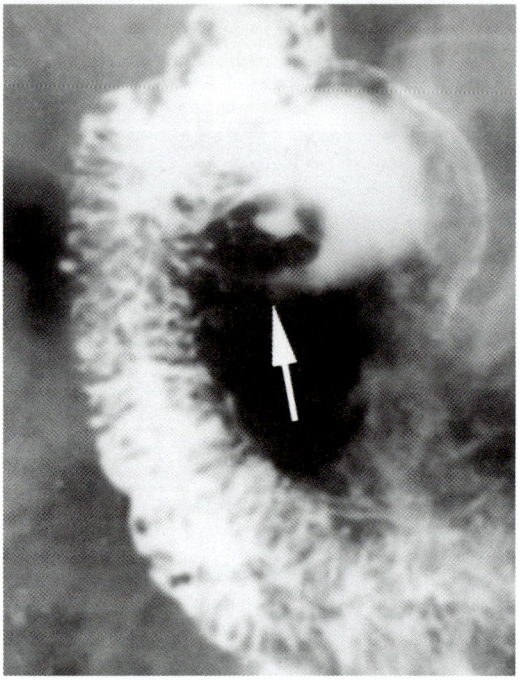

Fig. 42a–e. Female patient G., age 59. Diagnosis: gastric cancer. From anamnesis: patient complained of epigastric discomfort, regurgitation, persistent glossitis. Primary endoscopy revealed eroded mucosa on the posterior wall of the antral part of the stomach. Histological examination of tissue specimens revealed signs of chronic gastritis with sites of epithelialization and large number of helicobacteria. Tumor cells were not found. During subsequent 9 months the patient underwent repeated endoscopic examinations, the last of which revealed a saucer-like growth to 2 cm in diameter on the posterior wall of the antral part. Histological examination of numerous tissue specimens revealed signs of active inflammation with degenerative reconstruction and metaplasia of columnar epithelium. Three specimens had severe dysplasia of epithelium; no tumor cells were revealed. Progressive nature of the symptoms suggested compulsory X-ray examination, which was declined during the initial hospital stay and during subsequent months of observation and treatment. **a** Stomach X-ray (double contrast, horizontal position, right half-oblique projection): erosion of mucosal surface is seen in the antral part of the stomach; peristalsis is seen over the entire length. **b, c** Series of stomach X-rays (double contrast, horizontal position, anterior projection): during the absence of a peristaltic wave in the prepyloric part, a spider-like depot of contrast medium is seen in the antral part. Conclusion: Infiltrative-ulcerous cancer of the antral part of the stomach. In the absence of tumor cells in the examined tissue specimens, radiological examination of the stomach was recommended (ultrasonography, MRI). **d** Ultrasonography of the stomach according to the standard method (the stomach is tightly filled with water): the echogram shows thickening to 1 cm of the stomach wall for about 2 cm with destructive changes in its five-coat structure (black arrows) and with an ulcer to 5 cm (white arrow) in the center. **e** MR tomogram of the stomach (coronary projection, T2 image): a new growth of irregular shape, 18–20 mm on the posterior wall of the antral part; uneven contours; a depot of water is seen in the center which emits a specific hyperintensive MR signal (arrow). The wall is thickened over a length of 1 cm. Mucosal folds are thickened over their entire length. Unfortunately, X-ray, ultrasonography, and MRI did not produce convincing evidence of blastomatous affection of the stomach. Radical surgery was not performed in the absence of histological confirmation. The operation was declined

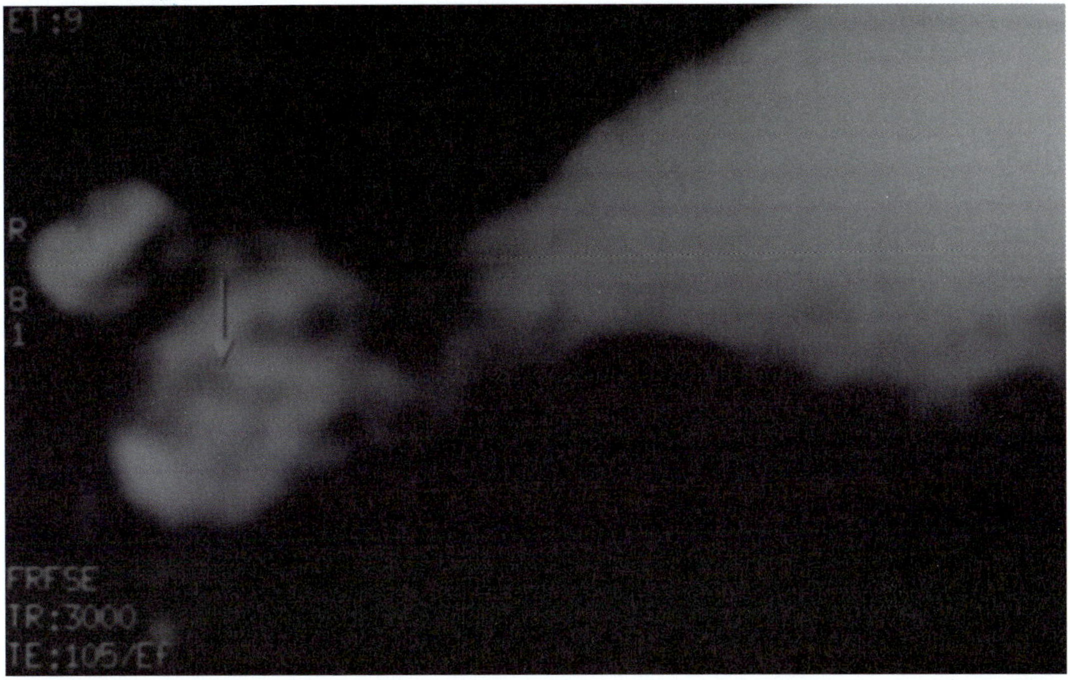

▲ **Fig. 42 e.**

sumed to be the basic tools. Unfortunately, the existing methodological and semiotic basis of endoscopy is the morphology of the intestinal forms of gastric cancer. Thus, it was only after a certain lapse of time that ultrasonography of the stomach departed from the signs characterizing the intestinal forms of gastric cancer. For many years, the main objectives of CT included estimation of expansion of the earlier diagnosed gastric cancer to the adjacent anatomical structures. Today, with the development of spiral CT, the emphasis is on gastric cancer staging. And again, this procedure relies mainly on endoscopic findings (◘ Figs. 42, 43).

We now have experience with MRI studies of the stomach. MRI is performed in patients with an empty stomach, in two stages, with no special preliminary preparation of the patient. The first stage includes the so-called native examination of the stomach, without distension, which displaces the stomach and changes relationships between the adjacent organs and structures. The patient is supine; the examined area extends from the dome of the diaphragm to the level of the kidneys. Section thickness is 9–12 mm, sections are spaced at 1–3 mm, with obligatory recording of T1 images, which more accurately correspond to the anatomical sections of the abdominal cavity. For special diagnostic indications, it is reasonable to acquire both T1- and T2-weighted images.

The following is assessed during examination of the stomach in the native state:

1. True anatomical and topographic relationships between adjacent organs and structures
2. The structure of parenchymatous organs (to rule out distant metastases, particularly into the liver)
3. Condition of regional and retroperitoneal lymph nodes, because their location can change during distension of the stomach cavity; this is especially important for perigastric and paravasal groups – N1 and N2 in accordance with the international TNM classification.

The second stage includes examination of the region extending from the upper border of the stomach fundus to the descending part of the duodenum with a filled stomach, which improves MR imaging. In its native state, stomach distension is uneven. In order to homogenize signal intensity inside the stomach

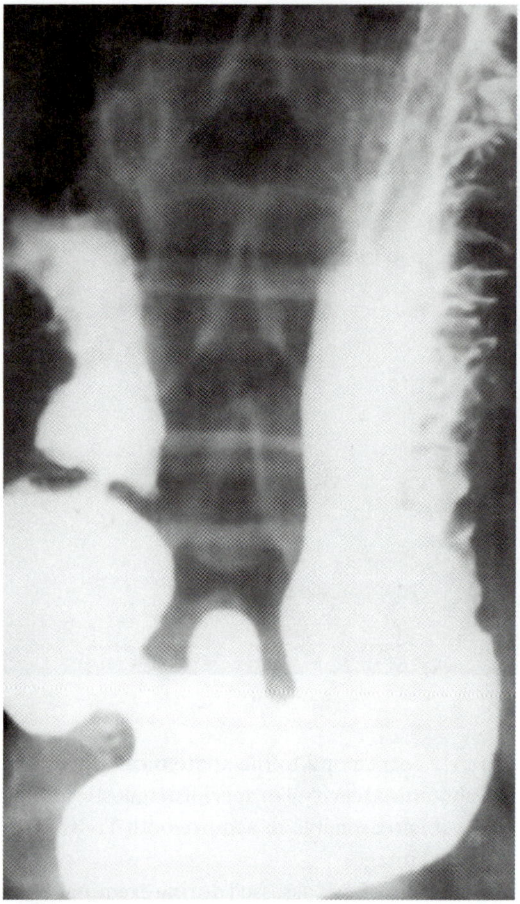

Fig. 43a–d. The same patient 2 months later. Patient's complaints persisted during subsequent 2 months. Control X-ray and endoscopic examinations were conducted. **a** Stomach roentgenogram (tight filling, vertical position, anterior projection): no organic changes can be seen. **b** Roentgenogram of the antral part of the stomach (double contrast, horizontal position, right quarter-oblique projection): growth as earlier, with same shapes but greater size, characterized by its specific atypical relief (spider type) is seen more distinctly. Control endoscopy and subsequent histological study of multiple tissue specimens failed to detect tumor cells. Based on radiological findings (traditional roentgenogram, ultrasonography, and MRI) and on the negative dynamics of the pathological process in conditions of anti-ulcer treatment, a decision was taken to operate on the patient despite the absence of tumor cells in numerous bioptates. **c** Macrospecimen: fragment of a resected part of the stomach: tumor infiltration of the wall in the antral part with ulceration (arrows) is determined. **d** Fragment of a macrospecimen (strip): the stomach wall is thickened due to white intramural infiltration (arrows). Histologically, a non-differentiated cancer

◄ **Fig. 43 a.**

▼ **Fig. 43 b.**

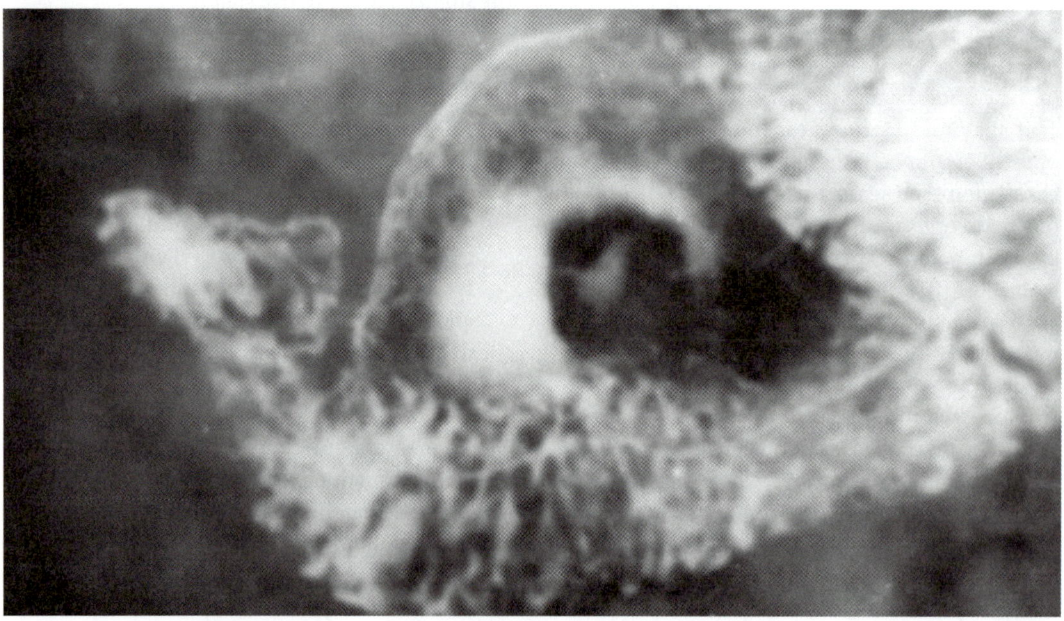

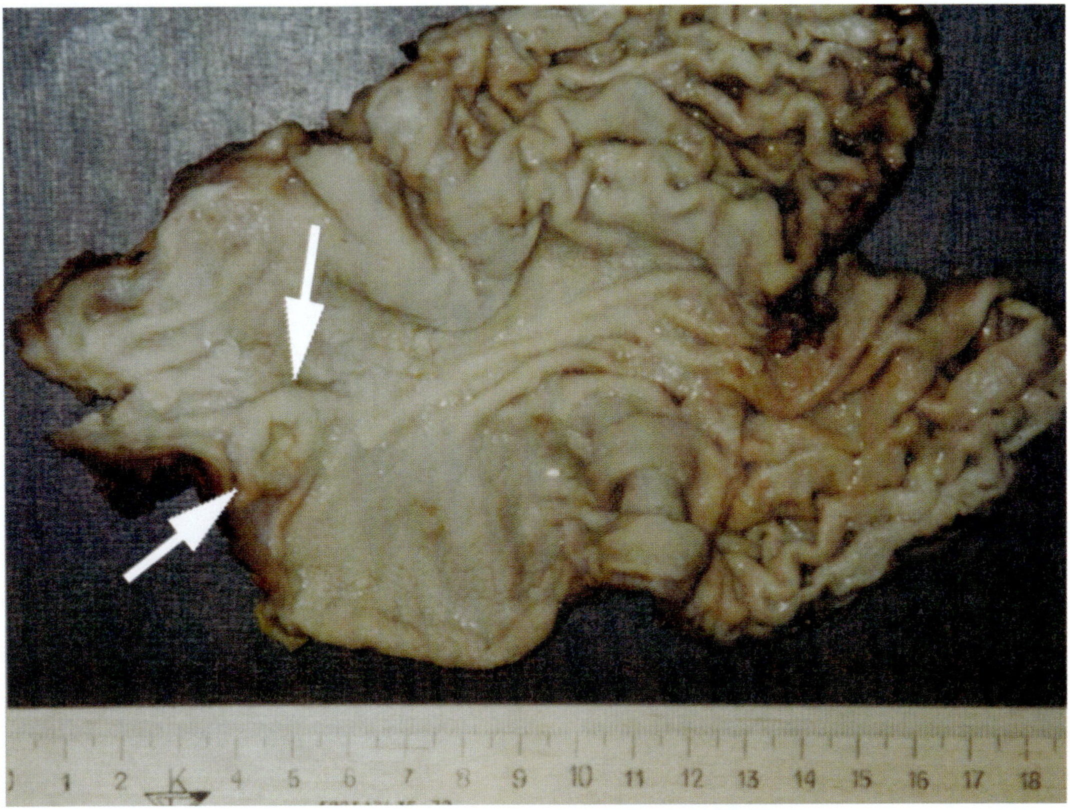

▲ **Fig. 43 c.**

▼ **Fig. 43 d.**

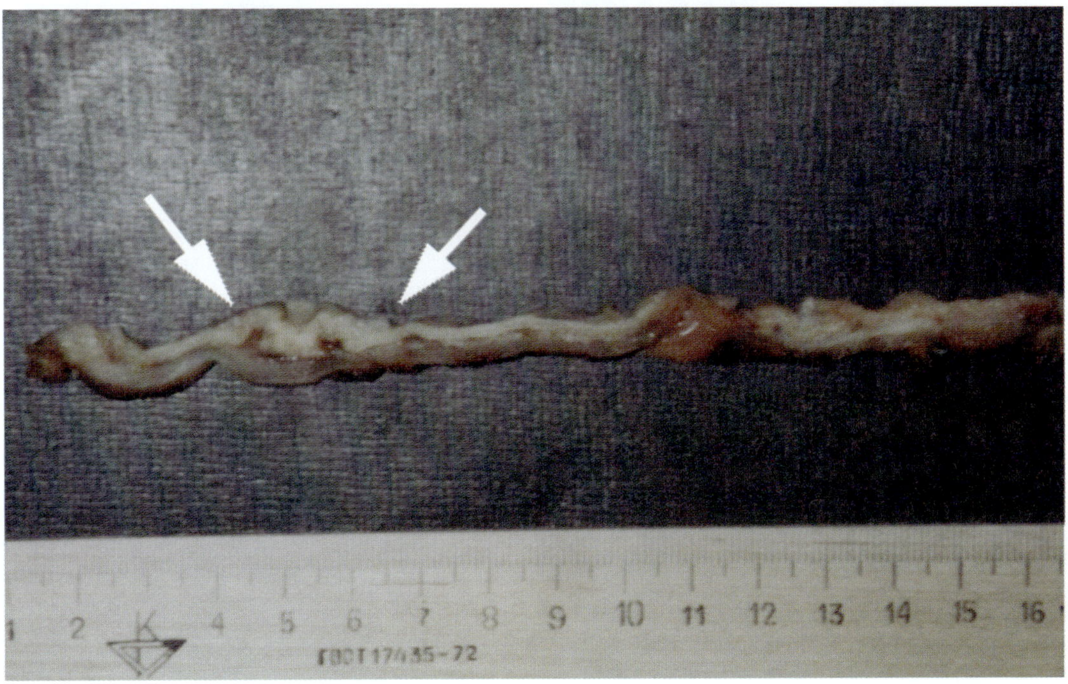

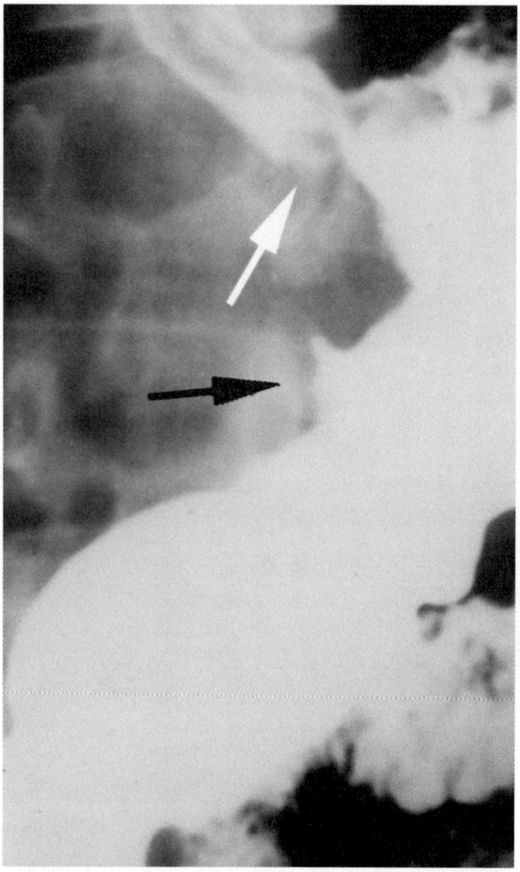

▲ Fig. 44 a.

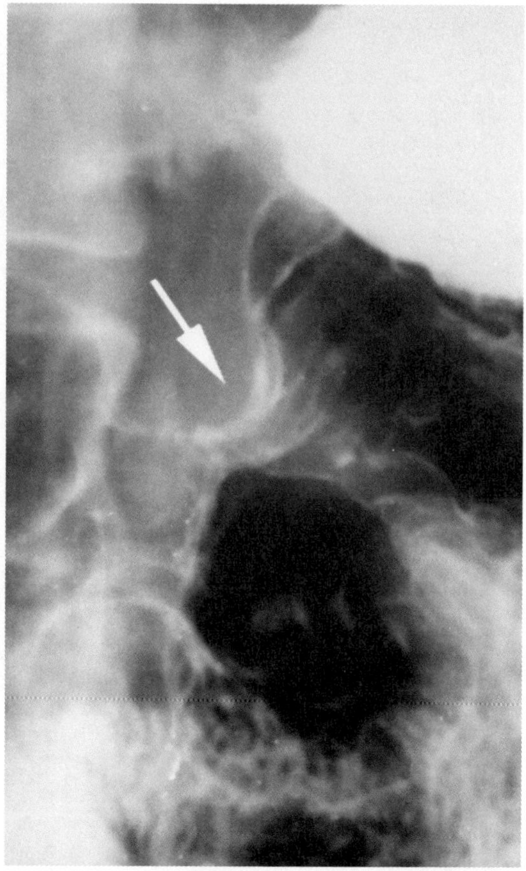

▲ Fig. 44 b.

▼ Fig. 44 c.

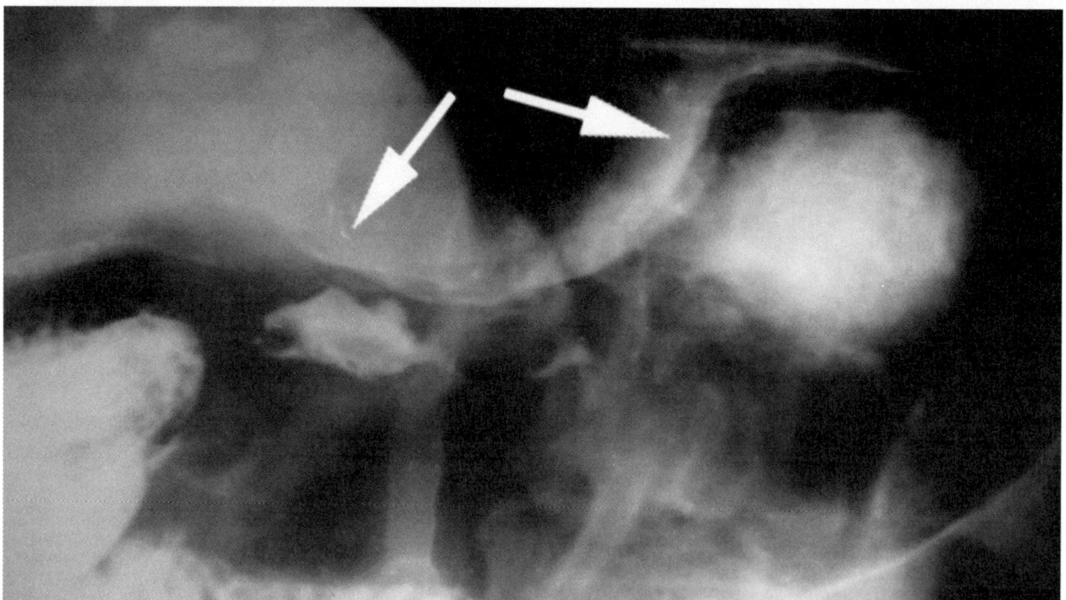

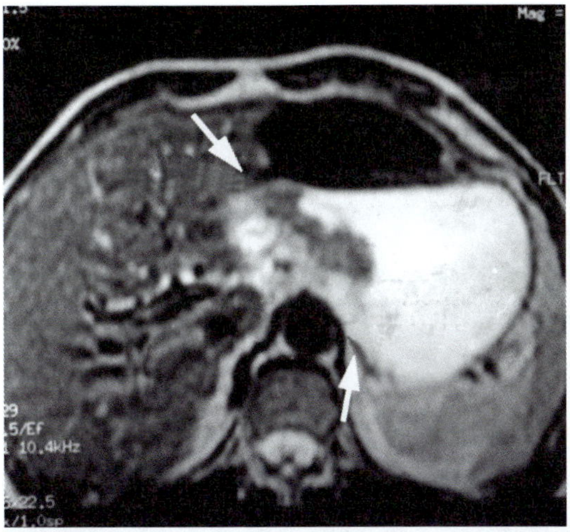

▲ **Fig. 44 d.**

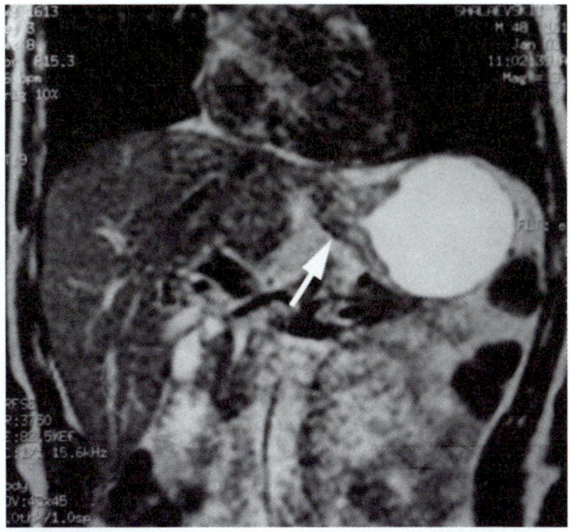

▲ **Fig. 44 f.**

▼ **Fig. 44 e.**

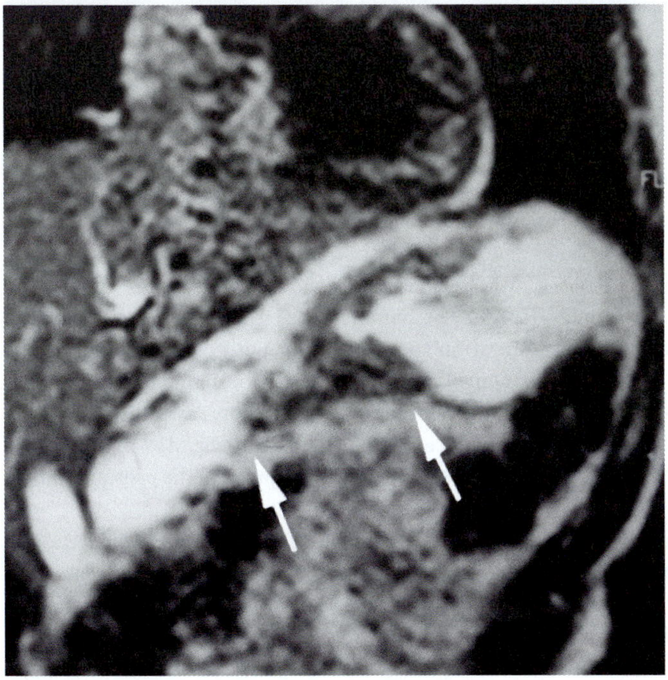

Fig. 44a–g. Patient D., age 67. Diagnosis: gastric cancer. **a** Stomach roentgenogram (tight filling, vertical position, anterior projection): uneven contour of the lesser curvature; an ulcer niche in the middle third (black arrow); disfigured and uneven contours of the abdominal segment of the esophagus (white arrow). **b** Stomach roentgenogram (double contrast, horizontal position, anterior projection): stomach body wall is thickened due to intramural infiltration (arrow). **c** Stomach roentgenogram (double contrast, horizontal position, left oblique projection): the anterior wall closer to the lesser curvature is thickened and rigid due to intramural infiltration spreading onto the upper part (arrows). Conclusion: Infiltrative-ulcerous cancer spreading to the abdominal segment of the esophagus. To verify spread of tumor infiltration to the neighboring anatomical structures, the patient underwent MRI examination. **d** MRI of the stomach (axial protection, T2 image): markedly thickened lesser curvature at the level of the upper part of the stomach extending to the anterior and posterior walls with heterogeneously reflected MR signal, ulcer crater, and overhanging edges of the infiltration ridge (arrows). **e** MR tomogram of the stomach (coronary projection, T2 image): tumor infiltration of the antral part wall (arrows); the pyloric part of the stomach is not changed. The inner contours of the stomach wall are uneven due to the presence of the ulcer (to 20 mm) located in the infiltrated wall of the stomach. Smaller foci emitting the hyperintensive MR signal are seen in the depth of the tumor infiltration. The outer contours of the stomach in its upper half are uneven and indistinct. Infiltration spreads to the region of the lesser omentum, the diaphragm (the region of the esophageal opening), the pancreas body, and the gastrocolic ligament. **f** MRI of the stomach (coronary projection, T1 image): thickened walls of the upper part with spread of intramural infiltration to the gastroesophageal junction zone. MR signal from the altered wall is of moderate intensity, heterogeneous due to the small hyperintensive foci (arrow). Conclusion: Infiltrative-ulcerous cancer with propagation onto the abdominal segment of the esophagus, the lesser omentum region, the diaphragm (the zone of the esophageal opening), the pancreas body, and the gastrocolic ligament. **g** Fragment of a macrospecimen (strip): stomach wall is thickened due to white tumor infiltration growing through all its layers (arrows)

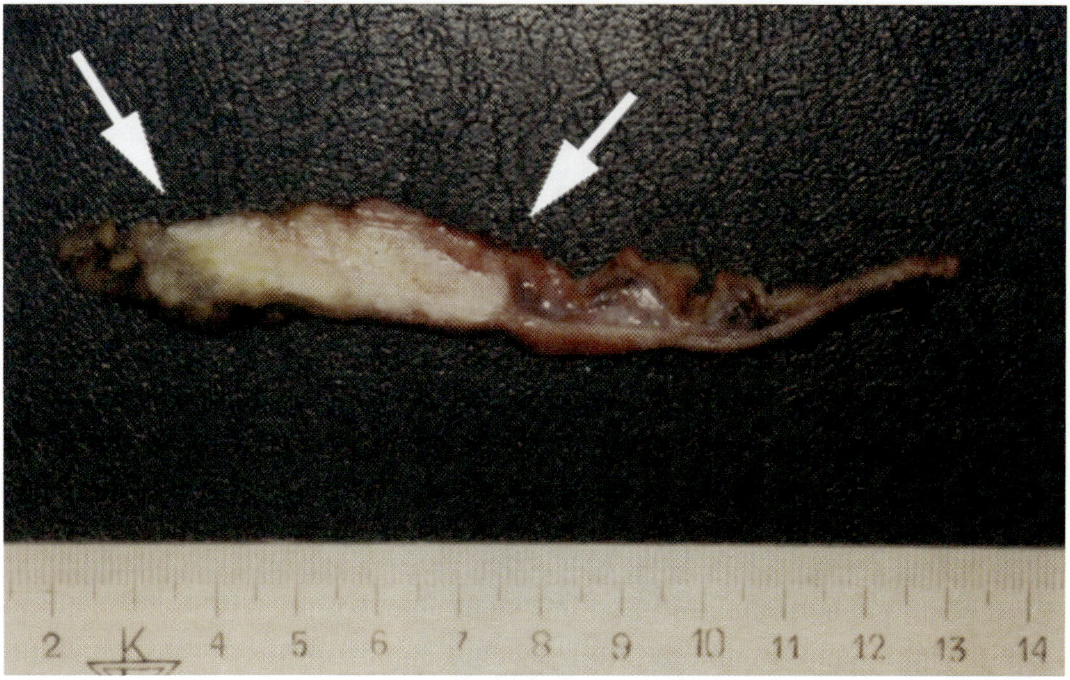

▲ Fig. 44 g.

lumen and also to distend its cavity, it is necessary that the patient ingest contrast medium. Many contrast media are now available. The choice depends on indications and the possible sequence of imaging. In cases with revealed or suspected spread of infiltration to the esophagus and adjacent organs and structures, the zone of examination is expanded (Fig. 44).

In order to rule out false results, MRI should be conducted at least 1 day (or two) after the X-ray examination, because the presence of minute traces of barium suspension in the stomach alters the signal (makes it less intensive) in spin echo pulse sequences, which may be mistaken for wall thickening. It must be noted here that the presence of barium sulphate in the intestinal loops does not cause artifacts (as is the case with computed tomography) and cannot be regarded as an absolute contraindication to MRI of the stomach on the day of X-ray examination in cases where this is necessary for diagnostic indications.

The intensity of signals received from various tissues during MRI depends on factors such as proton rotation speed, time constants of longitudinal (T1) and transverse (T2) relaxation, resonance signal frequencies characteristic of each particular tissue, chemical changes, magnetic sensitivity, associated current, perfusion, and other molecular processes. Signal intensity increases with the proton rotation speed or T2, or with decreasing T1; signal intensity decreases with proton movement speed or T2, or with increasing T1. Contrast substances thus influence signal intensity during MRI in the following three ways, viz., by changing the proton rotation speed, and also T1 or T2.

Water, the cheapest substance, increases the signal in T2 images homogeneously. Signal intensity in T1 images is intermediate. In order to distend the stomach adequately (depending on its size according to the findings of the traditional X-ray examination), the patient has to drink 500–800 ml of water in the horizontal position with his head tilted slightly upwards. It should be remembered that the rate of stomach evacuation slows down in a supine patient.

Air is a negative contrast medium immiscible with other substances. Air can be blown into the stomach through a thin elastic gastric tube or using special granulated powders. However, air intensifies peristalsis of the stomach and can therefore produce significant artifacts. When air is used as the contrast

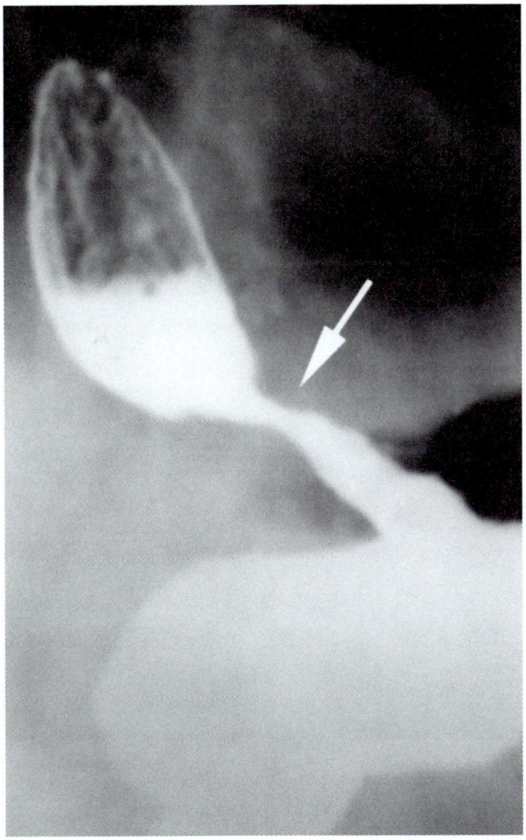

▲ **Fig. 45 a.**

Fig. 45a–d. Patient T., age 62. Diagnosis: gastric cancer. Anamnesis: The patient had complained of difficult swallowing for 3 months. Endoscopy revealed an infiltrative tumor in the abdominal segment of the esophagus, which significantly narrowed its lumen. It was impossible to examine the stomach because of the marked narrowing. In order to establish the initial location of the process, X-ray examination was recommended. **a** Stomach roentgenogram (tight filling, vertical position, anterior projection) at the moment of contrast medium passage through the gastroesophageal junction: marked narrowing of the abdominal segment of the esophagus due to circular infiltration (arrow). **b** Stomach roentgenogram (double contrast, horizontal position, left lateral projection): the anterior wall of the upper part of the stomach is thick, rigid; the relief of the cardiac rosette (cardioesophageal junction) is leveled, its specific radial pattern is absent (arrows). Conclusion: Infiltrative cancer of the upper part of the stomach with expansion to the esophagus. To verify the spread of the process, MRI was indicated. **c** MRI of the stomach (coronary projection, at level of upper part of the stomach, T2 image): uneven thickening of the fundus walls (black arrow) due to intramural infiltration with transition to the abdominal segment of the esophagus. The involved walls of the esophagus are markedly thickened due to circular infiltration (white arrow). **d** MRI of the stomach (sagittal projection, level of the upper part of the stomach and its body, T2 image): intramural infiltration of the anterior wall of the stomach body (arrows) with heterogeneous MR signal. In this particular case, diagnostic information was obtained only by radiological methods of examination in view of the objective infeasibility of adequate endoscopy with sampling of the necessary amount of material. MRI helped to detect the primary location of the tumor in the stomach and its spread to the esophagus

▼ **Fig. 45 b.**

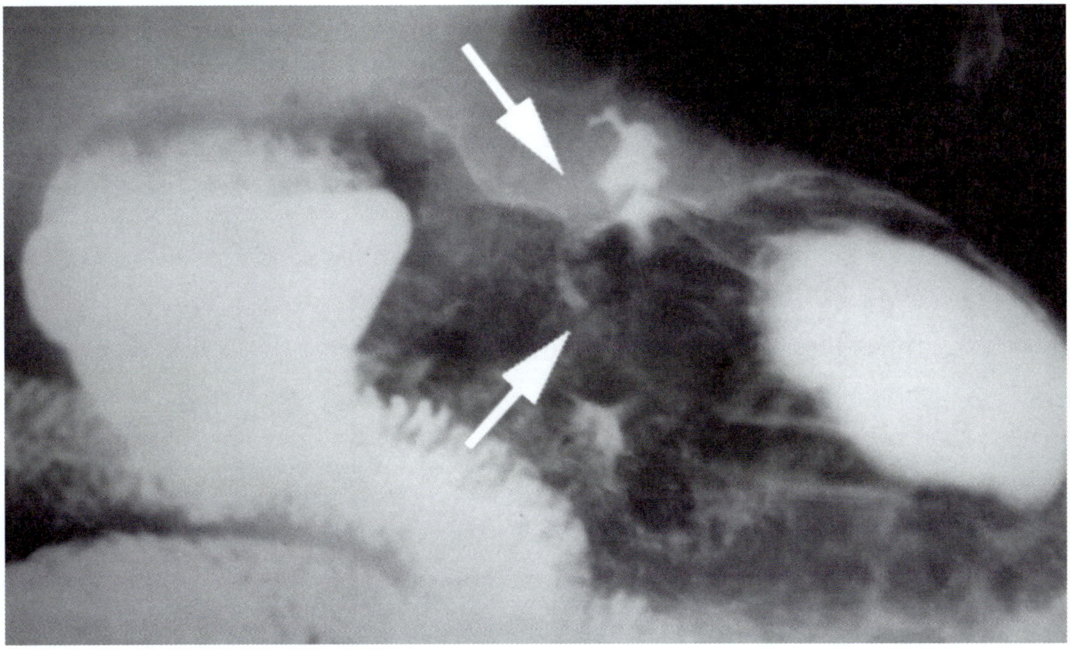

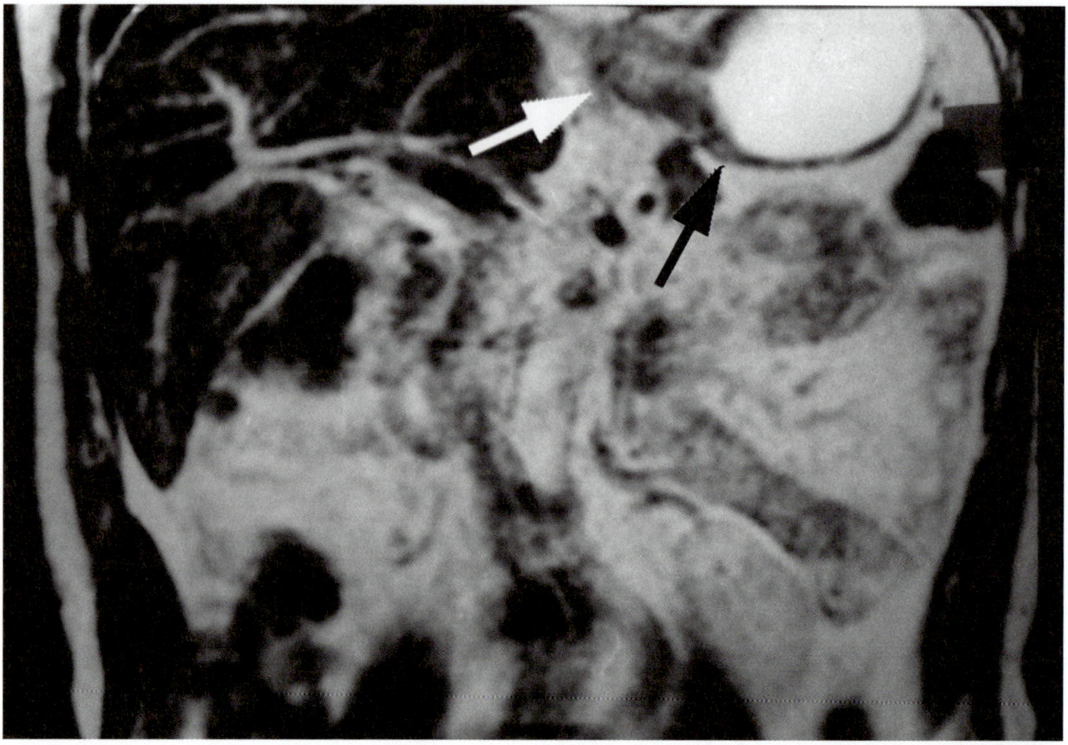

▲ Fig. 45 c.

▼ Fig. 45 d.

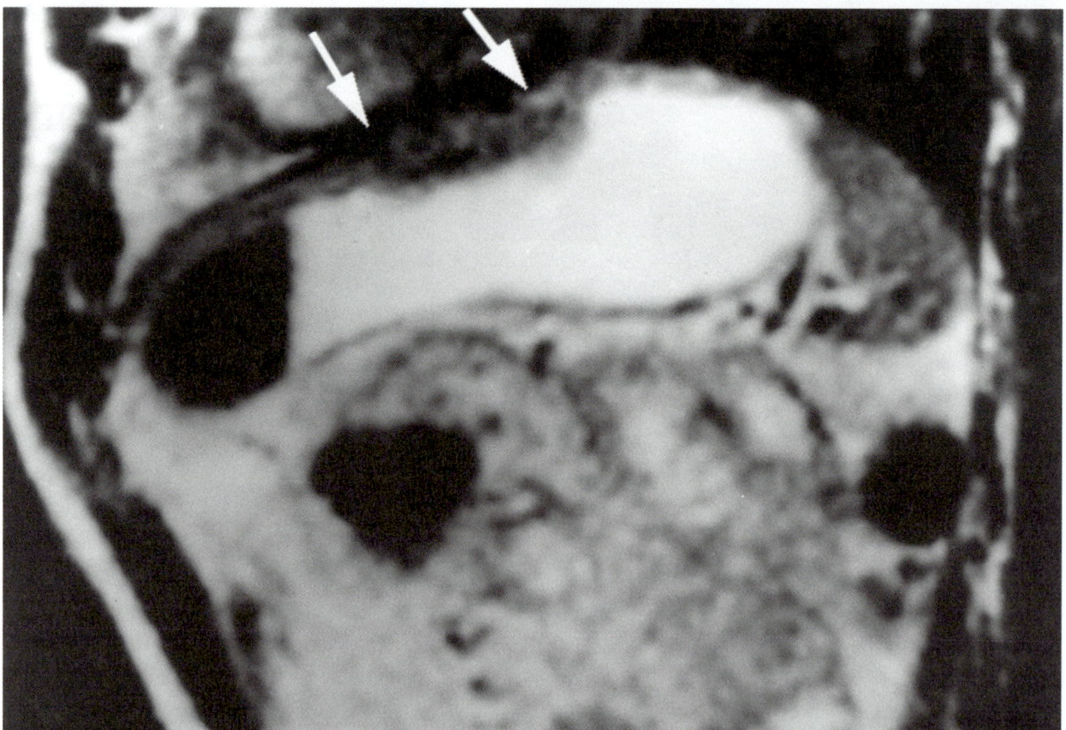

medium, it is necessary to medicate the patient in order to decrease peristalsis. Thus, the clinical use of air as a contrast medium in MRI is limited.

Solutions of contrast substances (1 ml/100 ml water) used in MRI are suitable for drinking because they are stable in the highly acid stomach conditions. Omniscan and Magnevist are not absorbed in the stomach walls, nor do they have any appreciable effect on peristalsis.

The second stage should be started with axial projection in conditions of T1 and T2 (the standard study protocol). For evaluation of the upper part of the stomach, the examination is supplemented with the coronary projection, and in order to estimate changes in the posterior and anterior walls in more detail, the study also includes an additional projection in the sagittal plane using the program with a delay, synchronization of respiration, and high-speed programs. For better visualization of the pyloric part, the sagittal projection with the patient in supine position is best; also good is positioning on the right side with an axial scanning plane, usually with administration of an additional portion of water for better filling of this part of the stomach. The section thickness and section spacing are selected in each individual case depending on the size and volume of the tumor (▣ Fig. 45) [69, 216].

Radiological diagnosis has been enriched with many new techniques which have significantly strengthened the potential of diagnosing gastric cancer. Ultrasonography, CT, and MRI are among these. Traditional X-ray methods also have high diagnostic potential owing to technical developments in digital X-ray technology. They should be returned to their rightful role in gastroenterology and, together with endoscopy, become the basic method of diagnosing gastric cancer.

In view of the changed accents in morphogenesis of gastric cancer and also in the location of primary cancer in various parts of the stomach, and above all, in view of an increased incidence of proximal cancer, new technologies – ultrasonography, CT, and MRI – must be actively employed as additional methods in verifying the diagnosis of gastric cancer. Each of these methods has its own advantages, which can help to clarify many cases.

While new technologies inevitably raise the problem of additional expenses, we and our colleagues have actively used new technologies in the radiological diagnosis of gastric cancer, and our experience shows that diagnostic problems can be solved by simple technologies at reasonable expenses.

Radiological Signs of Gastric Cancer

(jointly with O.V. Vyatchanin and G.A. Stashuk)

Introduction

In this chapter we describe in detail the corrections that we feel are necessary in the current semiotic principles of traditional gastroenterology for gastric cancer. Traditional X-ray methods are still the main tools of gastric cancer diagnosis. We will compare ultrasonography, computed tomography, and magnetic resonance imaging with X-ray technologies in the visualization of gastric cancer.

First of all, it is necessary to assess current views regarding so-called early gastric cancer. All current interpretations of the early gastric cancer concept, particularly the one based on the endoscopic classification of 1962, require verification. Nothing definitive can be said about early gastric cancer using radiological diagnosis alone. Likewise, this question cannot be answered using endoscopy. It becomes feasible only with microscopic examination of a resected stomach (Fig. 46) [64].

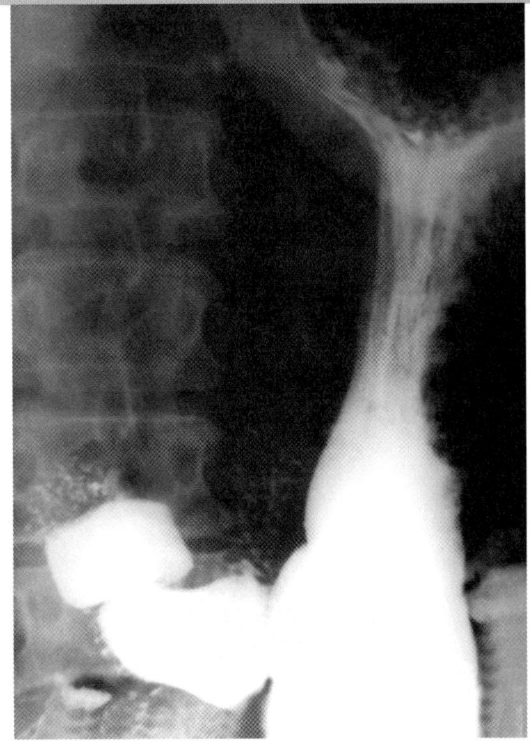

Fig. 46 a.

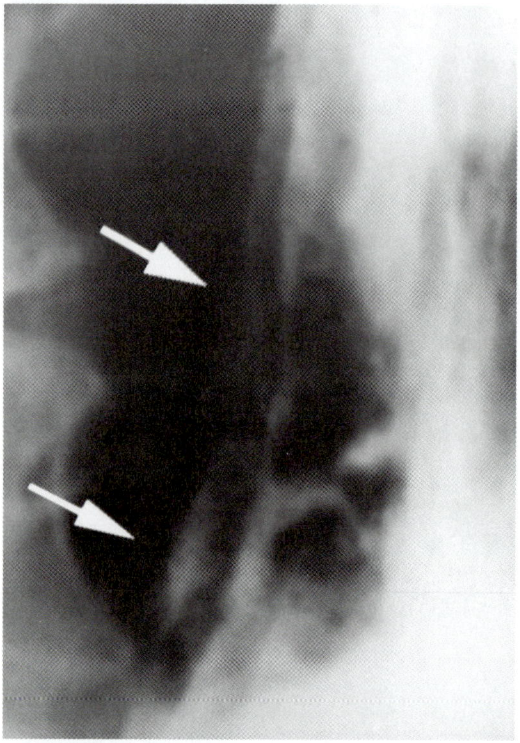

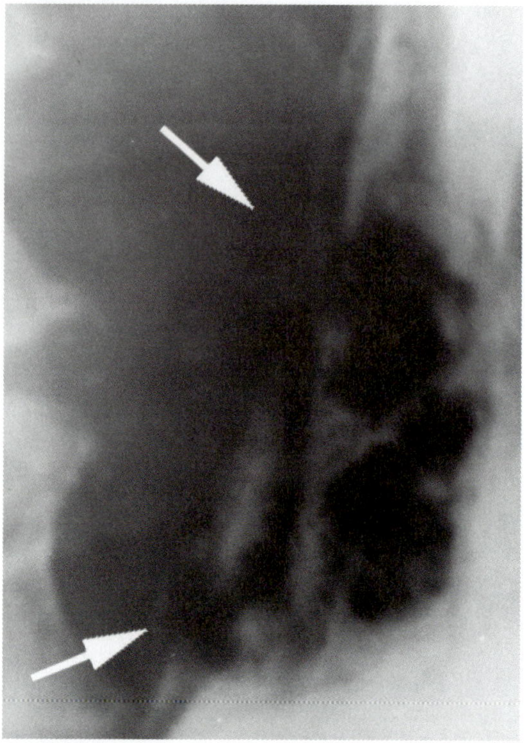

▲ Fig. 46 b. ▼ Fig. 46 d. ▲ Fig. 46 c.

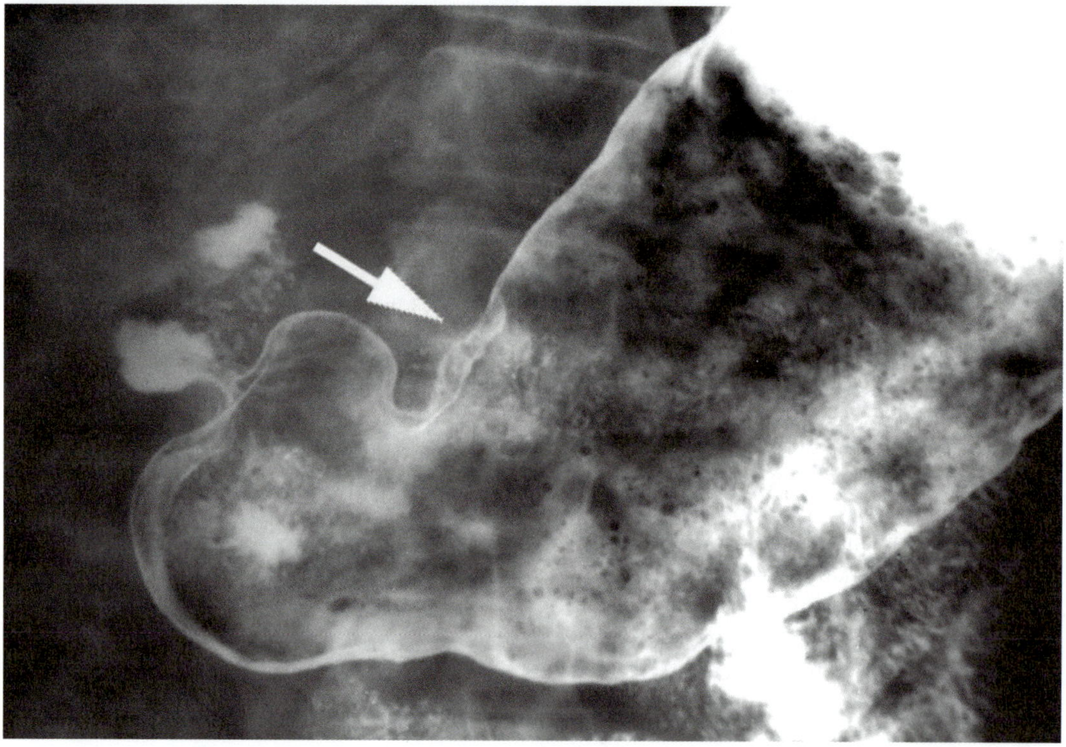

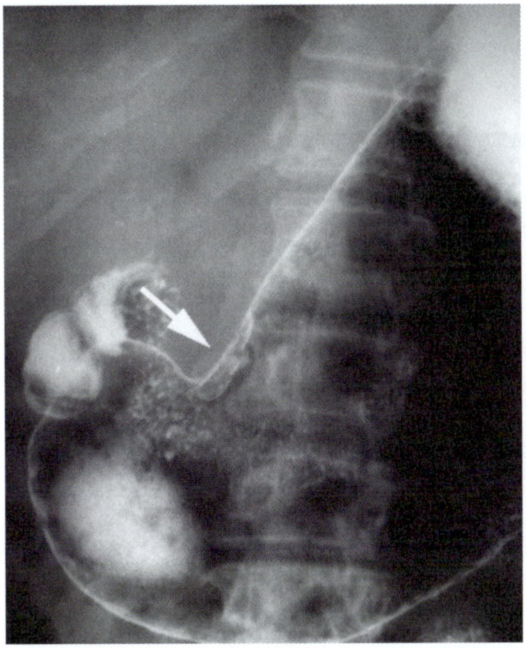

▲ **Fig. 46 e.**

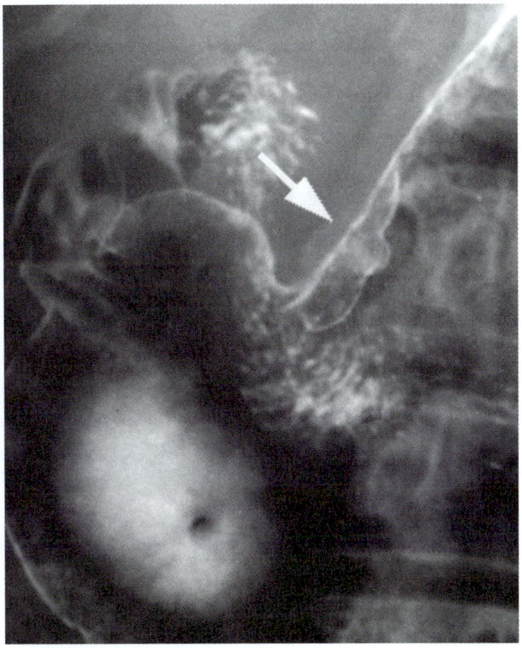

▲ **Fig. 46 f.**

▼ **Fig. 46 g.**

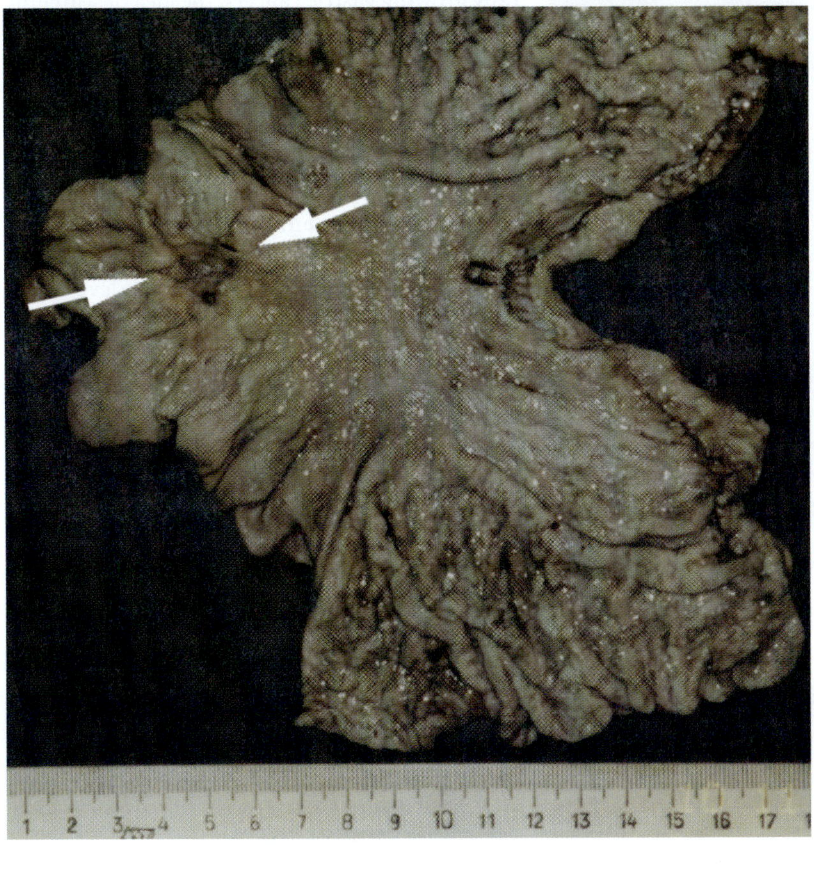

Fig. 46a–h. Patient S., age 55. Diagnosis: gastric cancer. **a** Stomach roentgenogram (tight filling, vertical position, anterior projection): the distal part is tightly filled with barium sulfate suspension; uneven contours, no visible organic changes, distinct peristalsis over the entire length. **b, c** Stomach roentgenograms (tight filling, vertical position, anterior projection), dosed compression: uneven and eroded contour of the lesser curvature of the lower third of the stomach body; flat ulcer niche not extending beyond the contour, with folds terminating at the periphery (arrows). **d, e, f** Stomach roentgenograms (double contrast, horizontal position, anterior projection): thickened stomach wall on the lesser curvature of the lower third of the stomach body, near the angular notch, due to intramural infiltration (arrow).

Conclusion: Minor infiltrative cancer of the lower third of the stomach body. **g** Macrospecimen of a resected stomach; the lesser curvature of the lower third of the stomach is firm; ulceration with atypical surrounding relief (arrows). **h** Fragment of the macrospecimen (strip): the stomach wall is thickened due to white intramural infiltration within the confinements of the mucous and submucous coats (white arrows); invasion of the muscular coat is not detectable visually (black arrows). Histologically, signet-ring cell carcinoma

▼ **Fig. 46 h.**

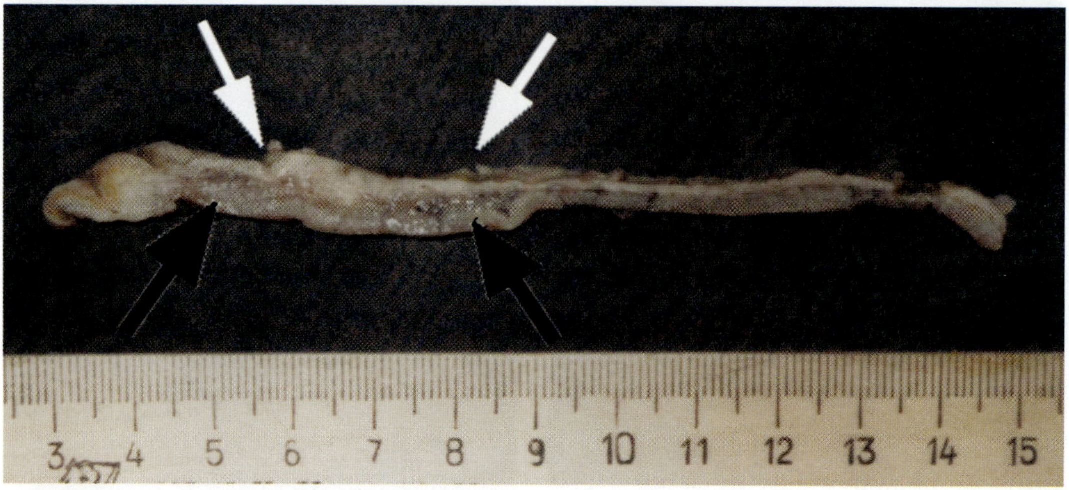

▼ **Fig. 47 a.**

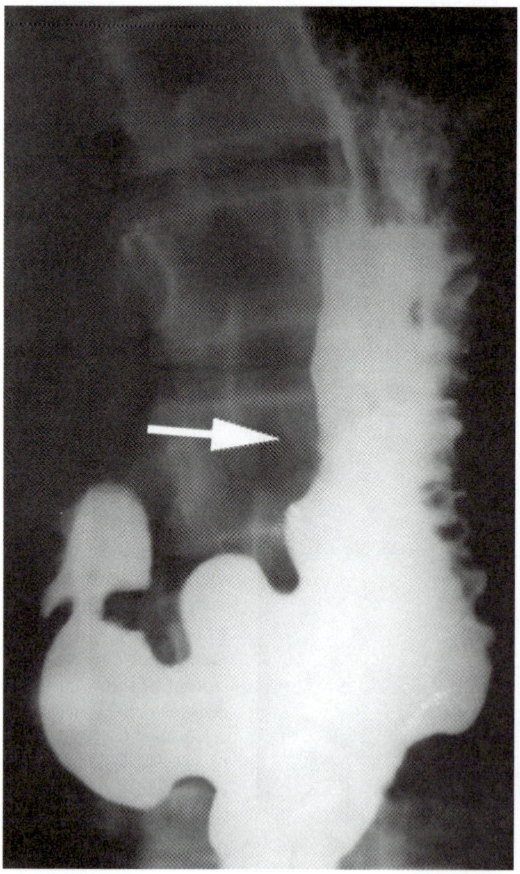

In consideration of the great prevalence of intramurally growing gastric cancers, the idea of searching for early cancer as it is classically understood – according to the endoscopic classification of 1962, as affection of the mucous membrane alone – is no longer valid and also requires correction (◘ Figs. 47, 48). We propose a definite symptom complex of early gastric cancer characterized by infiltrative growth, which we call intramural blastomatous infiltration. Its basic sign is uneven contours of the stomach over 1–3 cm with thickening of its wall at this level due to tumor infiltration (◘ Fig. 49) [31].

We will also discuss the need to radically revise the existing list of radiological signs of gastric cancer and clinical symptoms.

◘ **Fig. 47a, b.** Patient N., age 60. Diagnosis: gastric cancer. The patient had no complaints. Two relatives had had gastric cancer. Endoscopy revealed ulcer on the posterior wall of the stomach. Histological examination failed to detect tumor cells. **a** Stomach roentgenogram (tight filling, vertical position, anterior projection): uneven contour of the lesser curvature (depression); the wall is rigid (arrow). **b** Stomach roentgenogram (double contrast, horizontal position, left anterior oblique projection): the wall of the lesser curvature is thick and rigid due to intramural infiltration (white arrow); a depot of contrast medium on the posterior wall of the stomach body with converging folds (black arrow). Conclusion: Infiltrative-ulcerous cancer of the stomach body. Repeat endoscopy was conducted and many tissue specimens were taken. Histological studies verified non-differentiated cancer in two specimens.

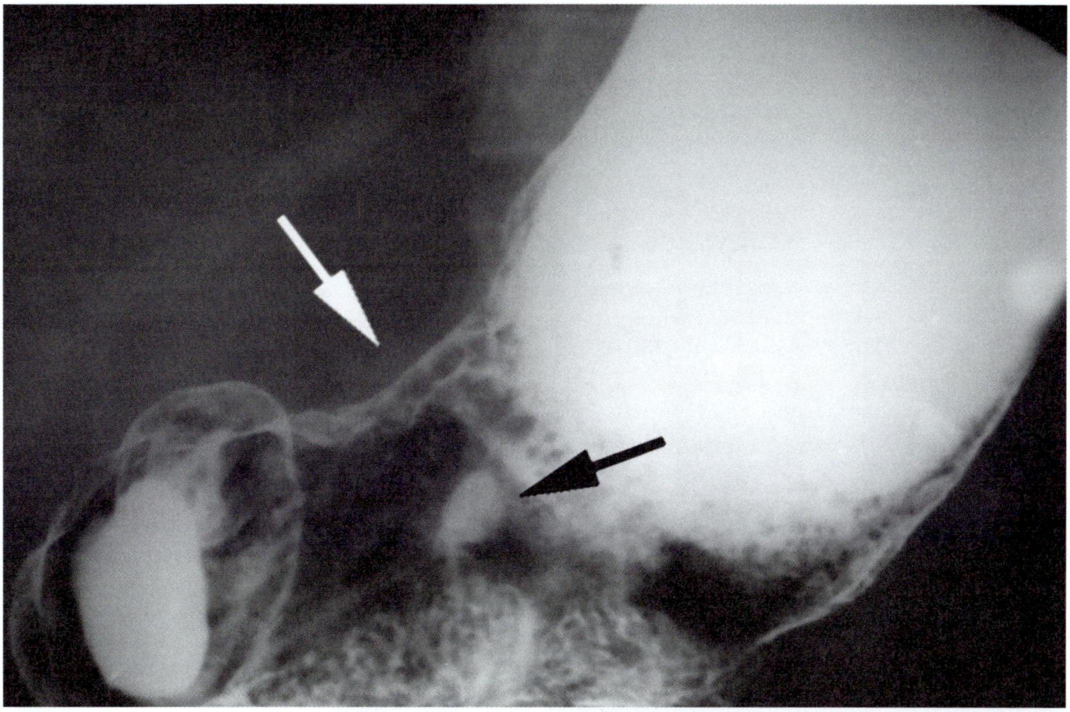

▲ **Fig. 47 b.**

► **Fig. 48.**

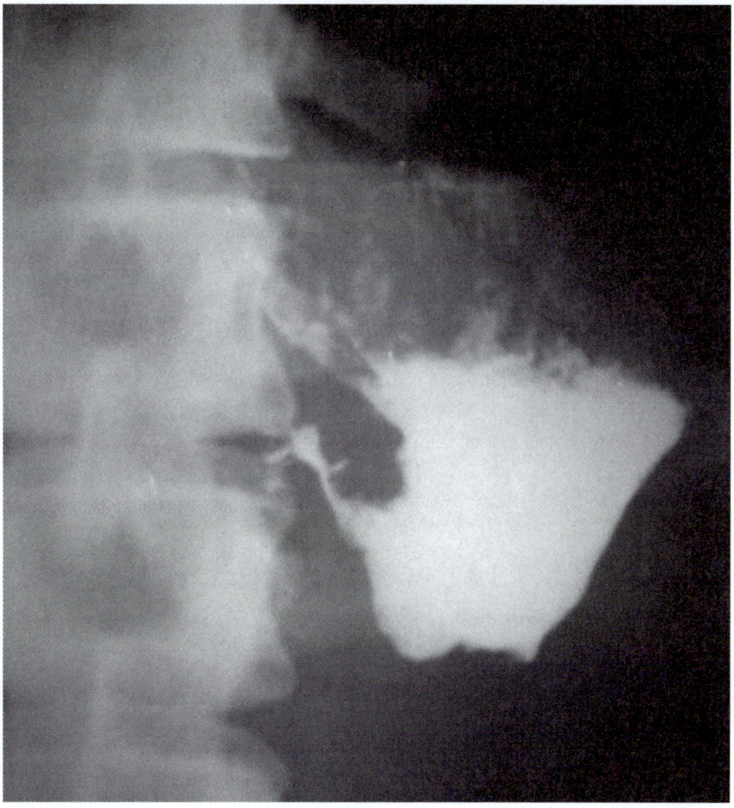

Fig. 48. The same patient, 6 months following stomach resection. X-ray of the stomach stump (tight filling, vertical position, anterior projection): the stump of irregular tapered shapes contains much fluid; evacuation is difficult due to pronounced narrowing of the gastrojejunal anastomosis affected by recurrent tumor as a result of intraoperative underestimation of the extent of intramural growth of the tumor discovered by radiological examination.

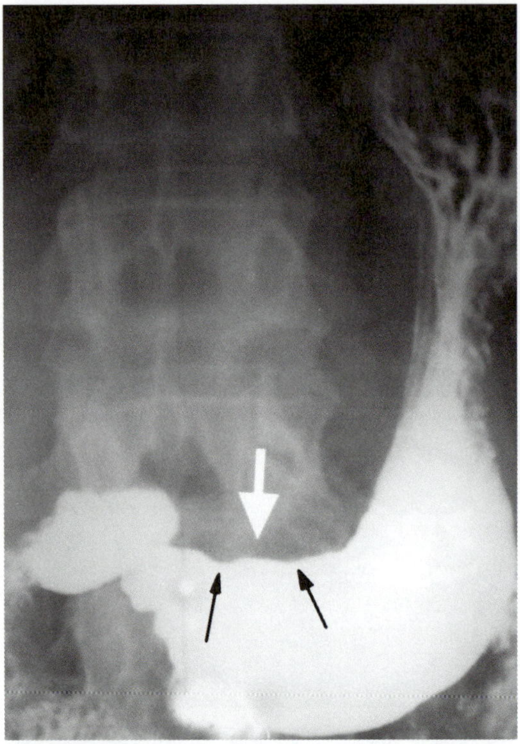

▲ Fig. 49 a.

▼ Fig. 49 b.

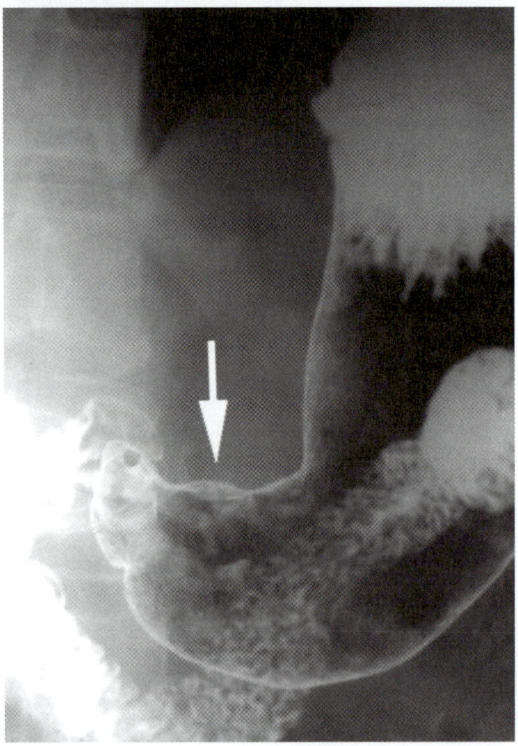

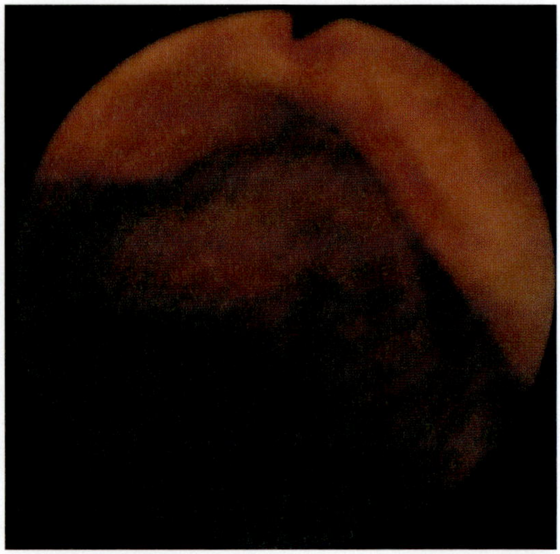

▲ Fig. 49 c.

Fig. 49a–c. Patient S., age 52. Diagnosis: gastric cancer. **a** Stomach roentgenogram (tight filling, vertical position, anterior projection): the lesser curvature of the antral part of the stomach is short, its contour is uneven due to the presence of a flat ulcer niche (white arrow) and the ridge of infiltration (black arrows). **b** Stomach roentgenogram (double contrast, horizontal position, left oblique projection): the wall of the lesser curvature of the antral part is thickened due to intramural infiltration (arrow). Conclusion: Infiltrative-ulcerous cancer of the distal part of the stomach. **c** Endophotograph: ca. 1.5-cm ulcer on the lesser curvature with firm and rigid edges; the surrounding mucosa is hyperemic and infiltrated. Histological examinations of the tissue specimen verified non-differentiated cancer.

Traditional Radiological Signs

In order to enable the reader to objectively assess the need for changes in the currently used set of traditional radiological signs of gastric cancer, we wish to give a concise history of the problem. There are a lot of signs that we think are connected only with far-advanced symptoms of cancer: The so-called filling defect corresponds mainly to far-advanced symptoms of intestinal and mixed forms of cancer. It is a sign of exophytic growth which is seen against the background of an air bubble during X-ray examination and it is typical of cancer of the upper part of the stomach. Other signs are peristaltic activity of the stomach walls, indicating that there is no tumor infiltration of the stomach, and the so-called floating splinter on the stomach contour. Much later (in the 1960s) the sign of an uneven stomach contour was described, and this remains important today. Unfortunately, it is given the least consideration in the general symptom complex of gastric cancer.

Of special importance are the various manifestations of gastric mucosal relief, which are indispensable for the diagnosis of the initial signs of gastric cancer [144, 145]. This also concerns those signs which were proposed by Japanese radiologists for the study of the so-called fine relief with double contrast. Unfortunately, there are publications which propose examination of the so-called pleated relief and areolar pattern of the tunica mucosa. However, it is not necessary to study the relief of the stomach mucosa with double contrast to detect the so-called bald sites of microrelief, finest irregularities, depressions, and only slightly noticeable elevations. If the mucosa is well impregnated with highly concentrated barium sulfate suspension, the image of the relief on the opposite side will always blur the image obtained for study, no matter how distinct it is. Hence, the image will be inadequately interpreted. A very good method exists for studying the relief of the inner surface of the stomach. This is endoscopy. Moreover, endoscopy is also used to take tissue specimens for histological studies, which makes this method especially valuable in the diagnosis of tumors which manifest themselves on the mucous membrane. Study of the relief of the gastric mucosa may be useful only in an examination of the cardiac rosette (cardioesophageal junction), where the condition of the relief is of primary diagnostic importance owing to its anatomical properties, in particular, the absence of the submucous coat (■ Figs. 50, 51).

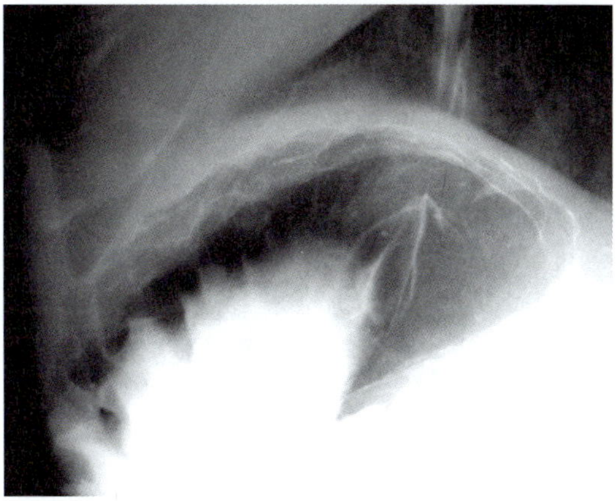

▲ **Fig. 50 a.**

■ **Fig. 50a–d.** Versions of normal structure of the cardiac rosette (cardioesophageal junction) relief. A series of X-rays of the upper part of the stomach (double contrast, horizontal position, left oblique projection): folds of the cardiac mucosa are continuation of the esophageal mucosal folds, symmetrically radiating from the medial wall of the upper part and uniformly unfolding as they reach the submucous coat (visually detectable asymmetry is due to projection distortions); very distinct impregnated interfold spaces.

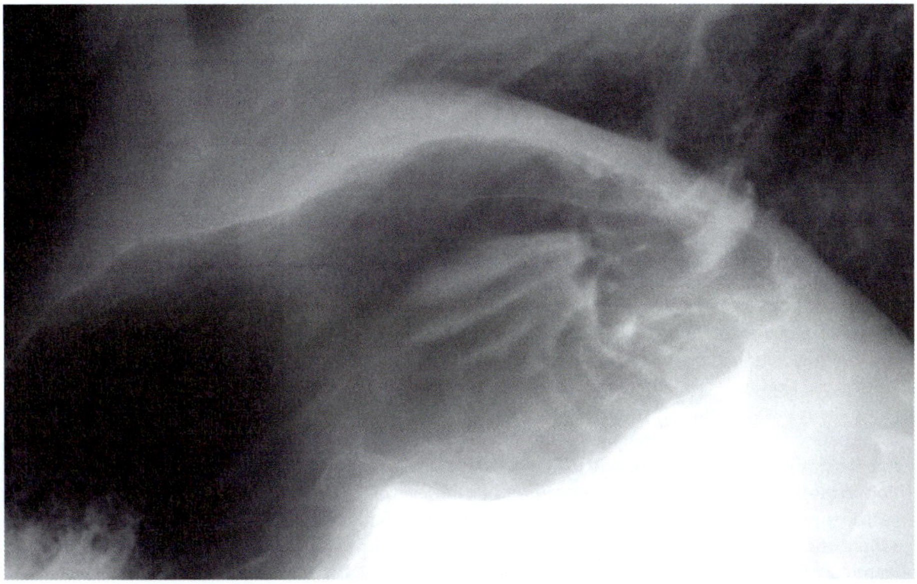

◀ **Fig. 50 b.**

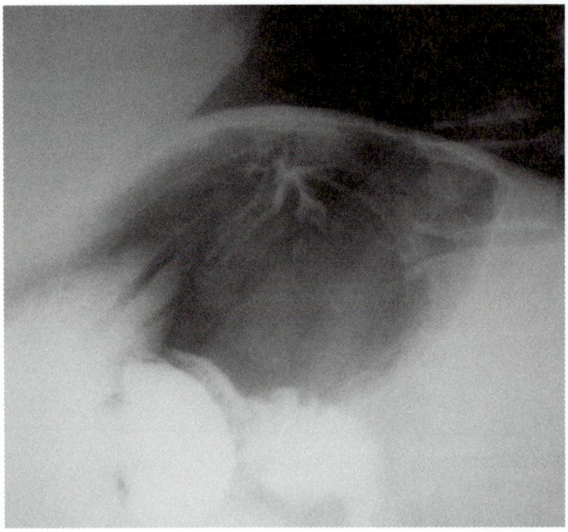

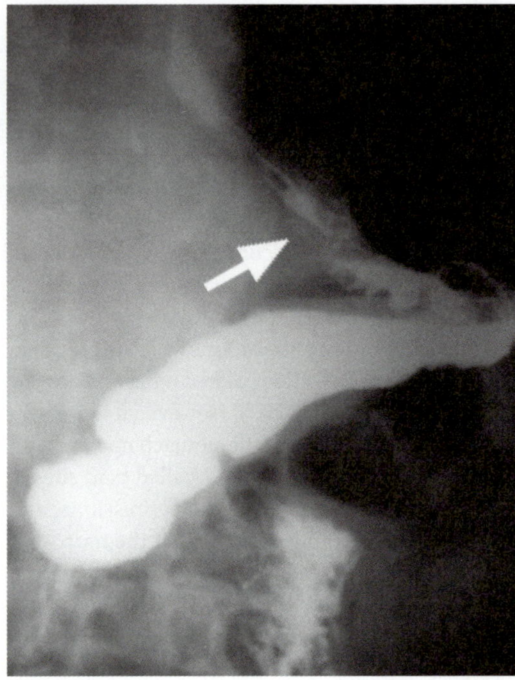

▲ Fig. 50 c. ▼ Fig. 50 d.

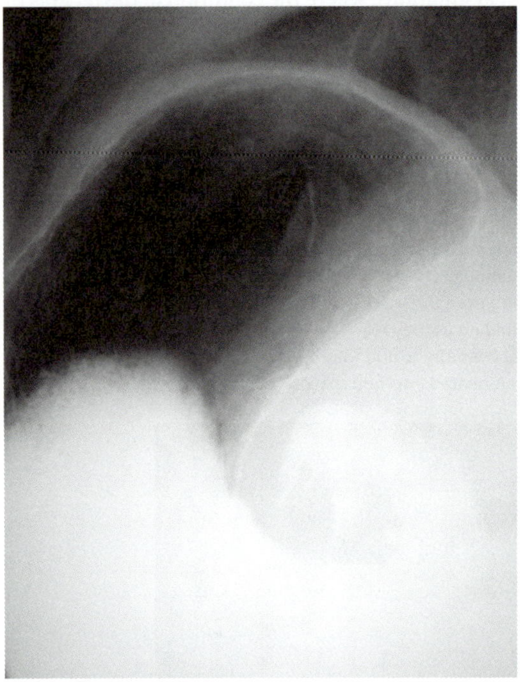

▲ Fig. 51 a. ▼ Fig. 51 b.

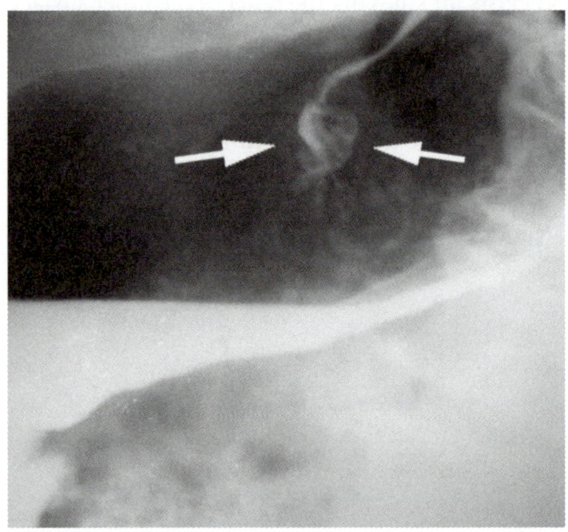

Fig. 51a–e. Female patient I., age 70. Diagnosis: gastric cancer. **a** Stomach roentgenogram (tight filling, vertical position, anterior projection): uneven contour in the cardiac projection (arrow). **b** Stomach roentgenogram (double contrast, vertical position, left oblique projection): changed relief of the cardiac rosette (cardioesophageal junction); the specific radial pattern is absent (arrows), uneven esophageal walls. Conclusion: Infiltrating cancer of the upper part of the stomach. To rule out infiltration spreading onto the esophagus, the patient was examined by computed tomography. **c, d** Computed tomograms of the stomach (the stomach is inflated with air, the patient is positioned on her right side; the level of the abdominal segment of the esophagus): the walls of the abdominal segment of the esophagus are thickened to 13 mm (arrow) due to intramural infiltration. **e** Computed tomogram of the stomach (position on the right side, the stomach is inflated with air, the level of the cardia): distinct visualization of the thickened wall of the stomach in the region of the cardiac rosette due to intramural infiltration (arrow), which spreads onto the abdominal segment of the esophagus. Conclusion: Infiltrative cancer of the upper part of the stomach with invasion of the abdominal segment of the esophagus.

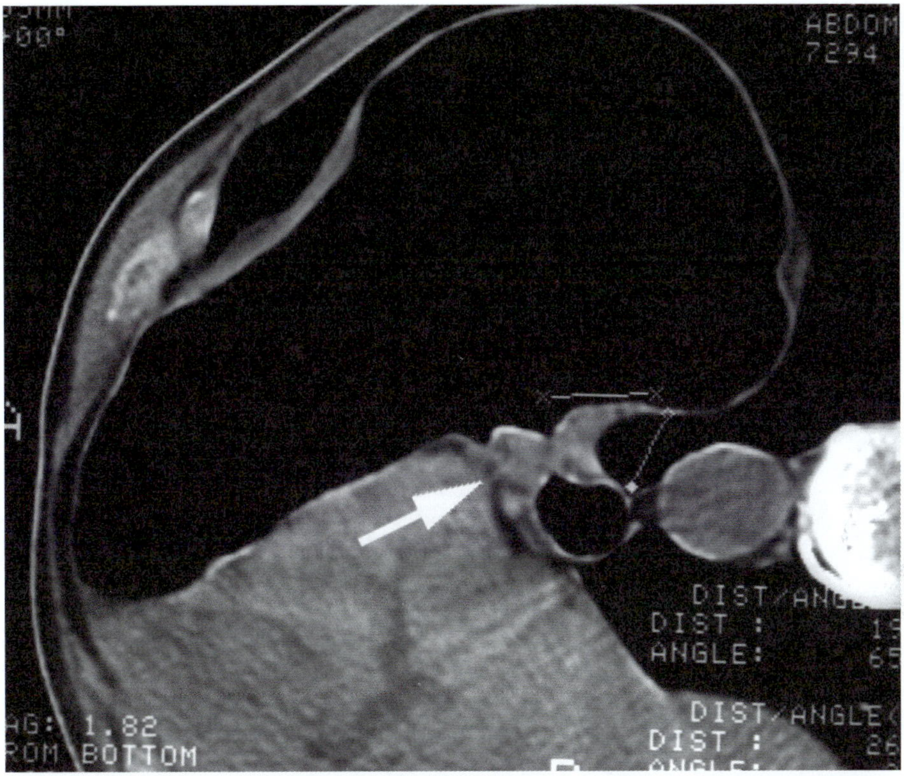

◀ **Fig. 51 c.**

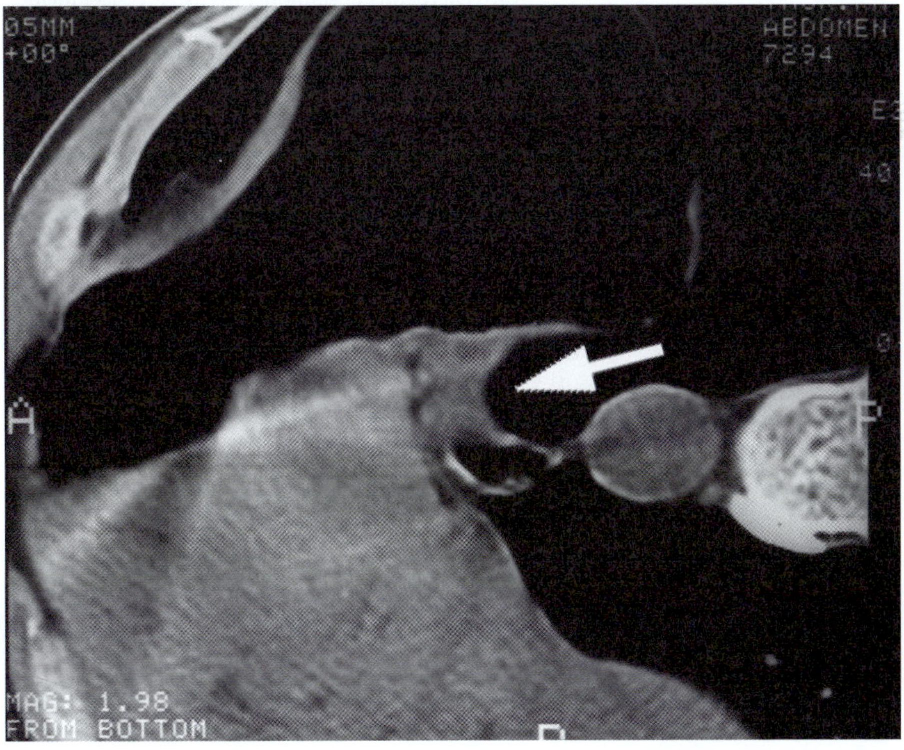

◀ **Fig. 51 d.**

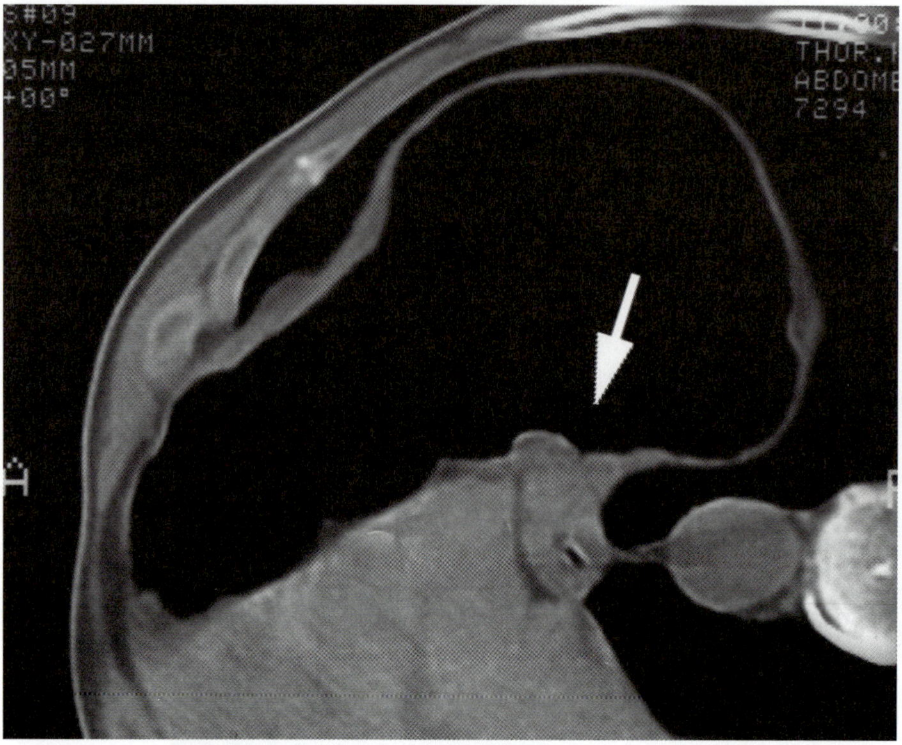

▲ **Fig. 51 d.**

▼ **Fig. 52 a.**

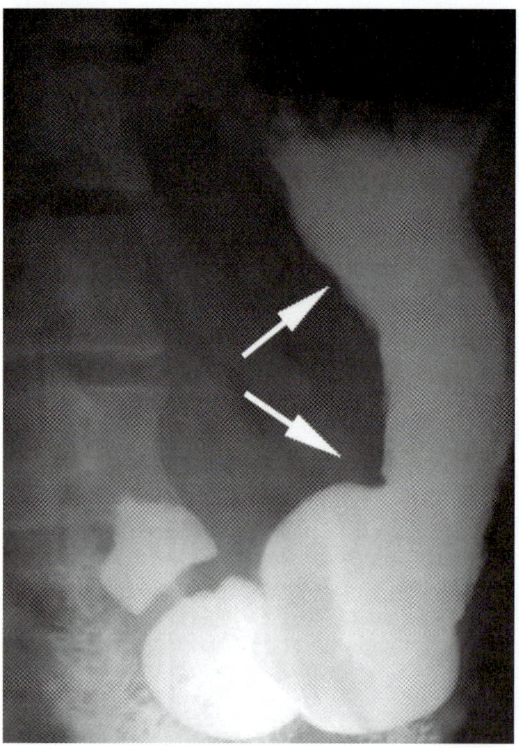

Current roentgenosemiotics of gastric cancer include the »old« sign – retention of residual barium sulfate suspension in the stomach 24 h after its intake, which occurs in cancer of the prepyloric part and the pylorus proper. Unfortunately, the so-called filling defect remains the main X-ray sign in the symptom complex of gastric cancer in its different versions (cup-shaped cancer, etc.).

In other words, the entire set of former X-ray signs was, and still is, based on the intestinal forms of gastric cancer. Its main anatomical signs were the results of prevailing changes mostly on the gastric mucosal surface [14, 65]. The outdated roentgenosemiotics of gastric cancer is based on the concept that the most common initial localization of the tumor is in certain parts of the stomach, viz., posterior wall, lesser curvature, the antral part (◘ Fig. 52). The greater curvature and the anterior wall were regarded as the sites where primary cancer tumors were unlikely to occur (◘ Fig. 53).

As a matter of fact, the same principle underlay the whole structure of the methodological approach to radiological examination of the stomach. The relief of the gastric mucosa was visualized with the

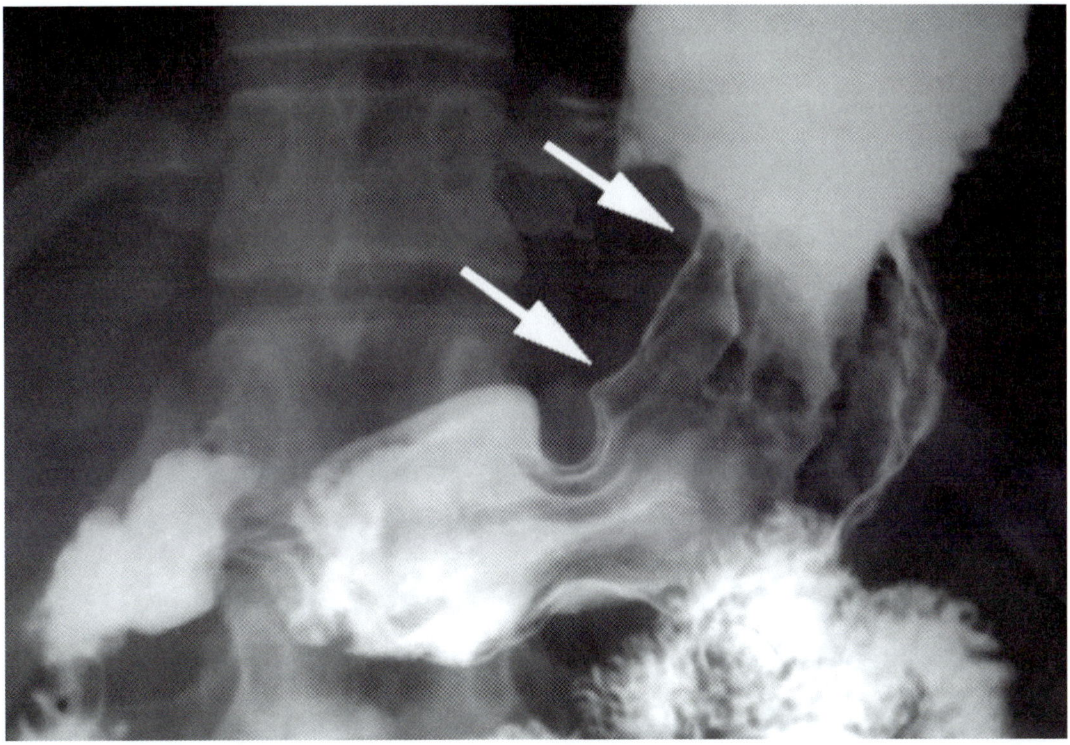

first gulps of the barium meal with dosed compression; next, as the stomach gradually filled with barium suspension, peristalsis of the gastric walls was studied, while less weight was given to characteristics of the stomach contours.

▲ **Fig. 52 b.**

▼ **Fig. 52 c.**

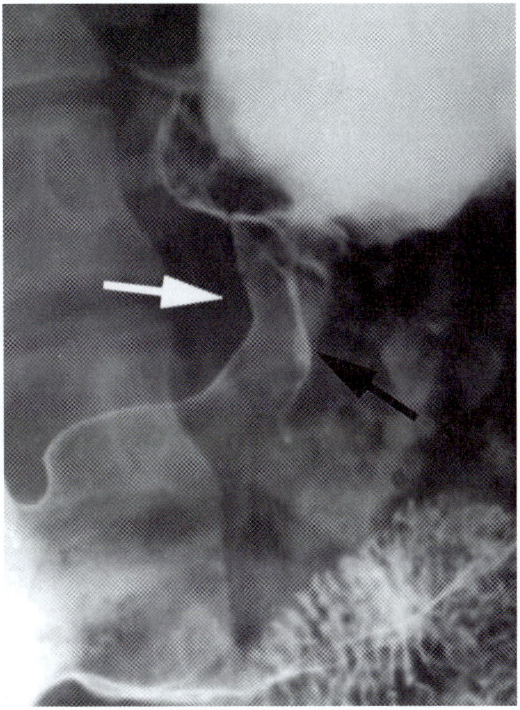

Fig. 52a–e. Patient R., age 57. Diagnosis: gastric cancer. **a** Stomach roentgenogram (tight filling, vertical position, anterior projection): the lesser curvature is depressed, its contour is uneven (arrows). **b** Stomach roentgenogram (pneumo-relief, horizontal position, anterior projection): the relief of the lesser curvature of the stomach body presents as a single thickened fold (arrows); mucosal folds terminate near the last fold of the lesser curvature. **c** Stomach roentgenogram (double contrast, horizontal position, anterior projection): infiltration of the wall of the lesser curvature is seen more distinctly; the wall is thickened and rigid (white arrow); a depot of barium sulfate is seen on the anterior wall as a fissure (black arrow). Conclusion: Infiltrative-ulcerous cancer of the lesser curvature of the stomach body. **d** Macrospecimen of a resected stomach: the stomach wall is dense; ulcers on the mucosal surface (arrow) with the surrounding relief changed due to tumor infiltration. **e** Fragment of a macrospecimen (strip): the stomach wall is thickened due to white intramural tumor infiltration (arrows)

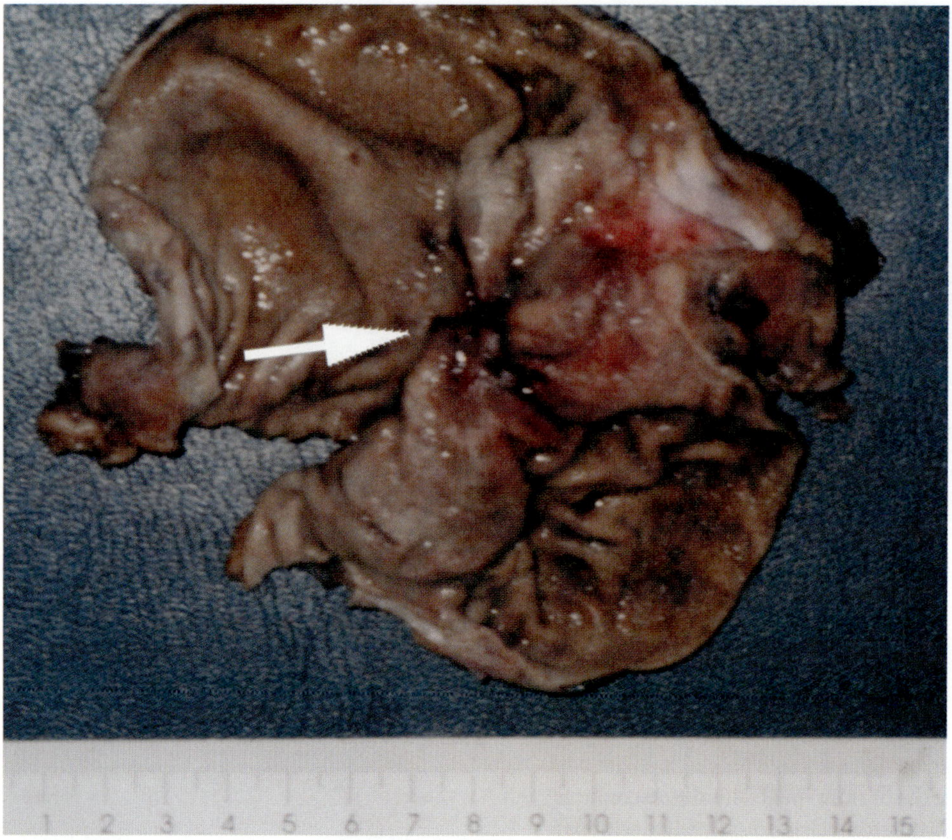

▲ Fig. 52 d.

▼ Fig. 52 e.

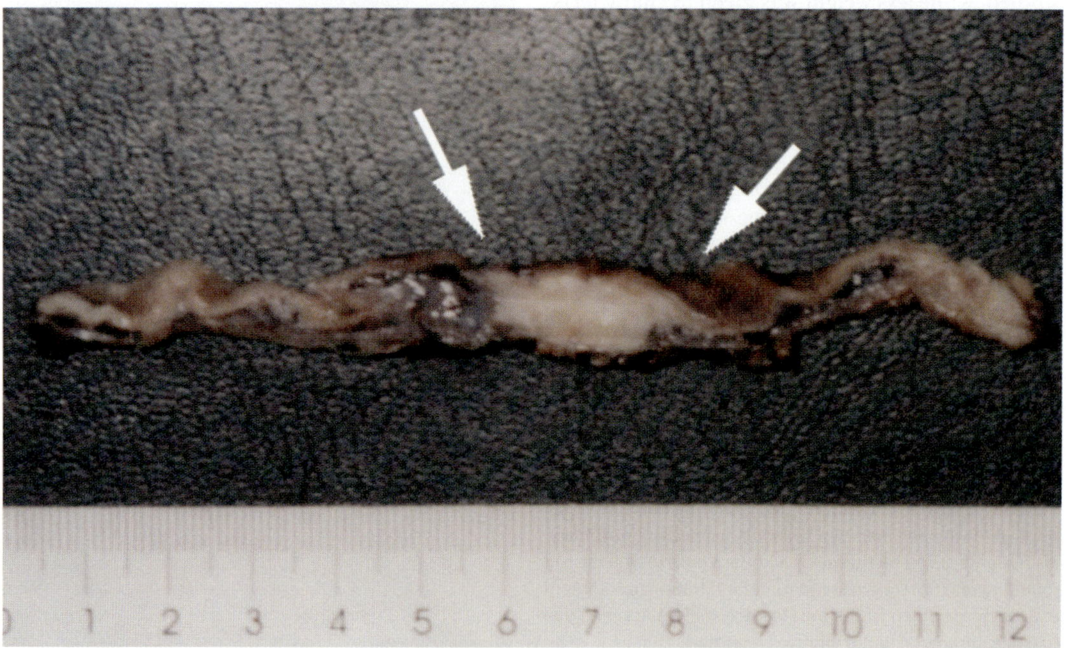

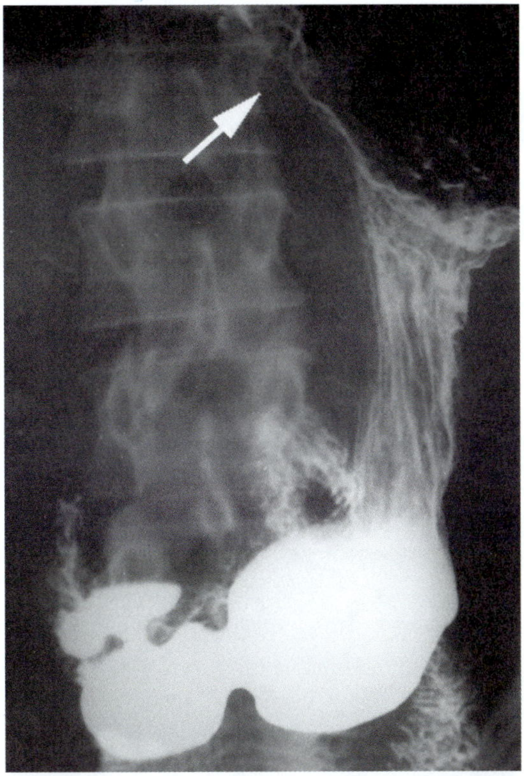

▲ **Fig. 53 a.**

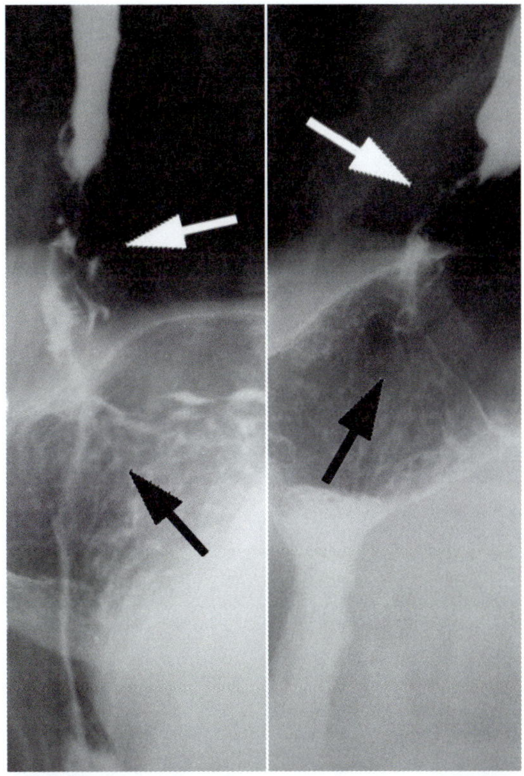

▲ **Fig. 53 c.**

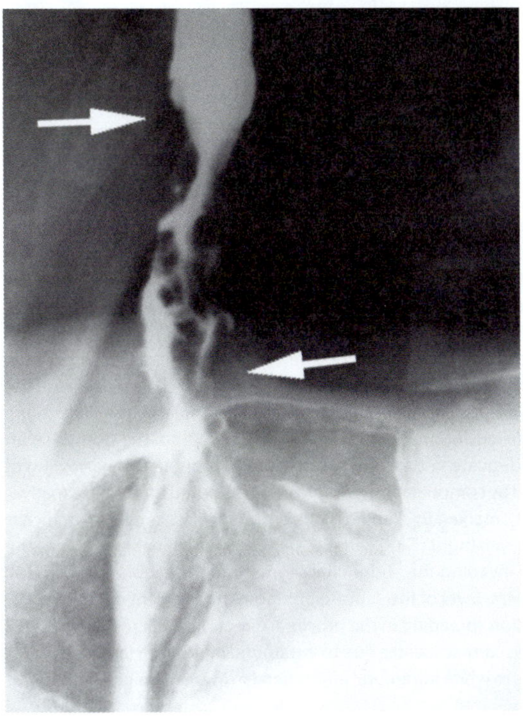

▼ **Fig. 53 b.**

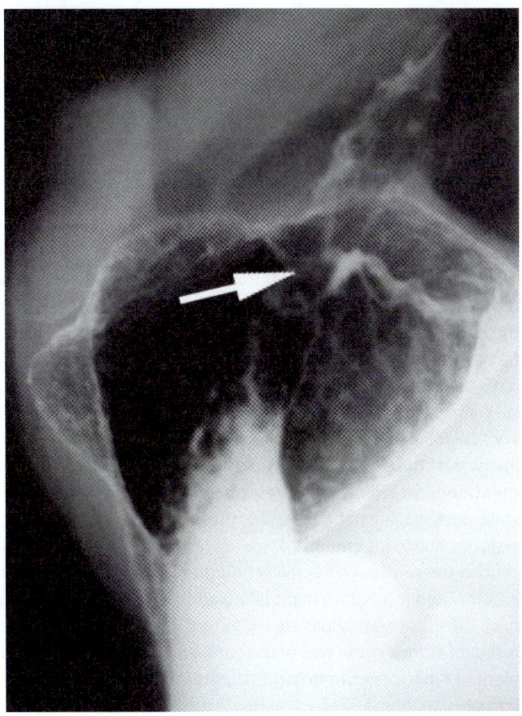

▼ **Fig. 53 d.**

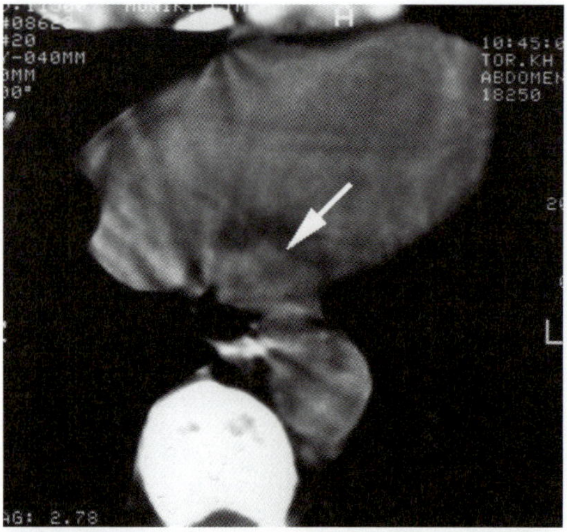

▲ **Fig. 53 e.**

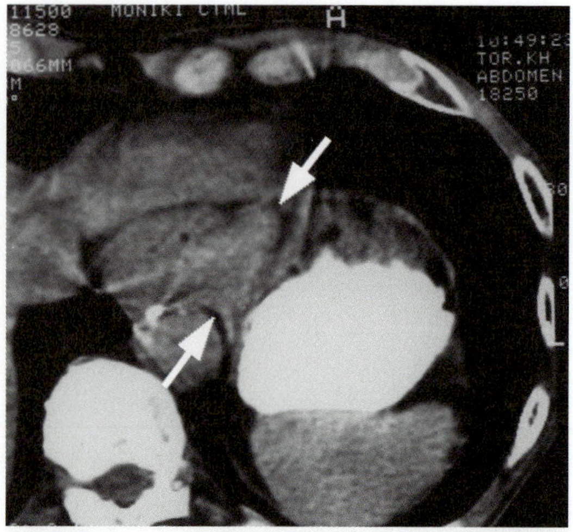

▲ **Fig. 53 g.**

▼ **Fig. 53 f.**

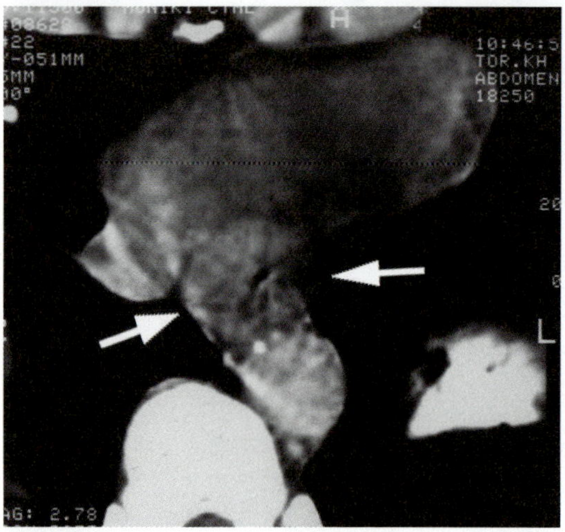

▼ **Fig. 53 h.**

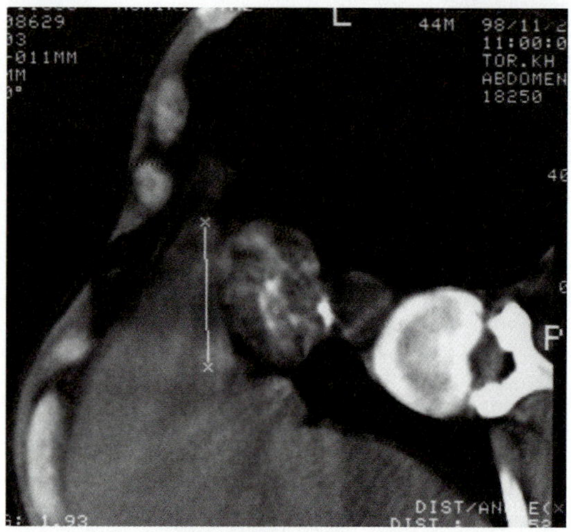

Fig. 53a–j. Patient M., age 61. Diagnosis: gastric cancer. **a** Stomach roentgenogram (tight filling, vertical position, anterior projection): the abdominal segment of the esophagus is disfigured, its walls are uneven, the rectilinear character of its mucosal folds is absent due to intramural infiltration (arrow). **b** Anterior projection (tight filling, vertical position, left lateral projection) at the moment of contrast medium passage through the gastroesophageal junction: marked deformation of the abdominal segment of the esophagus; uneven narrowing of the lumen due to intramural infiltration (arrows). **c** Stomach roentgenograms (double contrast, vertical position, left anterior oblique and left lateral projections) at the moment of contrast medium passage through the gastroesophageal junction: uneven narrowing of the abdominal segment of the esophagus (white arrows), changed relief of the cardiac rosette (black arrows). **d** Stomach roentgenogram (double contrast, horizontal position, left posterior oblique projection): atypical relief of the cardiac rosette is more distinct (arrow). Conclusion: Infiltrative cancer of the upper part of the stomach with invasion of the esophagus. In view of infeasibility of conducting adequate endoscopy because of the pronounced narrowing of the abdominal segment of the esophagus, the patient was examined by computed tomography. **e, f** Computed tomograms (native-state study, supine patient, level of the lower third of the esophagus): marked thickening of the esophageal walls over a significant distance due to intramural infiltration (arrows). **g** Computed tomogram (tight filling with E-Z-CAT DRY, supine patient, level of the cardia): the cardiac wall is thickened due to intramural infiltration invading the abdominal segment of the esophagus (arrows). **h** Computed tomogram (tight filling with E-Z-CAT DRY, supine patient, level of the supra-diaphragmatic segment of the esophagus): the esophageal walls are thickened due to intramural infiltration spreading in the proximal direction. **i** Macrospecimen of a resected stomach: the wall of the cardia is firm; atypical relief of the cardiac rosette due to intramural infiltration (arrows). **j** Fragment of a macrospecimen (strip): the stomach wall is thickened due to white intramural infiltration (arrows). Histologically, signet-ring cell carcinoma

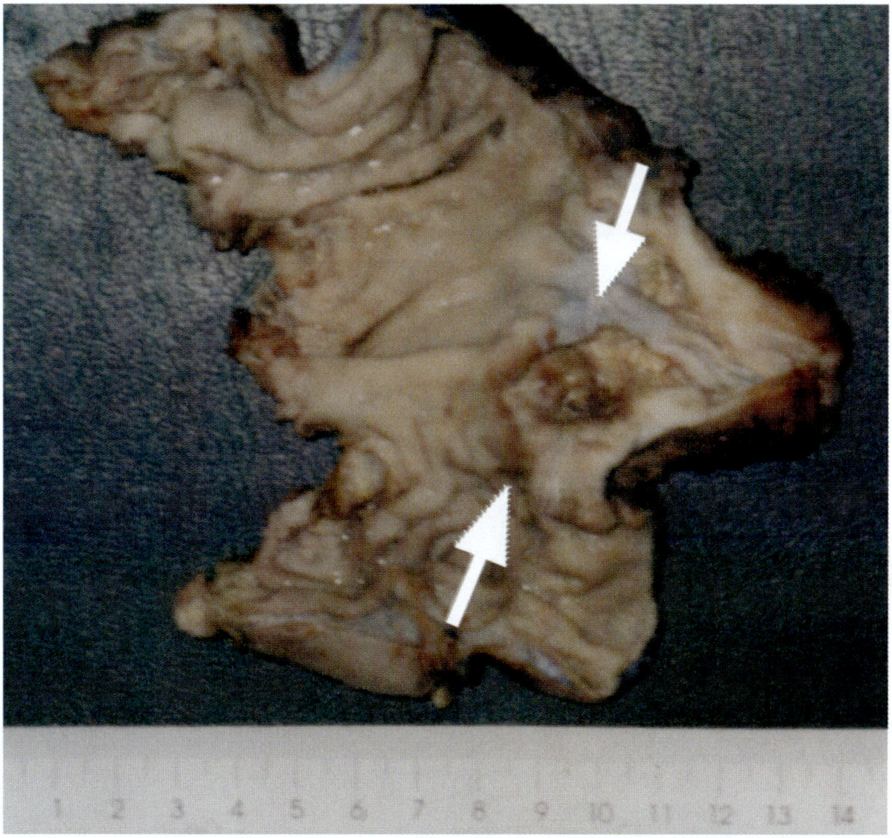

◄ **Fig. 53 i.**

▼ **Fig. 53 j.**

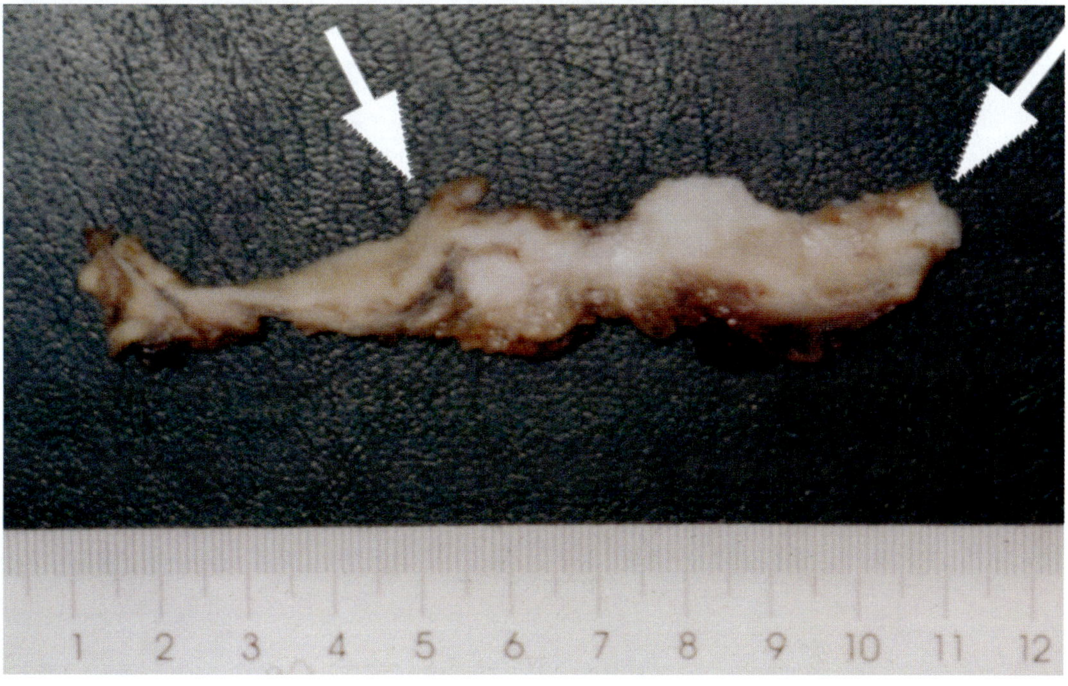

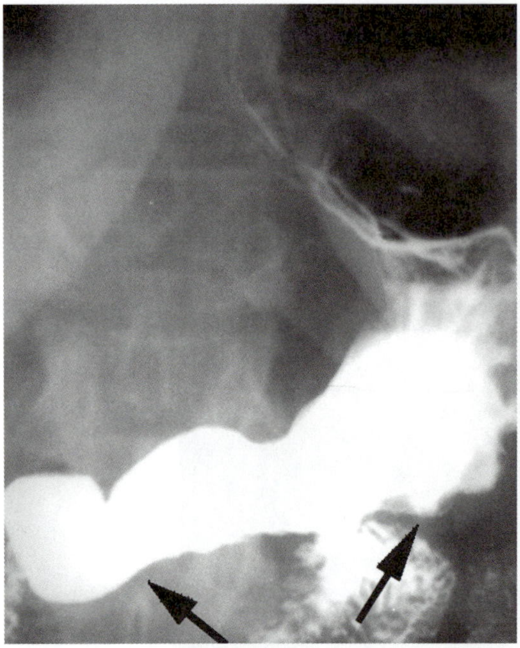

▲ Fig. 54 a.

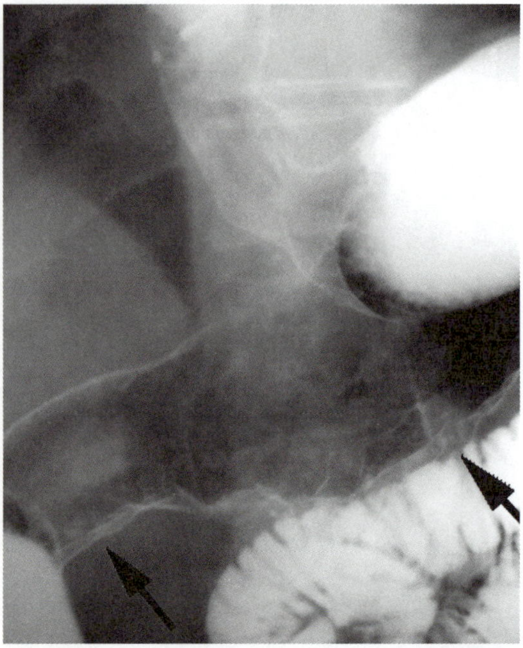

▲ Fig. 54 b.

▼ Fig. 54 c.

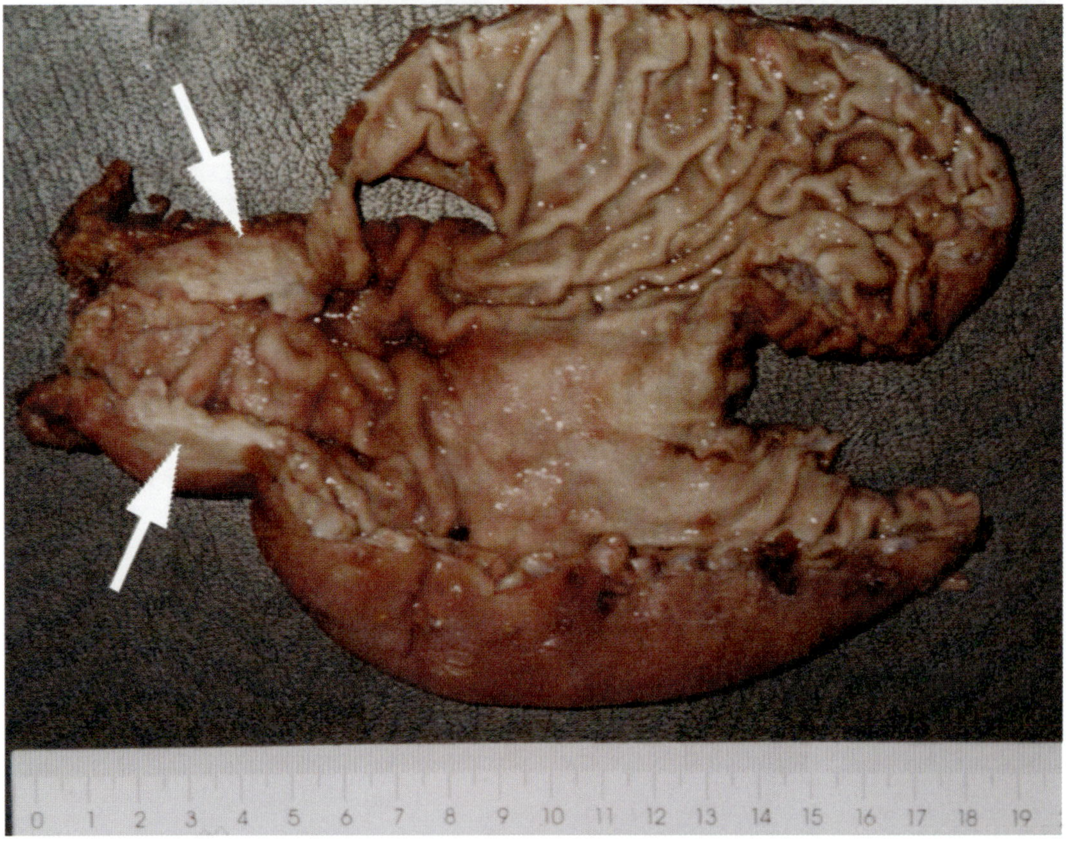

► **Fig. 54 d.**

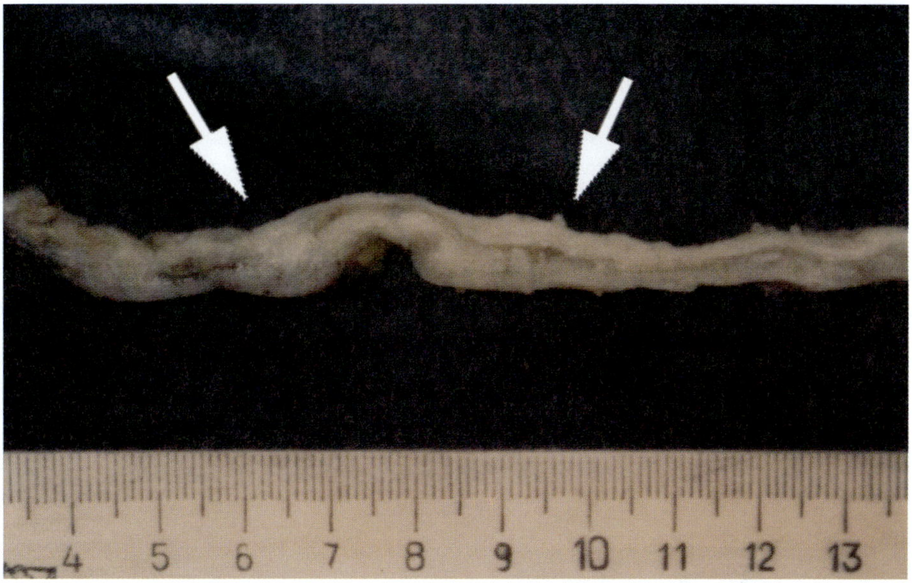

Fig. 54a–d. Female patient Sh., age 61. Diagnosis: gastric cancer. **a** Stomach roentgenogram (tight filling, vertical position, anterior projection): the wall of the greater curvature of the distal part is disfigured and rigid, its contour is uneven (arrows). **b** Stomach roentgenogram (double contrast, horizontal position, anterior projection): the wall of the greater curvature of the distal part of the stomach is rigid and thick due to intramural infiltration (arrow). Conclusion: Infiltrative cancer of the greater curvature of the distal part of the stomach. **c** Macrospecimen: a fragment of a resected part of the stomach: the wall of the greater curvature of the distal part is firm and thick due to tumor infiltration (arrows). **d** Fragment of a macrospecimen (strip): the stomach wall is thickened due to white intramural infiltration (arrows). Histologically, signet-ring cell carcinoma

▼ **Fig. 55 a.**

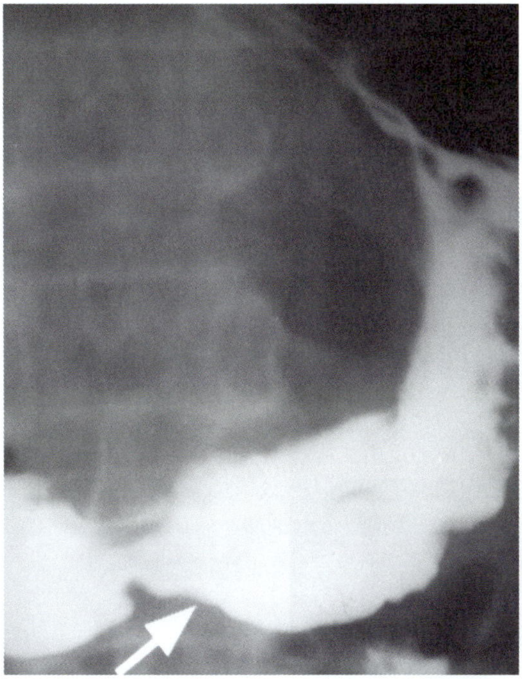

Thus, the analysis of condition of the greater curvature, of the anterior wall was inadequate. The specific functional and anatomical properties of the greater curvature were not taken into consideration during development of the methods for X-ray examination of the stomach, and hence in compiling a roentgenosemiotics of cancer affections (Fig. 54). The situation is the same with primary localization of cancer on the anterior wall of the stomach body and its antral part. It is common knowledge that in almost every radiological examination the mucosal relief, including those employing compression at the phase of tight filling (a full cup of the barium meal), the relief of the posterior was inspected. In order to visualize the anterior wall at tight filling, the stomach cavity should be filled with a large amount of contrast medium. Only in this way can we see the pleats on the anterior wall by applying the slightest compression (Figs. 55, 56). A large amount of barium sulfate is necessary to examine the greater curvature, especially at the level of the sinus, owing to its specific anatomical and functional properties [28, 31, 58, 223].

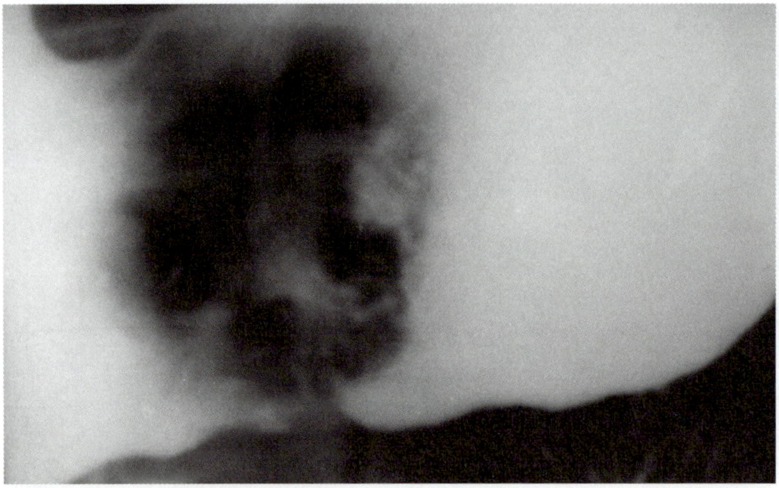

▲ **Fig. 55 b.**

▼ **Fig. 55 c.**

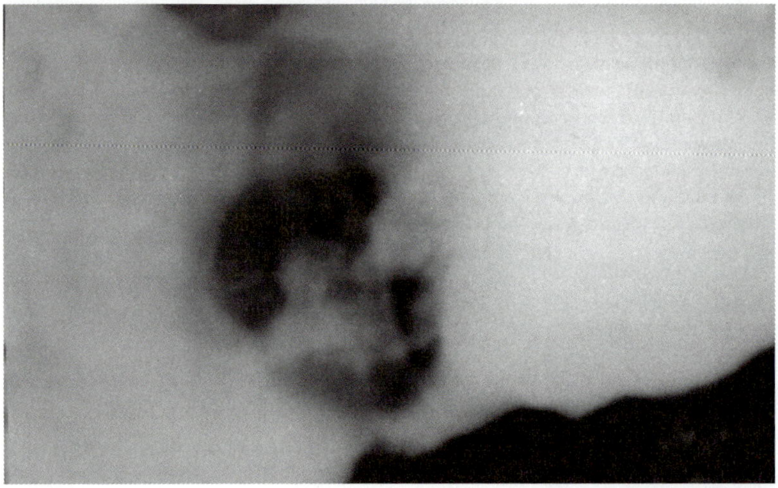

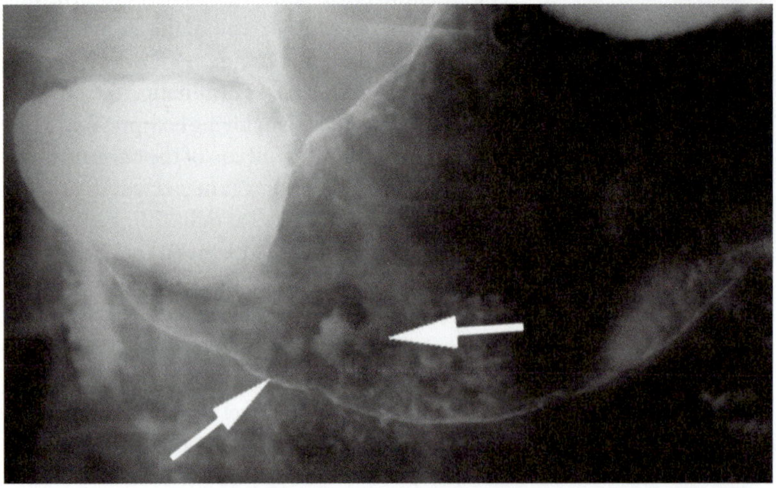

◄ **Fig. 55 d.**

Fig. 55a–d. Female patient G., age 58. Diagnosis: gastric cancer. **a** Stomach roentgenogram (tight filling, vertical position, anterior projection): contour of the greater curvature of the antral part is uneven (arrow). **b, c** Stomach roentgenograms (more tight filling, vertical position, anterior projection) after intake of an additional portion of the contrast medium, mild dosed compression: a depot of the contrast medium in the form of a spider with a ridge of infiltrated tissue is seen on the anterior wall of the antral part of the stomach. **d** Stomach roentgenogram (double contrast, horizontal position, anterior projection): impregnated ulcer crater of irregular shapes with the surrounding ridge of infiltrated tissue (arrows). Histological studies of tissue specimen taken during endoscopy failed to reveal tumor cells. Conservative anti-ulcer therapy was given

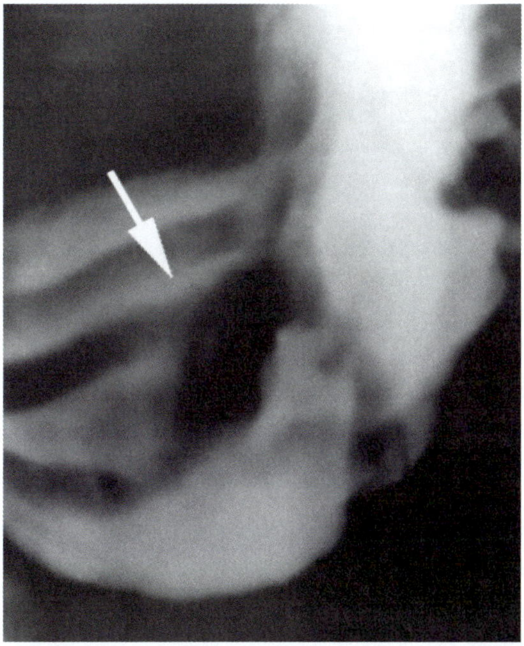

▲ **Fig. 56 a.**

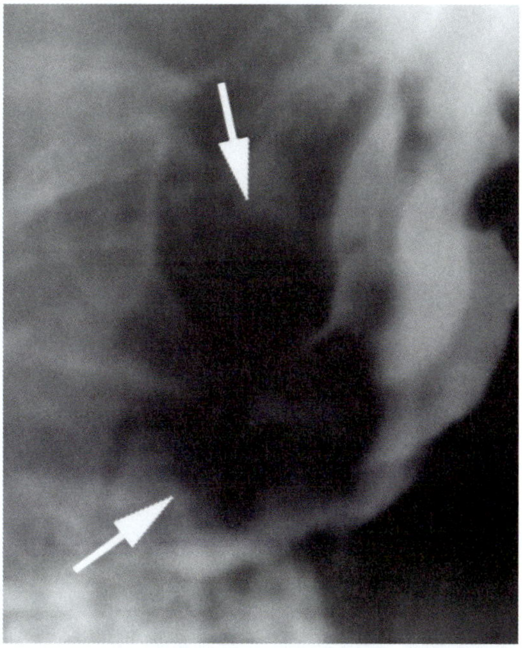

▲ **Fig. 56 b.**

► **Fig. 56 c.**

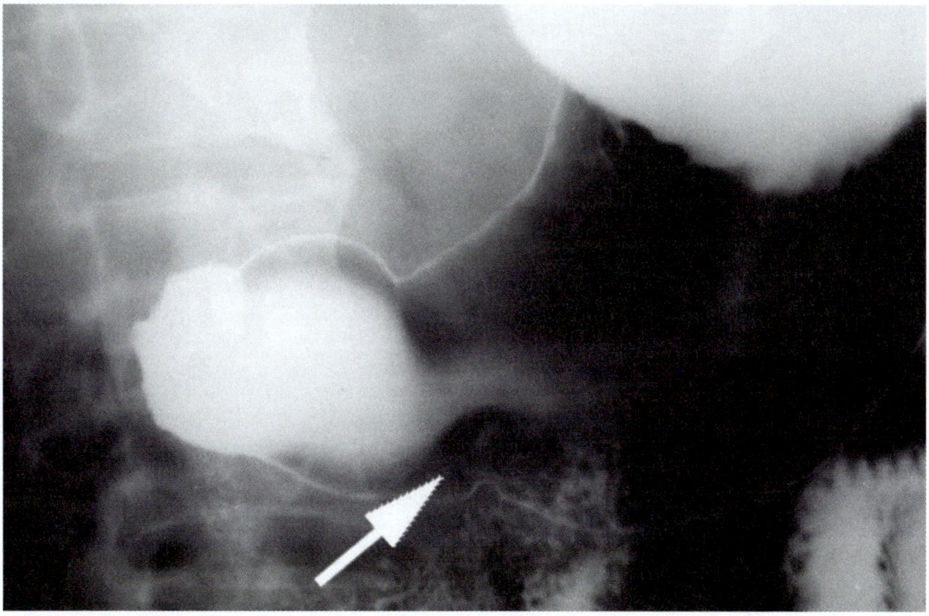

Fig. 56a–f. Same patient, 45 days later. **a, b** Stomach roentgenograms (tight filling, vertical position, anterior projection), dosed compression with application of pressure of varied strength: despite the active anti-ulcer treatment, the spider-like ulcer on the anterior wall persists; the ridge of infiltrated tissue increases, folds terminate by the periphery (arrows). **c, d** Stomach roentgenograms (double contrast, horizontal position, anterior projection): infiltration of the anterior wall of the antral part is ulcerated (arrow). Conclusion: Infiltrative-ulcerous cancer of the anterior wall of the antral part of the stomach. **e** Macrospecimen of a resected stomach: ulceration of the anterior wall of the antral part with a ridge of infiltration; the wall is firm due to intramural infiltration (arrows). **f** Fragment of a macrospecimen (strip): the stomach wall is thickened due to intramural infiltration (arrows). Histologically, a non-differentiated cancer.

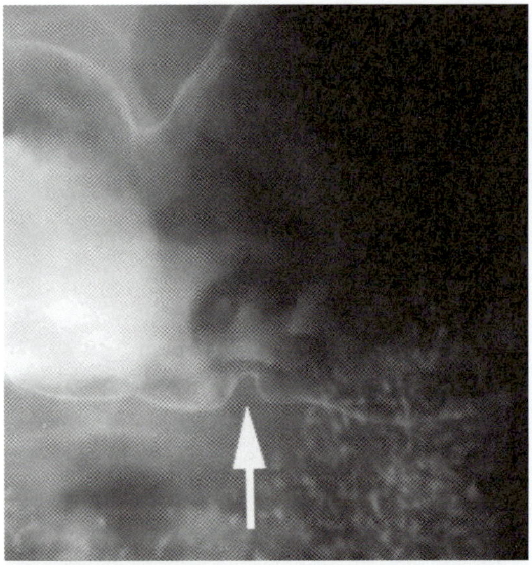

▲ **Fig. 56 d.**

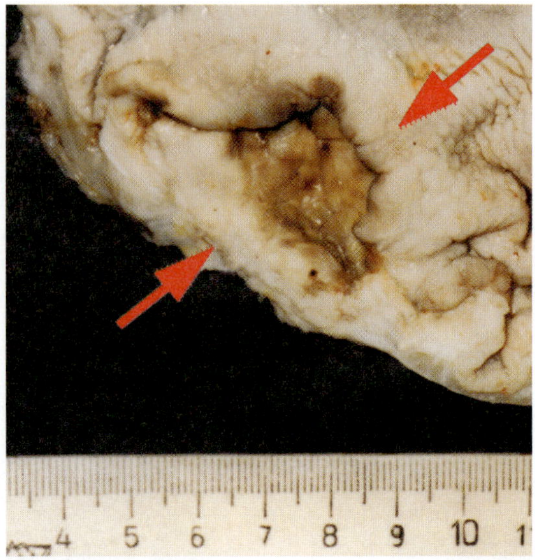

▲ **Fig. 56 e.**

▼ **Fig. 56 f.**

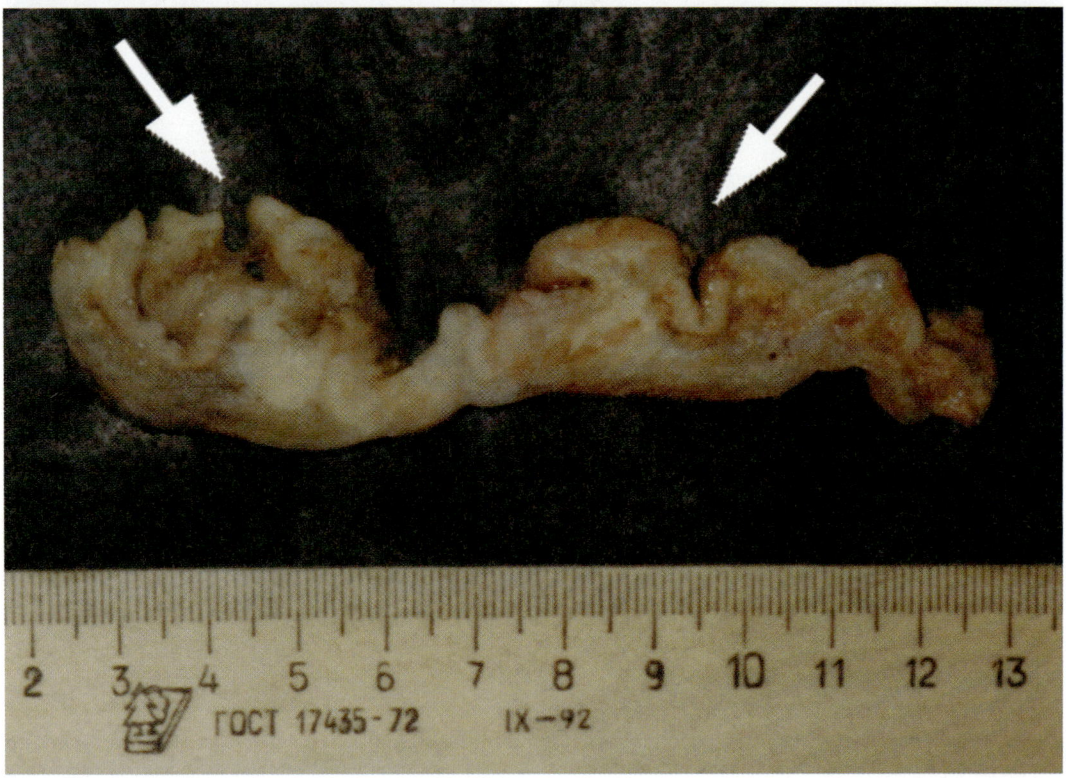

Fig. 57a–d. Patient B., age 73. Diagnosis: gastric cancer. **a** Stomach roentgenogram (tight filling, vertical position, anterior projection): the stomach cavity is diminished, the notch is straightened, the lesser curvature is short, depressed, uneven contours; the walls are rigid (arrows). **b** Stomach roentgenogram (double contrast, horizontal position, anterior projection): diffuse thickening of the stomach walls due to intramural infiltration, invading the upper part (arrows). Conclusion: Infiltrative cancer of the stomach. **c** Macrospecimen of a resected stomach: the wall is firm, mucosal relief is smoothed down due to intramural infiltration (white

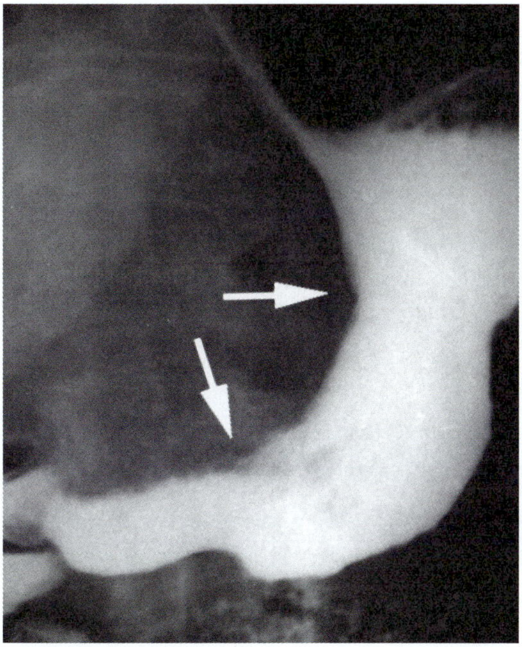

▲ **Fig. 57 a.**

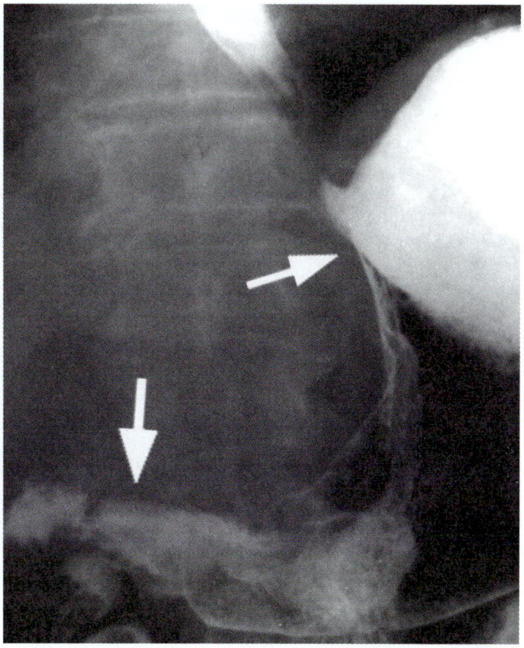

▲ **Fig. 57 b.**

▼ **Fig. 57 c.**

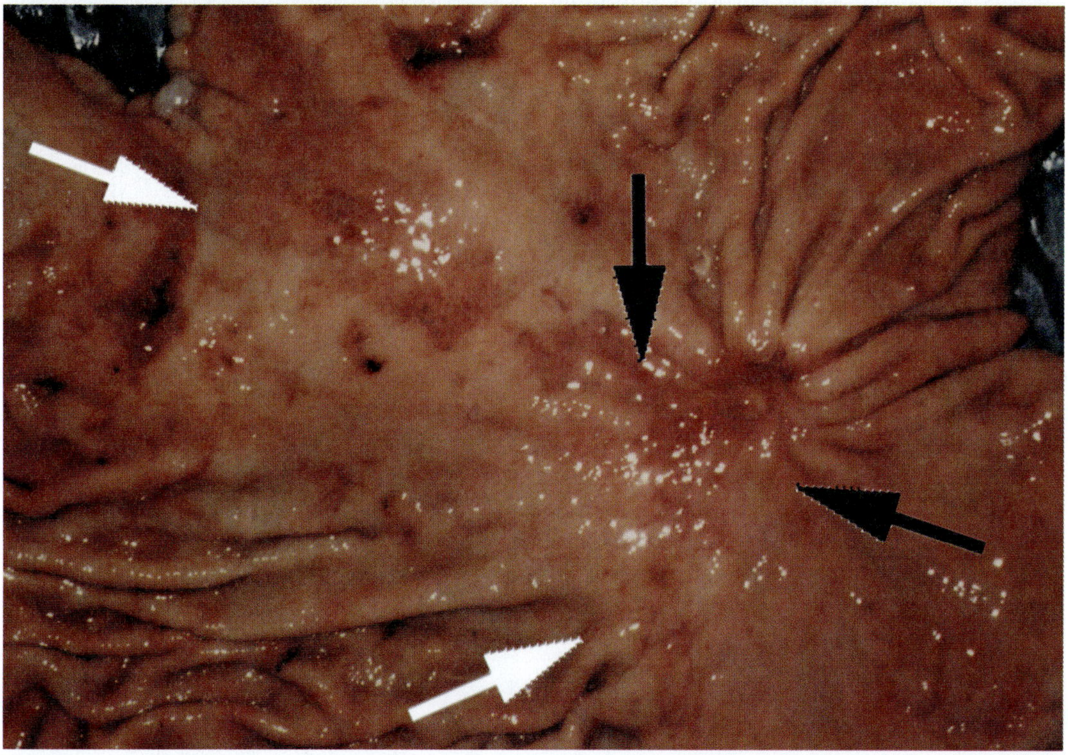

arrows); the relief of the cardiac rosette (cardioesophageal junction) is also leveled (black arrows). **d** Fragments of a macrospecimen (strips): the stomach wall is thickened due to intramural infiltration (arrows). Histologically, signet-ring cell carcinoma

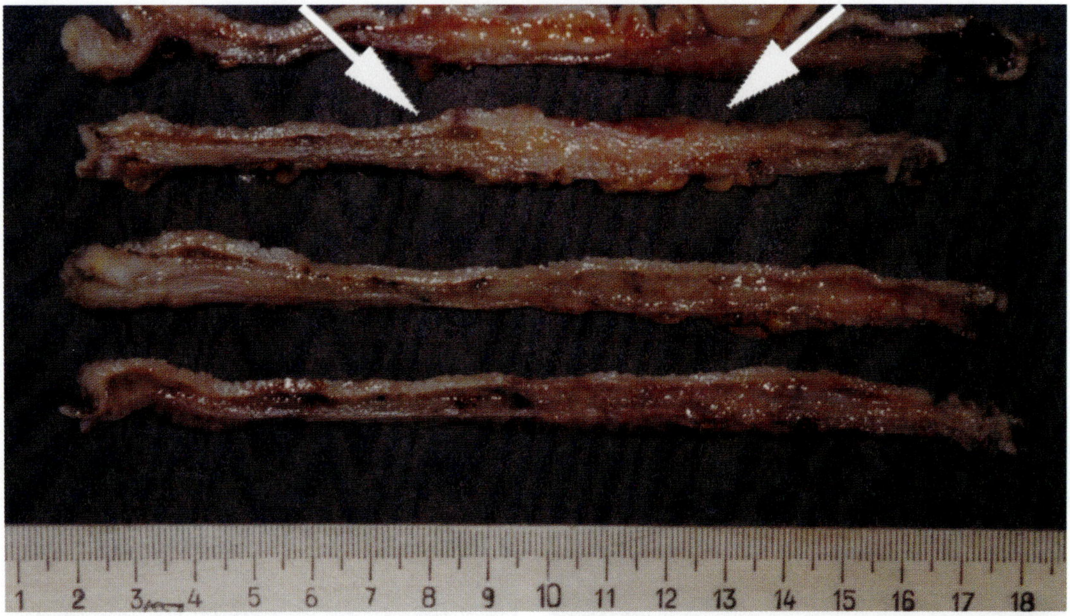

▲ Fig. 57 d.

▼ Fig. 58 a.

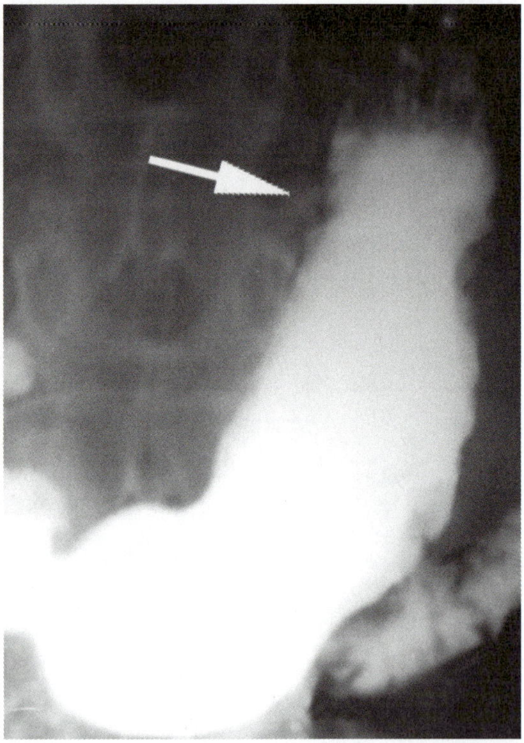

There is now a significant prevalence of diffuse and mixed forms in morphogenesis of cancer, predominantly with intramural submucous growth of the tumor (◘ Fig. 57). There is also an almost complete disappearance of purely exophytic forms of gastric cancer. At least, they occur so rarely that it is hardly reasonable to account for them while compiling radiological semiotics. And the existing classification of gastric cancer (including the endoscopic classification of 1962) also requires revision.

Thus, in view of the changes that have taken place in the morphological manifestations of cancer (the most important aspect) and also in view of the changed accents in the frequency of primary tumor locations in various parts of the stomach, we will discuss the two major radiological signs of gastric cancer. These include uneven contours of the stomach at the phase of its tight filling with barium sulfate suspension and thickening of its wall, which is detectable by the double-contrast technique (◘ Fig. 58). Naturally, while placing special emphasis on these two symptoms, we do not rule out consideration of the stomach mucosal relief, which is also requisite. Two aspects will be considered here. First, the condition of the relief should be assessed not at the beginning of the examination (with the first gulps of the contrast medium, as is commonly recommended) but rather during evacuation of the contrast medium from the stomach after its examination at the phase of tight filling. Second, the mucosal relief

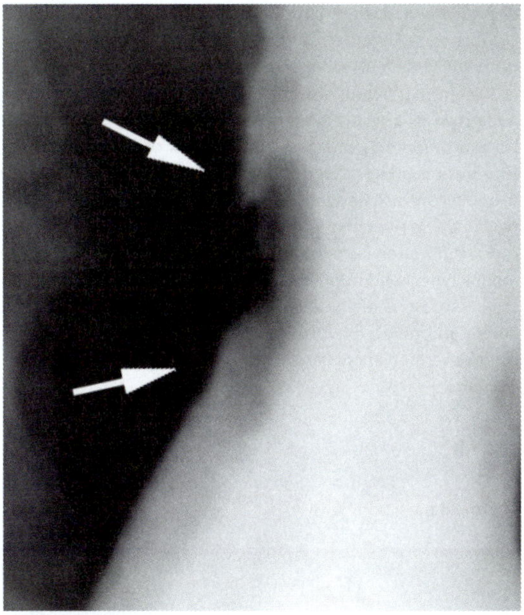

▲ **Fig. 58 b.** ▼ **Fig. 58 c.**

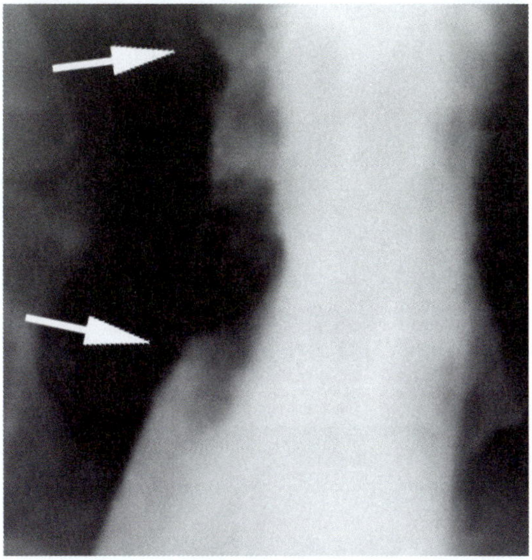

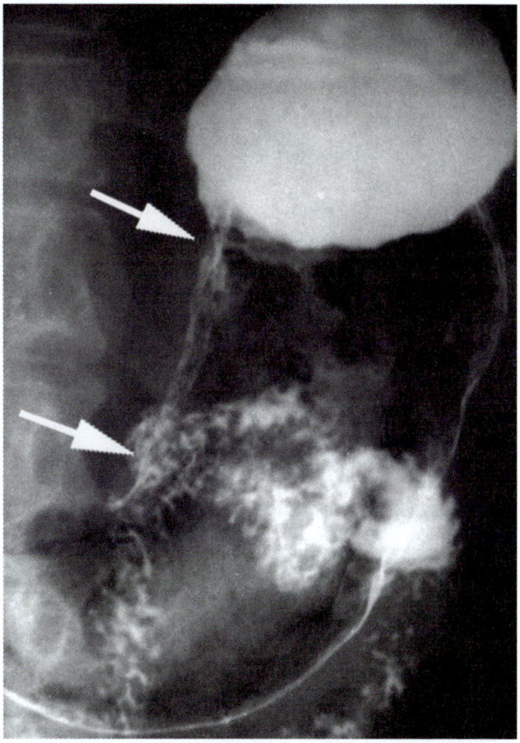

▲ **Fig. 58 d.**

should manifest changes. The most important characteristics are those obtained by the double-contrast technique owing to incomplete stretching of the mucosal folds in the presence of hyperplasia or the presence of two to three folds converging toward the part of the stomach wall which is thickened or has uneven contours. This is confirmed today by acknowledgement of the existence of the so-called hyperplastic or gigantic-fold forms of diffuse gastric cancer (◘ Fig. 59). In other words, the study of the mucosal relief must concentrate on the two major signs which we propose to consider, namely, uneven contours of the stomach and thickening of its wall (◘ Fig. 60). Our vast experience suggests that assessment of these two signs makes it possible to rule out the existing scheme of their recognition. The two symptoms are characterized by the variety of their manifestations – from minute irregularities of the stomach contours and insignificant thickening of the stomach wall over very small areas, detectable with the double-contrast technique, to large affections of 3–4 cm. We have cases illustrating dynamic growth of these two symptoms. As a rule, this occurred in patients in whom endoscopic examinations (both visual inspection and microscopy of tissue specimens) failed to discover the initial signs of diffuse infiltration for a considerable length of time. According to modern regulations, however, only endoscopic verification – to be more particular, only histological verification of the diagnosis of gastric cancer – may be regarded as a sort of official indication for radical surgery [72, 178, 259].

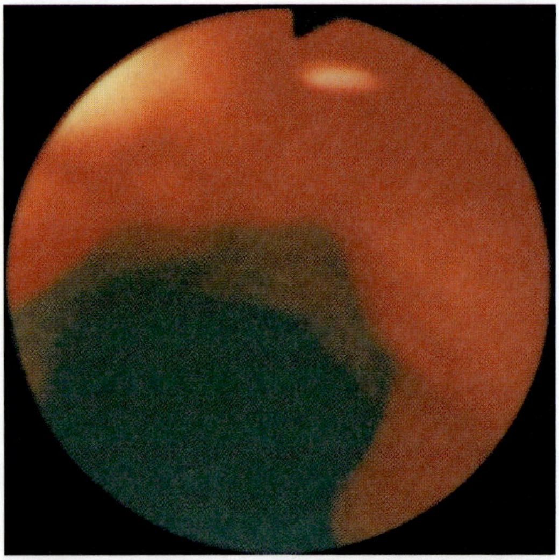

Fig. 58a–e. Patient V., age 54. Diagnosis: gastric cancer. **a** Double contrast (tight filling, vertical position, anterior projection): the lesser curvature of the body is depressed, its contour is uneven, in the form of a small prolapse into the stomach cavity (arrow). **b, c** Stomach roentgenograms (tight filling, vertical position, anterior projection): the contour of the lesser curvature is uneven and eroded (arrows). **d** Stomach roentgenogram (double contrast, horizontal position, anterior projection): the wall of the lesser curvature is thickened and rigid due to intramural infiltration (arrows). Conclusion: Infiltrative cancer of the stomach body. **e** Endophotograph: the lesser curvature of the stomach body is straightened, rigid, with rough surface; the mucous membrane is grayish pink. Histological examinations of bioptates verified adenocarcinoma with the signet-ring cell component

◂ **Fig. 58 e.**

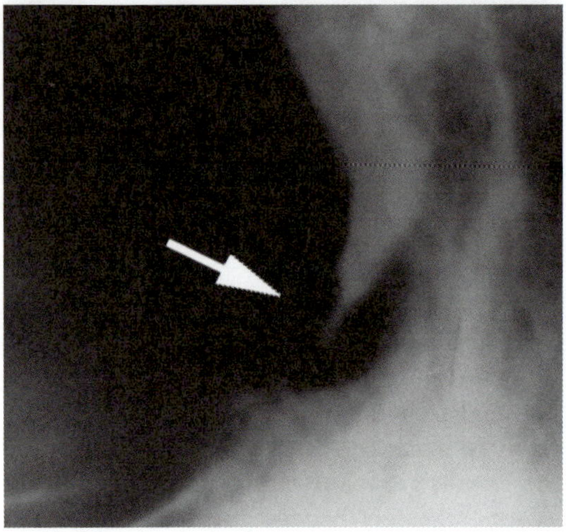

▴ **Fig. 59 a.**

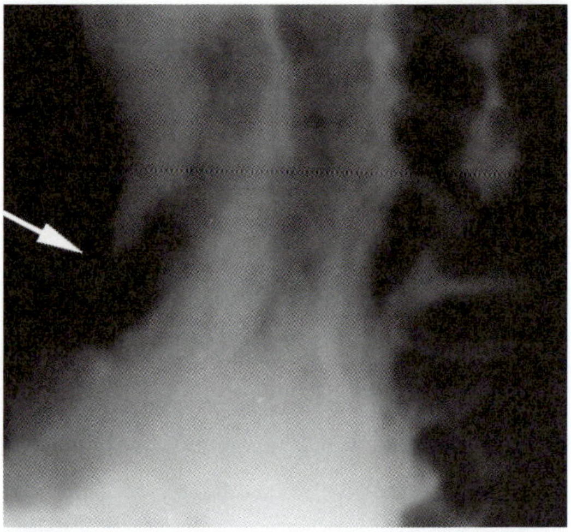

▴ **Fig. 59 c.**

▾ **Fig. 59 b.**

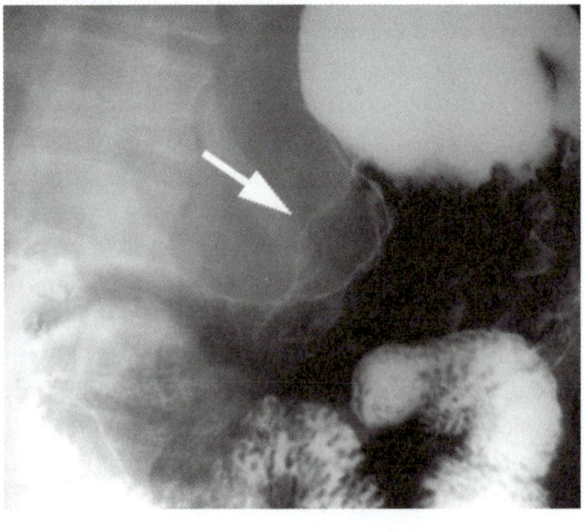

▾ **Fig. 59 d.**

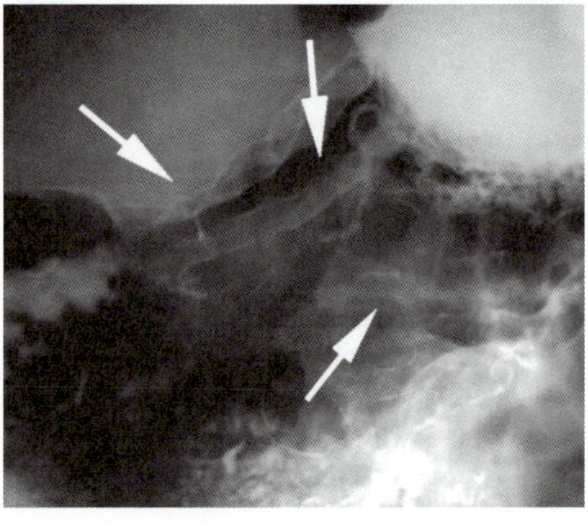

Fig. 59a–e. Patient A., age 61. Diagnosis: gastric cancer. **a, b** Stomach roentgenograms (tight filling, vertical position, anterior projection): contour of the lesser curvature is uneven (arrow). **c** Stomach roentgenogram (double contrast, horizontal position, anterior projection): wall of the lesser curvature is thickened and rigid due to infiltration (arrow); body folds are hyperplastic, unable to unfold completely with double contrast. **d** Stomach roentgenogram (double contrast, horizontal position, left oblique projection): hyperplasia and infiltration of the stomach body folds (arrows). Conclusion: Infiltrative cancer of the stomach body. **e** Endophotograph: gigantic folding (hyperplastic) type of infiltrative gastric cancer. Histological study of bioptates confirmed signet-ring cell carcinoma

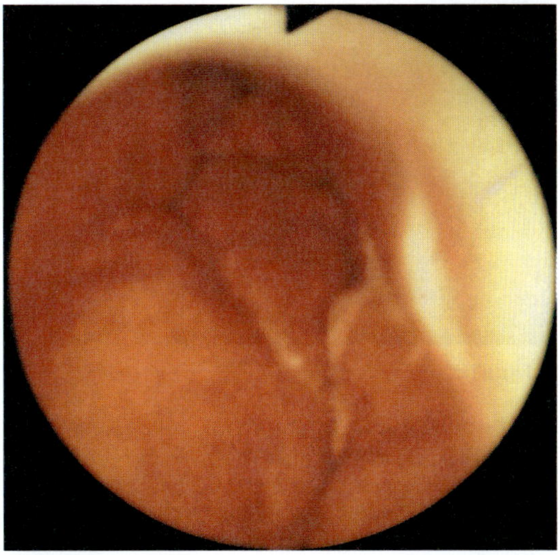

▲ **Fig. 59 e.**

▼ **Fig. 60 a.**

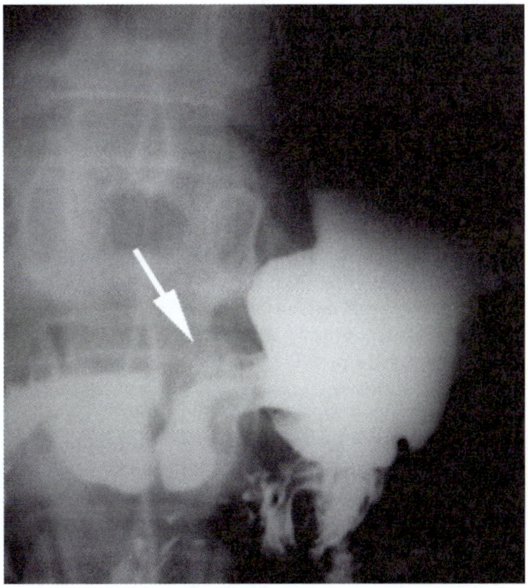

▶ **Fig. 60 b.**

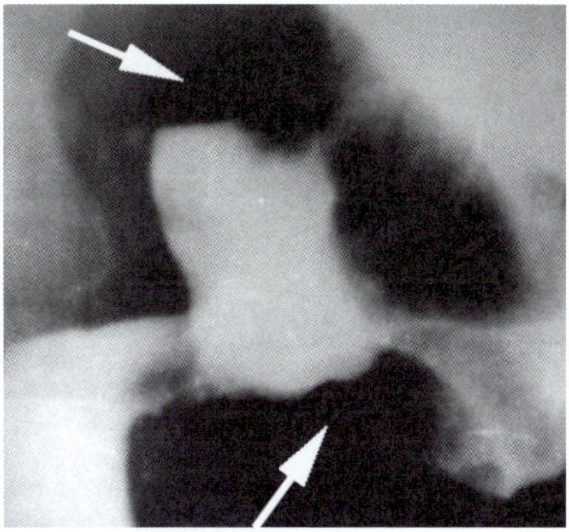

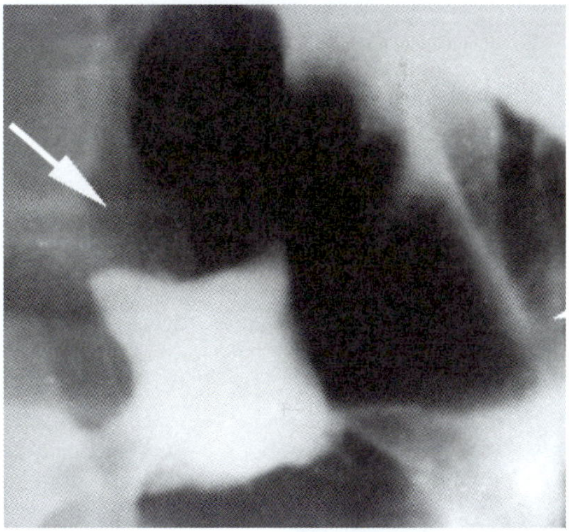

▲ **Fig. 60 c.**

▼ **Fig. 60 d.**

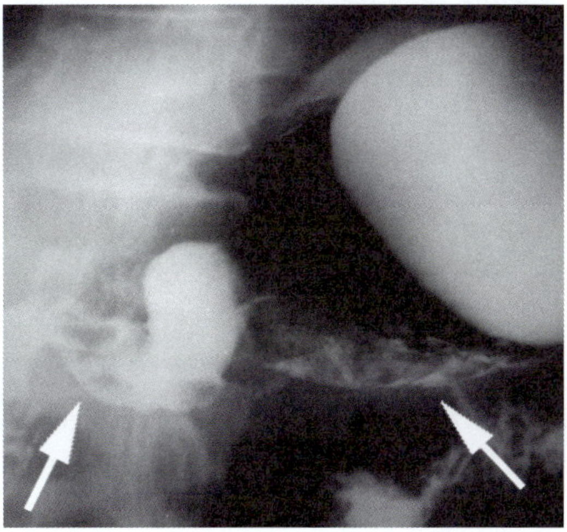

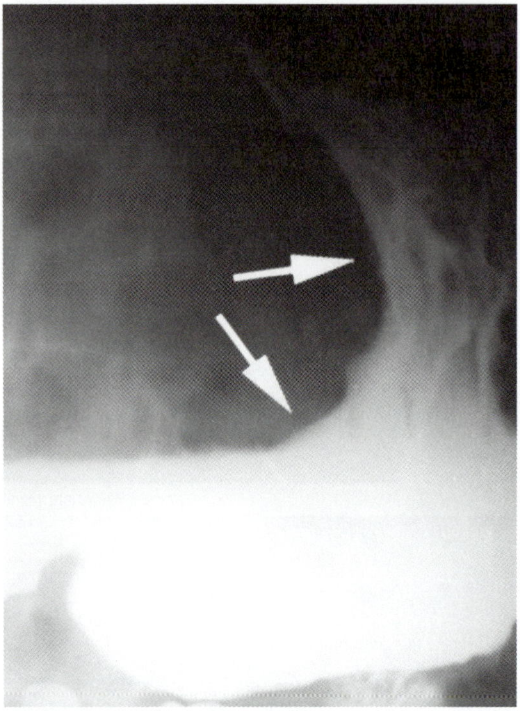

▲ Fig. 61 a.

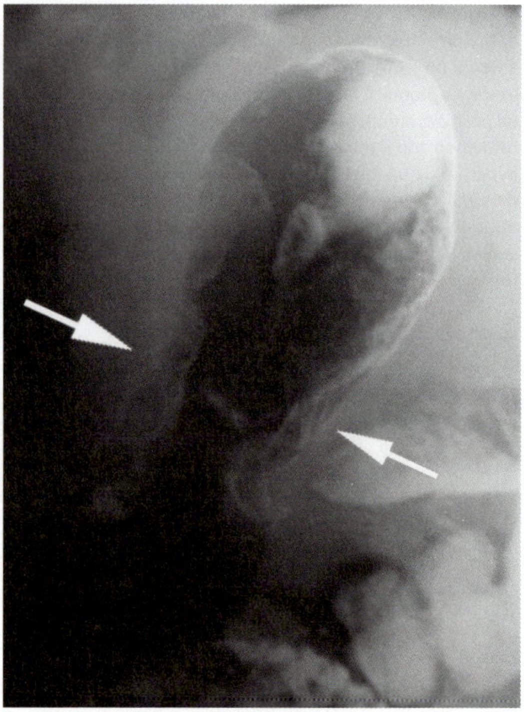

▲ Fig. 61 c.

▼ Fig. 61 b.

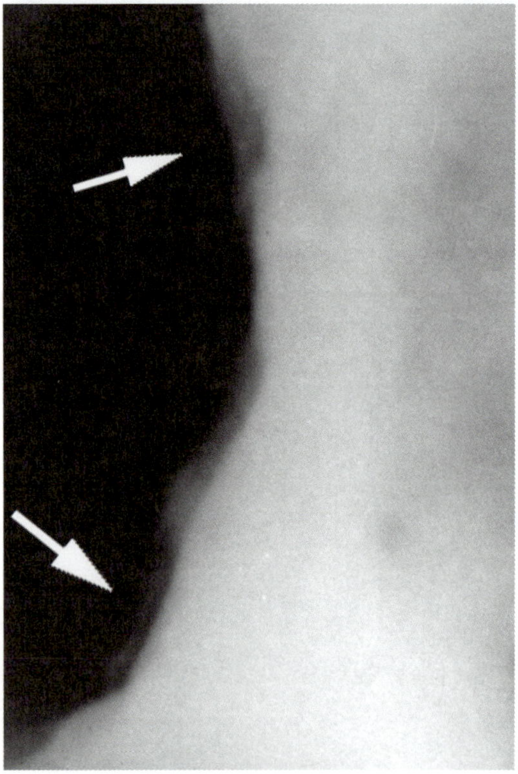

Fig. 60a–d. Patient I., age 58. Diagnosis: gastric cancer. **a** Stomach roentgenogram (tight filling, vertical position, anterior projection): the distal part is disfigured, the inner cavity decreased significantly, the walls are rigid, the contour of the lesser curvature of the middle third of the stomach body is uneven (arrow). **b, c** Stomach roentgenograms (tight filling, vertical position, right oblique projection): a large depot of contrast medium with a surrounding ridge of infiltrated tissue (arrows). **d** Stomach roentgenogram (double contrast, horizontal position, anterior projection): diffuse thickening of the walls of the distal part and the body of the stomach due to circular intramural infiltration (arrows). Conclusion: Infiltrative-ulcerous cancer of the distal part of the stomach with invasion of the stomach body. The patient was operated. Histologically, a non-differentiated cancer

Fig. 61a–c. Female patient L., age 66. Diagnosis: gastric cancer. **a** Stomach roentgenogram (tight filling, vertical position, anterior projection): the lesser curvature of the stomach body is short, its contour is uneven (arrows). **b** Stomach roentgenogram (tight filling, vertical position, anterior projection) after taking an additional portion of barium sulfate suspension: uneven contour of the lesser curvature of the stomach body (arrows). **c** Stomach roentgenogram (double contrast, horizontal position, left lateral projection): distinct visualization of the thickened anterior and posterior walls of the stomach body and its upper part due to circular intramural infiltration (arrows). Conclusion: Infiltrative cancer of the stomach body with invasion of the upper part. The patient was operated. Histologically, adenocarcinoma with the signet-ring cell component

It should be remembered that assessment of the stomach contours at the phase of tight filling and of its thickened wall by the double-contrast technique can be regarded as reliable only on condition that a sufficient number of X-ray images are taken. We discussed this point in our description of the methodological aspects of radiological examination of the stomach in ▸ Chap. 4.

We emphasize the importance of these two signs because they can point to intramural tumor infiltration of the stomach, both at the early and at appreciably advanced stages. It must be remembered that when we speak about stomach contours, we mean the inner contours, as if viewed from inside the wall, rather than from the side of the serosa, i.e., at the site where the process of tumor infiltration occurs (◘ Fig. 61).

While proposing these as the two main signs of gastric cancer detectable by the traditional radiological examination (at the tight filling phase and with double contrast), we understand that the reader may disagree, because, under existing conditions, the radiologist cannot always conduct the double-contrast examination correctly. It is necessary here to point out that tight filling of the stomach with barium sulfate suspension often gives more information on the condition of its contour than adequately conducted double-contrast examination. This may happen in the presence of initial signs of infiltration of the greater curvature, the prepyloric part, and the pylorus (◘ Fig. 62). Therefore, if it is impossible to adequately conduct a double-contrast examination of the stomach, the sign of uneven contour of a tightly filled stomach should be accepted, because it gives sufficiently objective information on the presence of infiltration in the stomach wall. At the same time, it should be noted that in order to obtain reliable information using this sign, some other factors should be considered.

These include proper selection of the time for taking a picture, at the phase when the peristaltic wave does not pass, and observation of technical requirements for taking pictures: maximum short exposure with correspondingly increased voltage, etc. This problem can be solved partly by using the »green« film/screen system, because owing to the high sensitivity and contrast of the film, the exposure can be reduced 2–4 times. The improved quality of X-ray pictures combines with a decreased radiation load on the patients and the medical personnel.

◘ Fig. 62a, b. Patient D., age 60. Diagnosis: gastric cancer. **a** Stomach roentgenogram (tight filling, vertical position, anterior projection): uneven and eroded contour of the lesser curvature of the prepyloric part of the stomach (arrow). **b** Target stomach roentgenogram (pneumorelief, horizontal position, anterior projection): thickened wall of the lesser curvature of the prepyloric part of the stomach (arrow); peristalsis can be seen over the entire length. Conclusion: Minor cancer of the prepyloric part of the stomach. The patient was operated. Histologically, adenocarcinoma with the signet-ring cell component.

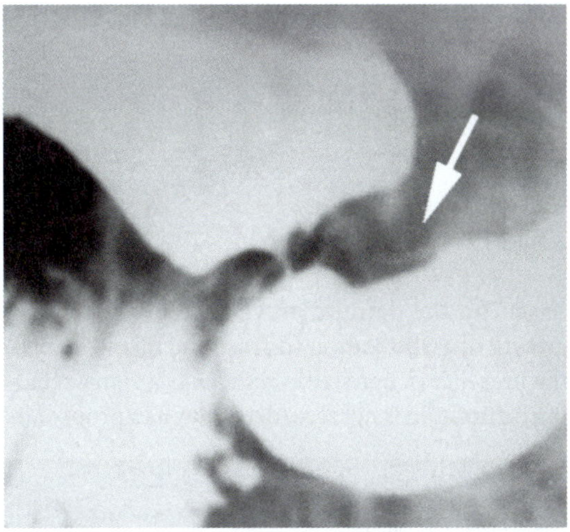

▲ **Fig. 62 a.**

▼ **Fig. 62 b.**

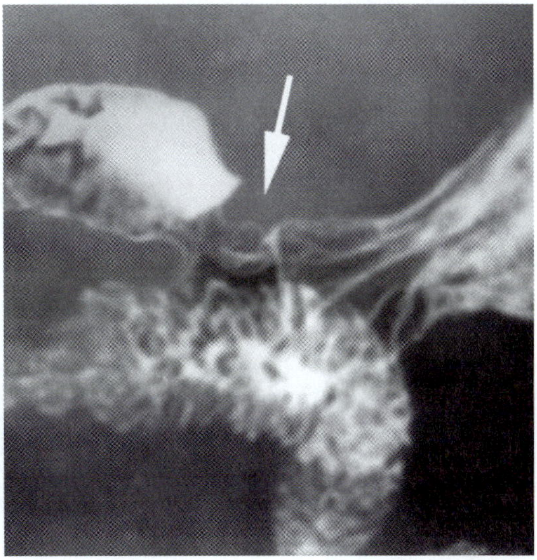

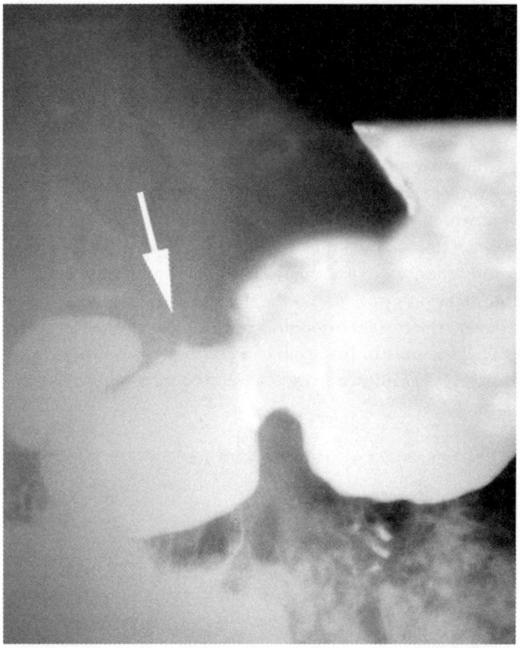

▲ Fig. 63 a.

Based on the definite prevalence of intramural growth of gastric cancer (diffuse and mixed forms), the presence of peristaltic activity as a sign excluding infiltration is not regarded today as a proof of its absence. Our experience shows that the intramural infiltration (not exceeding 3–4 cm) is often somewhat leveled owing to vigorous peristaltic activity of the neighboring parts of the stomach wall [33, 34, 58].

It is from these same standpoints that it is necessary to evaluate the various pharmacological drugs now widely used in radiological studies of the stomach to intensify or suppress peristaltic activity of the stomach walls. We conduct radiological examinations of the stomach based on a physiological approach which rules out any pharmacological drugs.

Using a contrast medium, and based on our experience with traditional radiological examination of the stomach, which combines the elements of tight filling and double contrast, we decided to use the double-contrast examination as the basic and the only suitable method. However, as we gained experience in combining tight filling of the stomach with double-contrast examination, we became convinced that the optimal method of radiological examination of the stomach is the one which allows visualization of the stomach contours at the phase of tight filling and estimation of stomach wall thickness using double contrast. Double contrast of the stomach

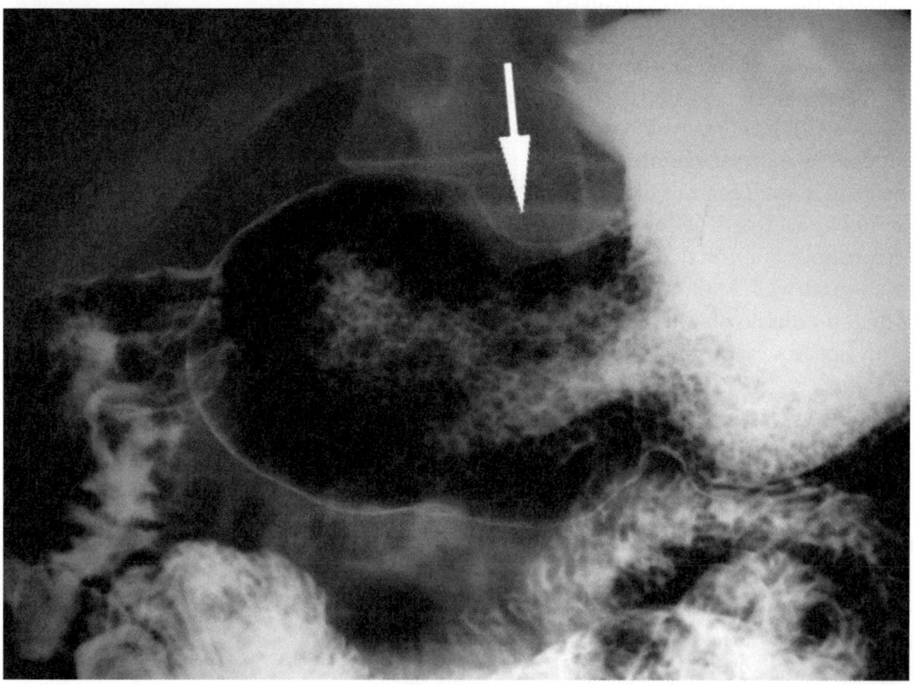

◄ Fig. 63 b.

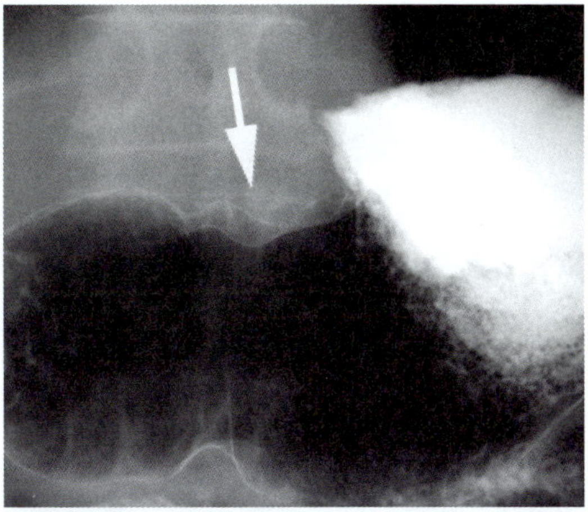

▲ **Fig. 63 c.**

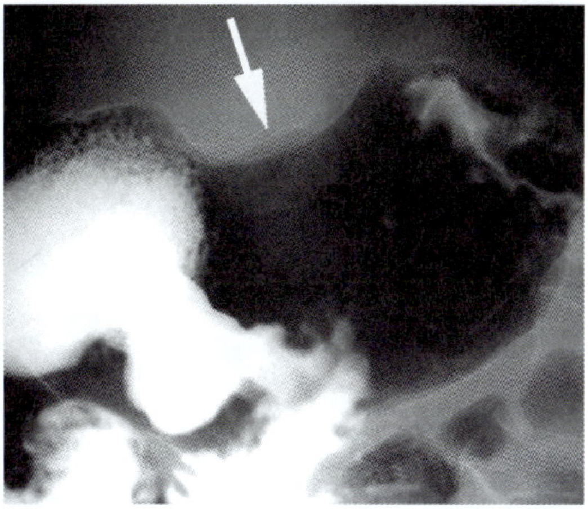

▲ **Fig. 63 e.**

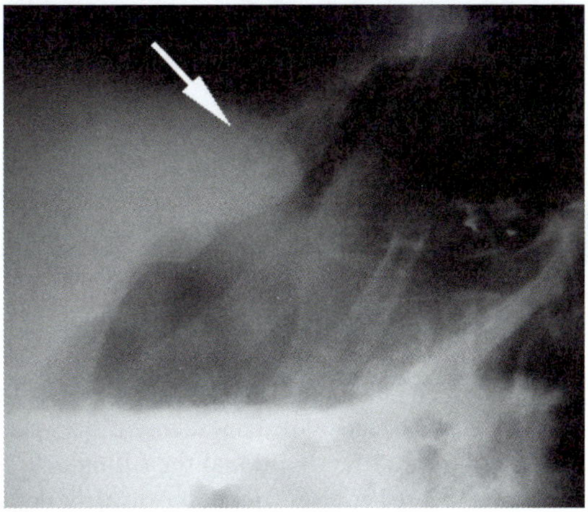

▼ **Fig. 63 d.**

can sometimes give wrong information on the presence of infiltration of the wall at its relatively early stage (2–3 cm). This is most typical for the prepyloric part of the stomach and the greater curvature. Today, tight filling of the stomach must be a prerequisite element of examination by traditional radiology [28].

While using contrast media for double contrasting of the stomach, we always examine a tightly filled stomach first; to this end, the patient often has to take two portions of the medium. Then we can examine a tightly filled stomach and obtain adequate double contrast [31].

Let us name some X-ray signs of gastric cancer which were established by researchers in the first half of the twentieth century. It is known that the X-ray picture of gastric cancer is quite varied and depends on the macro-morphological type of the tumor, the phase of growth, and localization of the lesion. Holzknecht and Jonas were the authors of the first book dedicated to the roentgenosemiotics of gastric cancer, published in Vienna in 1908. The filling defect, the classical sign of gastric cancer, was first described in detail in this monograph. The authors also described another specific sign of blastomatous affection of the stomach wall – the absence of peristalsis in the involved zone – but they did not fully appreciate its diagnostic importance [147]. The third sign, the so-called atypical relief associated with cancer, was established much later, when the method of studying mucosal relief was established. In 1911, Elischer made the first attempt to obtain an X-ray picture of the tumor surface in gastric cancer patients. But it was only at the end of the 1920s and in the early 1930s that the method of examining relief was acknowledged as an obligatory component of examination of the stomach where gastric cancer is suspected [117].

Beginning with the first publications dealing with X-ray examination of the stomach, the so-called filling defect was believed to be the direct sign of new growth as a result of visualization of the tumor node against the background of the stomach cavity filled with a contrast medium according to the classical methodology. For many decades the filling defect remained the main sign of exophytic tumors as well as of the mixed forms. It was only after the appearance of publications describing early cancer that the term polypoid formation started to replace the term

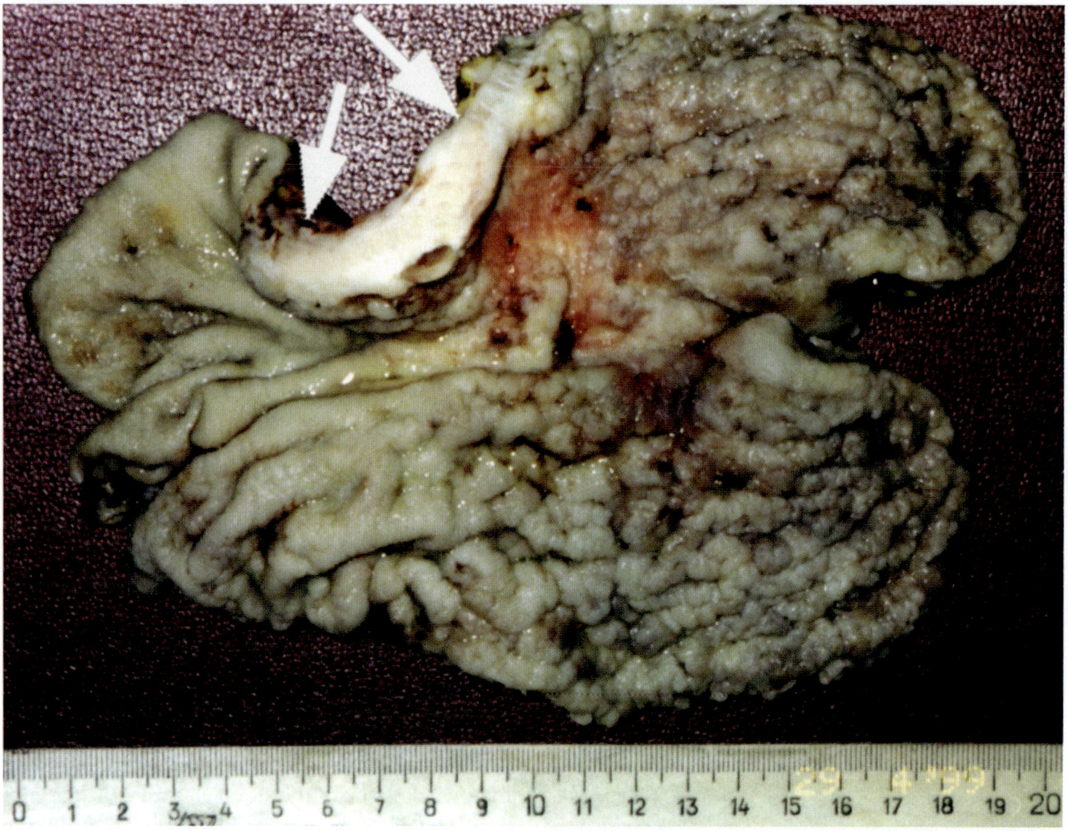

▲ Fig. 63 f.

Fig. 63a–h. Patient K., age 53. Diagnosis: gastric cancer. Complaints of epigastric discomfort after small meals, rapid satiability during the preceding 6 months. The patient lost 8 kg over a 3-month period. Roentgenological examination: **a** Stomach roentgenogram (tight filling, vertical position, right half-oblique projection): uneven contour of the lesser curvature of the antral part of the stomach (arrow); peristalsis over the entire length. **b, c** Stomach roentgenogram (double contrast, horizontal position, anterior projection): the walls are thickened due to intramural infiltration (arrow); peristalsis is visible. **d** Stomach roentgenogram (double contrast, vertical position, left oblique projection): the anterior wall of the stomach is thickened due to intramural infiltration (arrow). **e** Stomach roentgenogram (double contrast, horizontal position, left lateral projection): the anterior wall of the stomach is thickened and rigid due to intramural infiltration (arrow). Conclusion: Infiltrative gastric cancer. Despite considerable length of the lesion, peristalsis is seen on a series of X-rays. **f** Macrospecimen of a resected stomach: the wall is firm due to intramural tumor infiltration (arrows). **g** Fragment of a macrospecimen (strip): the wall is thickened due to tumor infiltration (black arrow). The muscular coat of the wall is unchanged (white arrows). **h** Microspecimen of a fragment of the stomach wall: non-differentiated cancer with initial invasion of the muscular coat

filling defect, because of disagreement between small lesions and the traditional the filling defect concept, and also because of development of the double-contrast technique.

Although we regard the filling defect as one of the most important signs of gastric cancer in the diagnosis of infiltrative tumors, we must admit that its use is limited. It is decisive in determining mostly the exophytic component of the tumor, which, in the current concept of gastric cancer morphology, is of limited importance. Every tumor has an exophytic component, but the infiltrative forms, with a much higher incidence than expansive tumors, are manifested by such insignificant changes on the mucosal surface that it is practically impossible to detect them. As radiological methods of studying the stomach gradually improved, these limitations, which were characteristic of the traditional method of tight filling, were gradually removed. With introduction of the double-contrast technique, the filling defect lost its former significance. And it

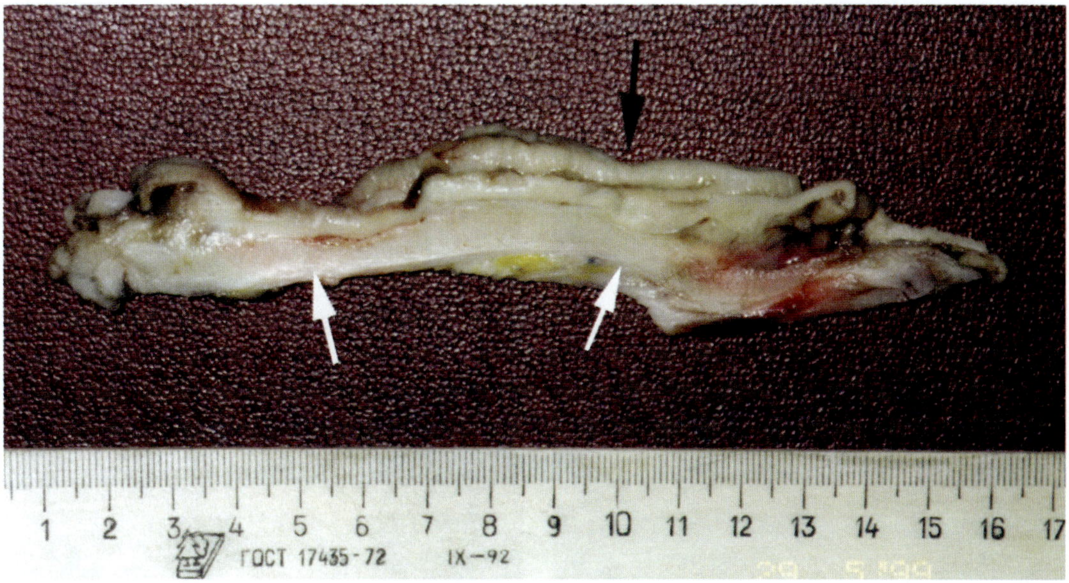

▲ Fig. 63 g.

▼ Fig. 63 h.

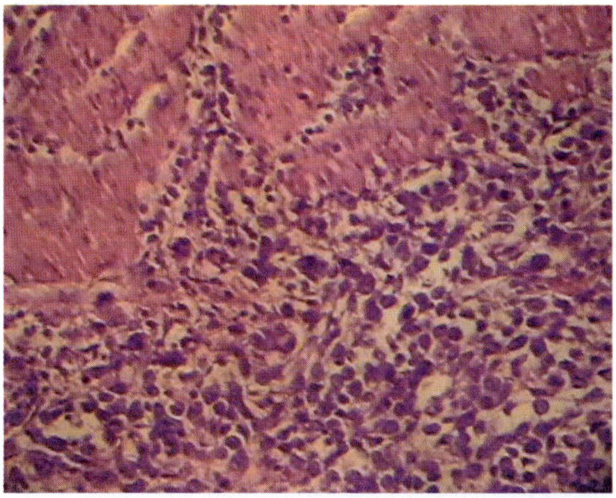

acquires a completely new meaning when the elements of the classical methods (tight filling) and double contrast are combined. Ingestion of barium suspension in a slightly greater amount for a greater contrast helps reveal an insignificant depression or unevenness of the stomach contour. This is an important addition to the other manifestations of infiltrative cancer and facilitates diagnosis to a greater degree of reliability.

Let us point out once again that the absence of peristalsis is a threatening sign, suggesting a considerable (as regards depth and area) affection of the stomach wall with involvement of the muscular coat. Minor endophytic cancer, located mostly in the submucous coat, does not invade the muscular coat and therefore does not affect peristalsis. For this reason, the presence of peristalsis does not rule out endophytic cancer (◘ Fig. 63).

The main relief element characteristic of gastric cancer is the so-called relief defect. But this term should not be likened to the filling defect. As stated above, the requisite condition for visualizing the filling defect is tight filling of the stomach with a contrast medium. What is necessary for a relief defect is adequate impregnation of the mucous membrane with a thin layer of contrast medium. In some cases, a relief defect is devoid of any pattern; in others it has its own pathological pattern, which in most cases is connected with impregnation of the ulcer crater. Each defect is a limited elevation on the inner surface of the stomach wall due to protrusion of the tumor into the stomach lumen. In essence, this is a tumor which is more or less elevated over the surface of the mucous membrane (exophytic or mixed tumor).

When the inner surface of the stomach is examined using a thin layer of contrast medium, the ordinary pattern of folds and furrows is absent. Instead, multiple indistinct defects appear on the relief; they are of various shapes and not isolated but, on the contrary, fuse (merge) to a lesser or greater extent. They are not fully separated, and there may be narrow or broad stripes of barium sulfate suspen-

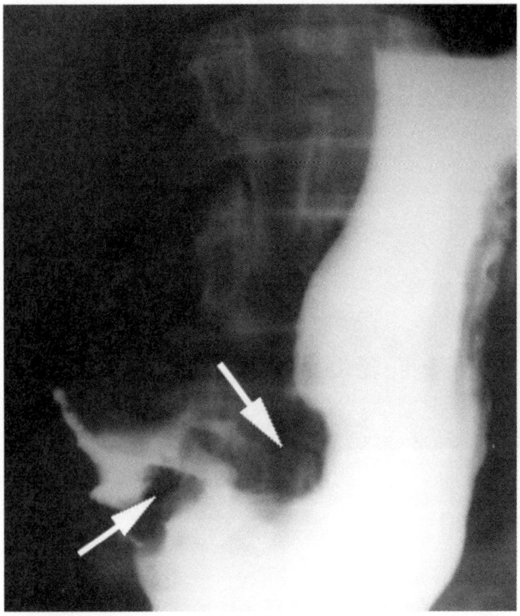

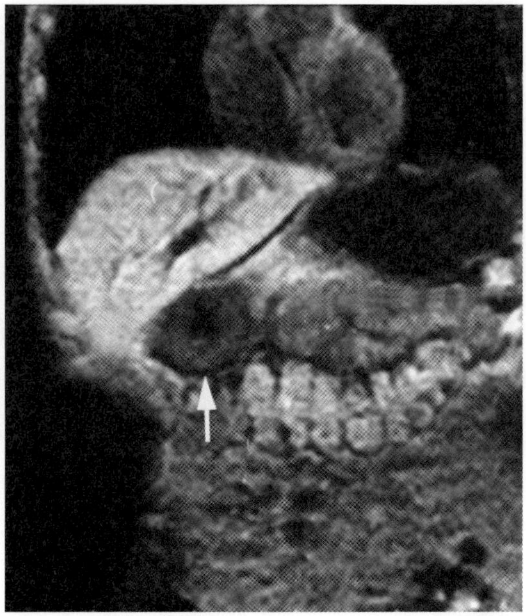

▲ **Fig. 64 a.** ▼ **Fig. 64 b.** ▲ **Fig. 64 c.**

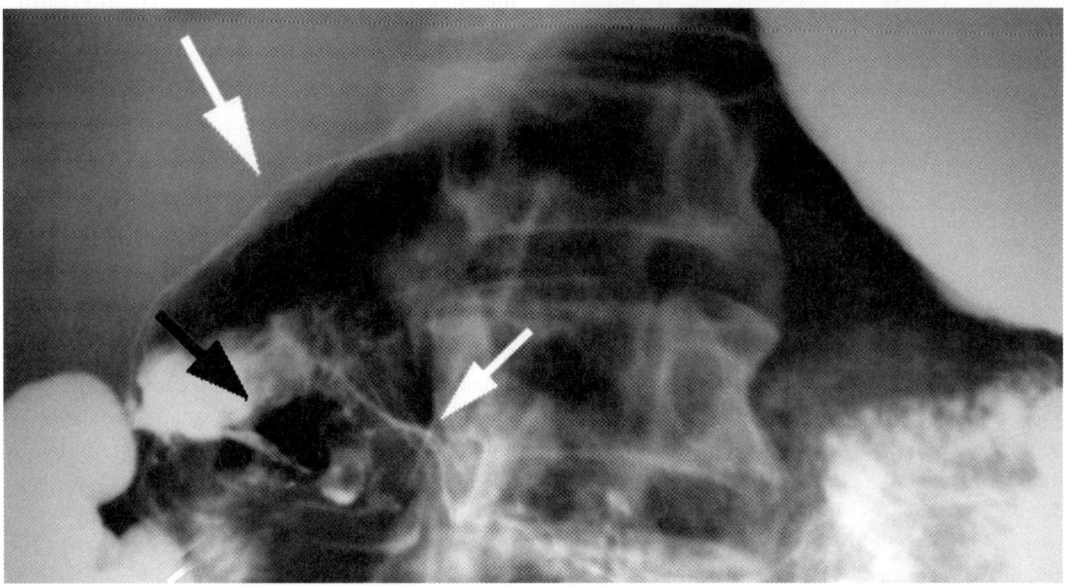

Fig. 64a–e. Patient R., age 67. Diagnosis: gastric cancer. **a** Stomach roentgenogram (tight filling, vertical position, anterior projection): markedly disfigured pyloric part of the stomach; uneven and eroded contours, the angular notch straightened (arrows); **b** Stomach roentgenogram (double contrast, horizontal position, anterior projection): the walls of the distal part and thickened due to intramural infiltration (white arrows). Ulceration on the greater curvature of the antral part (black arrow). Conclusion: Infiltrative-ulcerous cancer of the distal part of the stomach. Histological examination of bioptates taken from the edges of the ulcer crater did not reveal the presence of tumor cells. The patient was examined by MRI. **c** MRI of the stomach (coronary projection, T1 image): the »ring« sign in the antral part, heterogeneous MR signal from the infiltration ridge (arrow). **d** MRI of the stomach (coronary projection, T2 image): hyperintensive signal from water in the ulcer crater (arrow). **e** MRI of the stomach (sagittal projection, T2 image): circular thickening of the antral part wall to 14 mm; heterogeneous MR signal from the wall (arrow). The patient was operated. Histologically, a non-differentiated cancer

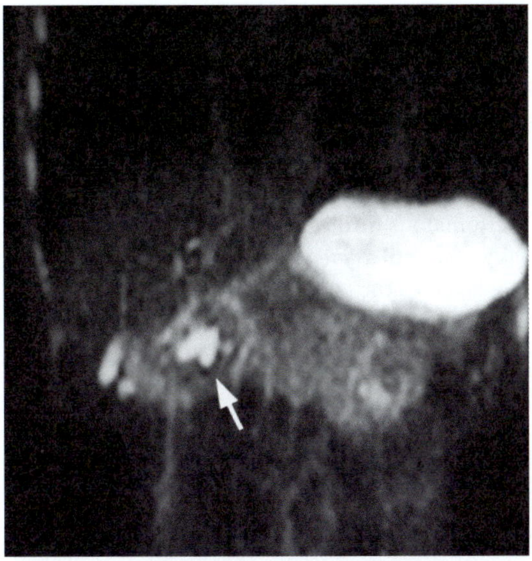

▲ **Fig. 64 d.**

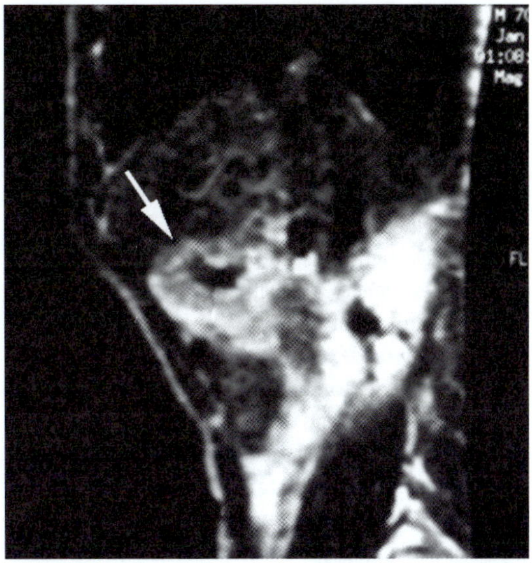

▲ **Fig. 64 e.**

sion which sort of trim the defects on the relief, to show their irregular contours (Fig. 64). Uneven in width and intensity, these stripes sometimes terminate, then appear again, before they finally disappear. They can narrow or widen to form stable shapeless spots of contrast medium resembling deep lacunas of sophisticated configuration. Regardless of the specificity of the pattern or the prevalence of this or that detail, the pathological relief is characterized by stability.

It is necessary to note again that this briefly described X-ray picture of the relief of the inner stomach surface is characteristic above all of the exophytic forms of cancer, the proportion of which is quite insignificant today, and also of its mixed forms. Unfortunately, in most cases it characterizes advanced forms of cancer, in which the tumor protrudes into the stomach lumen and has an irregular tuberous form, which interferes with studies at the pneumorelief phase. From the current standpoint of epidemiology and morphogenesis of gastric cancer, the study of the surface relief alone during X-ray examination does not meet the modern requirements of gastroenterology and must be regarded by radiologists only as an additional source of information supplementing the two basic radiological signs, namely, uneven contours with tight filling and thickening of the stomach walls with the double-contrast technique (Fig. 65).

Nevertheless, practical radiological diagnosis still often tends to be based upon the known triad of signs, count today, unfortunately, as the so-called general roentgenosemiotics of gastric cancer. The triad includes the filling defect, due to sufficiently large exophytic tumor; the absence of peristaltic activity of the stomach walls in the region of blastomatous infiltration; and, finally, atypical mucosal relief. The practitioners examine the patient for the presence of these three signs without considering the morphological form or stage of the cancer.

We think that the three main signs mentioned above provide no valuable diagnostic information. In the overwhelming majority of cases, these signs indicate only the presence of a tumor in the advanced stage. Moreover, they are sometimes not detectable even in patients with advanced disease. For example, circular affection of the antral part of the stomach completely rules out the symptom of atypical relief, and affection of the posterior wall is often accompanied by almost complete absence of an aperistaltic zone.

Generally speaking, the signs which were described later, such as termination of folds at the tumor border or the »hoop« symptom, described by Knothe, are characteristic only of exophytic forms of gastric cancer, which occur far less frequently. If we want to be more objective, we should point out that purely exophytic forms do not exist today. The

X-ray picture of diffuse (endophytic) cancer, especially of its early manifestations, has little in common with the »classical triad« of signs; to be more exact, it has nothing in common [31, 37].

Only some of the earlier established symptoms of gastric cancer remain significant today. They have been described in the literature sufficiently well, and therefore we mention some only to remind the reader of their existence. These include microgastria, various deformities of the stomach (hourglass, rigid tube, rigid cascade, cancer canal, etc.), limited displacement of the stomach, depressed and short lesser curvature, increased or decreased angle of the gastric notch, increased stomach–spinal column and stomach–diaphragm distances, disordered (accelerated or slowed down) evacuation, rigidity of the stomach walls, stronger contour contrast, ulcer niche in a »dry« stomach, bald or leveled mucosal relief, rigid relief, floating splinter, resilient »corset bone«.

It has long been known that only radical operative treatment can help the patient, and this concept is not disputed. For this reason, roentgenooncology in the second half of the twentieth century developed in the direction of revealing minor forms of gastric cancer.

Tight filling of the stomach has become an indispensable component of any modern X-ray examination of the stomach. Supplemented by the double-contrast technique, it markedly increases the chance of obtaining the necessary diagnostic information and significantly aid in forming the diagnosis. We are convinced that with a tightly filled stomach, one can reveal the specific signs of gastric tumor, including its initial forms. This becomes especially important in patients with endophytic cancer, but it requires complete rejection of the principles aimed exclusively at searching for intestinal forms of cancer. Under certain conditions of X-ray examination, malignant infiltrations, which disfigure the contour of the stomach, can characterize spread of the new growth and its properties – the exophytic component, ulceration, the nature of infiltration (circular or a rigid spot, etc). In diffuse (mostly submucous) cancer, the relief pattern of the mucosa is normal, or nearly normal, depending on individual properties. Blastomatous infiltration spreads mostly intramurally, and until a given moment does not involve surface layers of the mucous membrane proper. In this case, the mucosal relief which is visualized by an

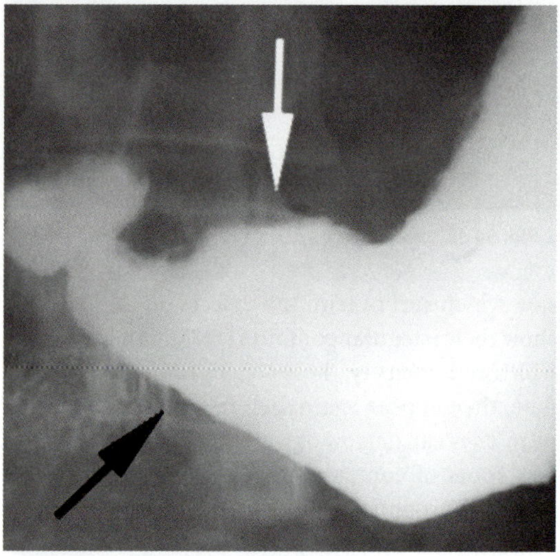

▲ **Fig. 65 a.** ▼ **Fig. 65 b.**

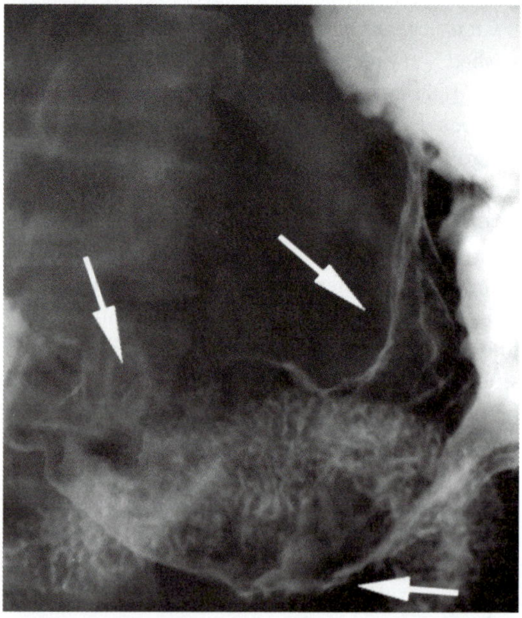

Fig. 65a, b. Patient B., age 62. Diagnosis: gastric cancer. **a** Stomach roentgenogram (tight filling, vertical position, anterior projection): the wall of the greater curvature of the distal part of the stomach is straightened and rigid (black arrow), peristalsis is seen over the lesser curvature of the distal part, the symptom of a floating splinter (white arrow). **b** Stomach roentgenogram (double contrast, horizontal position, anterior projection): diffuse thickening and rigidity of the walls in the distal part due to circular intramural infiltration (arrows). Conclusion: Infiltrative cancer of the distal part of the stomach and its body

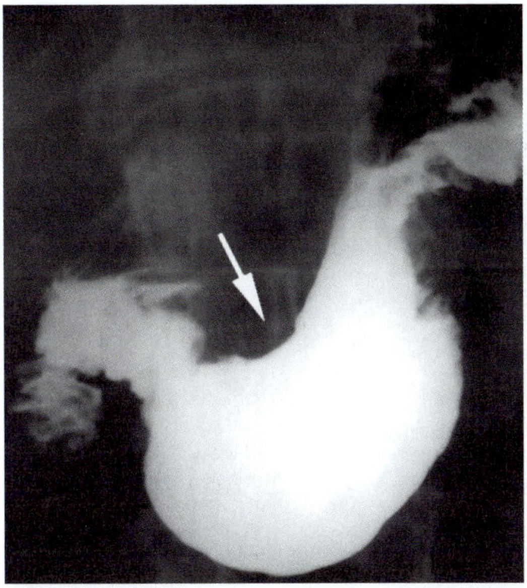

▲ **Fig. 66 a.**

endoscopist is formed at the expense of the mucous membrane proper, which overlies the tumor. The mucous membrane itself in such cases shows signs of dystrophy. As the tumor progresses, the mucosal cover thins, the dystrophic process increases, and all coats of the mucous membrane are eventually replaced by the tumor tissue. The relief pattern persisting on the inner surface of the stomach is characteristic of the early stages of infiltrative cancer. For a long time, these stages of infiltrative cancer were unknown to many roentgenologists, despite attempts to establish standard roentgenosemiotics (◘ Fig. 66).

We fully agree with R. Gutmann, who wrote in his monograph »Sur les cancers gastriques imiscibles a l'operation« (1960) that, contrary to common opinion, early X-ray diagnosis of gastric cancer is feasible in most cases [132]. He stresses that in some cases, early affection of the gastric mucosa can

◘ **Fig. 66a–d.** Patient A., age 67. Diagnosis: gastric cancer. **a** Stomach roentgenogram (tight filling, vertical position, anterior projection): uneven contours of the lesser curvature, depression in the form of a platform of about 2 cm with characteristic serration by the margins showing the borders of intramural infiltration (arrow). **b** Stomach roentgenogram (double contrast, horizontal position, anterior projection): wall of the stomach body is thickened over a length of about 3 cm, rigid due to intramural infiltration (arrow). Conclusion: Minor infiltrative cancer of the angular notch. **c** Macrospecimen of a resected stomach: stomach wall is thickened, a small navel-like depression with visually unaltered converging folds of the stomach mucosa (arrows). **d** Fragment of a macrospecimen (strip): the stomach wall is thickened over a distance of about 3 cm due to intramural infiltration of the submucous coat (arrows). Histologically, adenocarcinoma with the signet-ring cell component.

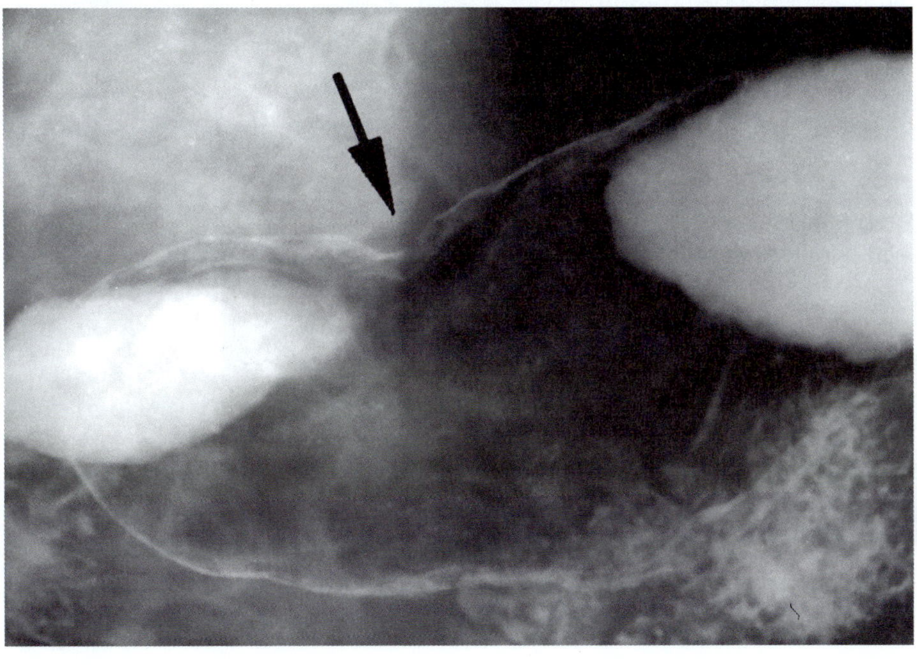

◄ **Fig. 66 b.**

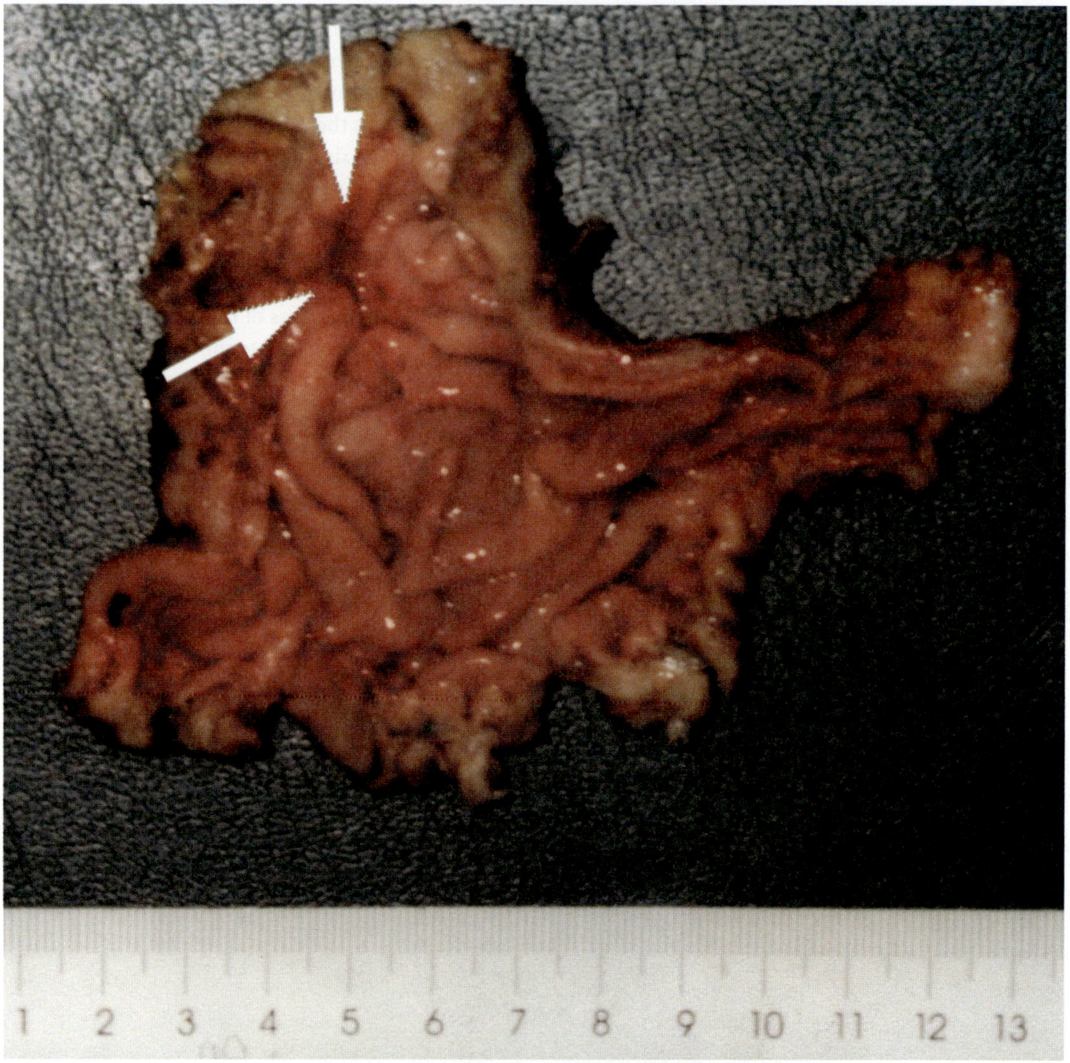

▲ **Fig. 66 c.**

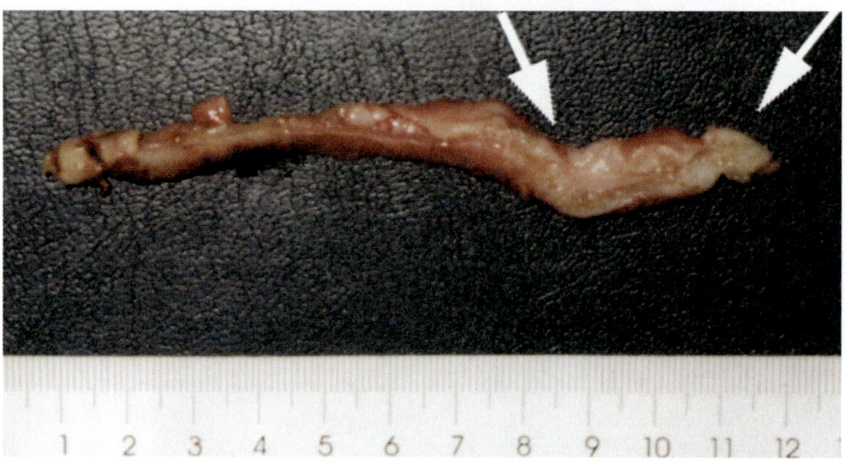

◂ **Fig. 66 d.**

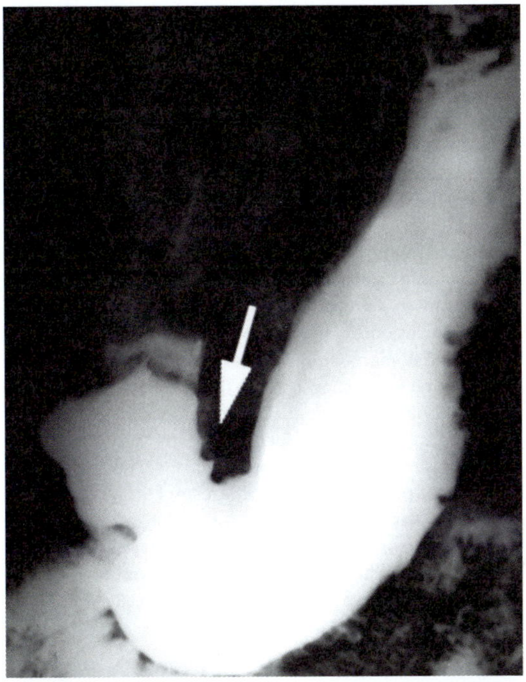

▲ **Fig. 67 a.** ▼ **Fig. 67 b.**

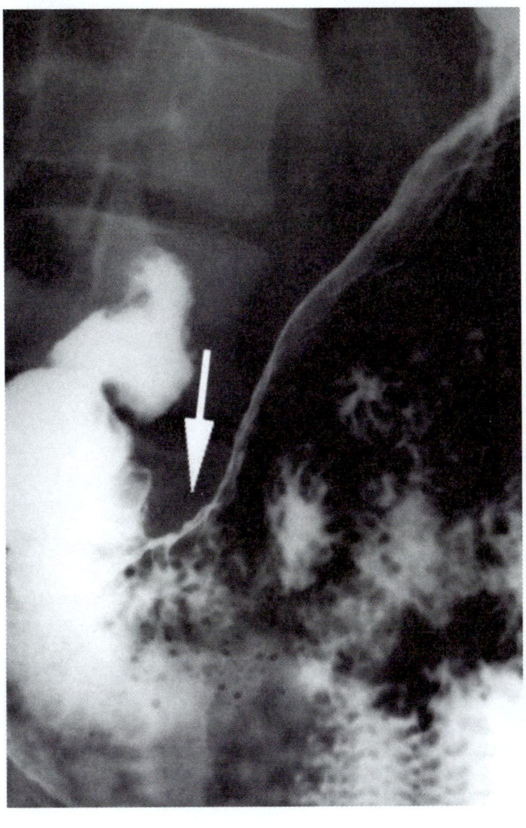

remain unnoticed by the surgeon during intraoperative palpation of the stomach walls and even during visual examination of its inner surface. We have also observed similar situations, where early signs of endophytic cancer detected by X-ray examination were impalpable during surgery. If the stomach was resected at the request of an X-ray expert, the intramural infiltration was verified only after thorough morphological examination of the resected material. If resection was declined, in several months it became necessary to perform another operation following endoscopic and mainly histological confirmation of gastric cancer. This gives us the right to state that, in such situations, radiological diagnosis is of greater diagnostic importance. It must be used as substantiation of radical surgical intervention (◘ Fig. 67). And this requires radical revision of some standards to establish relationships between radiological diagnosis and endoscopy in gastroenterology and gastro-oncology (◘ Fig. 68). ► chapter 6 deals with the objective evaluation of relationships between radiological diagnosis and endoscopy.

We have already noted that two basic X-ray signs of gastric cancer are recognized today:

1. The uneven contour of a tightly filled stomach: Sometimes this sign is revealed when a patient ingests contrast medium in a slightly greater amount than the standard recommendation.
2. A thickened stomach wall as visualized with double-contrast radiology. This is evidenced by the »ring« sign characteristic of the presence of intramural blastomatous infiltration (◘ Figs. 69, 70).

◘ **Fig. 67a, b.** Patient G., age 63. Diagnosis: gastric cancer. **a** Stomach roentgenogram (tight filling, vertical position, anterior projection): uneven contours of the lesser curvature of the antral part (arrow); peristalsis is seen over the entire length. **b** Stomach roentgenogram (double contrast, horizontal position, anterior projection): the wall of the lesser curvature of the antral part is thickened and rigid due to intramural infiltration (arrow). Conclusion: Minor infiltrative cancer of the lesser curvature of the antral part of the stomach. Endoscopy with subsequent histological examination of bioptates failed to reveal tumor. Traditional roentgenological examination using double contrast gave grounds for surgery in the absence of histological verification. The patient was operated. Histologically, signet-ring cell carcinoma.

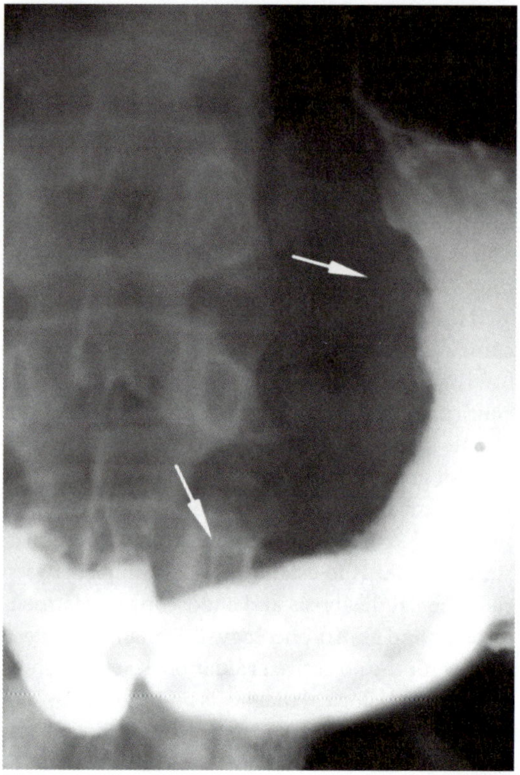

Fig. 68a–d. Patient Z., age 54. Diagnosis: gastric cancer. The patient had no complaints. From anamnesis: familial cases of gastric cancer. The primary roentgenological examination revealed gastric cancer. Endoscopy was performed several times within 2 months. Histological examinations of bioptates did not reveal tumor cells. **a** Stomach roentgenogram (tight filling, vertical position, anterior projection): the cavity of the antral part and the body of the stomach is reduced, the lesser curvature is short and depressed, uneven contours (arrows). **b** Stomach roentgenogram (double contrast, horizontal position, anterior projection): walls of the antral part and the body of the stomach are thickened due to intramural infiltration (arrows). Conclusion: Infiltrative cancer of the antral part and the body of the stomach. Histological examination of the bioptates taken during endoscopy failed to find tumor cells. Nevertheless, the convincing evidence of the presence of infiltrative affection of the stomach provided grounds for surgery in the absence of histological verification. **c** Macrospecimen: a fragment of a resected part of the stomach: the relief of the mucous membrane is leveled due to intramural infiltration (arrows). **d** Fragment of a macrospecimen (strip): the stomach wall is thickened due to tumor infiltration of mostly submucous and muscular coats of the stomach wall (arrows). Histologically, signet-ring cell carcinoma

▲ **Fig. 68 a.**

5

▼ **Fig. 68 b.**

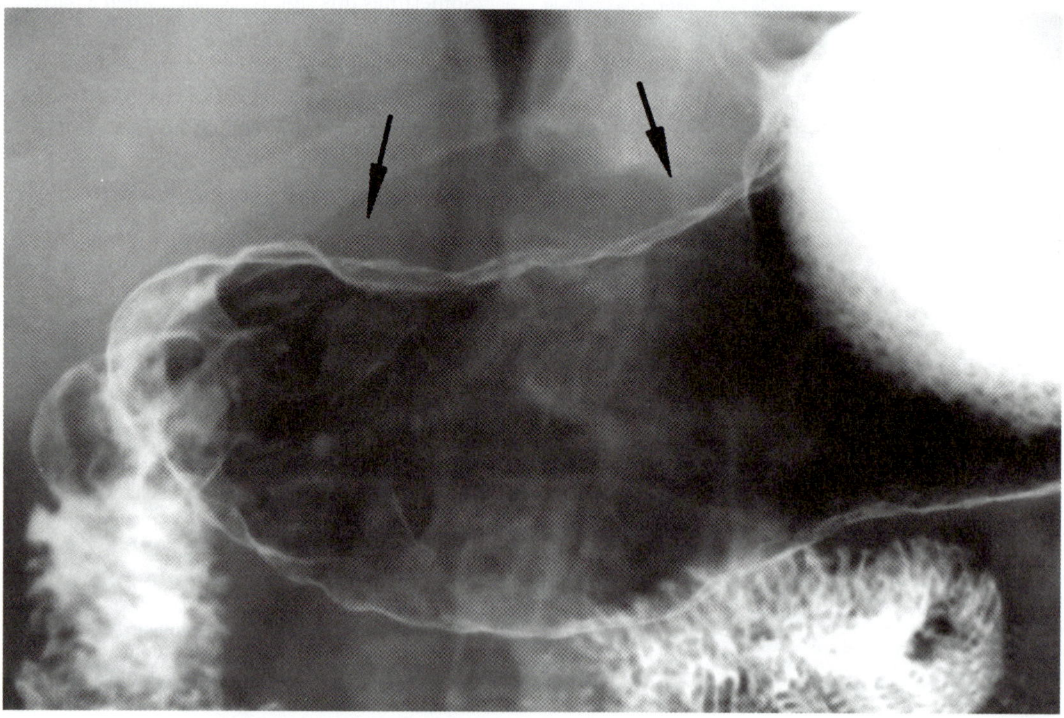

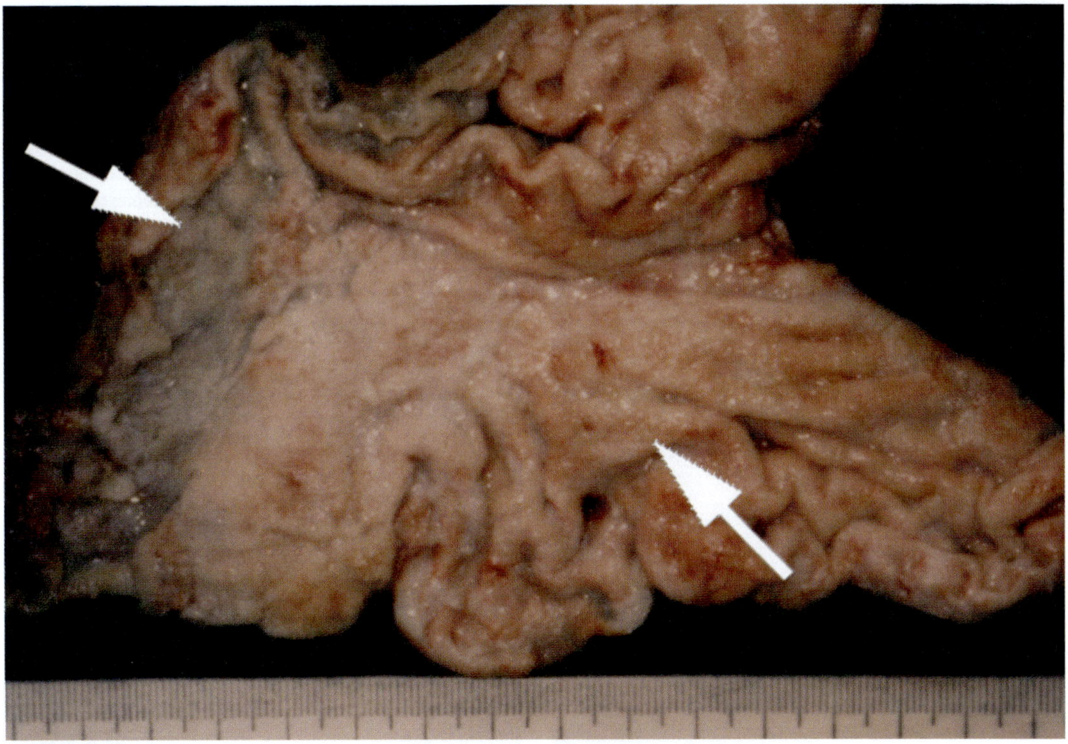

▲ **Fig. 68 c.**

▼ **Fig. 68 d.**

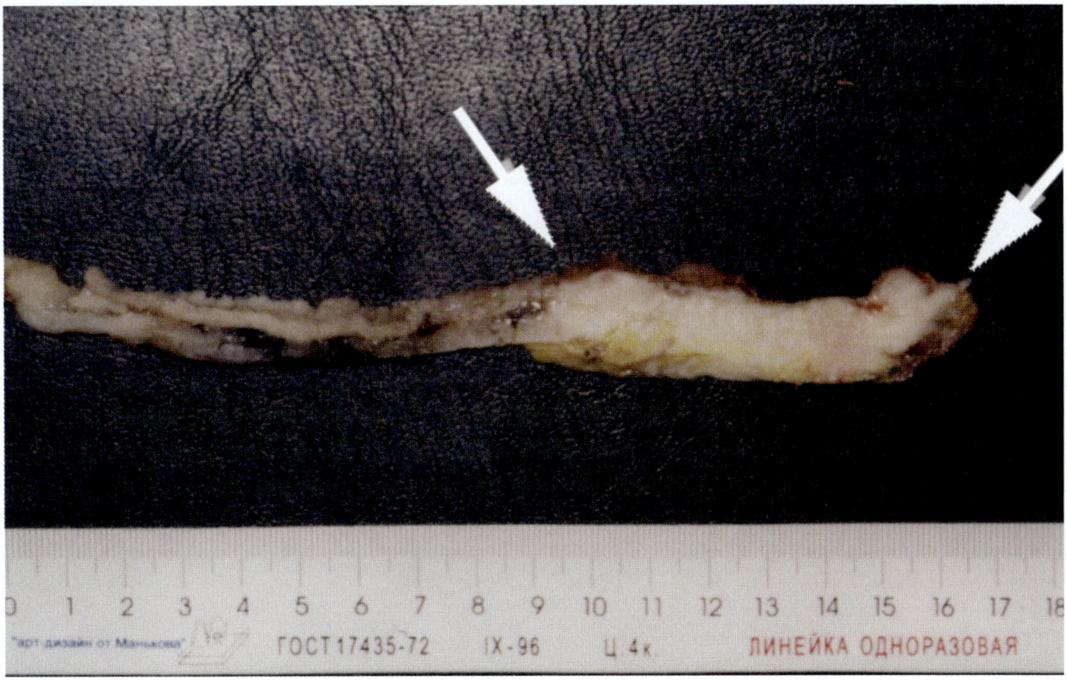

Fig. 69a–c. Patient K., age 65. Diagnosis: gastric cancer. **a** Stomach roentgenogram (vertical position, anterior projection): gas redistribution in the air bubble of the stomach; the stomach is stretched. **b** Stomach roentgenogram (tight filling, vertical position, anterior projection): the lesser curvature is short and depressed, the walls of the stomach are uneven and rigid (arrows). **c** Stomach roentgenogram (double contrast, horizontal position, anterior projection): the wall of the lesser curvature is thickened and rigid due to intramural infiltration (arrows), a depot of contrast medium with atypically changed relief of the inner surface of the stomach. Histological examination of the bioptates taken during numerous endoscopies failed to find tumor cells. Pneumogastography was used as an additional method of examination

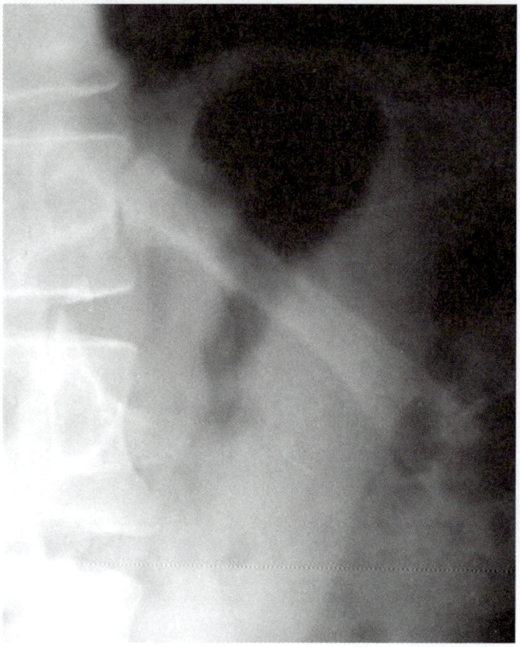

▲ **Fig. 69 a.**

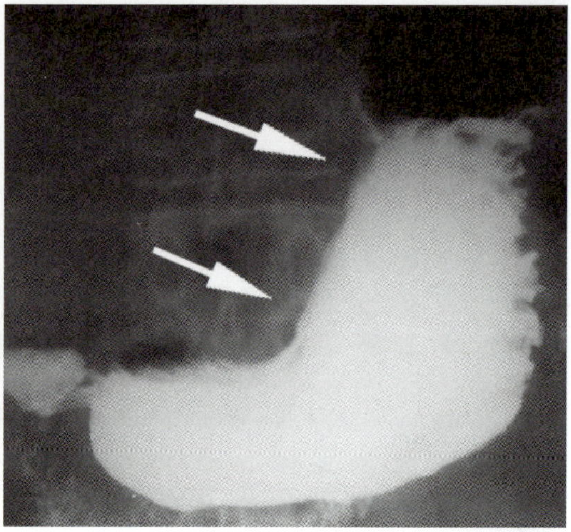

▲ **Fig. 69 b.**

▼ **Fig. 69 c.**

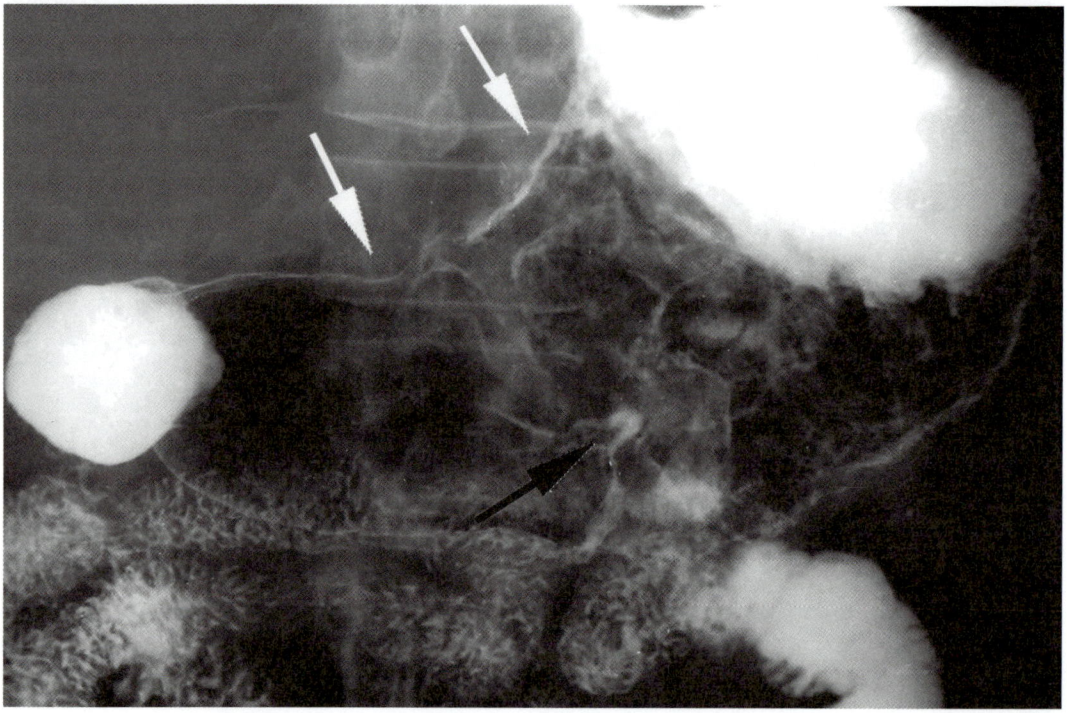

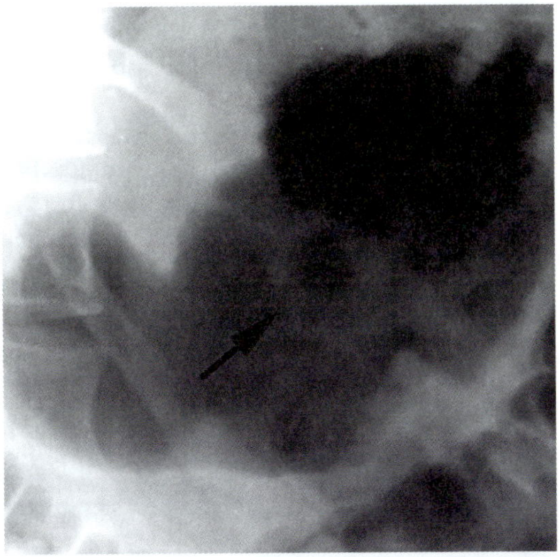

▲ **Fig. 70 a.**

▼ **Fig. 70 b.**

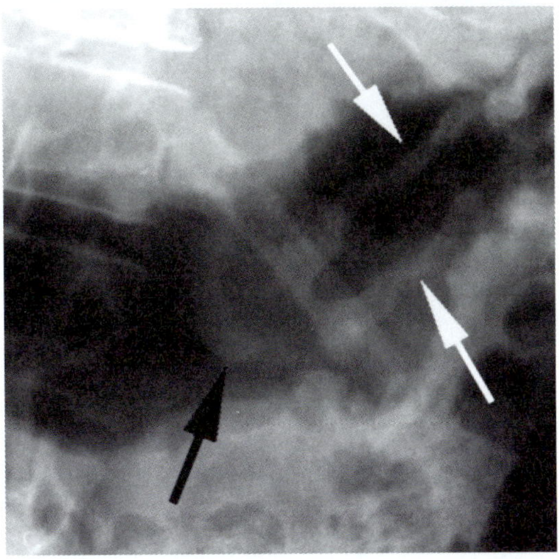

Fig. 70a–c. Same patient. Pneumogastrograms: distinctly seen is the 'ring' symptom due to the ridge of infiltration around the ulcer crater (black arrow) filled with air; converging folds are thick and outstretched due to the tumor spreading onto the upper part of the stomach (white arrows). Conclusion: Infiltrative-ulcerous cancer of the stomach body with invasion of the upper part. The patient was operated. Histologically, signet-ring cell carcinoma

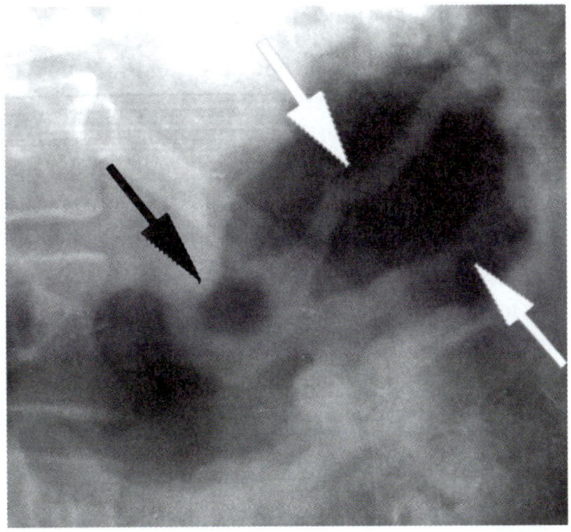

▲ **Fig. 70 c.**

The benefits of tight filling in infiltrative-ulcerous cancers of the stomach now become more apparent. The versatility of the tight-filling method helps correct the interpretation of the X-ray picture of the initial form of gastric cancer with uneven contours and protrusions in cases where double-contrast radiology fails to obtain the necessary information. Dosed compression in these situations makes it possible to examine a particular site of affection and to recognize reliable signs which may serve as criteria for a differential diagnosis of infiltrative-ulcerous cancer and peptic ulcer of the stomach. It is also possible to better visualize the specific changes in the stomach contour and deformities of the relief of the mucous membrane. While we consider tight filling very valuable, we do not want to say that it is better than double-contrast radiology: In order to detect endophytic forms of cancer and the early symptoms of any blastomatous process in the stomach, the greatest amount of information may be obtained using both methods.

The most important aim of research in the diagnosis of gastric cancer should be to reveal its minor forms. While the currently used definition of early gastric cancer is good from a purely practical standpoint, it should be noted that the potentials of radiological examination and endoscopy for verifying the depth of affection are limited. Deeper structures such as the muscular coat are often affected in tumor patients with typical signs of early gastric cancer. In other words, it can be considered proven that diagnosis of early cancer in its classical understanding (according to the endoscopic classification of 1962) is associated with certain difficulties of interpretation of the visible picture during preoperative determination of the depth of tumor invasion. To be more accurate, the diagnosis is not feasible. These circumstances, and the fact that surgery (the only radical way to treat the patient with subsequent pathomorphological examination) is the final method for determining the depth of invasion of the stomach wall, has led us to use the term »minor cancer« to characterize the initial manifestation [24, 25, 67, 68].

Minor cancer implies lesions of up to 1 cm. But the existing criteria of minor cancer of the stomach do not account for the specificity of the early manifestations of endophytic new growths. This is the weak point in our understanding of modern definition of gastric cancer signs, and hence in its diagnosis [25, 30].

There is, unfortunately, no consensus on the specific features of early blastomatous affection. Nor do we know what primary signs should be considered first by radiological diagnosis for early detection of cancer. The dispute is ungrounded. Again, it concerns the attempt to establish specific changes in the so-called fine relief of the mucosa, areolar zones, and the like. And again we want to declare that radiological diagnosticians should not be involved in this problem because the study of mucosal surfaces is the prerogative of endoscopists. The main objective of radiological studies, and especially of the traditional X-ray studies, should be to search for intramural blastomatous infiltration.

The characteristic radiological signs of minor cancer include uneven contours of the stomach over a short length of 1–3 cm, (which is detectable using tight filling) and thickening of the wall relevant to this part (detectable with double contrast). Rigidity of the stomach wall, which is characteristic of advanced forms of gastric cancer, is usually detectable with tumors 3–4 cm and larger. Such tumors are often affected by ulceration. In some cases, for more reliable results, it is necessary to swallow additional portions of contrast medium and to take a series of muti-projectional views. The usefulness of compression should also be noted: It facilitates the detection of converging folds, which are often found in patients with minor and mostly ulcerative cancer.

Double-contrast radiology is beneficial mainly for detection of minor cancer of the body and the upper part of the stomach. In some cases it gives detailed information on the character of changes in the distal part as well, especially in the presence of tumor infiltration resulting in thickening of the stomach wall, which is especially characteristic of endophytic cancer [58, 183].

Our experience in screening risk groups and asymptomatic persons for gastric cancer at MONIKI confirms the fact that a complex examination of the stomach, which includes tight filling and double contrast, should be regarded as the optimal method [58, 222].

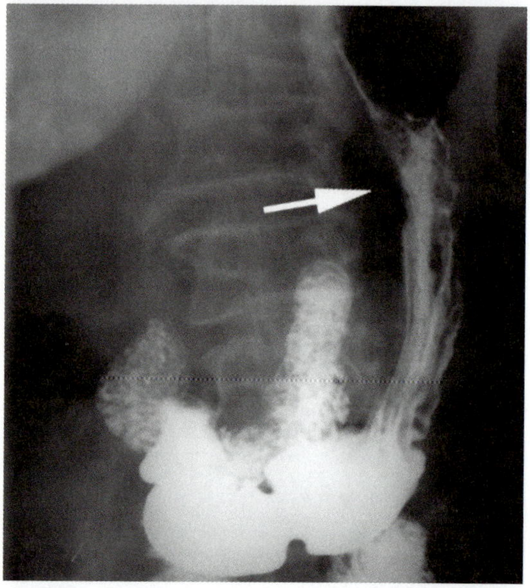

▲ **Fig. 71 a.**

For diagnosis of the early forms of infiltrative cancer, the accepted algorithm of examination must be directed not at endoscopic detection of disfiguring changes in the surface of the mucous membrane but at the search for an intramural blastomatous process, which is better detectable by X-ray examination. It has long been recognized that the complexity of forming a differential diagnosis only by the signs of pathological changes on the surface of the gastric mucosa makes it impossible in most cases to detect sufficiently specific differentiation criteria (Fig. 71).

Based on what has been said, we are now absolutely sure that the sign of intramural blastomatous infiltration (characterized by thickening of the stomach wall over a length up to 3 cm), which we proposed in 1993, should be considered the initial manifestation of gastric cancer [31].

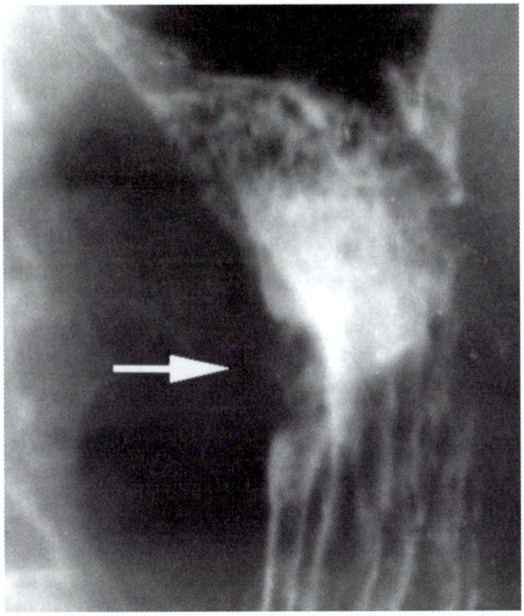

▲ **Fig. 71 b.**

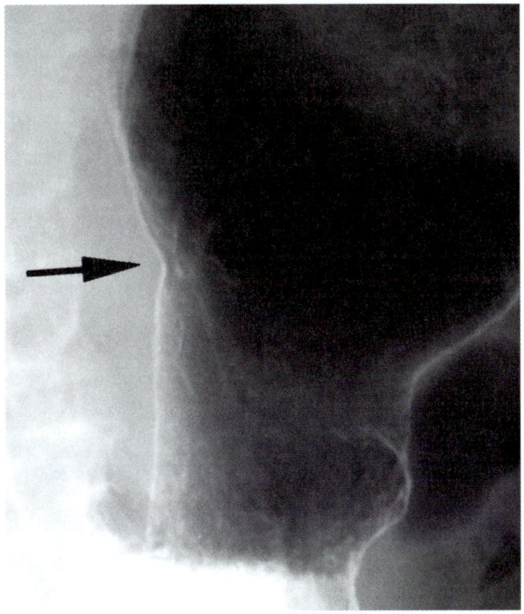

▲ **Fig. 71 d.**

▼ **Fig. 71 c.**

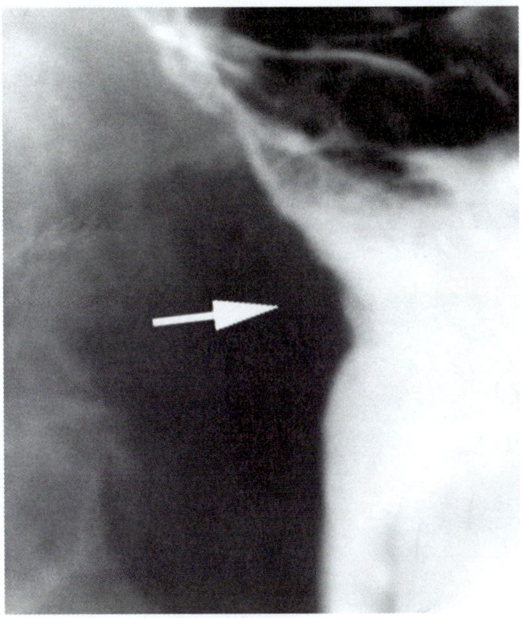

▼ **Fig. 71 e.**

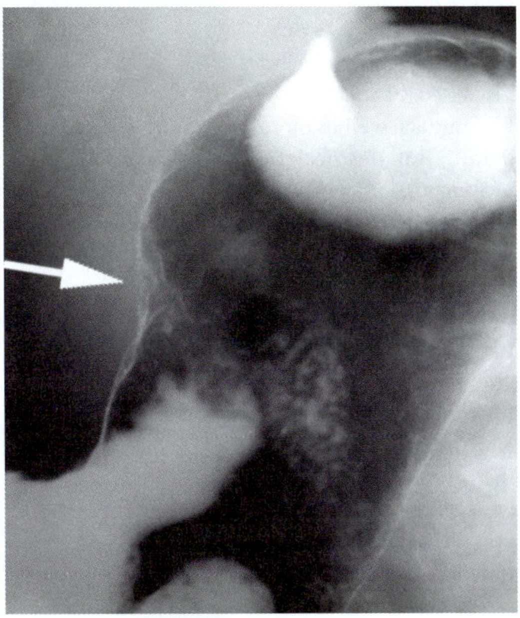

Fig. 71a–e. Female patient V., age 68. Diagnosis: gastric cancer. **a** Stomach roentgenogram (tight filling, vertical position, anterior projection): uneven contours of the lesser curvature of the upper third of the stomach body (arrow). **b, c** Stomach roentgenograms (tight filling, vertical position, anterior projection) after ingestion of an additional portion of barium sulfate suspension: more distinctly visualized are uneven and eroded contours of the lesser curvature of the upper third of the stomach body (arrow). **d** Stomach roentgenogram (double contrast, vertical position, anterior projection): the wall of the lesser curvature is rigid, the contour is slightly depressed into the stomach cavity (arrow). **e** Stomach roentgenogram (double contrast, horizontal position, left lateral projection): in the optimal projection, visualized is the thickened anterior wall due to intramural infiltration (arrow). Conclusion: minor infiltrative cancer of the anterior wall of the upper third of the stomach body. Histologically, adenocarcinoma with the signet-ring cell component.

Ultrasonographic Signs

In 1976, Lutz and Petzolt were the first to describe target ultrasonographic symptoms in a patient with gastric tumor: increased echogenicity of the central part of the stomach and decreasing echo toward the periphery [185]. The potentials of ultrasonographic studies in pathologies of the stomach were also studied by Russian researchers. Lemeshko proposed »the symptom of affection of a hollow organ« to designate the acoustic picture of changes in the gastrointestinal tract, in the stomach in particular [17]. However, sonographic signs (badge-cockade, target, affection of a hollow organ, etc) are characteristic of advanced forms of cancer and mostly of the intestinal type. Few publications of this period discussed the condition of the stomach wall in more detail. But despite the proven possibility of visualization of the stomach wall coat, appropriate significance was not attached to the new signs because the approach to sonographic diagnosis of gastric cancer was oriented to endoscopy, which was then dominant. It was only 10–15 years later, when morphological studies were started (in which diffuse cancer, characterized mostly by intramural growth, was given special importance) that publications appeared which evaluated the potentials of sonography under this new aspect. These publications radically changed the general attitude toward known signs of gastric cancer. Their authors tried to estimate the potential of sonography for characterizing the walls of an intact and affected stomach; and they proved that it was possible to visualize all coats of the stomach wall using ultrasound (Fig. 72) [31, 42, 49].

The known ultrasonographic signs of intramural tumor infiltration are based on the sonographic picture of an intact liquid-filled stomach which

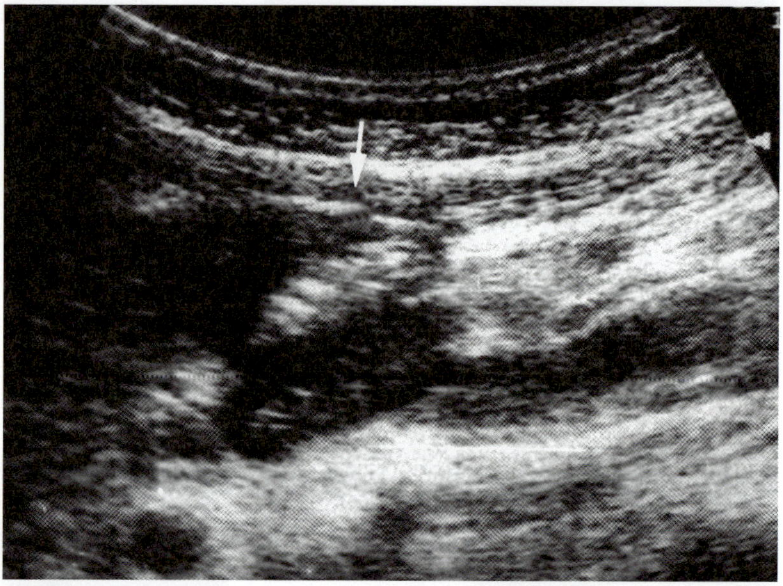

▲ Fig. 72 a.

▼ Fig. 72 b.

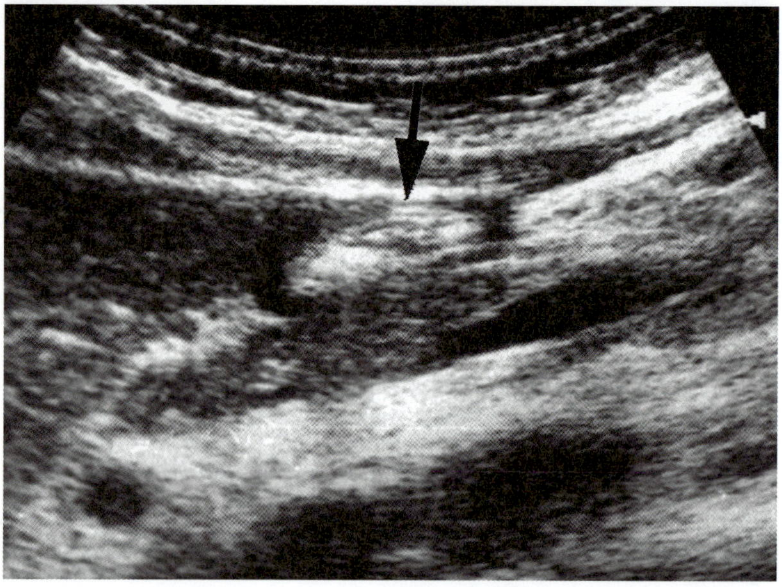

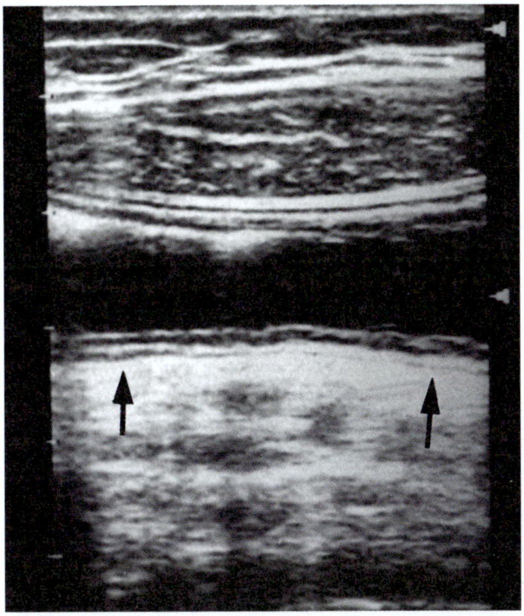

▲ Fig. 72 c.

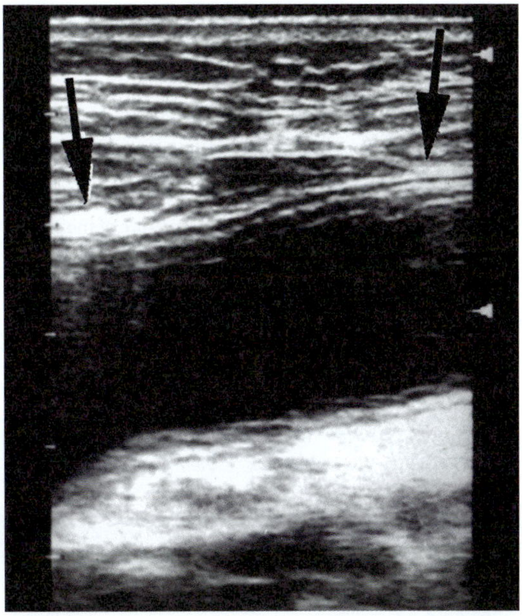

▲ Fig. 72 e.

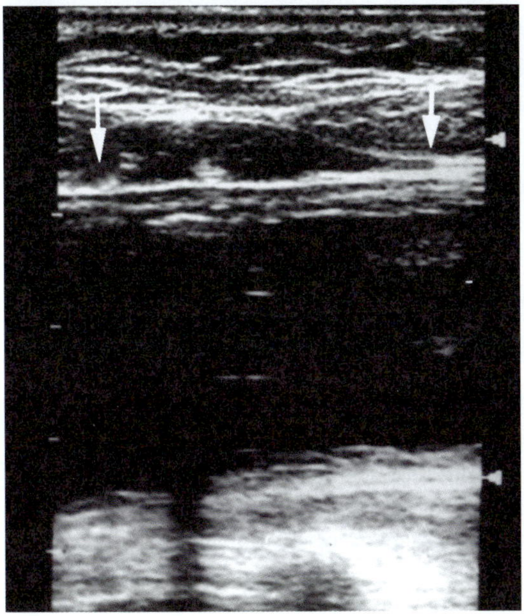

▼ Fig. 72 d.

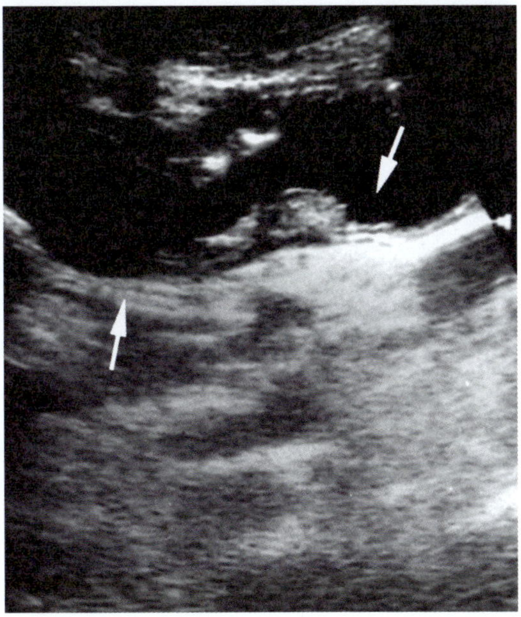

▼ Fig. 73.

appears as a five-layered structure with even contours and a thickness of 6–7 mm in the pyloric part and of 4–7 mm in the stomach body and its upper part [28, 38, 50, 53].

The main ultrasonographic symptoms of intramural blastomatous infiltration include thickened walls of the stomach in the involved region and a significantly changed five-layered structure at this level (Fig. 73). During ultrasound examination, wall thickness remains constant (absence of pseudo-thickening due to passage of a peristaltic wave). Thickness of the wall in the region of infiltration can be even or uneven. If the wall is to 8–10 mm thick it is normally uniform with even and distinct contours,

Fig. 72a–e. Ultrasonogram of a normal stomach. **a** Transverse echotomogram of the stomach (without filling with water, section at the level of the antral part): visualized are intact walls of the antral part of the stomach, to 6 mm thick (arrow). **b** Transverse echotomogram of the stomach (without filling with water, section at the level of the stomach body): intact wall of the stomach body, to 5 mm thick; the signal from the wall is hypoechogenic and homogeneous (arrow). **c** Transverse echotomogram of the stomach (the stomach cavity is filled with water, section at the level of the antral part): distinctly visualized in a five-layered structure of the stomach wall (arrows). **d** Transverse echotomogram of the stomach (the cavity of the stomach is filled with water, section at the level of the stomach body): distinctly visualized are all the five coats of the intact stomach wall (arrows). **e** Transverse echotomogram of the stomach (the stomach cavity is filled with water, section at the level of the upper part of the stomach, an additional projection): the five-layered structure of the stomach wall is intact (arrows)

Fig. 73. Patient N., age 62. Diagnosis: gastric cancer. Echotomogram of the stomach (the stomach cavity is filled with water, longitudinal section relative the stomach axis): the posterior wall is thickened to 9–12 mm over a length of 5 cm; the five-layered structure is absent (arrow)

Fig. 74. Patient R., age 68. Diagnosis: gastric cancer. Echotomogram of the stomach (the stomach cavity is filled with water, oblique section at the level of stomach body): local thickening of the stomach wall to 7–8 mm with disordered echo structure due to intramural infiltration over a length of 3 cm (arrows)

▼ Fig. 74.

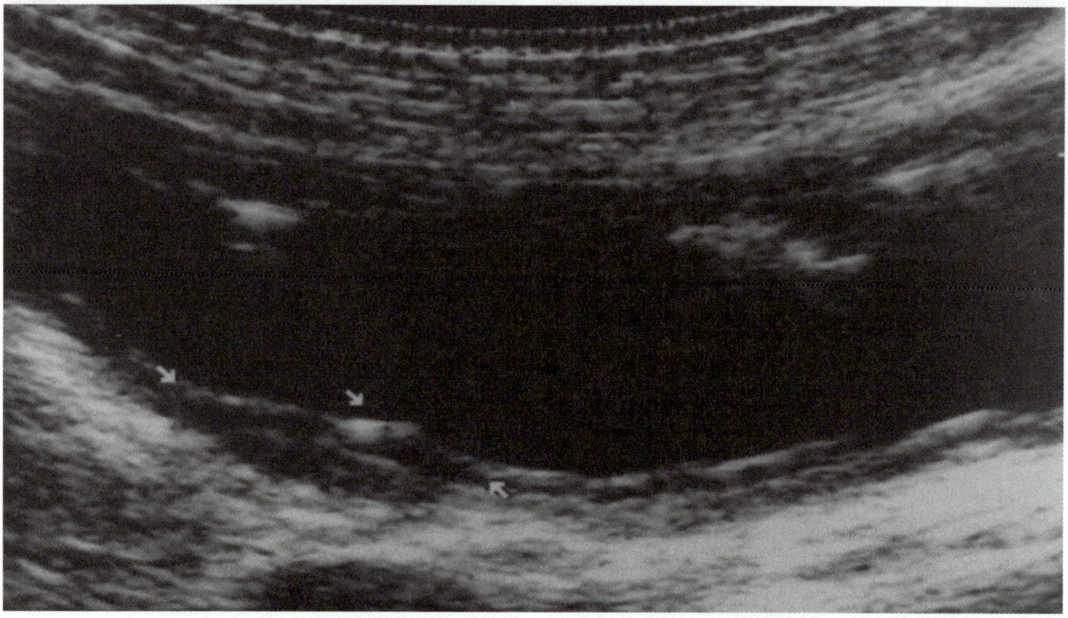

which is characteristic of a relatively early gastric cancer (Fig. 74). If the tumor spreads over a large area, the wall thickens to 15–20 mm; its inner contour is uneven and tuberous. Some patients, in addition to thick walls and changes in the five-layer structure, may also have a distinct exophytic component of the tumor protruding into the lumen of the stomach. If the tumor is located in the antral part of the stomach with involvement of all its walls, the ultrasonographic picture of the walls corresponds to the picture of the cancer canal (Fig. 75).

An important advantage of ultrasonography is that it can detect relatively early signs of gastric cancer extending over about 3 cm. Initial affection of the stomach wall attended by moderately pronounced but stable thickening and destruction of the layered structure is thus revealed (Fig. 76) [43, 50, 98]. While we value the potentials of ultrasonography in the diagnosis of gastric cancer, we nevertheless think that its staging potentials are limited; determination of stages I and II is best accomplished by morphological study of material from the resected stomach.

Our research showed that ultrasound reliably and distinctly recognized ulcers in the infiltrated wall of the stomach in patients in whom ulceration was discovered by X-ray and endoscopic examinations of the stomach (Fig. 77). In the presence of an ulcer crater greater than 10 mm, accumulated air can be determined in its central parts (Fig. 78).

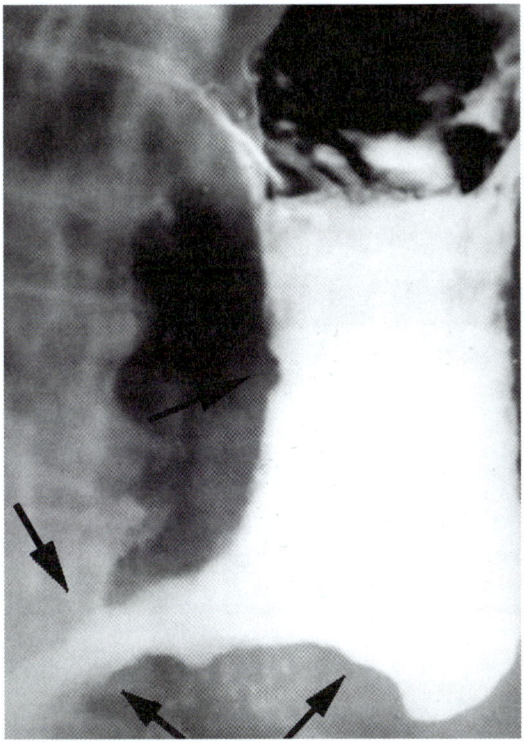

▲ Fig. 75 a.

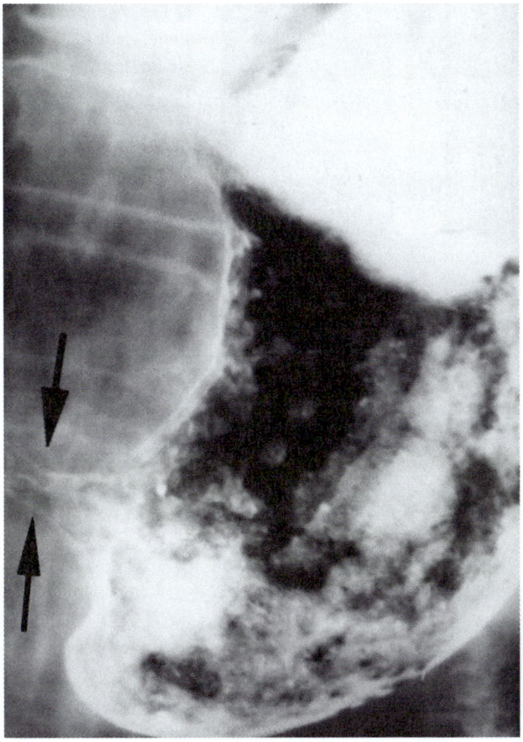

▼ Fig. 75 b.

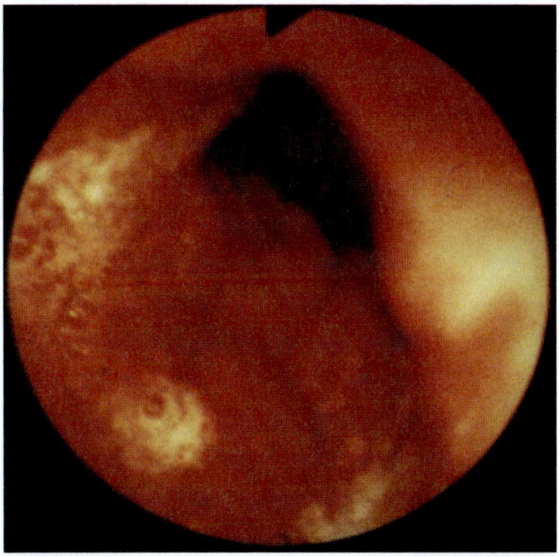

▲ Fig. 75 c.

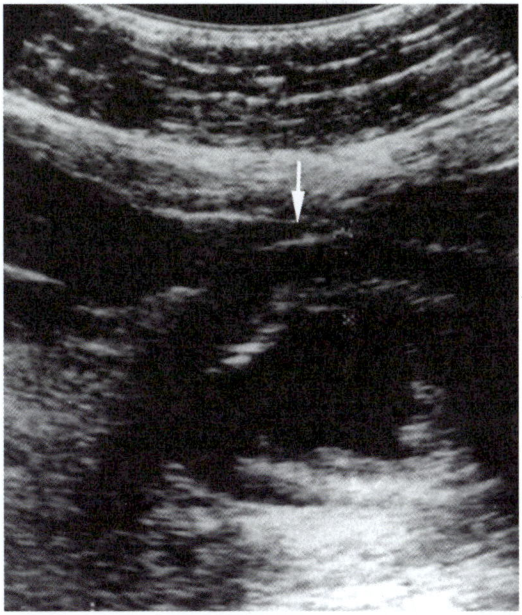

▼ Fig. 75 d.

Fig. 75a–e. Patient L., age 73. Diagnosis: gastric cancer. **a** Stomach roentgenogram (tight filling, vertical position, right quarter-oblique projection): the distal part unevenly narrowed, uneven contours due to a circular intramural infiltration, invading the stomach body by the lesser curvature (arrows).
b Stomach roentgenogram (double contrast, horizontal position, anterior projection): walls of the distal part are thickened and rigid due to circular intramural infiltration (arrows). Conclusion: Infiltrative cancer of the distal part of the stomach.
c Endophotograph: the mucous membrane of the greater curvature of the stomach sinus is strongly disfigured and tuberous, protrudes into the stomach lumen to narrow its lumen.

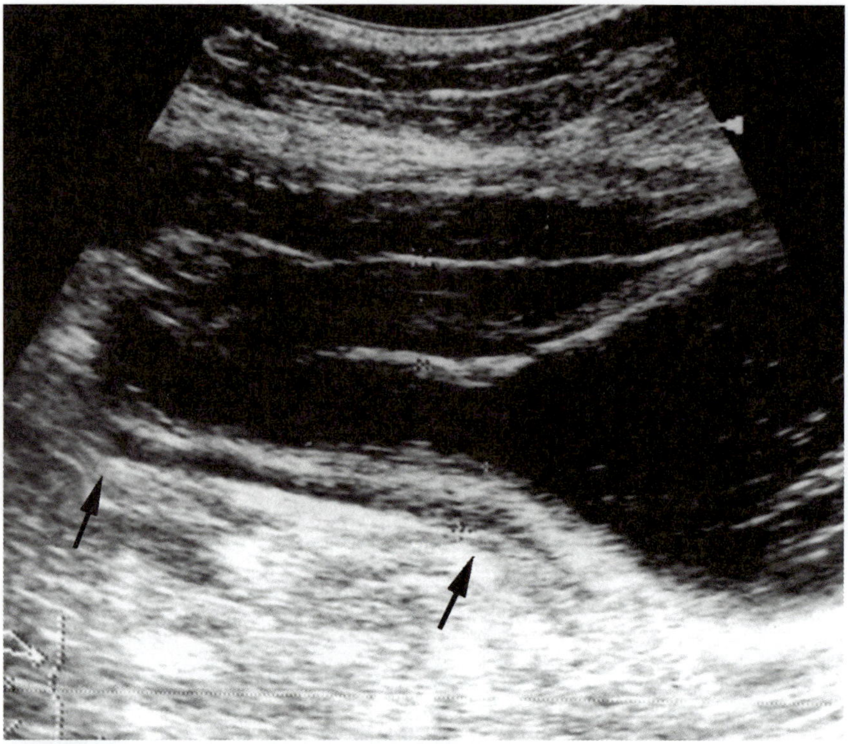

▲ Fig. 75 e.

Histological examination verified adenocarcinoma with the signet-ring cell component. **d** Echotomogram of the stomach (the stomach cavity is filled with water, the sagittal section at the level of the antral part of the stomach): the walls are thickened circularly and unevenly, the five-layered structure is disordered at this level (arrow). **e** Echotomogram of the stomach (the stomach cavity is filled with water, transverse section at the level of the pyloric part of the stomach): the lumen of the pyloric part is narrowed with formation of a cancer canal to 6 cm long, the walls are thickened to 7–5 mm (arrows)

▼ Fig. 76.

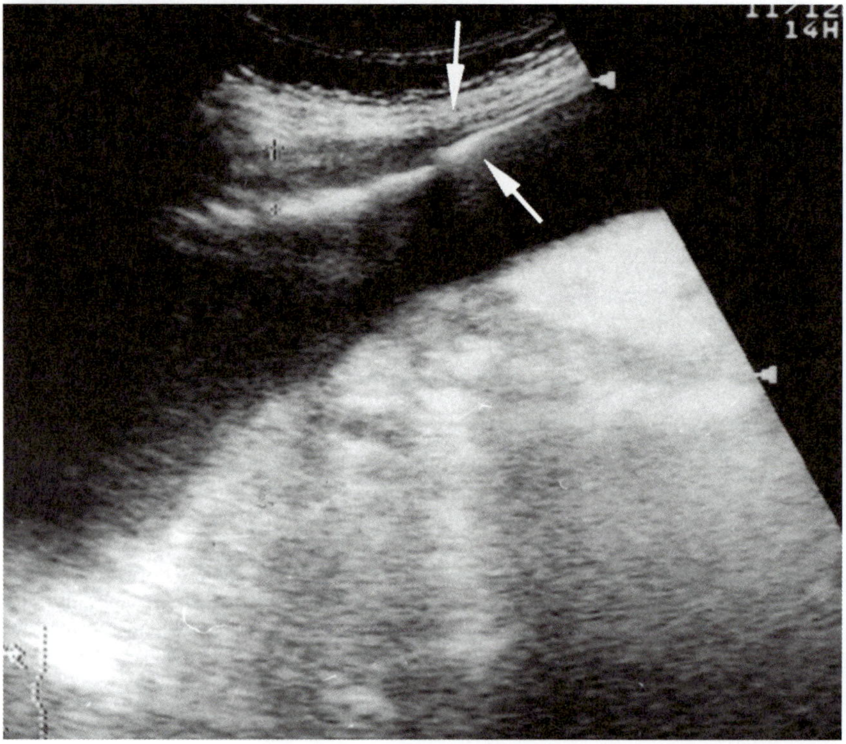

Fig. 76. Female patient U., age 71. Diagnosis: infiltrative cancer of the stomach. Echotomogram of the stomach (longitudinal section relative to the stomach axis): the anterior wall is thickened to 11 cm with corresponding disorder in the layered structure at this level. Border between the intact and the involved wall of the stomach is distinctly visualized (arrows)

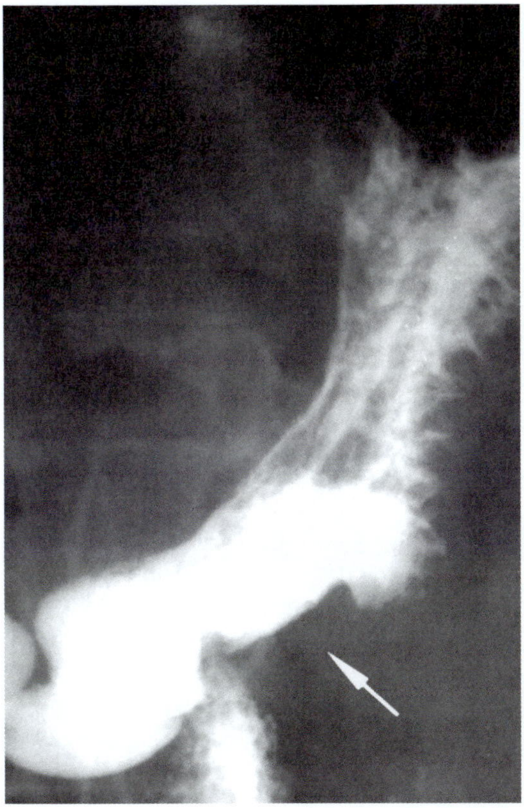

▲ Fig. 77 a.

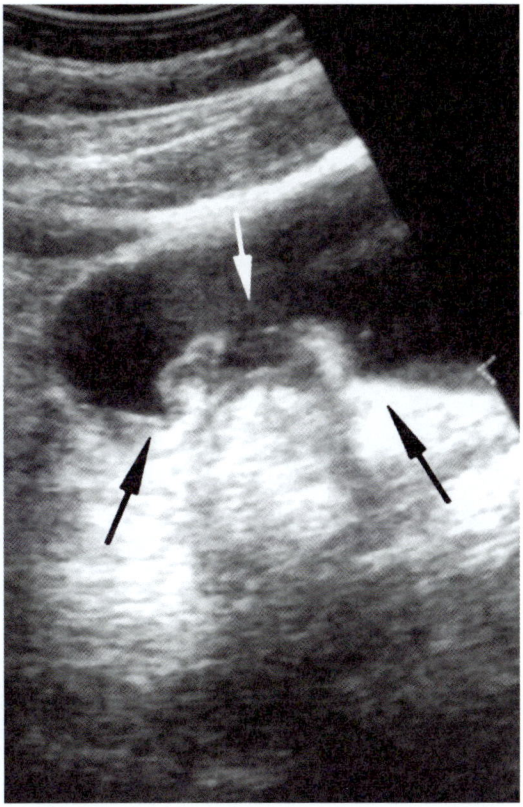

▼ Fig. 77 b.

▲ Fig. 77 c.

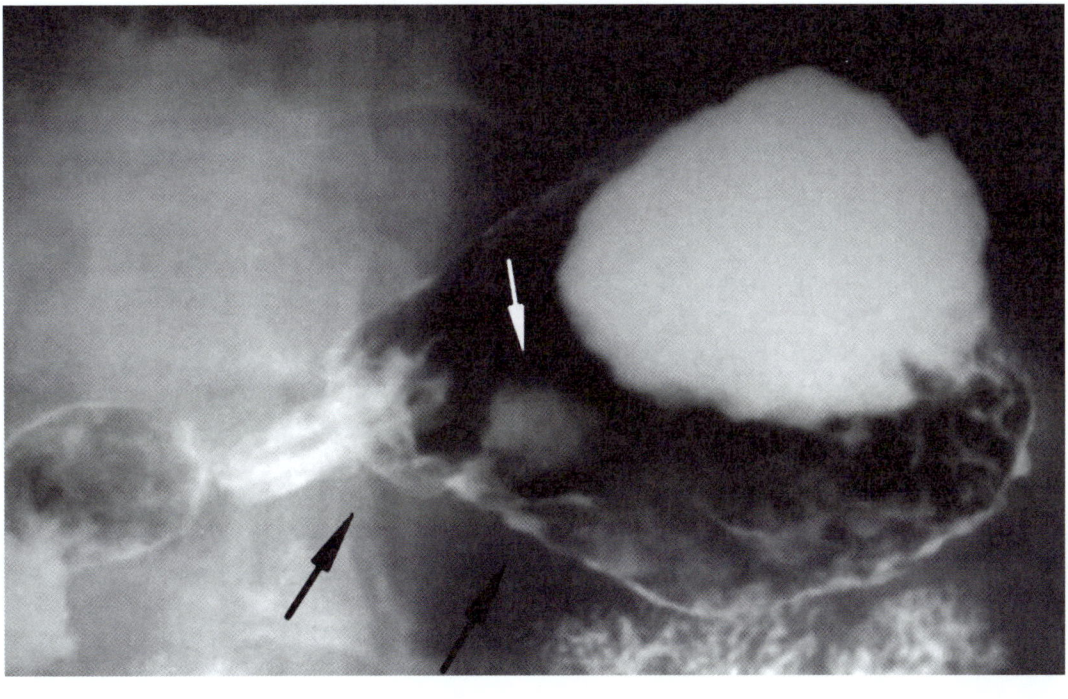

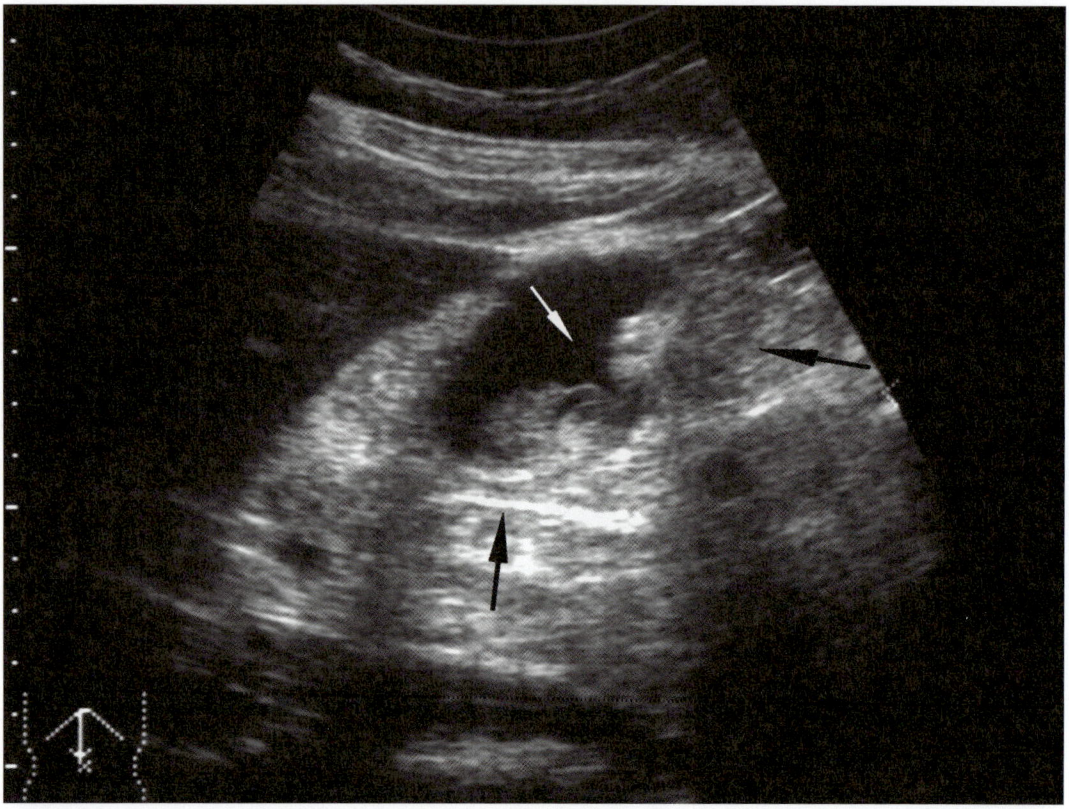

▲ Fig. 77 d.

▼ Fig. 77 e.

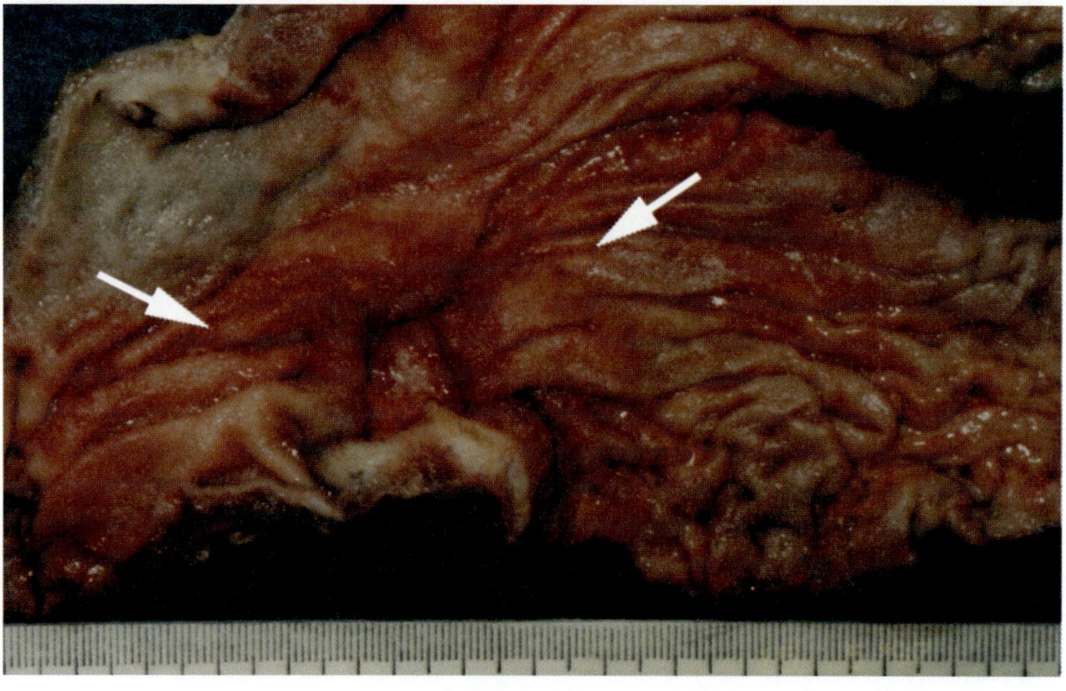

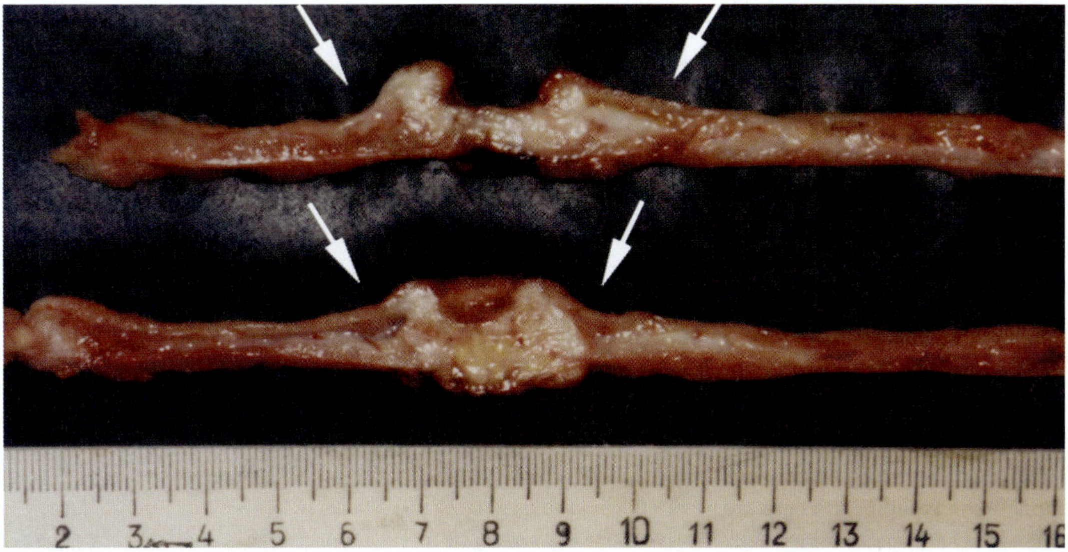

▲ **Fig. 77 f.**

▼ **Fig. 78.**

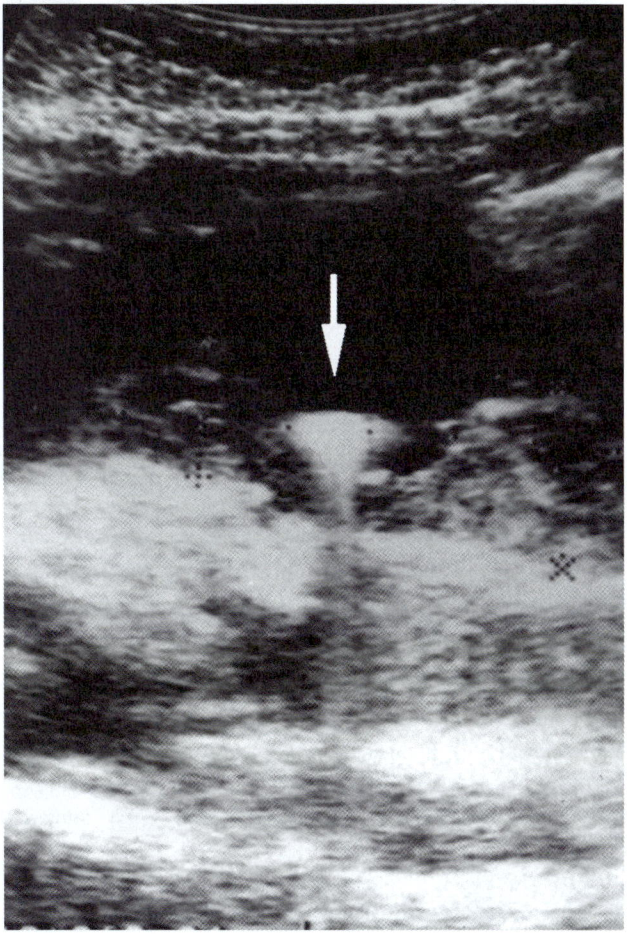

Fig. 77a–f. Patient T., age 64. Diagnosis: gastric cancer. **a** Stomach roentgenogram (tight filling, vertical position, anterior projection): uneven and eroded contours of the greater curvature of the stomach sinus is depressed into the stomach cavity (arrow). **b** Stomach roentgenogram (double contrast, horizontal position, anterior projection): the wall of the greater curvature of the stomach sinus is thickened due to intramural infiltration (black arrows); in the center a rounded depot of contrast medium is visualized, corresponding to reflection of the ulcer crater (white arrow). **c, d** Ultrasonogram of the stomach: a series of echotomograms shows local thickening of the wall of the greater curvature of the sinus over a length of 5 cm due to intramural infiltration with the corresponding disorder in the five-layered echo-structure at this level (black arrows). Ulcer crater in the depth of the infiltrated wall (white arrow). Conclusion: Infiltrative-ulcerous cancer of the stomach sinus. **e** Macrospecimen of a resected stomach: a crater-like depression with an overhanging ridge of infiltrated tissue (arrows); the wall is thickened; white tissue infiltrating the stomach wall is seen. **f** Fragments of a macrospecimen (strips): stomach wall is thickened due to white ulcerated tumor infiltration (arrows). Histologically; adenocarcinoma with the signet-ring cell component

Fig. 78. Patient E., age 61. Diagnosis: infiltrative-ulcerous cancer of the stomach. Echotomogram of the stomach (longitudinal section at the level of the upper third of the stomach body): the walls are unevenly thickened from 7 to 25 mm over a length of 12–13 cm: the absence of differentiation of the layers. A large ulcerous defect sizing 2x1 cm in the center of the thickening; air is present (arrow). Histologically; a non-differentiated cancer.

The set of ultrasonographic signs currently used to diagnose gastric cancer can also be used to establish accurately the boundaries of the tumor, which is very important for diagnosis of the infiltrative forms. Margins of infiltration are determined more accurately in patients with endophytic cancer of the stomach. More commonly, it is possible to visualize only one border in patients with diffuse cancer (◘ Fig. 79).

Most therapeutic and prophylactic institutions today have ultrasonographic equipment. Therefore, when X-ray and endoscopic examinations (with subsequent histological studies) fail to verify gastric cancer, ultrasonography should be used as an additional method at the pre-hospital stage.

While we value the potentials of sonography in the diagnosis of gastric cancer highly, we still adhere to the opinion that it is only an additional diagnostic method. The primary and basic instrumental methods of revealing gastric cancer are the traditional X-ray and endoscopic examinations.

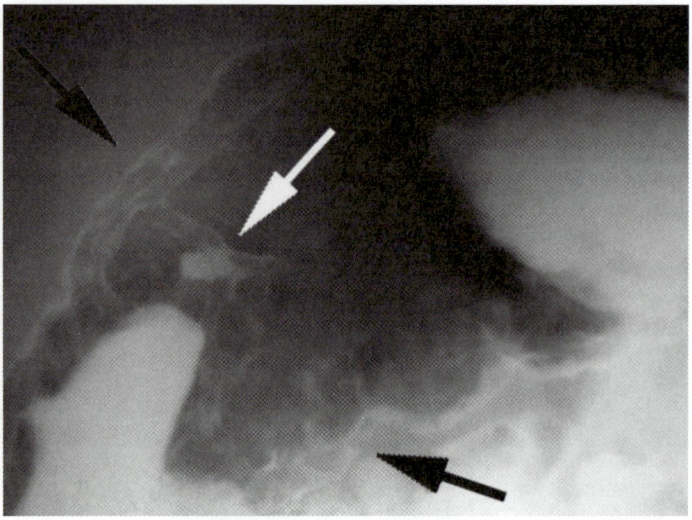

▲ **Fig. 79 b.**

▼ **Fig. 79 c.**

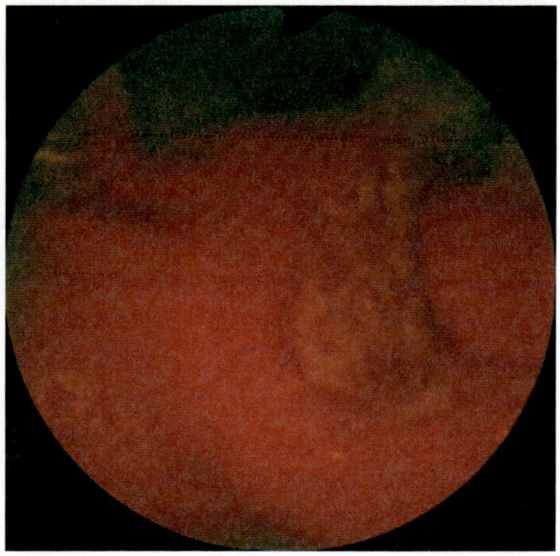

▼ **Fig. 79 a.**

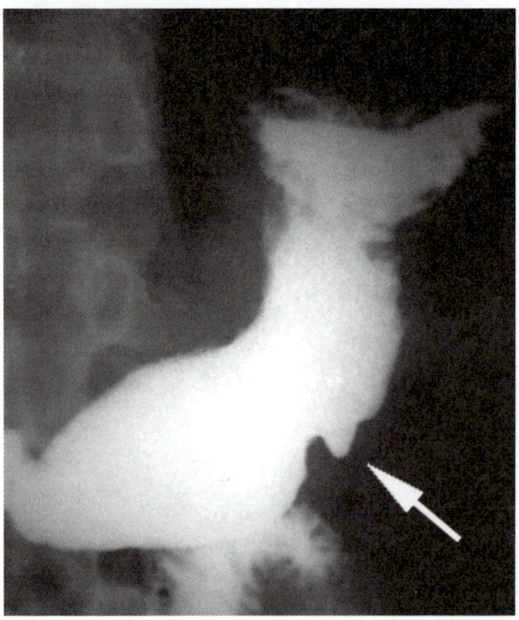

◘ **Fig. 79a–e.** Patient N., age 68. Diagnosis: gastric cancer. **a** Stomach roentgenogram (tight filling, vertical position, anterior projection): the lesser curvature of the stomach body is short and depressed; ulcer niche on the greater curvature of the stomach body (arrow). **b** Stomach roentgenogram (double contrast, horizontal position, left lateral projection): the stomach walls are thickened due to intramural infiltration (black arrows) with a depot of contrast medium (white arrow). Conclusion: Infiltrative-ulcerous cancer of the stomach body. **c** Endophotograph: ulcer with a flat irregular floor and tuberous and eroded edges, and also periulcerous ridge are seen in the lower third of the stomach body on the posterior wall with invasion of the greater curvature; some mucosal folds converge toward the ridge periphery. Histologically; signet-ring cell carcinoma. **d, e** Ultrasonograms of the stomach distinctly visualize the border between the intact and involved stomach wall (arrow)

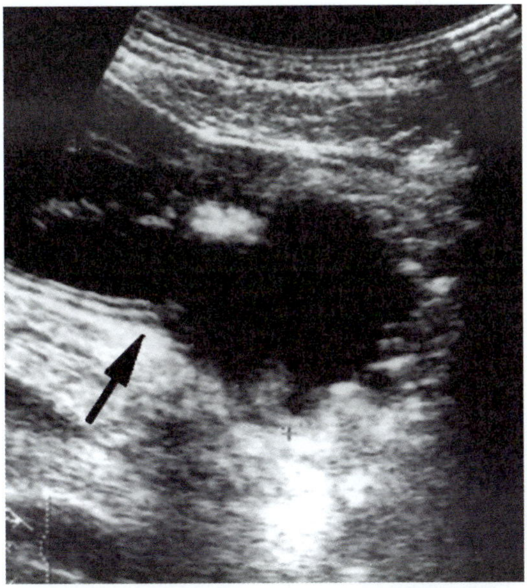

▲ Fig. 79 d. ▼ Fig. 79 e.

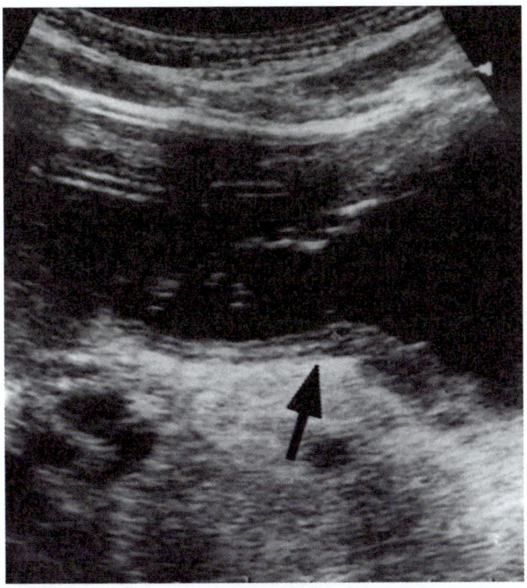

Computed-Tomography Signs

Computed tomography is commonly used to study those anatomical structures characterized by a relative homogeneity of structure and by the absence of permanent peristaltic contractions. Modern CT made it possible to study internal organs regardless of the presence of peristalsis. This stimulated the elaboration of methodological instructions for the use of CT in diagnosing diseases of the stomach, particularly tumors. Signs of gastric cancer detected by computed tomography were then established (Fig. 80) [33, 35, 81, 235, 251].

As experience with CT accumulated, its disadvantages became apparent. The main one was its limited potential for revealing intramural infiltration of the stomach. Some authors spoke of possible hyperdiagnosis due to the so-called pseudo-thickening of the stomach wall. Hence, the opinion was expressed that computed tomography might be used only as the source of additional information on the extent of affection and the spread of the process onto the adjacent anatomical structures.

▼ Fig. 80 a.

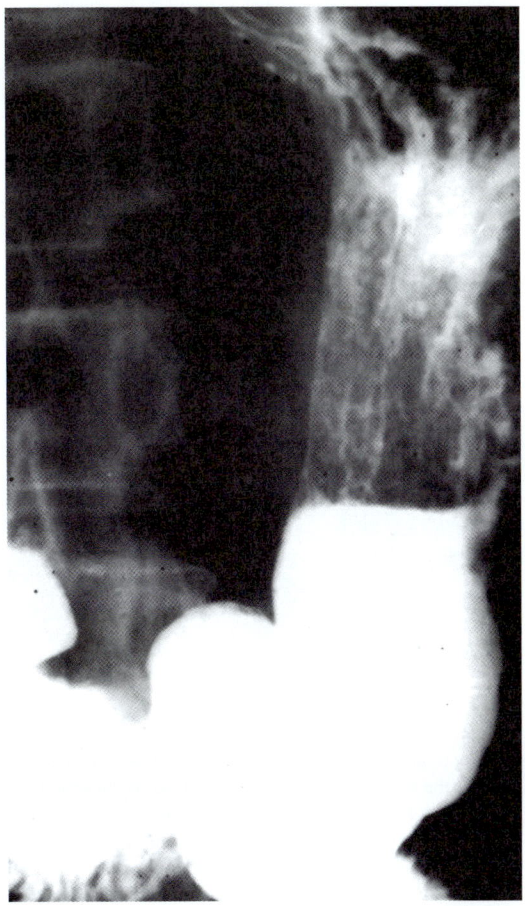

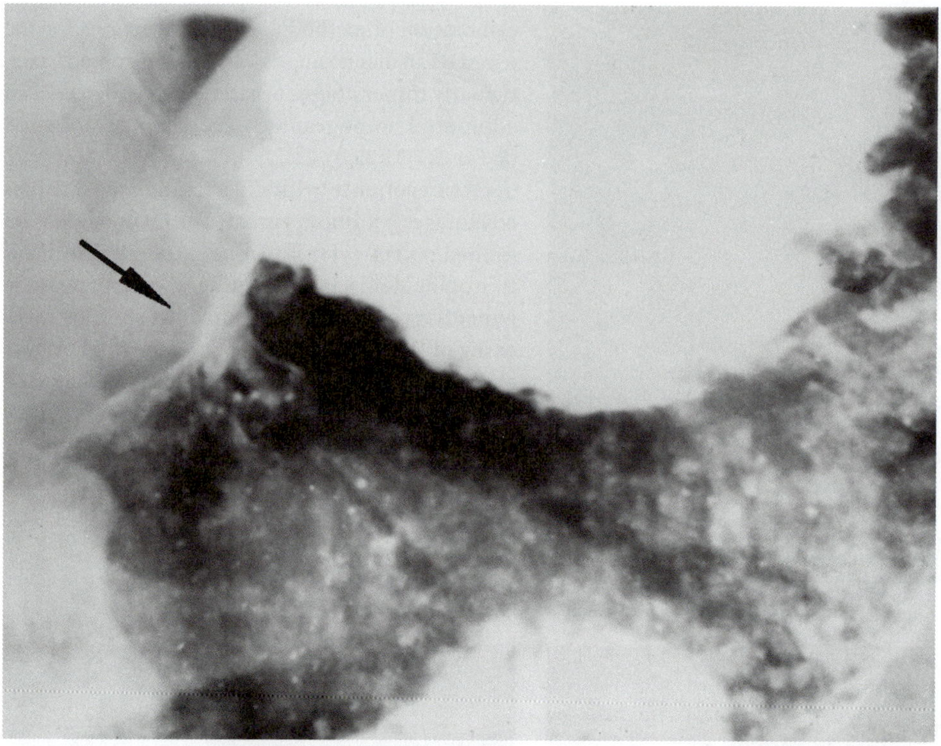

◀ **Fig. 80 b.**

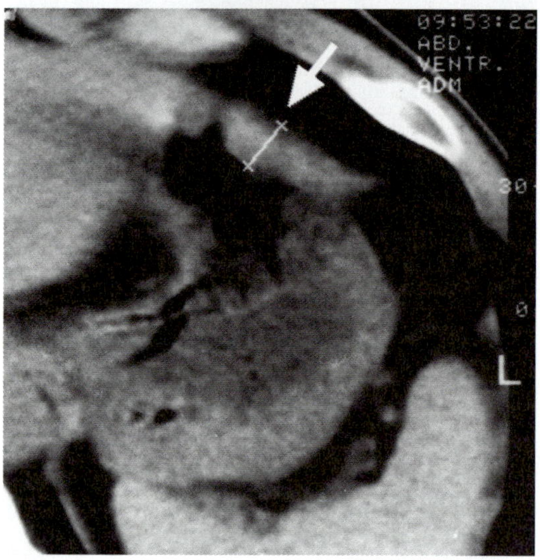

▲ **Fig. 80 c.**

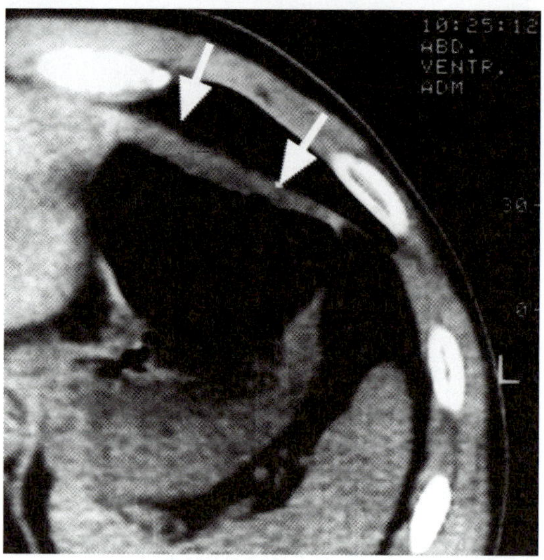

▲ **Fig. 80 d.**

Fig. 80a–e. Patient M., age 55. Diagnosis: gastric cancer. **a** Stomach roentgenogram (tight filling, vertical position, anterior projection): organic changes are not visible. **b** Stomach roentgenogram (double contrast, horizontal position, left half-oblique projection): the anterior wall of the stomach body is thickened due to intramural infiltration (arrow). Conclusion: Infiltrative cancer of the stomach. Histological examination of bioptates taken during endoscopy verified signet-ring cell carcinoma. **c, d, e** Tomograms of the stomach (stomach inflated with air, supine patient): thickening of the wall due to intramural infiltration, which remains stable on repeated inflation of the stomach. Depending on the amount of insufflated air, thickness of the infiltrated stomach wall varies from 13 to 9 mm; the wall remains thick with the stomach inflated to the maximum (arrows).

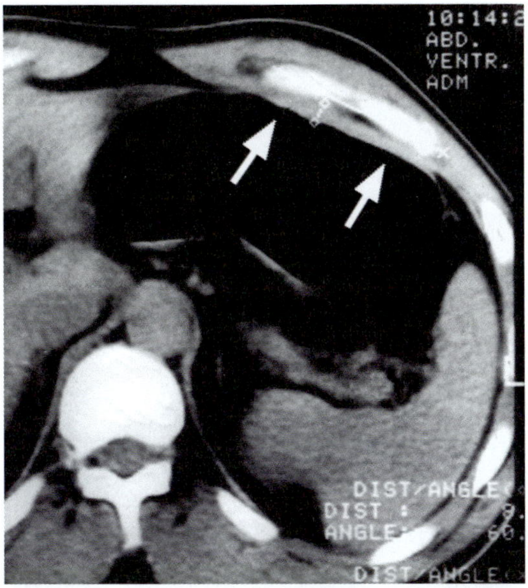

▲ **Fig. 80 e.**

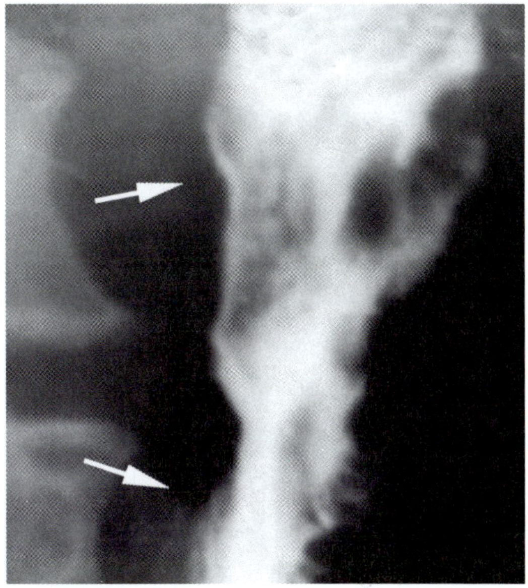

▲ **Fig. 81 b.**

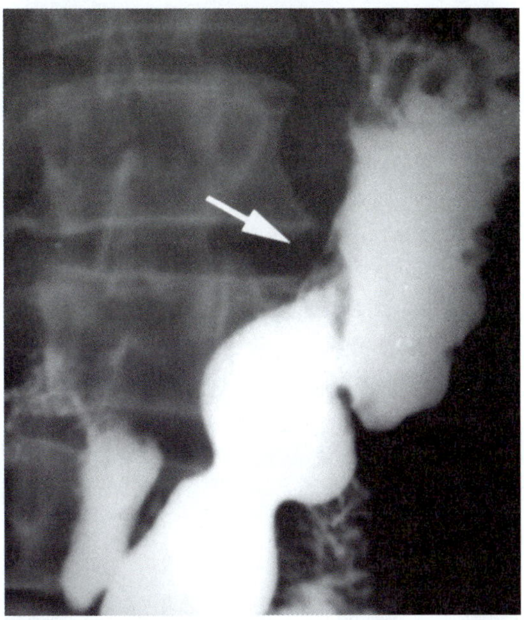

▼ **Fig. 81 a.**

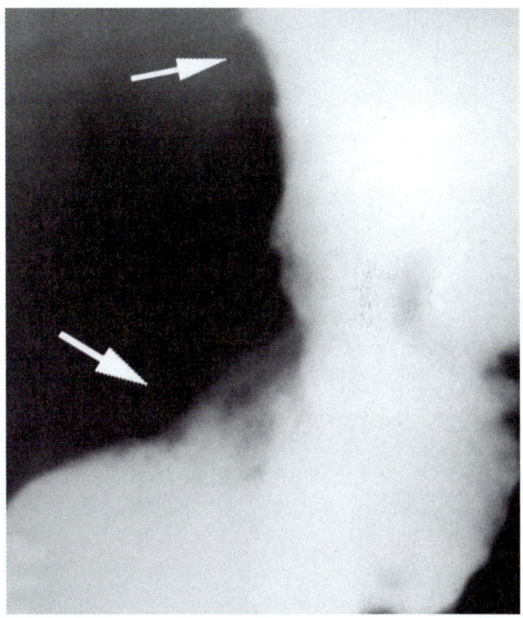

▼ **Fig. 81 c.**

Fig. 81a–j. Patient G., age 72. Diagnosis: gastric cancer. **a** Stomach roentgenogram (tight filling, vertical position, anterior projection): uneven contours of the lesser curvature of the stomach body; the lesser curvature is depressed (arrow). **b, c, d** Target stomach roentgenograms (tight filling, vertical position, anterior projection) as the stomach is filled with barium sulfate suspension: uneven contours of the lesser curvature (arrows). **e** Stomach roentgenogram (double contrast, horizontal position, anterior projection): wall of the lesser curvature is rigid and thickened due to intramural infiltration (arrows). Conclusion: Infiltrative cancer of the stomach body. Histological examination of bioptates taken during endoscopy failed to detect tumor cells. The patient was examined by computed tomography. **f** Computed tomogram of the stomach (tight filling with E-Z-CAT DRY, supine patient): visualized are the walls of the lesser curvature, thickened due to intramural infiltration. **g, h, i, j** Computed tomograms (dosed inflation of the stomach with air, supine position): wall is thickened unevenly, inner contour is uneven, sometimes tuberous due to intramural infiltration (arrows). The patient underwent surgery. Histologically; adenocarcinoma with signet-ring cell component.

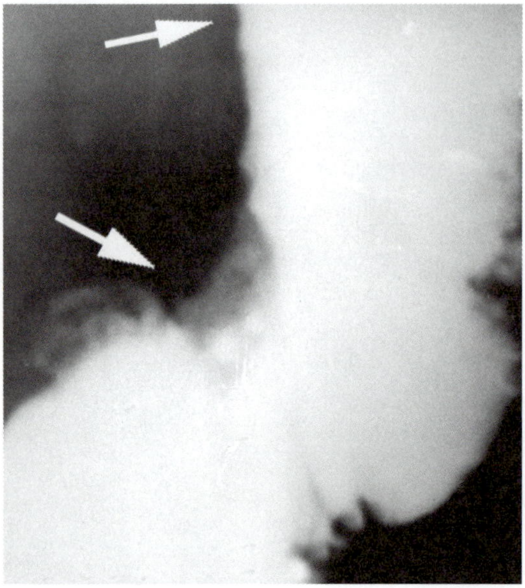

▲ Fig. 81 d.

▼ Fig. 81 e.

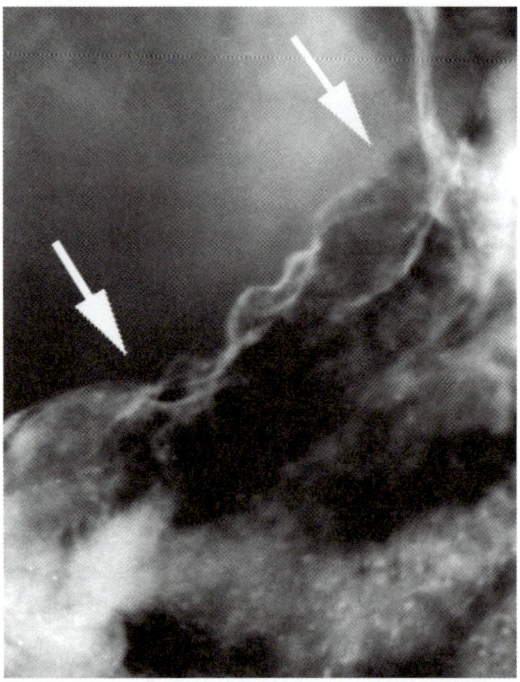

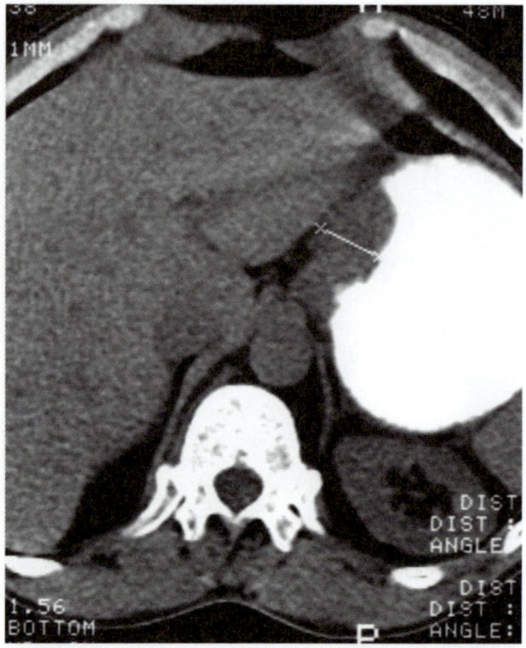

▲ Fig. 81 f.

▼ Fig. 81 g.

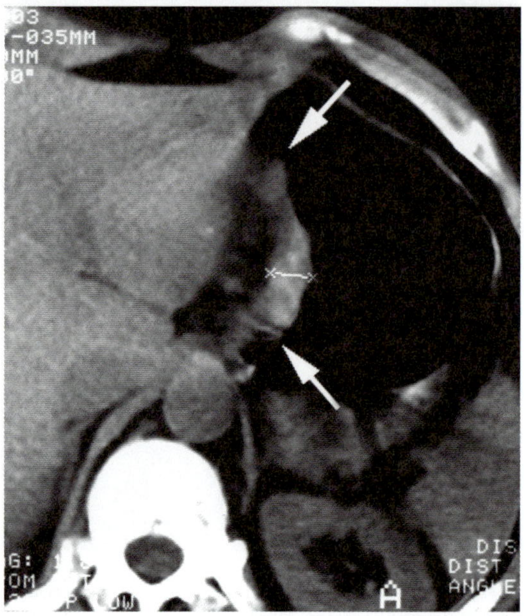

The two methods of computed tomography proposed by us and our colleagues and described in the previous chapter are based on determination of thickness of the stomach wall (◻ Fig. 81). The methods can give a significant amount of information on the condition of the stomach wall (◻ Fig. 82). One of the proposed methods (pneumotomography) helps avoid mistakes connected with pseudo-thickening and distorted information on wall thickness during CT using water as the contrast medium. Thus, pneumotomography markedly broadens the diagnostic potentials of the method. Moreover, data obtained

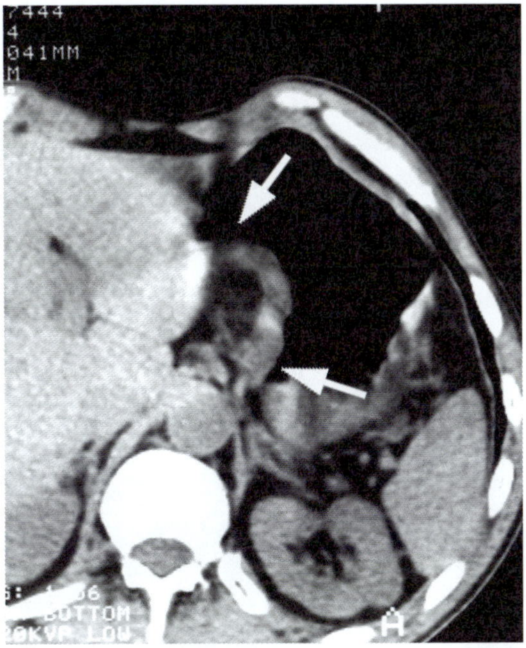

▲ **Fig. 81 h.**

▼ **Fig. 81 i.**

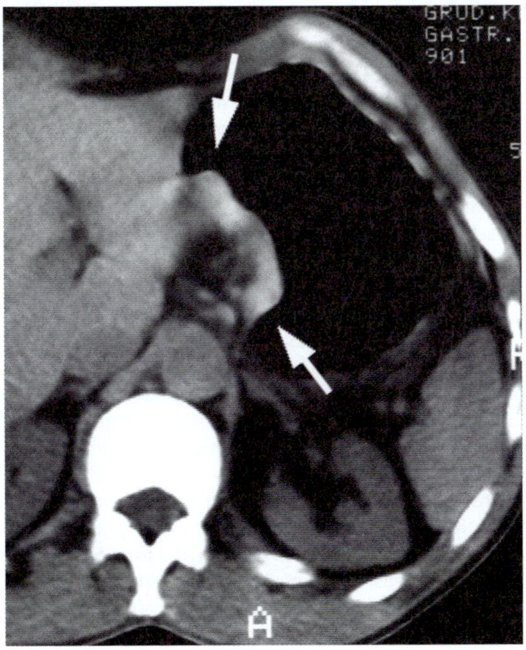

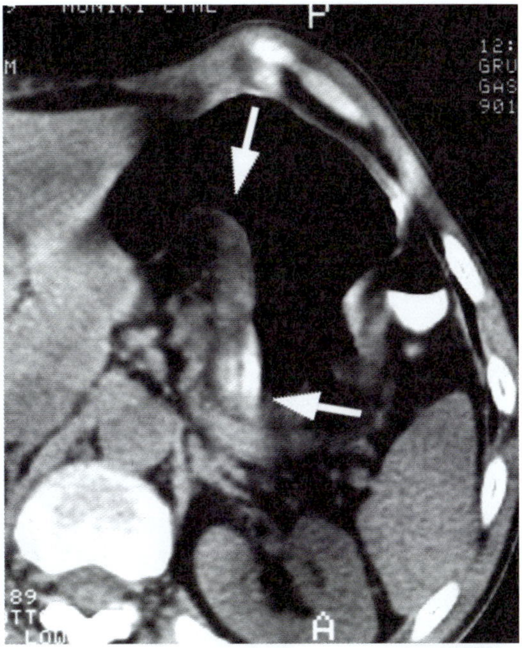

▲ **Fig. 81 j.**

▼ **Fig. 82 a.**

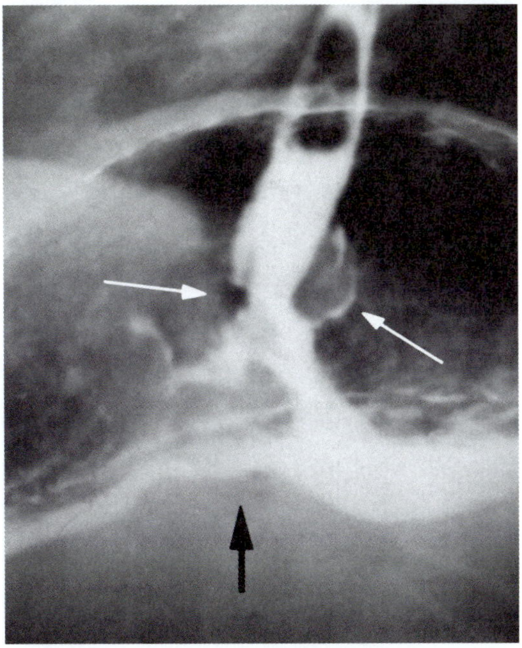

with this method can completely change our understanding of the character of tumor infiltration based on the results of the traditional X-ray and endoscopic examinations, especially in patients with cardioesophageal cancer. Data obtained using pneumotomography confirm our main concept: that intramurally spreading carcinomas predominate among the malignant tumors of the stomach (Fig. 83) [44].

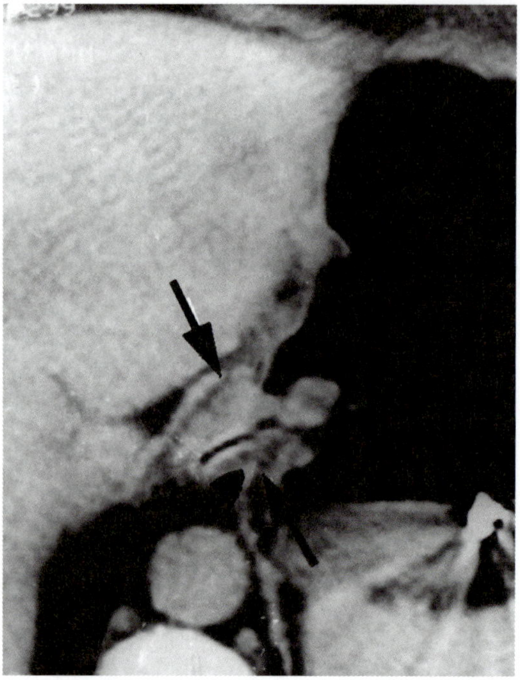

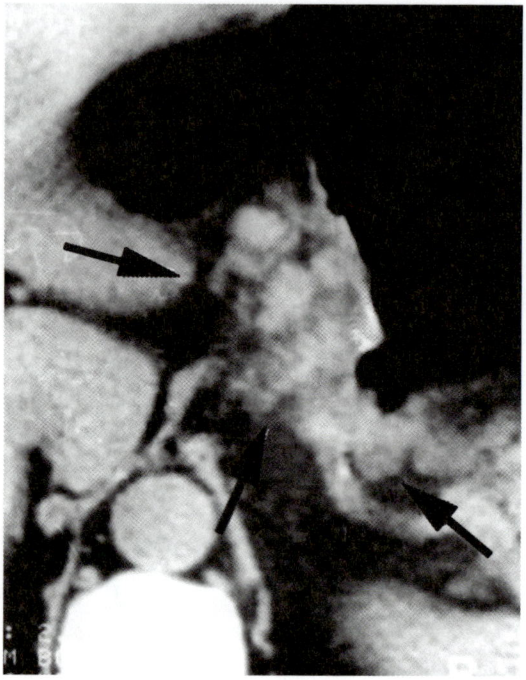

▲ Fig. 82 b. ▼ Fig. 82 c. ▲ Fig. 82 d.

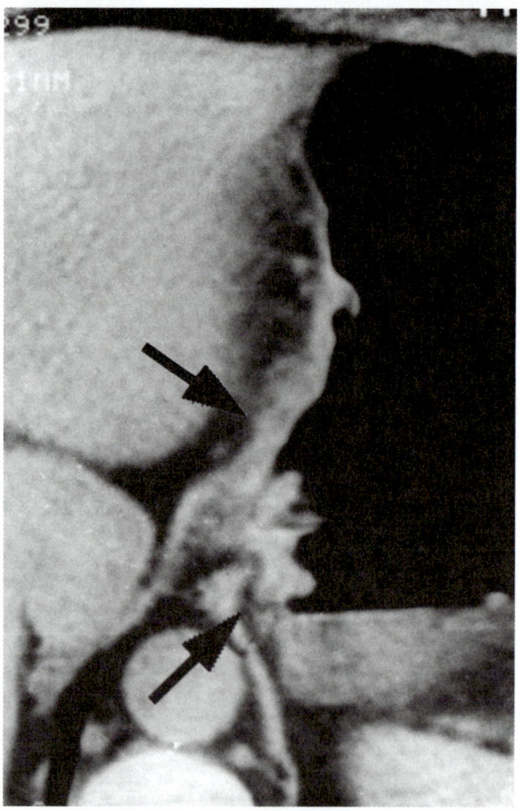

Fig. 82a–d. Female patient K., age 63. Diagnosis: gastric cancer. **a** Stomach roentgenogram (tight filling, vertical position, left lateral projection) at the moment of contrast medium passage through the gastroesophageal junction: a limited portion of the infiltrated wall of the stomach with possible involvement in the process of the abdominal segment of the esophagus can be seen in projection of the cardiac rosette (black arrows). No changes are detected in the underlying parts of the stomach; the wall thickness is normal (white arrow). In order to verify the spread of infiltration onto the abdominal segment of the esophagus, the patient's stomach was examined by CT. **b** Computed tomography of the stomach (dosed inflation of the stomach with air, the level of the cardiac rosette, supine position): the cardiac wall is thickened due to intramural infiltration invading the abdominal segment of the esophagus (arrows). **c** Computed tomography of the stomach (dosed inflation of the stomach with air, the level of the cardiac rosette, supine position): following insufflation of additional air, thickening of the walls of the abdominal segment of the esophagus persists (arrows). **d** Computed tomogram of the stomach (dosed inflation of the stomach with air, the level of the stomach body, supine position): a group of enlarged lymph nodes with uneven contours and maximum diameter of 15–17 mm is seen in the projection of the lesser omentum (arrows). Conclusion: Infiltrative cancer of the upper part of the stomach with invasion of the esophagus; metastases to the lymph nodes of the lesser omentum. The patient was operated. Histologically; signet-ring cell carcinoma.

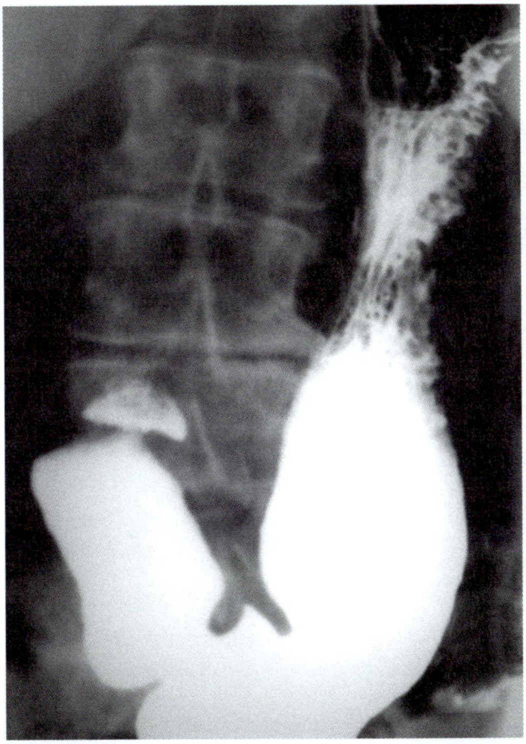

▲ Fig. 83 a.

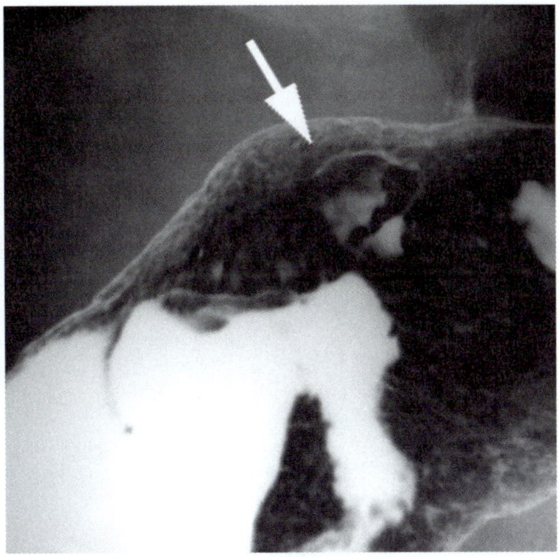

▲ Fig. 83 c.

▼ Fig. 83 b.

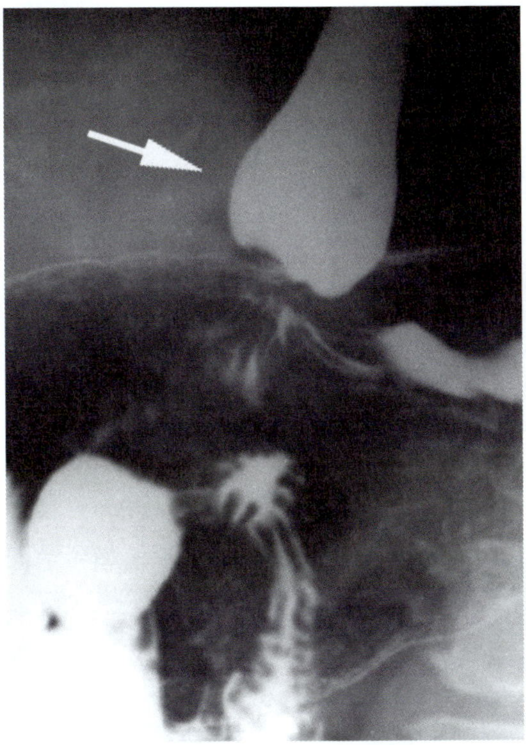

Fig. 83a–l. Female patient Z., age 73. Diagnosis: gastric cancer. **a** Stomach roentgenogram (tight filling, vertical position, anterior projection): no organic changes are observed. **b** Stomach roentgenogram (double contrast, horizontal position, left lateral projection) at the moment of contrast medium passage through the gastroesophageal junction at the inspiration phase: normal function of the gastroesophageal junction; formed esophageal ampulla (arrow). **c, d, e, f, g** Stomach roentgenograms (double contrast, horizontal position, left lateral projection): atypical relief of the cardiac rosette (cardioesophageal junction) with termination of the folds by the periphery (arrows). **h** Stomach roentgenogram (double contrast, vertical position, left lateral projection): atypical relief of the cardiac rosette (arrows); the specific radiating pattern is absent. Conclusion: Minor infiltrative cancer of the cardiac part of the stomach. Endoscopy with subsequent histological examination of bioptates failed to find organic changes. The patient's stomach was examined by computed tomography. **i, j** Computed tomograms of the stomach (double contrast, the level of the upper part of the stomach, supine position): the wall of the cardiac part of the stomach is thickened over a small length due to intramural infiltration as seen in projection of the cardiac rosette (arrow); **k,l** Computed tomograms of the stomach (double contrast, at the level of the upper part of the stomach, position on the right side): the wall of the cardiac part of the stomach is thickened over a short length due to intramural infiltration as seen in projection of the cardiac rosette (arrow); Conclusion: Minor infiltrative cancer of the cardiac part of the stomach. Repeated endoscopic examinations conducted later did not reveal organic changes. Tumor cells were not detected by histological examination of the bioptates either. In the absence of histological verification of gastric cancer, the patient was not operated despite the convincing evidence obtained by radiological examination. A year later, histological examination of the material taken during another endoscopy revealed the presence of signet-ring cells.

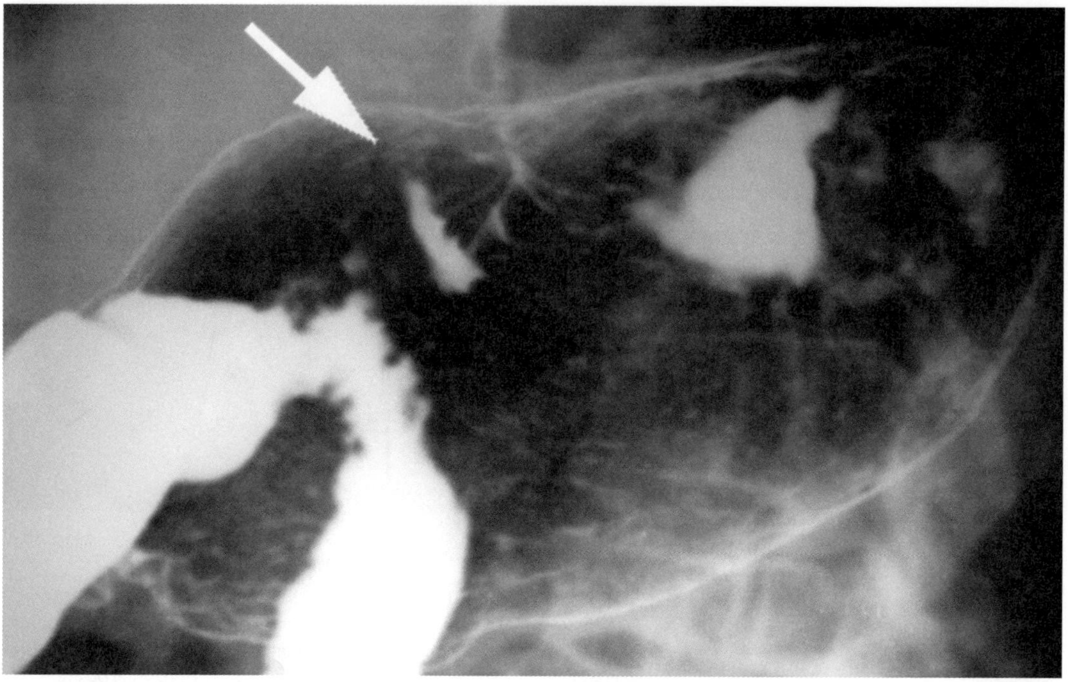

▲ Fig. 83 d.

▼ Fig. 83 e.

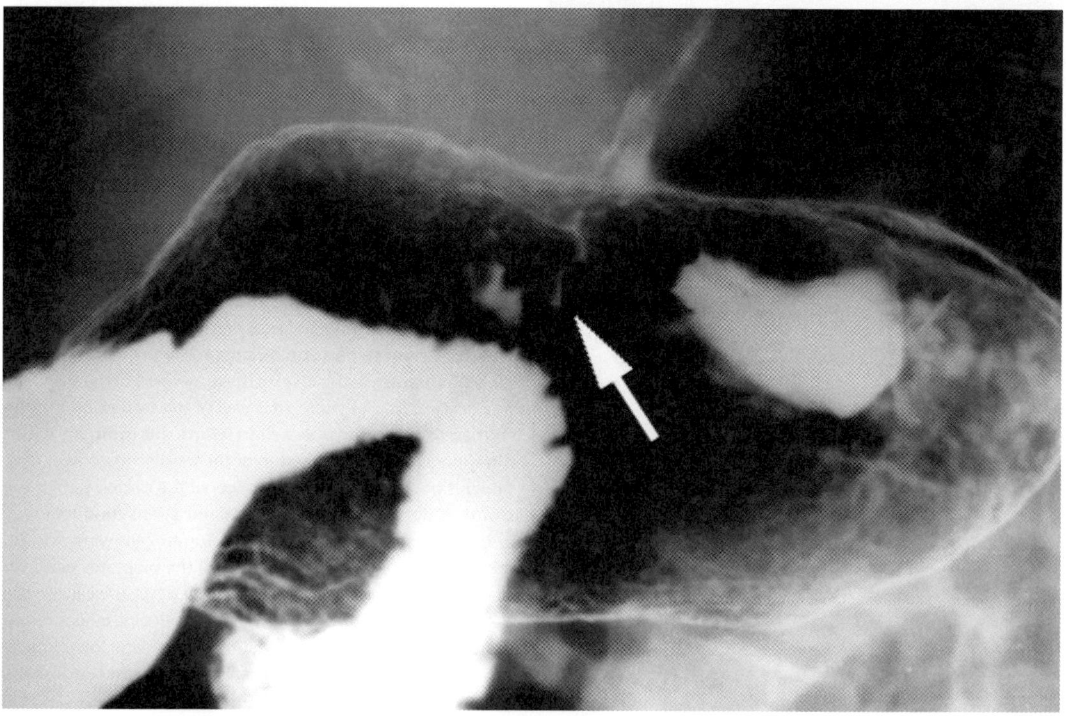

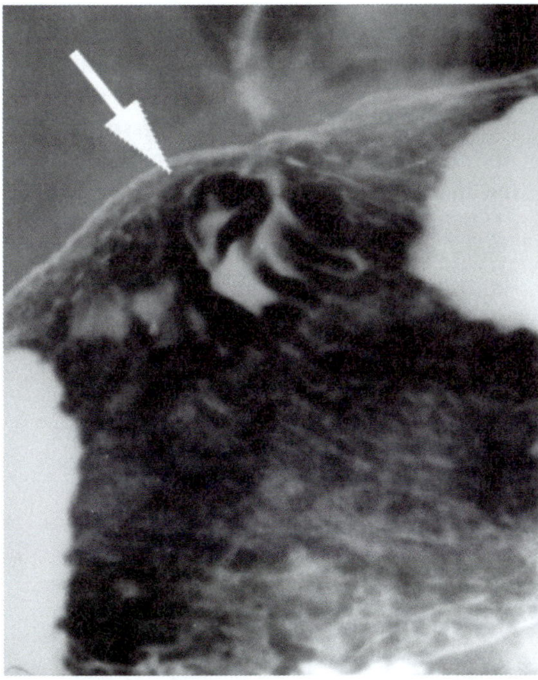

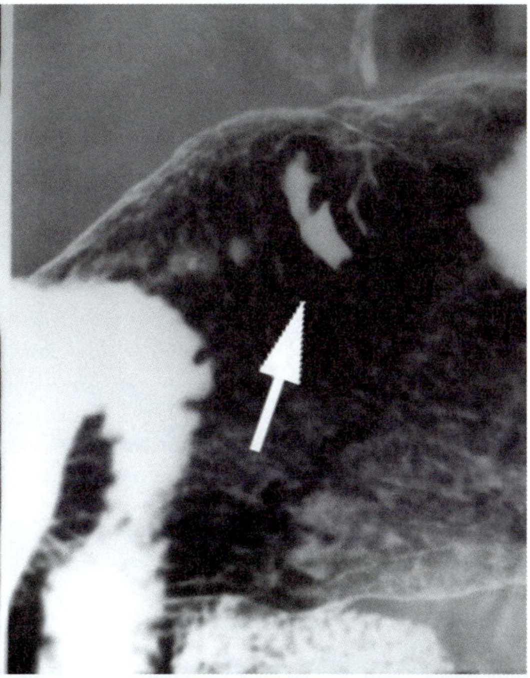

▲ **Fig. 83 f-g.**

▼ **Fig. 83 h.**

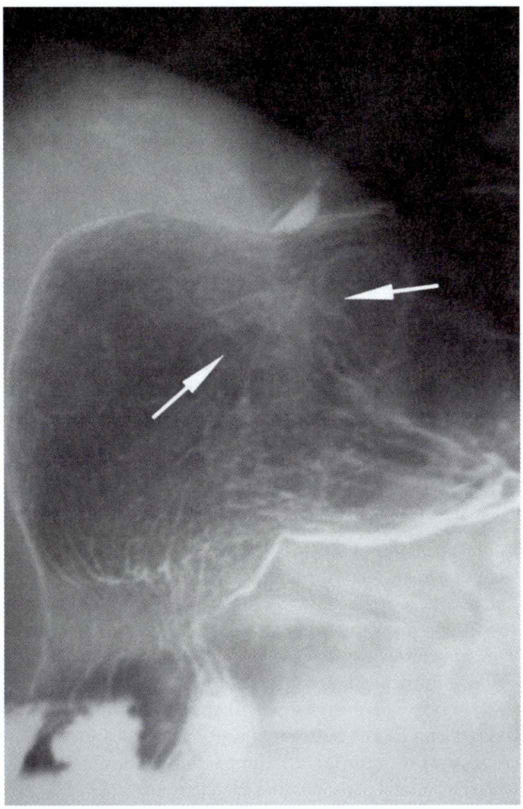

▼ **Fig. 83 i.**

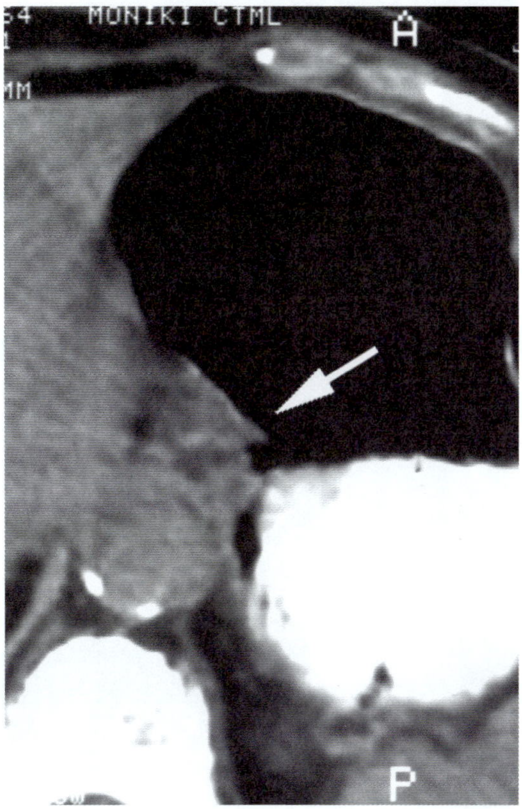

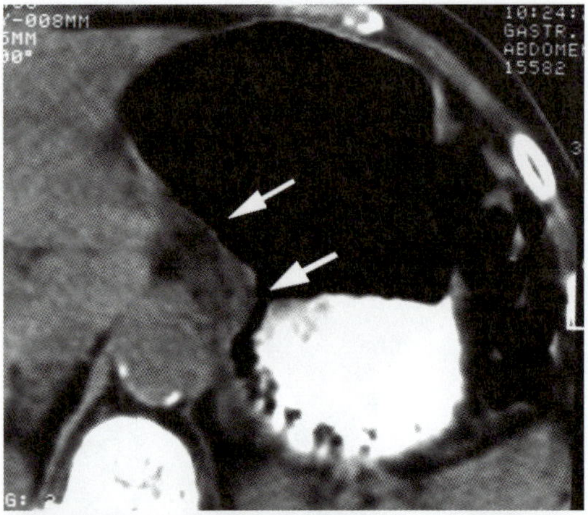

▲ **Fig. 83 j.**

▼ **Fig. 83 k.**

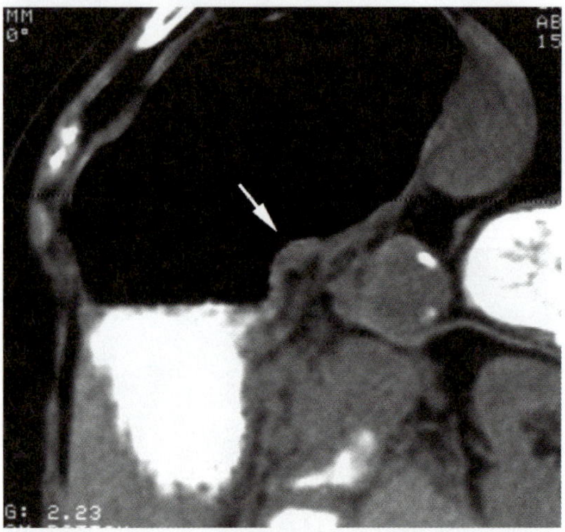

▼ **Fig. 83 l.**

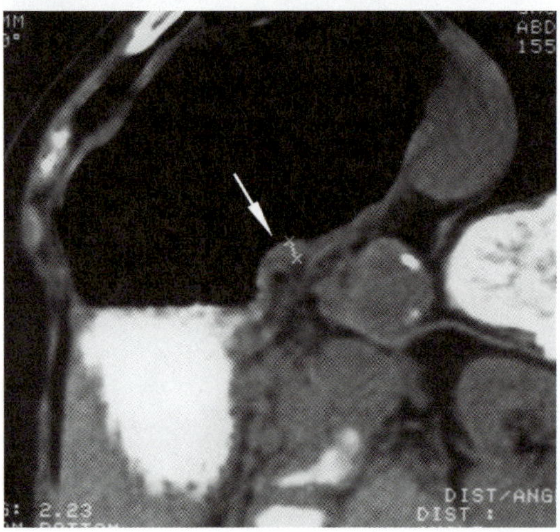

The orientation of CT toward the discovery of intramural growth explains the necessity of formulating more detailed computed tomographic semiotics, particularly for diffuse forms of gastric cancer. Above all, this depends on the possibility of estimating thickness of the stomach wall.

Using our methods, the symptoms of diffuse cancer are identical [38, 40, 47, 53]:

- Thickening of the stomach wall to various degrees (7–45 mm)
- Loss of wall elasticity at the site of tumor infiltration

As a rule, in addition to thickening of the stomach wall at the site of a blastomatous process, it is possible to reveal uneven (sometimes polygonal) contours, which persist after inflation of additional portions of air, suggesting rigidity of the wall (◘ Fig. 84). Intact portions of the wall remain elastic and their thickness is 1.5–2.5 mm on average, with distinct inner and outer contours, except in the prepyloric and cardiac parts of the stomach, where normal thickness is 5–6 mm (in conditions of adequate inflation) [160]. This is especially obvious when using pneumotomography.

◘ **Fig. 84a–g.** Patient P., age 58. Diagnosis: gastric cancer. **a** Stomach roentgenogram (vertical position, anterior projection): the sign of air redistribution in the bubble, which is elongated. **b** Stomach roentgenogram (tight filling, vertical position, anterior projection): the cavity volume decreased, the angular notch is straightened, the lesser curvature is shortened and depressed; its contours are uneven; the walls are rigid (arrows). **c** Stomach roentgenogram (double contrast, horizontal position, anterior projection): diffuse thickening of the walls due to intramural infiltration (arrows). Conclusion: Infiltrative cancer of the stomach. **d, e, f, g** Consecutive computed tomograms of the stomach (dosed stomach inflation with air, supine position): the walls are rigid and thickened over the entire length, the inner contours are polygonal. Retroperitoneal lymph nodes are enlarged, a hypodense stripe of irregular character is seen between the stomach wall and the pancreas over the entire length; commissure of the anterior wall with the parietal peritoneum is seen (arrows)

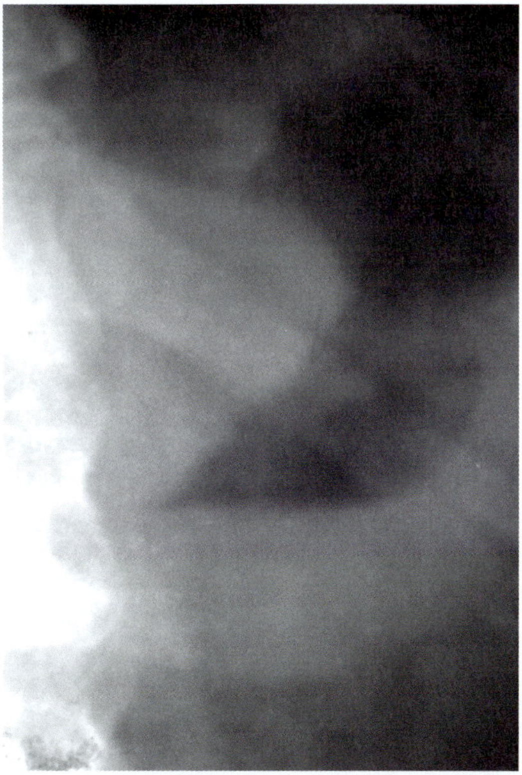

▲ Fig. 84 a.

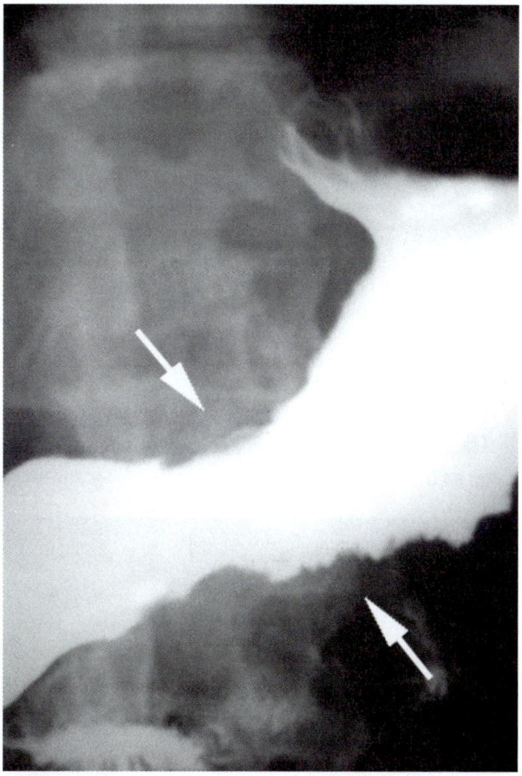

▲ Fig. 84 b.

▼ Fig. 84 c.

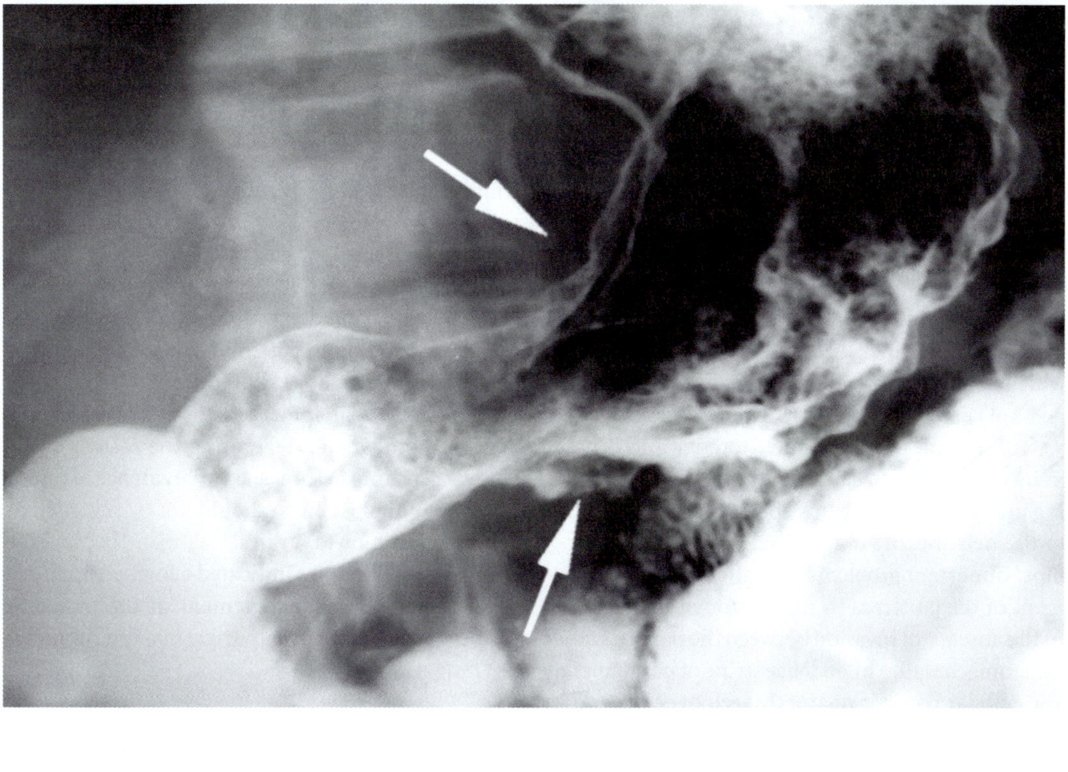

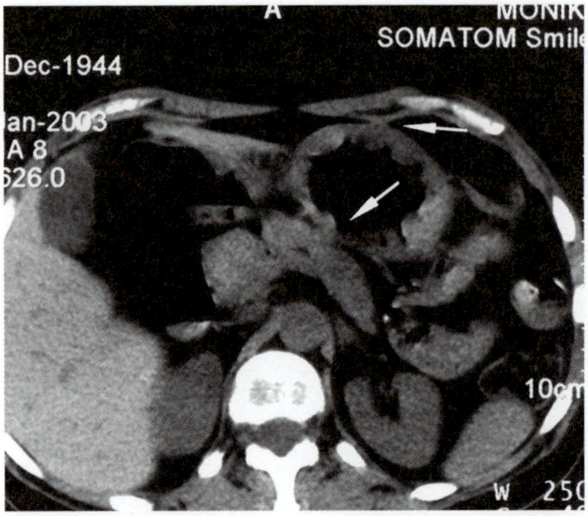

▲ Fig. 84 d.

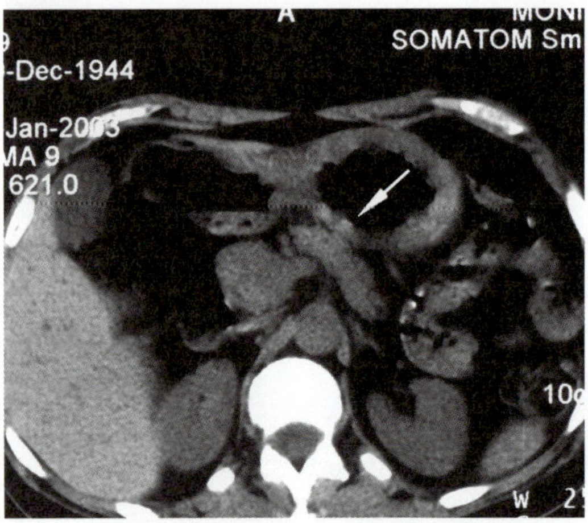

▼ Fig. 84 e.

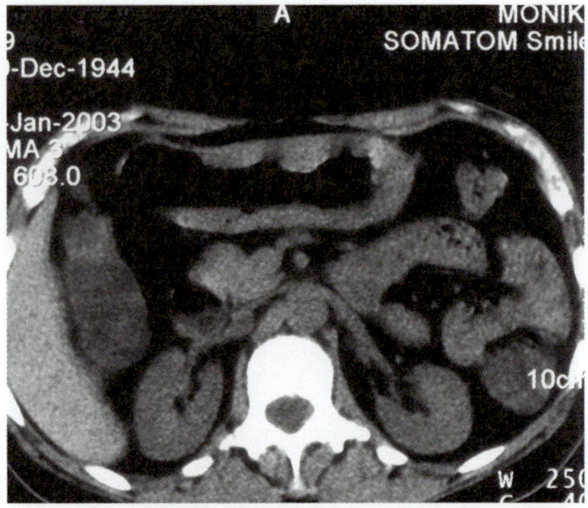

▲ Fig. 84 f.

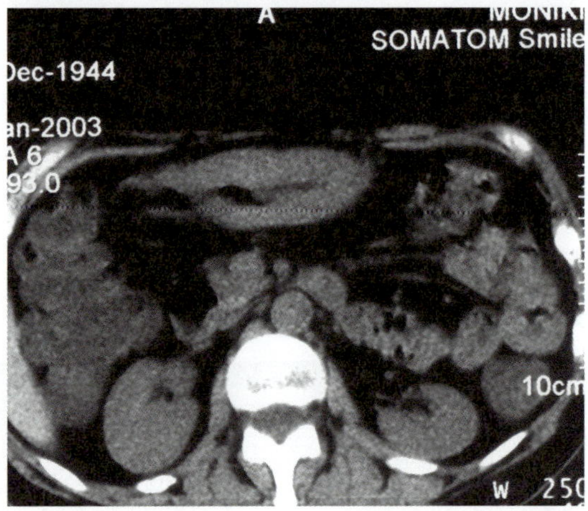

▼ Fig. 84 g.

While assessing the results of using computed tomography for the diagnosis of stomach tumors, especially its infiltrative forms, it is necessary to note that CT sometimes not only gives additional information on the intramural growth of tumors, but also helps discover a thickened wall over a short distance, which considerably facilitates the differential diagnosis of early forms of gastric cancer.

At the same time, computed tomography is used in its earlier known capacity to the full extent, giving information on the possible spread of tumor into the neighboring organs and tissues. One of the most important problems is verification of involvement of the pancreas in the blastomatous process. In the absence of invasion between the pancreas and the stomach wall, a hypodense stripe of parapancreatic cellular tissue is distinctly seen over the entire length, which is easily identifiable owing to CT densitometry parameters that are characteristic of fatty tissue (◘ Fig. 85). As gastric tumor grows into the pancreas, this stripe is not differentiated either partly or over the entire length (◘ Fig. 86). But it is necessary to note that in patients with cachexia due to cancer, parapancreatic cellular tissue may be absent on CT images of an intact pancreas. This should be kept in mind when interpreting the results of the study. According to Kim et al., CT evidence of tumor invasion of the pancreas should not be regarded as a contraindication to surgical treatment, because the results of their studies indicated a low sensitivity of CT in determining involvement of the pancreas proper (60%) and of the perigastric lymph nodes [3, 121, 167].

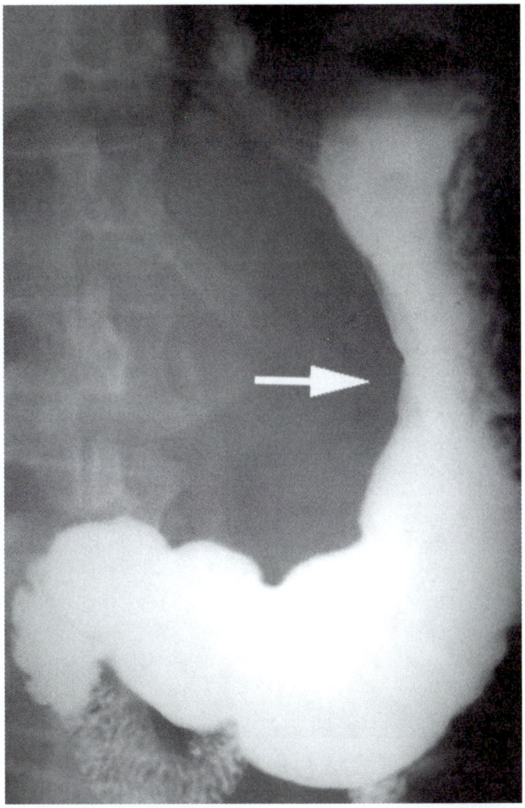

Fig. 85a–j. Patient L., age 64. Diagnosis: gastric cancer. **a** Stomach roentgenogram (tight filling, vertical position, anterior projection): uneven contours of the lesser curvature (arrow). **b** Stomach roentgenogram (double contrast, horizontal position, anterior projection): thickening of the lesser curvature due to intramural infiltration (arrows). In order to verify spread of the tumor to the adjacent anatomical structures, the patient was examined by computed tomography. **c, d, e, f, g** Consecutive computed tomograms of the stomach (tight filling with E-Z-CAT DRY, supine position, at the level of the upper part and the body of the stomach): the posterior wall is thickened due to intramural infiltration. Distinctly differentiated is the hypodense stripe of cellular fat tissue between the infiltrated wall of the stomach and the intact pancreas at the level of its tail and body (arrow). **h, i, j** Computed tomograms of the stomach (tight filling with E-Z-CAT DRY, position on the right side, the level of the antral and pyloric parts of the stomach): the posterior wall is thickened due to intramural infiltration. Distinctly differentiated is the hypodense stripe of cellular fat tissue between the stomach wall and intact pancreas at the level of its body and head (arrows). Conclusion: Infiltrative cancer of the stomach body. The patient was operated. Histologically, adenocarcinoma.

◄ **Fig. 85 a.** ▼ **Fig. 85 b.**

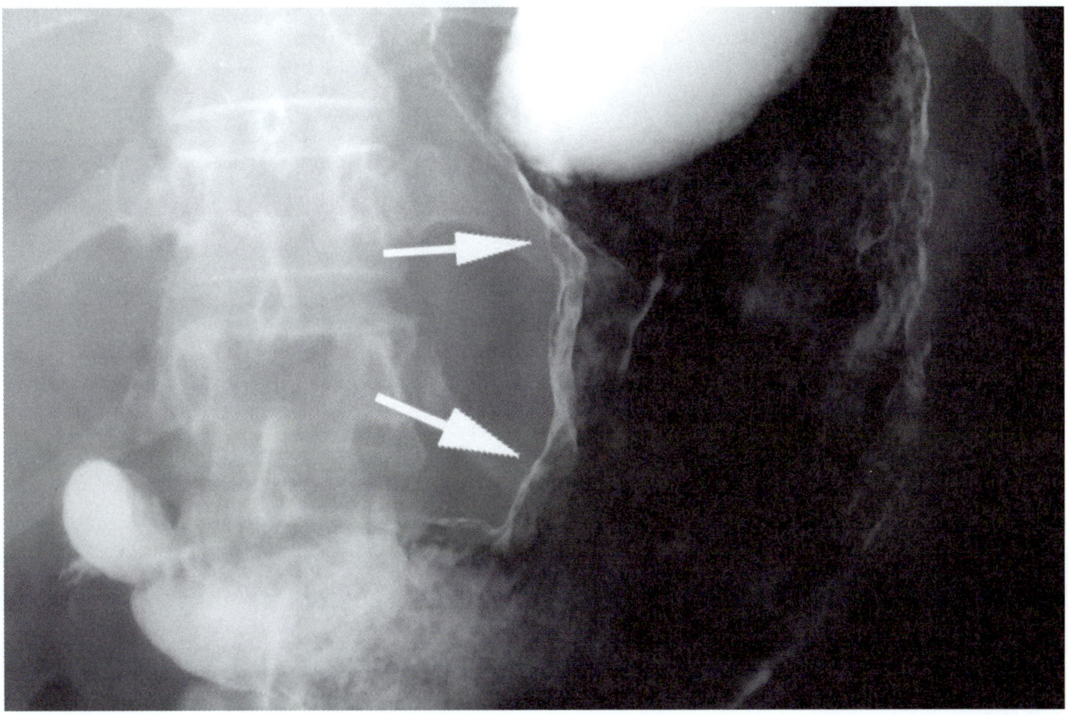

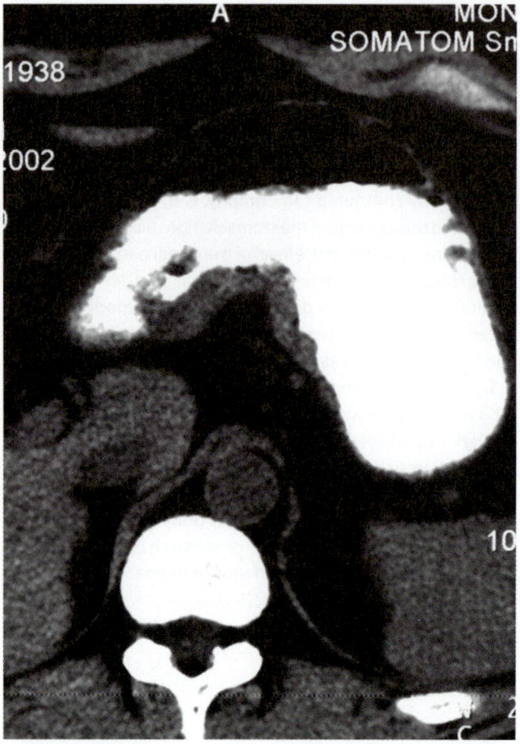

▲ Fig. 85 c.

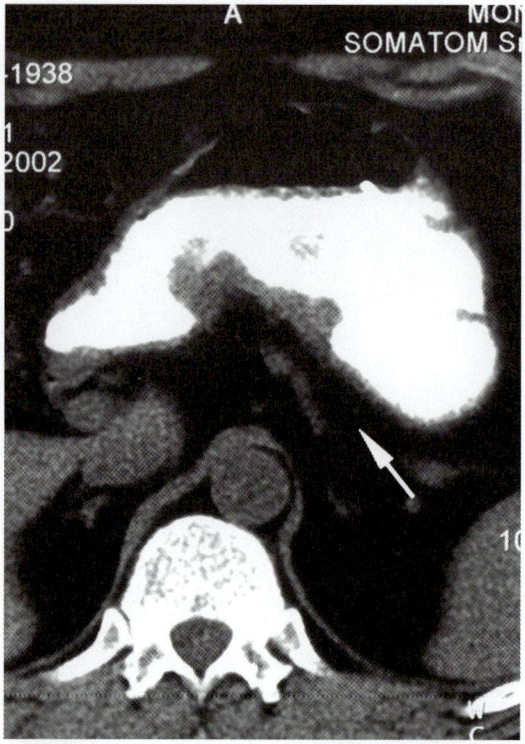

▲ Fig. 85 e.

▼ Fig. 85 d.

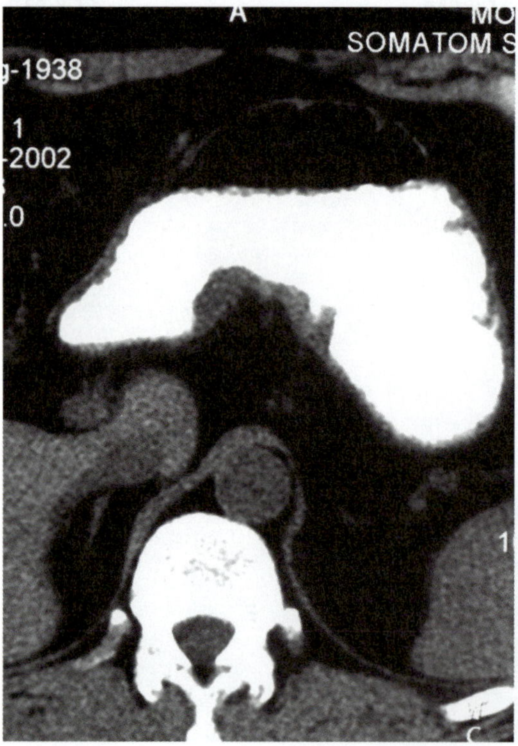

▼ Fig. 85 f.

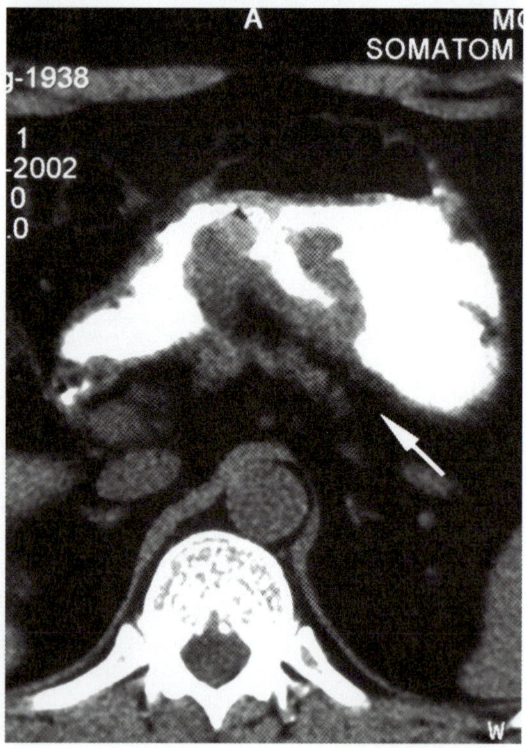

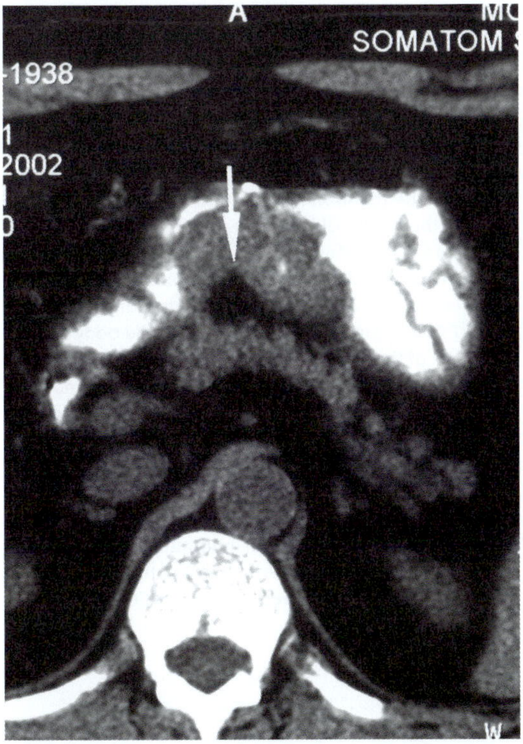

▲ **Fig. 85 g.**

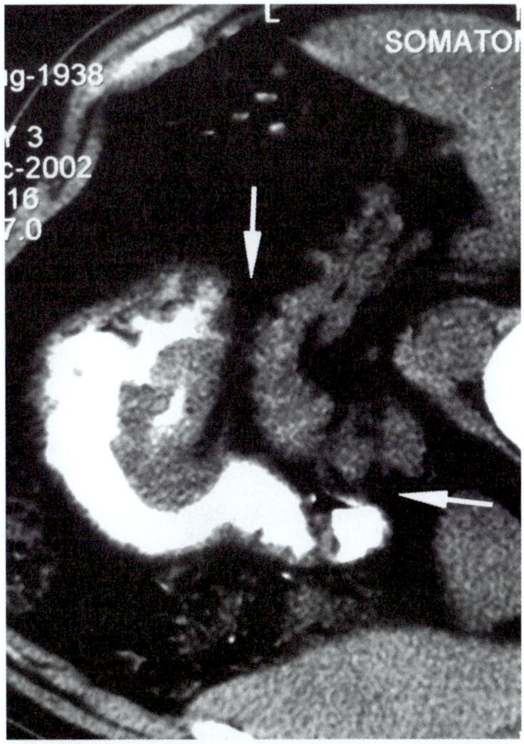

▲ **Fig. 85 i.**

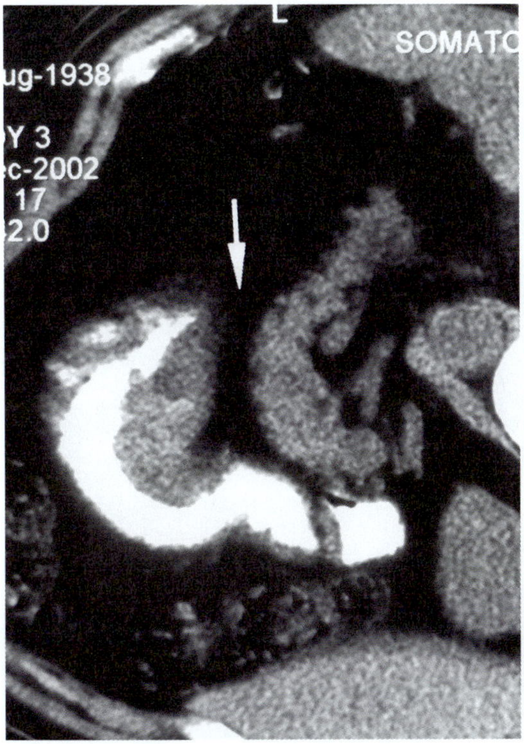

▼ **Fig. 85 h.**

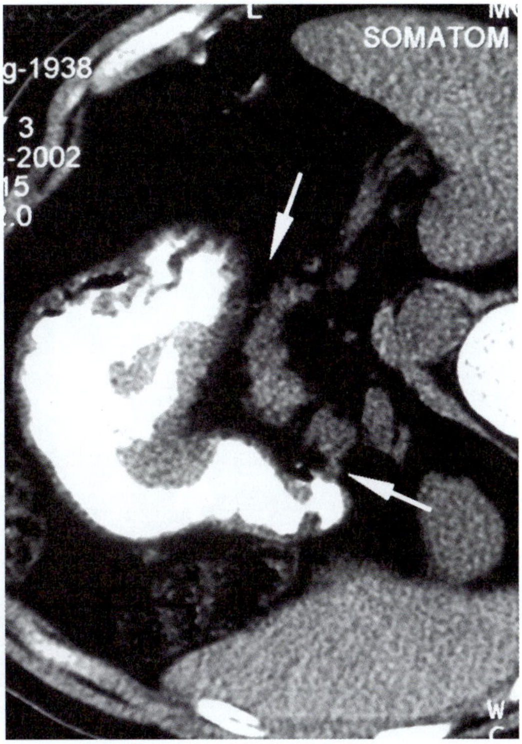

▼ **Fig. 85 j.**

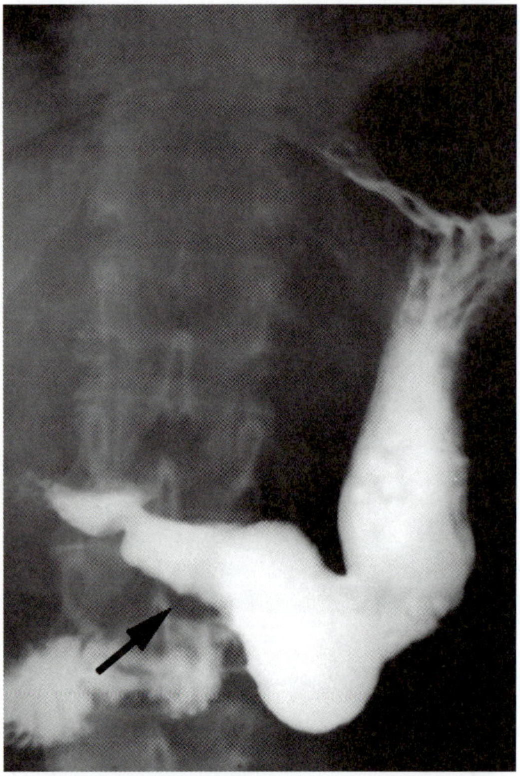

Fig. 86a–f. Female patient V., age 56. Diagnosis: gastric cancer. **a** Stomach roentgenogram (tight filling, vertical position, anterior projection): the antral part is narrowed and curved, the walls are rigid, the contour of the greater curvature is uneven (arrow), the stomach sinus sags. **b** Stomach roentgenogram (double contrast, horizontal position, anterior projection): the antral part is irregularly and circularly narrowed due to intramural infiltration; the walls are rigid (arrows); the duodenal loop is straightened. In order to verify the spread of the tumor to the adjacent anatomical structures, the patient was examined by computed tomography. **c** Computed tomogram of the stomach (tight filling with E-Z-CAT DRY, supine position, the level of the body and the distal part of the stomach): the walls are thickened unevenly due to circular intramural infiltration (white arrow indicates site of the maximum thickening). The hypodense stripe of a fat layer between the infiltrated stomach wall and the pancreas body is absent (black arrow). **d, e, f** Computed tomograms (tight filling with E-Z-CAT DRY, supine position, at the level of the body and the distal part of the stomach): the walls are thickened due to intramural infiltration. The hypodense stripe of fatty tissue between the infiltrated stomach wall and the pancreas head is irregular (arrow). Conclusion: Infiltrative cancer of the antral part of the stomach with invasion of the pancreas

◄ **Fig. 86 a.**

▼ **Fig. 86 b.**

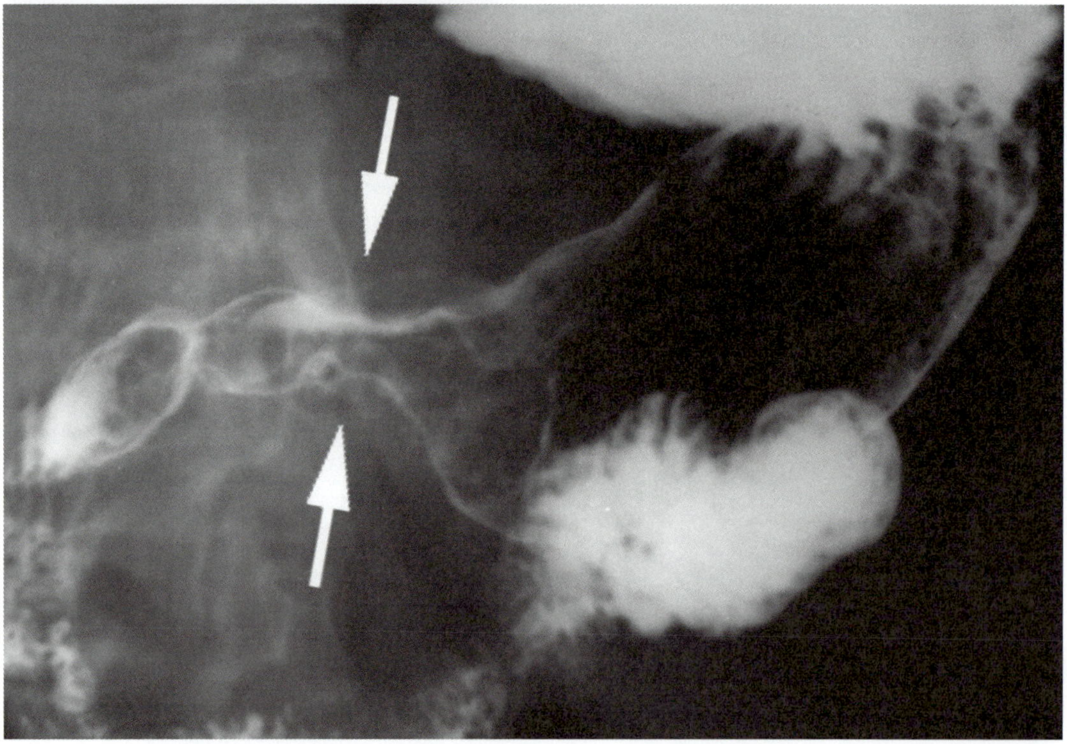

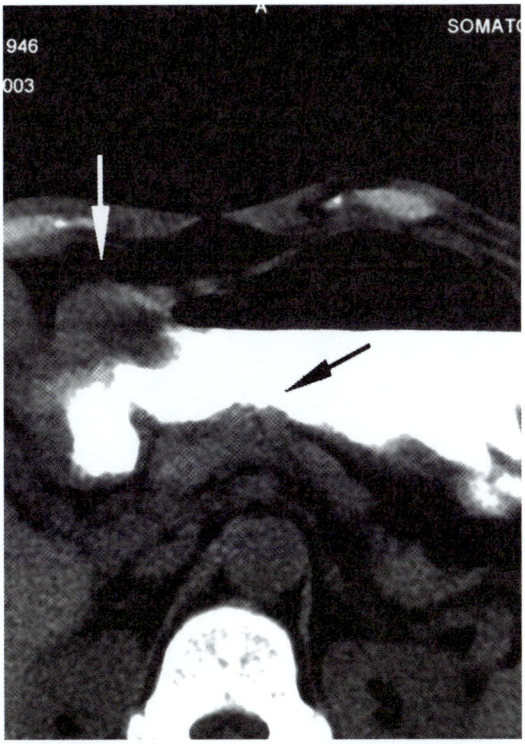

▲ **Fig. 86 c.**

▼ **Fig. 86 d.**

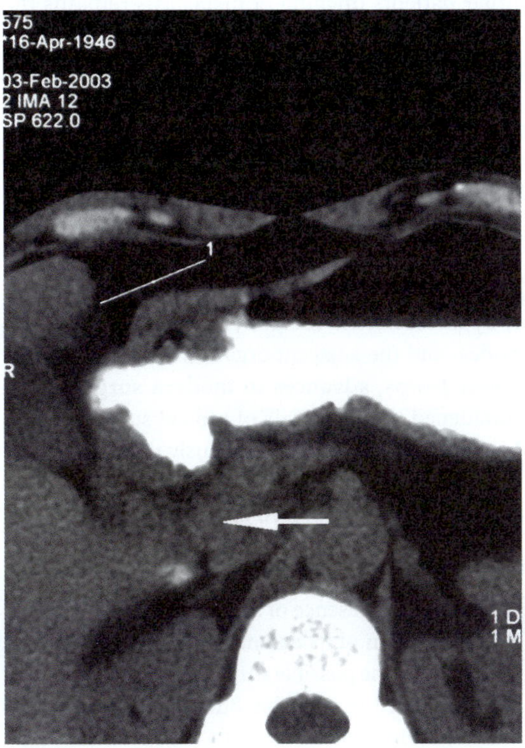

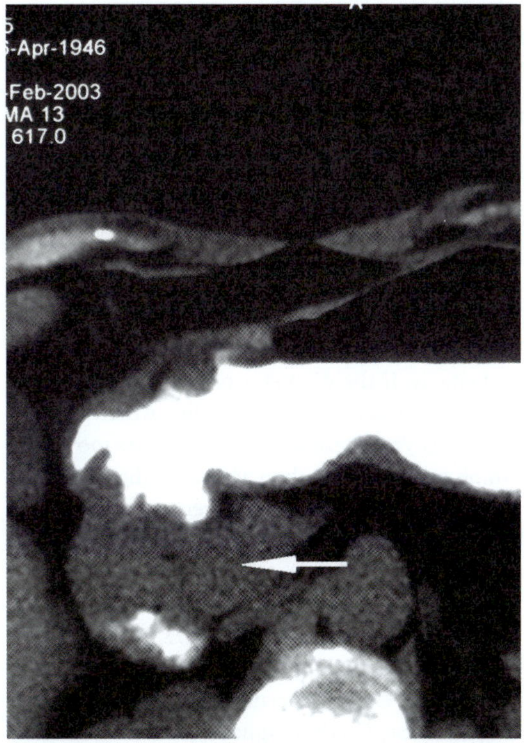

▲ **Fig. 86 e.**

▼ **Fig. 86 f.**

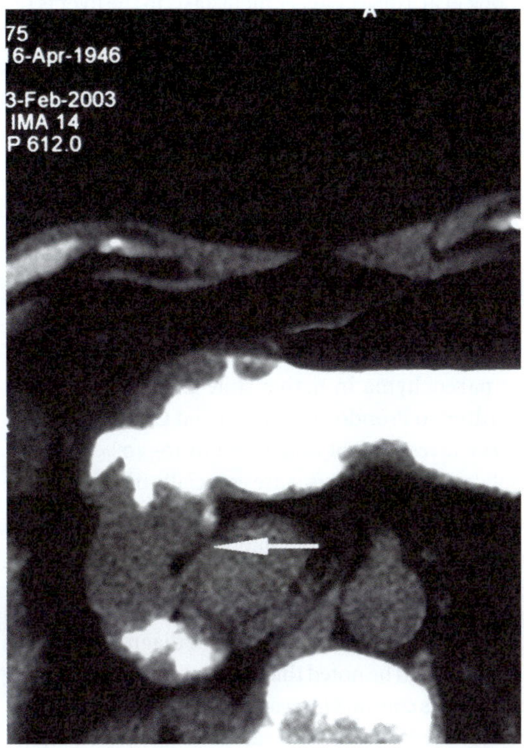

CT assessments of lymph node involvement in the tumor process reported by various authors are controversial. This is explained by the fact that CT only determines the size of the nodes without giving information on the nature of their enlargement. Meanwhile, tumor invasion of the lymph nodes is not always accompanied by their enlargement. Likewise, enlargement of even perigastric lymph nodes is not always connected with their affection by metastasis. Kitaev indicates that lymph nodes greater than 20 mm in diameter more definitely indicate metastasis. If the diameter of lymph nodes is between 11 and 20 mm, the probability of their involvement is 85.5%, whereas probability nears 100% with lymph nodes greater than 20 mm in diameter. The most reliable criterion of involvement of the lymph nodes is their conglomerates, in which the size of separate nodes exceeds 10 mm (Fig. 87). Fukuya et al. report that the efficiency of CT in determining metastases to the lymph nodes is 72.5% [125].

While the evaluation of metastases to lymph nodes using CT is associated with certain difficulties, its efficacy in the diagnosis of metastatic affection of the liver is sufficiently high. According to Cook et al. (1986), cancer metastasis to the liver is revealed in 85–96% cases; according to Karmazanovsky (1997), the accuracy of CT in diagnosing involvement of the liver is 86% [13].

The density of intact liver parenchyma is 50–75 Hounsfield units (Hu). In native-state studies, it is impossible to detect focal affections such as metastases, the density of which differs only insignificantly (by 5–10 Hu) from that of normal liver parenchyma. False-negative results may also be due to the small size of foci (less than 10 mm), which remain undifferentiated against the background of the liver parenchyma in native-state examinations. According to Prondo et al. (1979) and Oue et al. (1985), metastases are not diagnosed in 10–40% of cases; subcapsular metastases are especially difficult to detect.

It is known that computed tomography conducted before and after contrast intensification (potential administration of water-soluble contrast medium) is an important element of the diagnostic search. But it should be noted that such intensification of intravenous contrast improves visualization of metastases in only one third of cases because parenchyma density increases only by 20–30 Hu in such cases. In other patients imaging of metastasis remains the same or becomes less distinct. The latter is explained by leveling of the densitometric parameters of metastasis-affected and intact parenchyma, which masks the foci. Therefore, if metastasis to the liver is suspected, contrast medium should be given in bolus using automatic injectors.

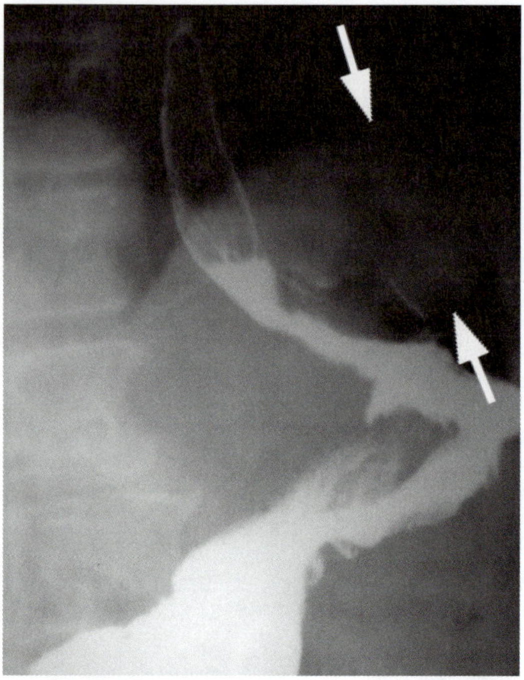

▲ **Fig. 87 a.**

Despite advances that have been made in diagnostic methods, the percentage of diagnostic laparotomies remains high. This is accounted for mostly by metastases to the liver, retroperitoneal lymph nodes, and the adjacent organs and major vessels. Nevertheless, advances in modern surgery have broadened the potentials of radical surgery. It has become popular to simultaneously remove the primary tumor and intraoperatively discovered metastases to the liver, provided only one lobe of the liver is involved. If both lobes are affected by metastasis, radical surgery is infeasible. Therefore, accurate detection of the presence of focal affection of the liver and estimation of its extent are of the greatest importance for the possible surgical removal of metastases localized in one lobe. But the resolution power of conventional CT and of CT with intravenous

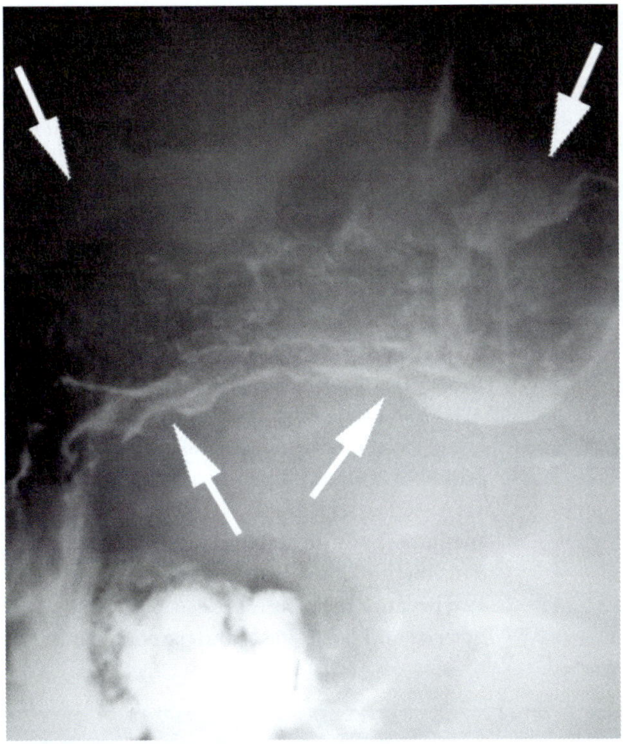

▲ **Fig. 87 b.**

Fig. 87a–e. Female patient D., age 58. Diagnosis: gastric cancer. **a** Stomach roentgenogram (tight filling, vertical position, anterior projection) at the moment of contrast medium passage through the gastroesophageal junction: the abdominal segment of the esophagus near the cardia is narrowed, uneven contours, marked deformation of the body and the upper part of the stomach, the stomach–diaphragm distance markedly increased (arrows). **b, c** Stomach roentgenograms (double contrast, horizontal position, left lateral position): the walls of the body and the upper part of the stomach are thickened and rigid due to diffuse circular intramural infiltration (arrows). Conclusion: Infiltrative cancer of the body and the upper part of the stomach with invasion of the abdominal part of the esophagus. In order to verify the extent of propagation of the tumor process to the adjacent anatomical structures, the patient was given a CT examination. **d, e** Computed tomograms (dosed inflation of the stomach with air, supine position, the level of the upper third of the stomach): uneven thickening of the walls due to intramural infiltration; uneven internal contours. Enlarged lymph nodes, with a diameter of 10–35 mm, are visualized in the projection of the spleen hilus, lesser omentum (arrows), and para-aortally. Conclusion: Infiltrative cancer of the body and the upper part of the stomach with metastases to the lymph nodes of the abdominal cavity and the retroperitoneal space.

▼ **Fig. 87 c.**

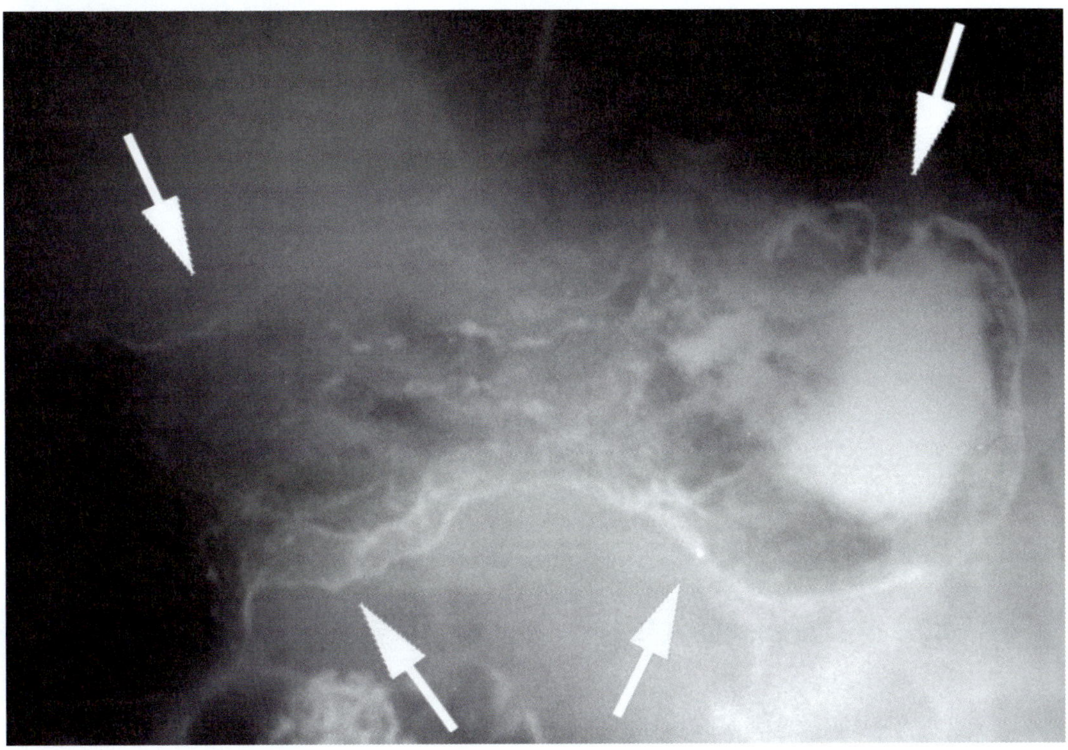

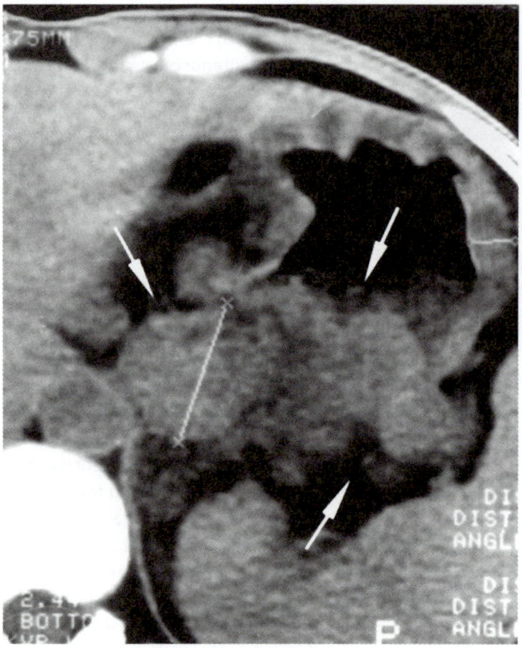

▲ Fig. 87 d.

intensification is insufficient; therefore, methods have been developed using selective intra-arterial administration of contrast medium.

There are three methods of intra-arterial enhancement of CT images:

1. CTAP – CT arterial portography, in which contrast medium is administered into the superior mesenteric artery. Intensification is obtained by contrast medium delivery through the portal vein.
2. CTA – CT arteriography, in which contrast medium is administered through the hepatic artery and the image is intensified largely in the arterial phase and to a lesser degree in the parenchymatous phase.
3. CTA – CT arteriography, in which contrast medium is administered into the iliac stem. This method has advantages over the former two because the results are estimated in both arterial and porto-vasal and parenchymatous

▼ Fig. 87 e.

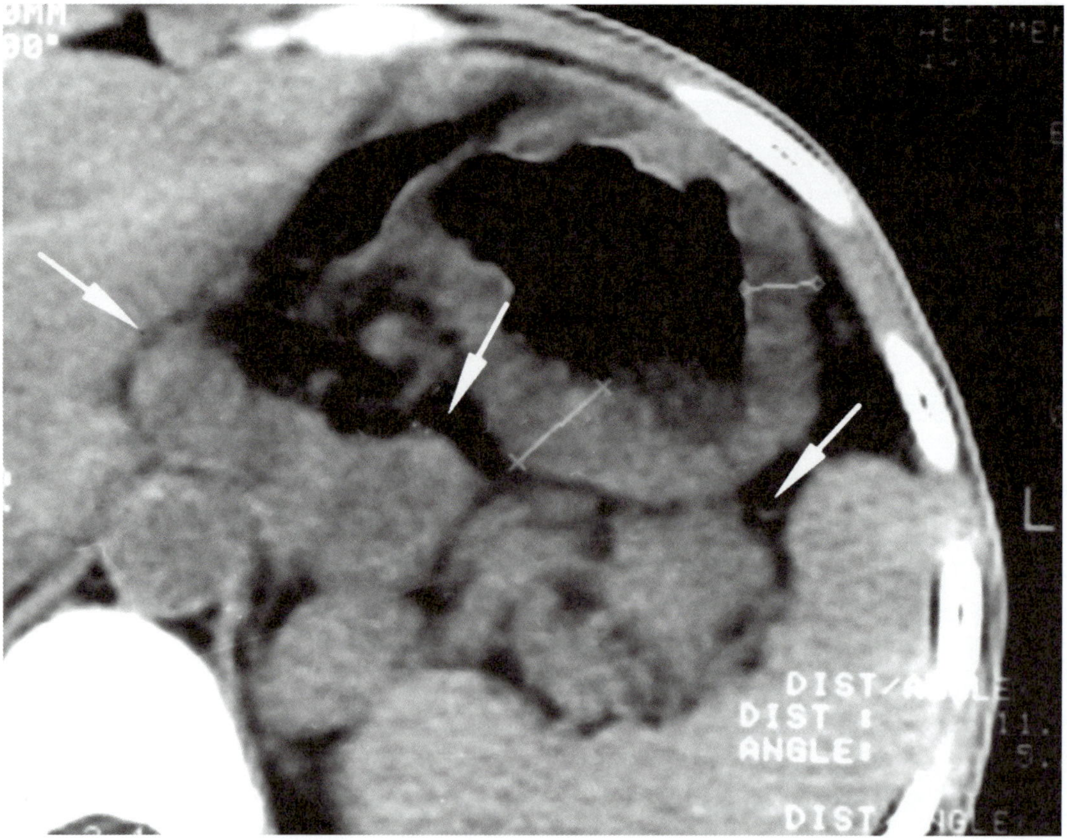

phases. However, the latter method is connected with the use of a catheter and performance of the procedure at one working post.

Intra-aortic enhancement of a CT image of the liver significantly increases density of the liver parenchyma, as contrast medium is consecutively accumulated in the parenchyma and in the foci of pathology; this helps to detect those foci which are undetectable by standard CT. Without going into much detail regarding CT arteriography, which is described in the monograph by Karmazanovsky, Vilyavin, and Nikitaev »Computed tomography of the liver and the bile ducts« (1997), we want to note that selective intra-arterial administration of radiopaque contrast medium increases density of the liver parenchyma 2.5–4.0 times to attain the value of 150–240 Hu. The significant difference in density and time of appearance of contrast between the focus and the liver parenchyma and the presence of a hypervascular rim are the main factors increasing the resolution power of CT. This helps detection of foci which have the same density as that of the parenchyma and are not therefore detectable by standard CT [13].

To summarize the data related to the use of computed tomography in the diagnosis of gastric cancer, several major factors can be emphasized: There is the possibility of CT to detect early endophytic cancer of the stomach (the wall-thickening sign), and there is verification of the extent of tumor spread (invasion of the neighboring organs and tissues, metastases). Computed tomography findings are another confirmation of the prevalence of the infiltrative form of cancer among malignant tumors of the stomach.

Magnetic Resonance Signs

There are two reasons for including MRI in the sections of this book describing our understanding of current methodological-semiotic possibilities of radiological diagnosis of gastric cancer. First, MRI of the stomach is now acknowledged as a common method for diagnosing gastric pathology in general and gastric cancer in particular. Second, recent publications imply that endoscopy is the foundation on which the characteristics of MRI of the stomach are based; the results of modern traditional radiology with tight filling and double contrast are completely disregarded. This approach inevitably interferes with a complete and objective estimation of the diagnostic role of MRI of the stomach.

In addition to endoscopic findings, while looking at the possibilities of MRI, we took the results of traditional X-ray examinations with double contrast and subsequent comparative studies of MRI, anatomical, and surgical data as the basic initial data. We used these basic data to study MRI signs of gastric cancer, which we will now discuss.

In order to evaluate the condition of the stomach wall and the basic MRI criteria of affection, the MRI characteristics of an intact stomach (without signs of pathology) were first established. As the stomach cavity is distended with water, the stomach contents are shown on a T1 image by the low-intensity signal; on a T2 image it is bright due to the long T1 and T2 of water. On a T1 image, the stomach wall at optimal distension is not visualized except in the zone of the gastroesophageal junction, the anteroposterior size of which does not exceed 10 mm (◘ Fig. 88). Visualization of the wall on a T1 image is always connected with tumor or inflammatory infiltration (◘ Fig. 89) [14, 111, 220, 235].

On a T2 image, the wall thickness at the level of the stomach body (anterior and posterior walls and the lesser curvature) is 2–4 mm; on the greater curvature and in the sinus region it is 3–4 mm, due to the specific character of the mucosal relief and the higher tone of the circular fibers of smooth muscles of the greater curvature compared with the other parts of the stomach. The signal from the intact stomach wall is homogeneous and has moderate intensity (◘ Fig. 90). The inner configuration of the wall may be somewhat uneven, as if serrated, due to incompletely stretched mucosal folds. The outer contours are distinct, excepting those of the greater curvature in the lower third of the stomach and its sinus. As on a TI image, the thickness of the gastroesophageal junction is 10 mm, signal intensity is lower than that from the stomach walls over the other parts, or identical to it. This is because of the large volume of muscle tissue in this zone, and because natural distension of the esophageal and stomach walls in this region is viewed in the oblique plane of scanning in the axial projection [136, 159].

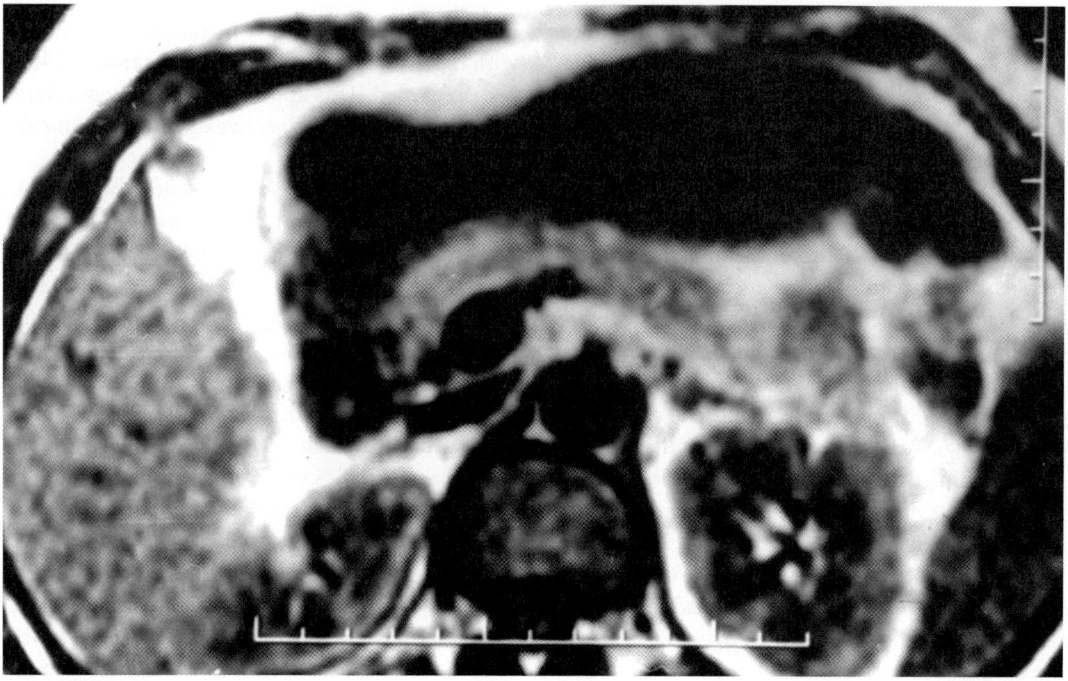

▲ **Fig. 88.** MRI of an intact stomach body on a T1 image: the wall is not visualized.

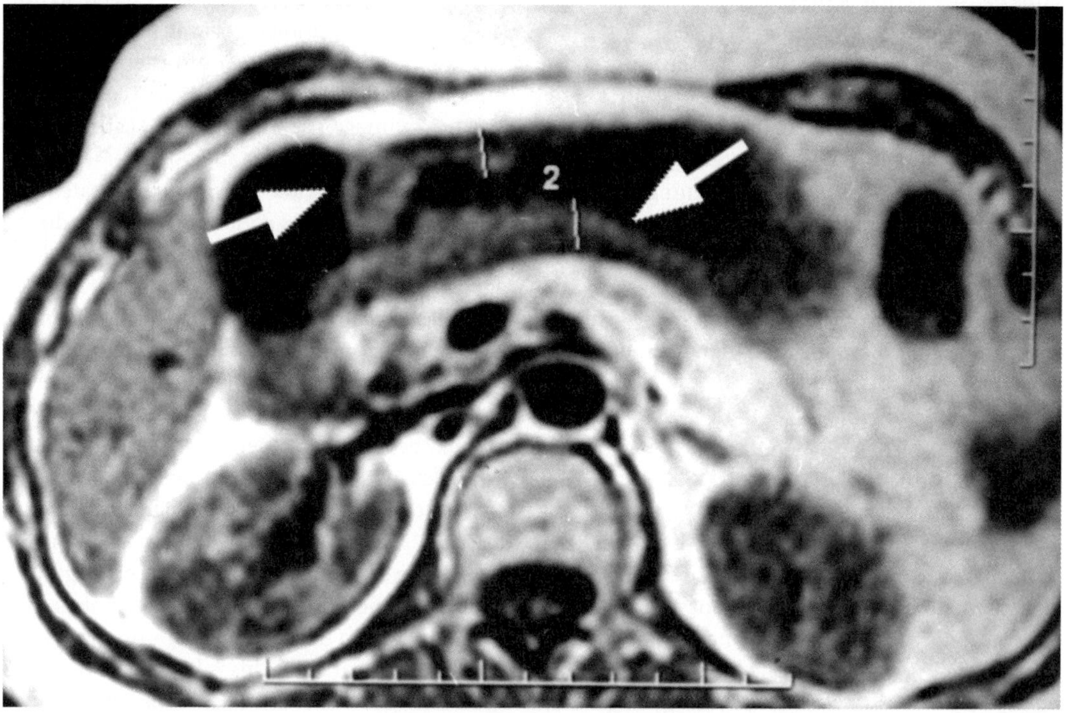

Fig. 89. Patient M., age 67. Diagnosis: gastric cancer. MRI of the stomach on a T1 image: uneven thickening of the anterior wall (1) and posterior wall (2) to 12 mm. The MR signal from the affected wall is heterogeneous, mostly of moderate intensity (arrows). The patient was operated. Histologically, adenocarcinoma

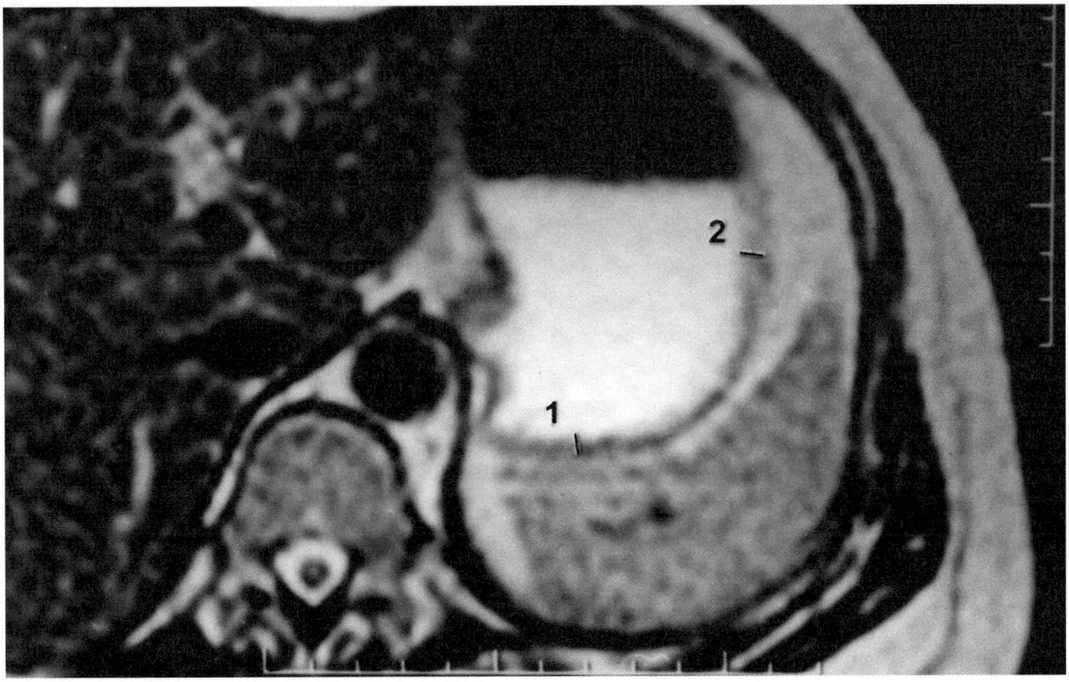

▲ **Fig. 90.** MRI of the upper part of an intact stomach as viewed on a T2 image: the posterior wall is 4 mm thick (1), the greater curvature wall is 5 mm thick (2)

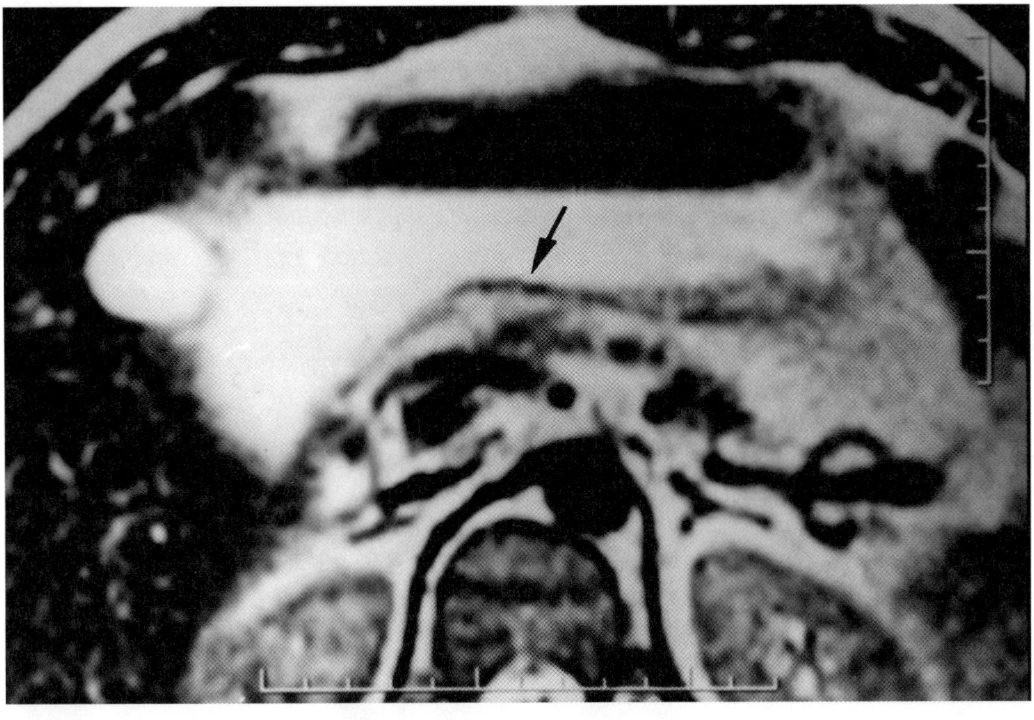

▲ **Fig. 91.** MRI of the pyloric part of the intact stomach on a T2 image: a distinct hypointense, uniform 1.5-mm stripe is seen along the posterior wall – the reflection of the serous membrane (arrow)

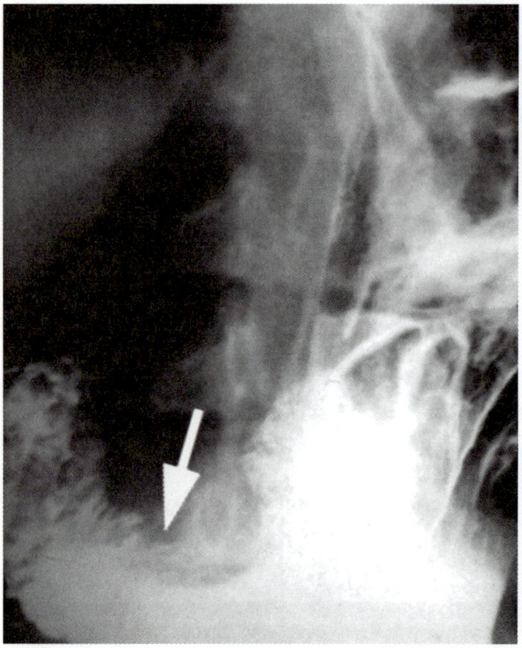

▲ **Fig. 92 a.**

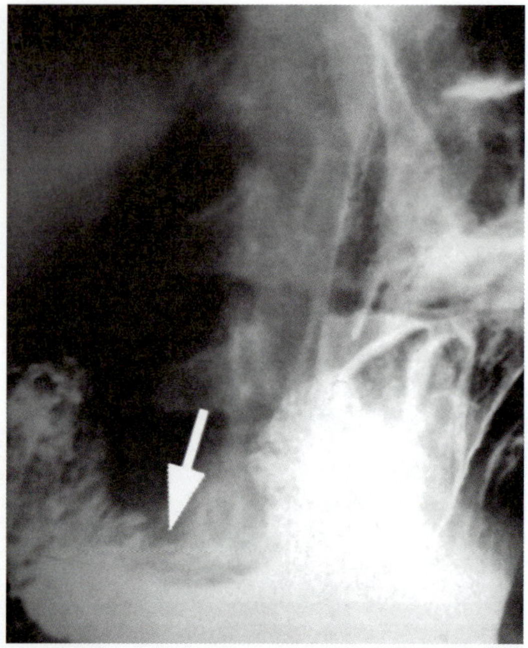

▲ **Fig. 92 b.**

▼ **Fig. 92 d.**

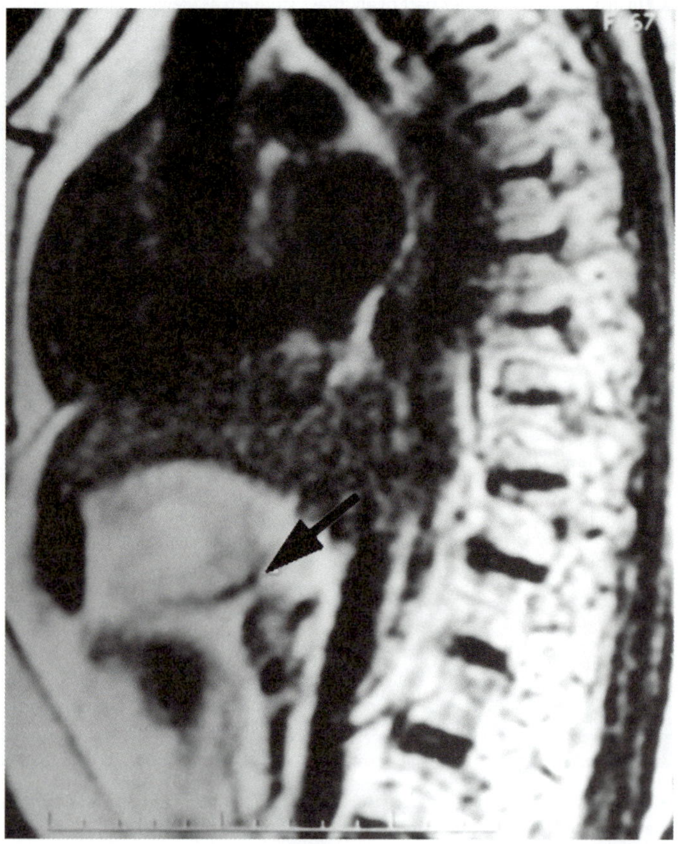

Fig. 92a–e. Female patient R., age 63. Diagnosis: gastric cancer. **a** Stomach roentgenogram (tight filling, vertical position, anterior projection): the distal part of the stomach is strongly disfigured, pulled upwards due to massive circular infiltration (arrow). **b** Stomach roentgenogram (double contrast, horizontal position, right half-oblique projection): walls of the antral part and the lower third of the stomach body are thickened and rigid due to intramural infiltration, invading the stomach body (arrows). Conclusion: Infiltrative cancer of the antral part and the body of the stomach. **c** MRI (stomach filled with water, axial projection, level of the pyloric part of the stomach, T2 image): the border between the infiltrative tumor of the stomach and the pancreas head is not detectable (arrows). **d** MRI of the stomach (stomach filled with water, sagittal projection, level of the pyloric part of the stomach, T2 image): distinctly visualized is the border between the infiltrated tumor of the stomach wall and the pancreas head (arrow). **e** Fragment of a macrospecimen (strip): stomach wall is thickened over a considerable length due to white intramural infiltration into the muscular coat (arrows). Histologically; signet-ring cell carcinoma with extracellular accumulation of mucus

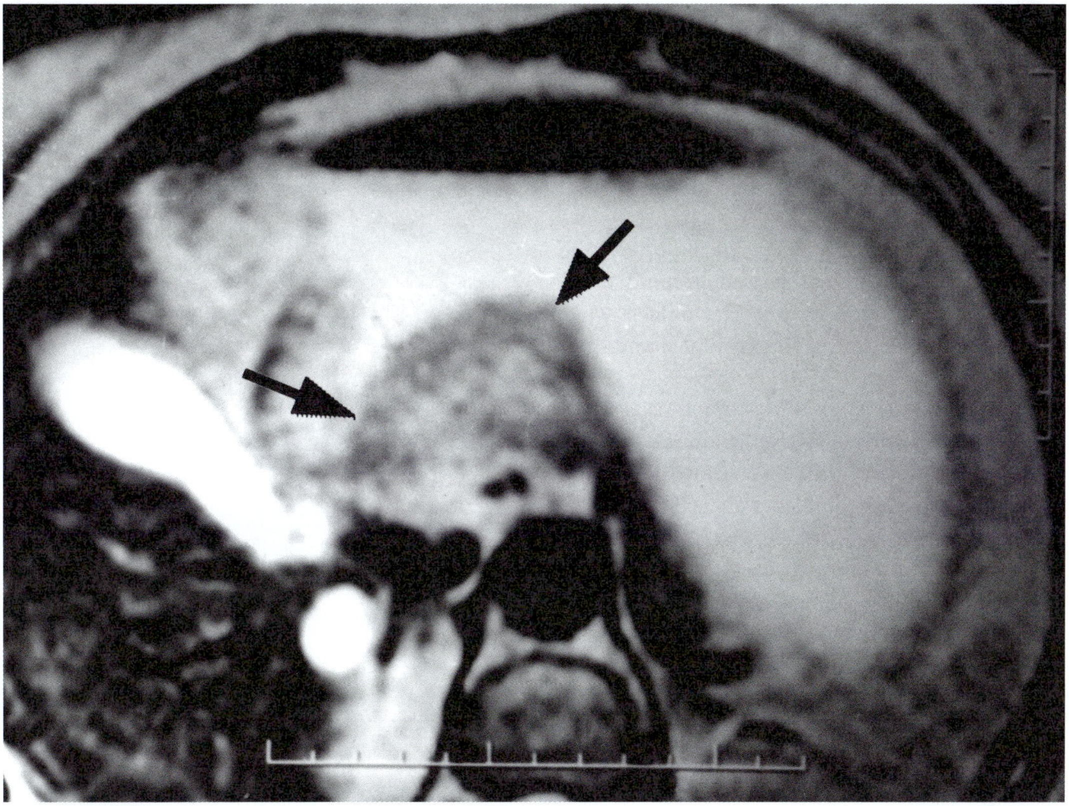

▲ **Fig. 92 c.**

▼ **Fig. 92 e.**

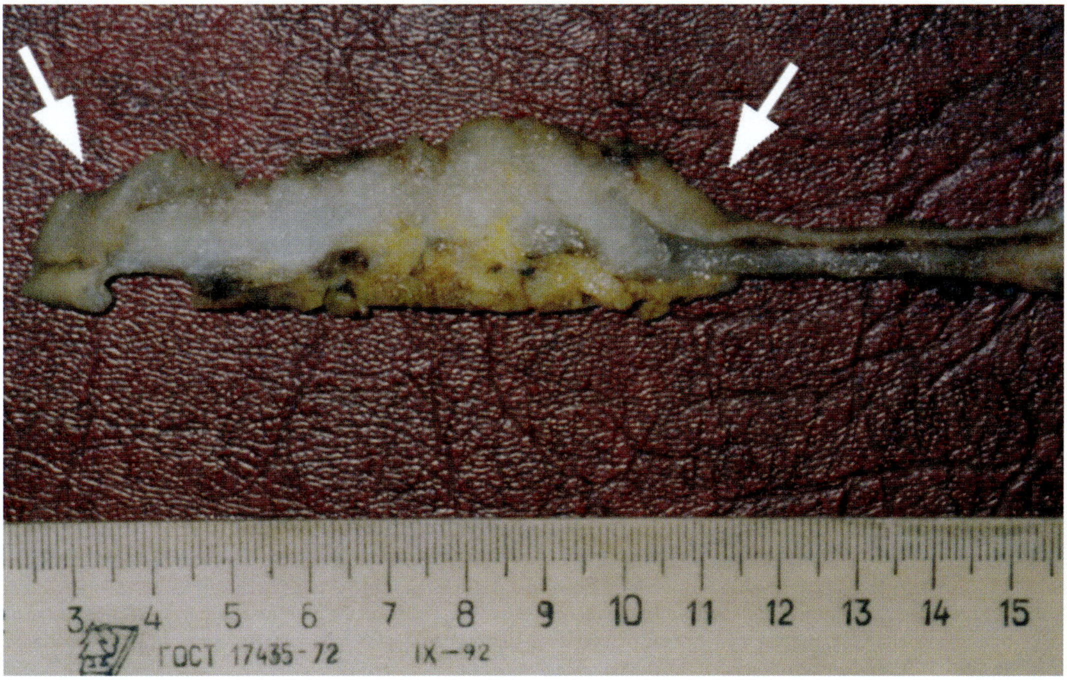

With good reflection of the pyloric part of the stomach in the axial plane of scanning, its wall thickness does not exceed 3 mm. The signal intensity is identical to that from the wall at the level of the stomach body. The outer contour of the stomach is distinct owing to a 1- to 1.5-mm-thick hypointensive stripe, which is the reflection of the serosa (Fig. 91). It is especially distinct in the pyloric part, probably because of the coincidence of the tomographic section and the position of this part of the stomach, which has its own reflection in the sagittal plane scans (Fig. 92).

The main MRI signs of blastomatous affection of the stomach, above all of the intramural spread of tumor infiltration, include thickening of the stomach wall, uneven contours, and also changes in the MR signal from the infiltrated wall (Fig. 93). Wall thickness with intramural tumors is 10–24 mm, with mixed tumors up to 40 mm. In case of intramural blastomatous affection, the signal from the stomach wall is usually of low intensity on the T2 image and intermediate on the T1 image. In some cases, the signal can be markedly heterogeneous in all scanning regimes or hyperintensive on the T2 image (in cases of signet-ring cell carcinoma with extracellular accumulation of mucus).

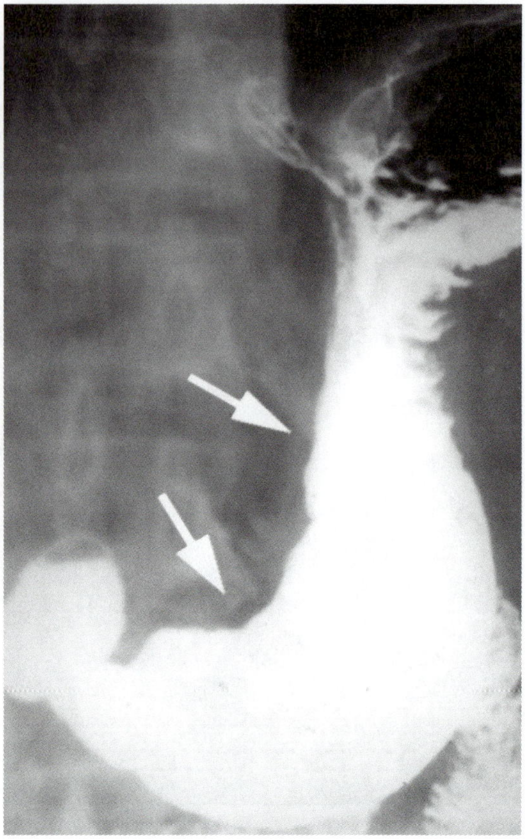

▲ **Fig. 93 a.**

Fig. 93a–d. Patient S., age 60. Diagnosis: gastric cancer. **a** Stomach roentgenogram (tight filling, vertical position, anterior projection): contour of the lesser curvature is uneven, the angular notch is straightened (arrows). **b** Stomach roentgenogram (double contrast, horizontal position, right half-oblique projection): the wall of the lesser curvature of the antral part and the body of the stomach is thickened and rigid due to intramural infiltration with marked convergence of the folds (white arrows) and a depot of contrast medium (black arrow). Conclusion: Infiltrative-ulcerous cancer of the antral part and the body of the stomach. Endoscopy revealed a 4x3-cm ulcer defect with rigid walls in the lower third of the stomach body on the lesser curvature. Histological examination of the bioptates taken from the floor of the granulating ulcer: sites of columnar epithelium; from the edges of the ulcer defect: small accumulation of proliferating epithelium against the background of inflammatory infiltration. Elements of yeast-like fungus. Tumor cells are not found. The patient was examined by MRI. **c** MRI of the stomach (stomach filled with water, axial projection, the level of the antral part and the body of the stomach, T2 image): anterior and posterior walls of the antral part are unevenly thickened, MR signal is heterogeneous, mostly hypointense due to intramural infiltration (arrows). **d** MRI of the stomach (stomach filled with water, sagittal projection, T2 image): infiltration spreads along the posterior wall to the angular notch, along the anterior wall to the middle third of the stomach body. The affection extends over 6.5 cm (arrows). Distal part of the thickened walls has eroded contours, the lumen of the pyloric part at this level is narrowed unevenly. Thickening of walls is uneven, maximum thickness to 12–15 mm. The inner contour of the affected wall is uneven, the outer contour is distinct and even. MR signal from infiltrated wall is mostly hypointense and heterogeneous. No signs of invasion of the adjacent cellular tissue. Enlarged lymph nodes are not detected. Conclusion: Infiltrative-ulcerous cancer of the antral part and the body of the stomach. Repeat endoscopy with subsequent histological examination of the bioptates revealed signet-ring cell carcinoma. This example is more evidence that one may not depend on the results of endoscopic examination alone.

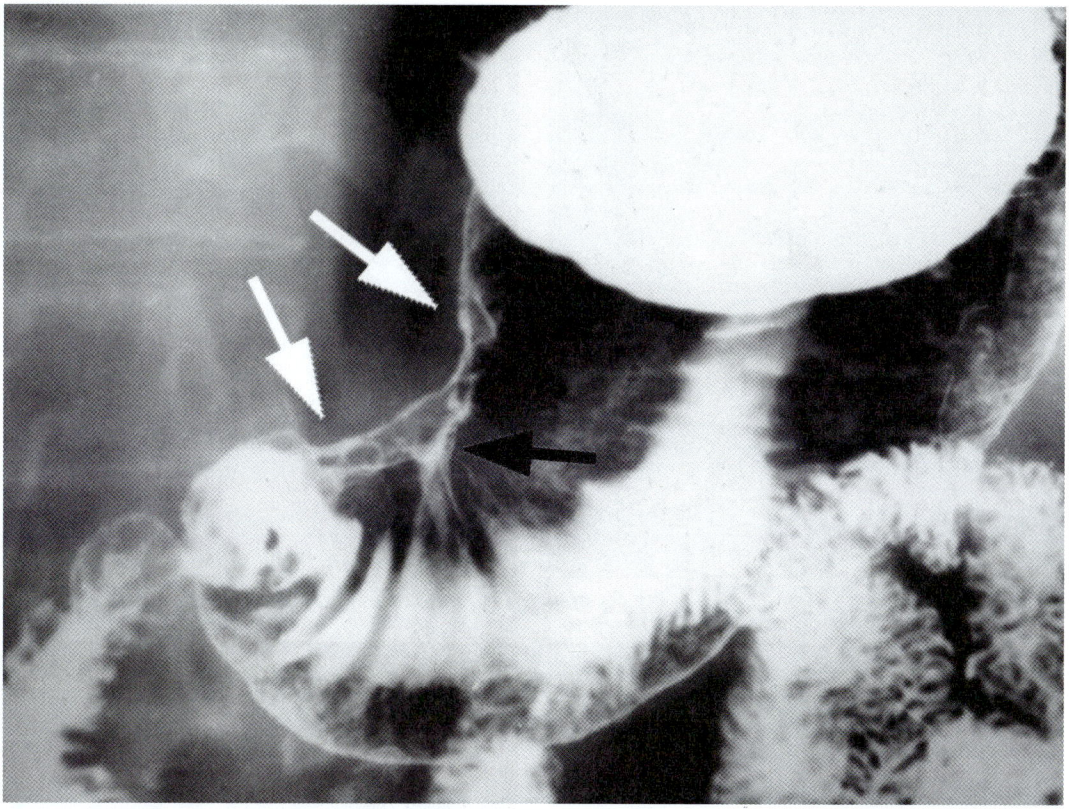

▲ **Fig. 93 b.**

▼ **Fig. 93 c.**

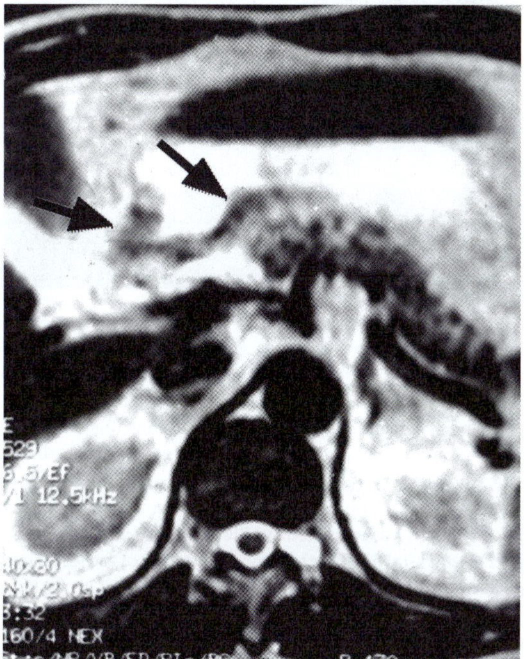

▼ **Fig. 93 d.**

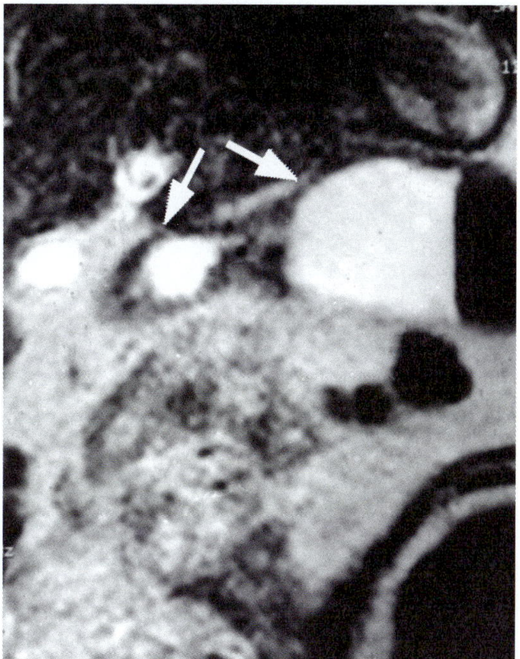

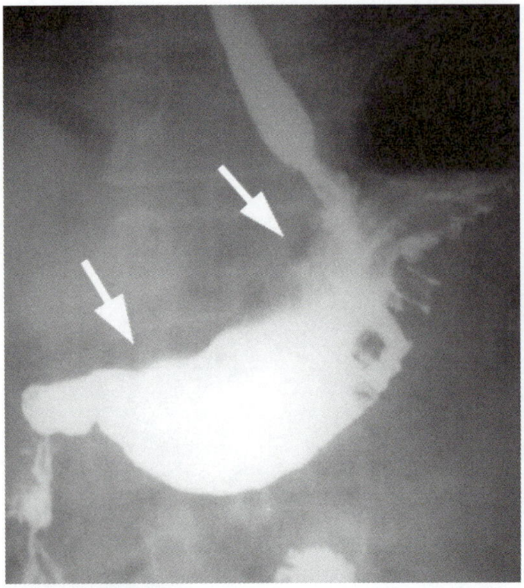

▲ **Fig. 94 a.**

▼ **Fig. 94 b.**

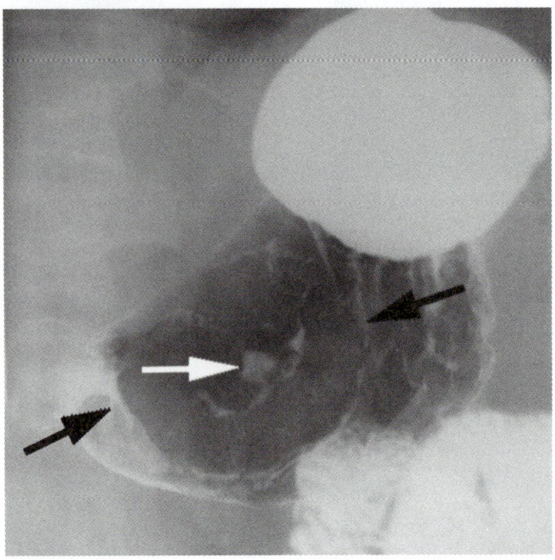

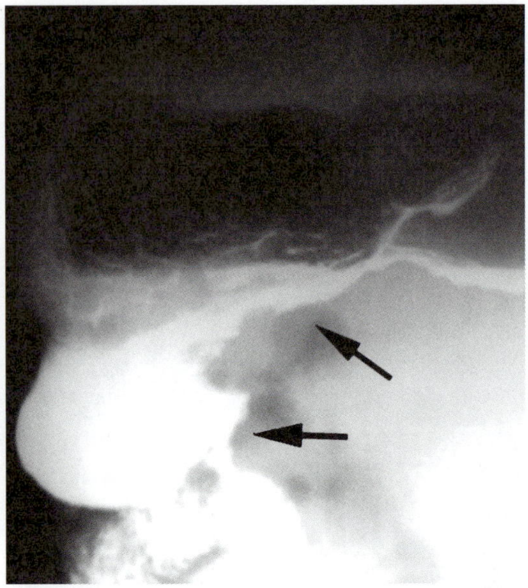

▲ **Fig. 94 c.**

▼ **Fig. 94 d.**

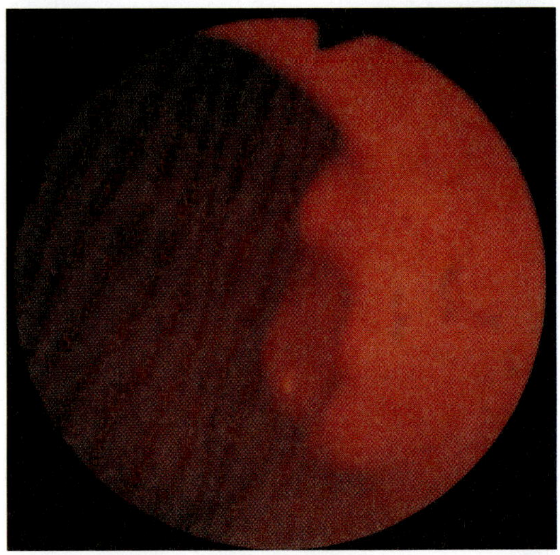

Fig. 94a–g. Patient A., age 64. Diagnosis: gastric cancer. **a** Stomach roentgenogram (tight filling, vertical position, anterior projection): the angular notch is straightened, markedly uneven contour of the lesser curvature of the stomach body (arrows). **b** Stomach roentgenogram (double contrast, horizontal position, anterior projection): a depot of contrast medium (white arrow) is distinctly visualized on the posterior wall of the lower third of the stomach body surrounded with marked infiltration (black arrows). **c** Stomach roentgenogram (double contrast, vertical position, left lateral projection): uneven contours of the posterior wall due to intramural infiltration with an ulcer niche (arrows). Conclusion: Infiltrative-ulcerous cancer of the stomach. **d** Endophotograph: a ridge of infiltrated tissue of about 3 cm with ulceration in the center is seen on the posterior wall of the lower third of the stomach body. Histological studies of bioptates did not reveal tumor cells. The patient was examined by MRI. **e, f** MR images of the stomach (coronary and axial projections, T2 SSFSE), the lumen is narrowed in the distal part due to tumor infiltration of the lesser curvature and the adjacent anterior and (more markedly) posterior walls (arrows). **g** MR image of the stomach (axial projection, T2 SSFSE), ulceration in the depth of tumor infiltration on the posterior wall; hyperintense MR signal from water (arrow). Conclusion: Infiltrative-ulcerous cancer of the stomach. Histological study of numerous bioptates taken during repeated endoscopies verified non-differentiated gastric cancer

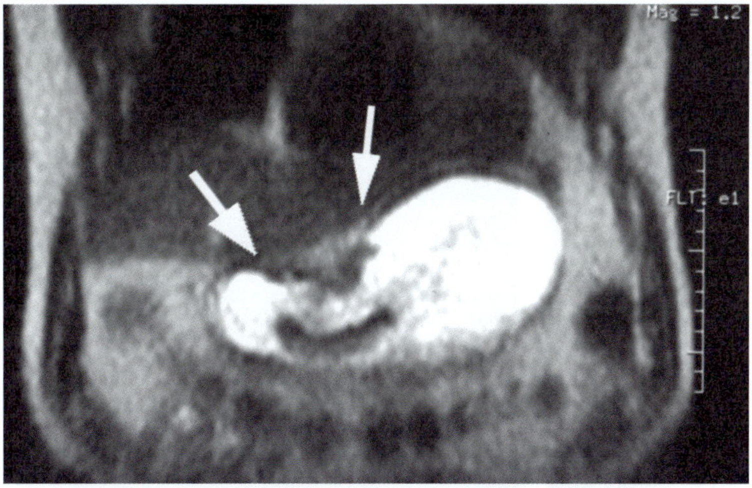

▲ **Fig. 94 e.**

▼ **Fig. 94 f.**

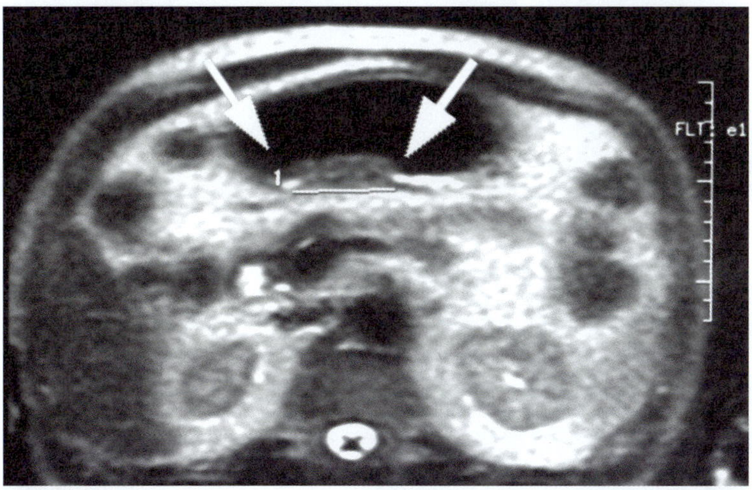

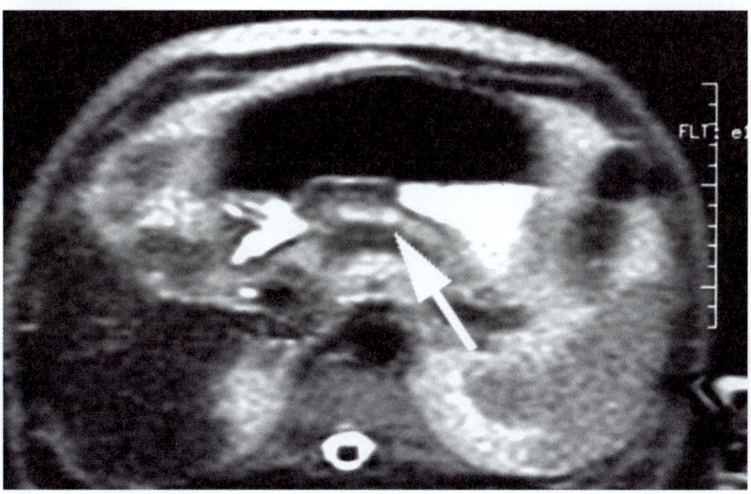

◄ **Fig. 94 g.**

The inner contours of the wall at the level of the affection are usually uneven and tuberous. The ulcerative form of gastric cancer is characterized by the niche or depot signs – a bright hyperintensive signal visualized in the depth of the affected wall of the stomach on the T2 image and a low-intensity signal on the T1 image are characteristic of water. Ulcers usually have irregular shapes and uneven contours (■ Fig. 94).

Tumor infiltration extending beyond the limits of the stomach wall to the perigastric cellular tissue is characterized by indistinct outer borders of the tumor and by a reticular and band-like pattern of the perigastric cellular tissue with a heterogeneous MR signal, which is more pronounced on the T1 image. The absence of a visualized hypointensive stripe (showing the serous membrane) in tumor affection of the pyloric part may suggest infiltration of the serous membrane (■ Fig. 95) [164, 216, 243].

As the tumor spreads to the adjacent organs and structures, the border between the affected stomach wall and the organ to which infiltration spreads is absent. The intensity of the signal from tumor invasion in the involved organ corresponds to the that of the infiltrated stomach wall (■ Fig. 96).

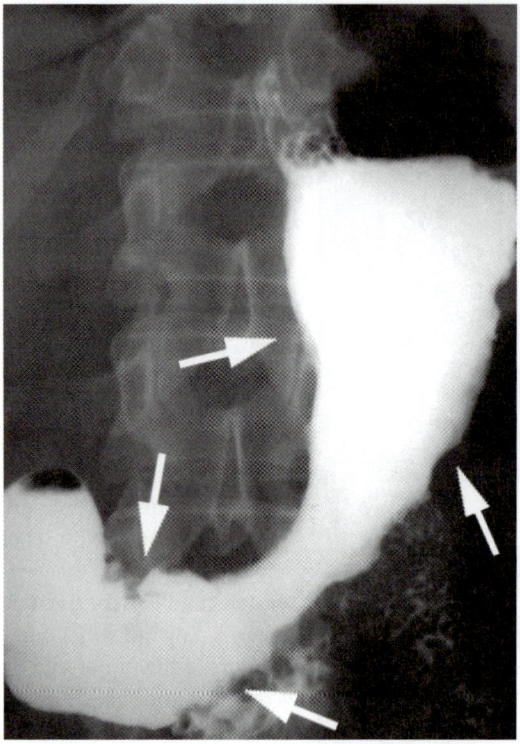

▲ **Fig. 95 a.**

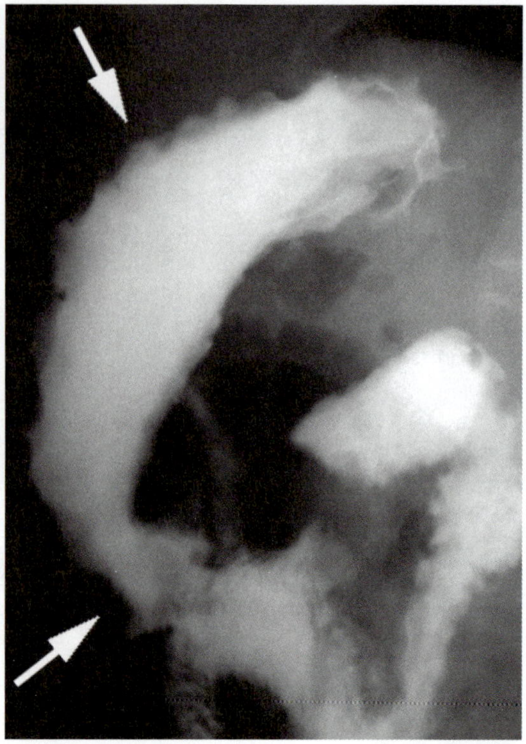

▲ **Fig. 95 b.**

▼ **Fig. 95 c.**

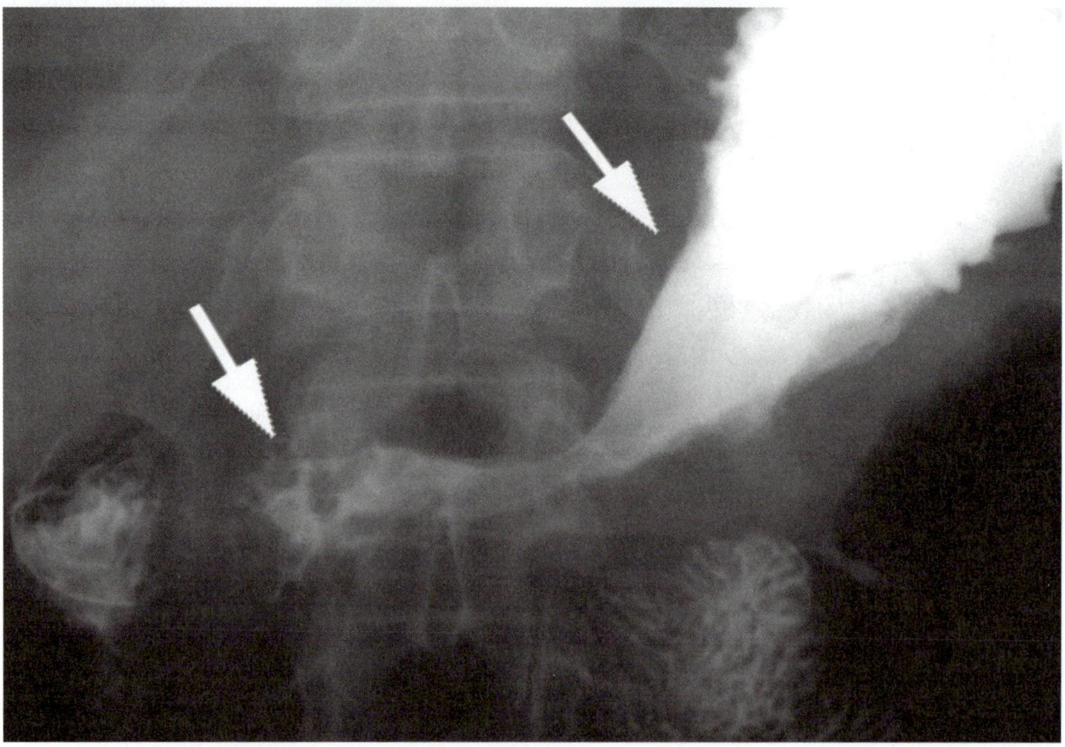

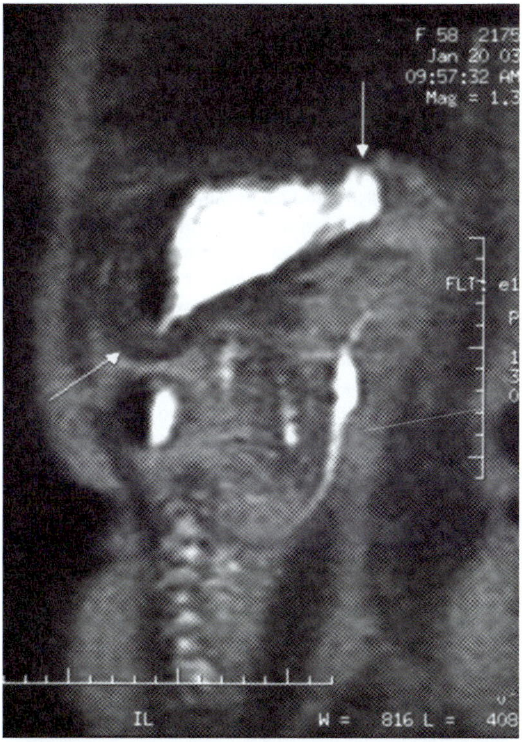

▲ **Fig. 95 d.**

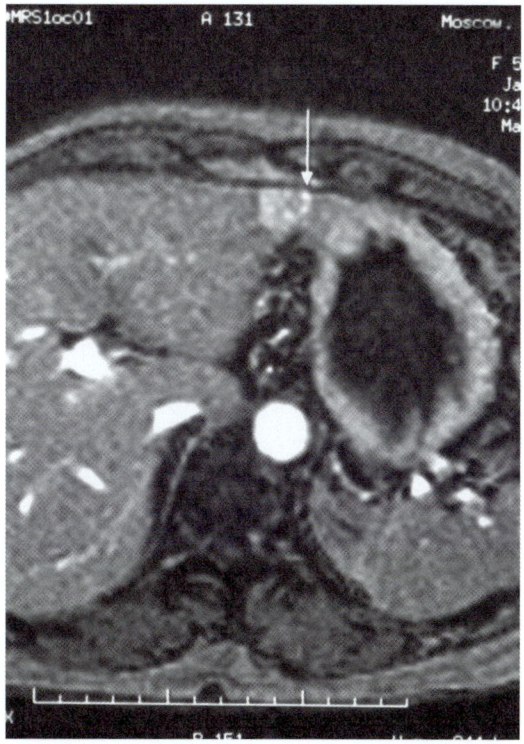

▲ **Fig. 95 f.**

▼ **Fig. 95 e.**

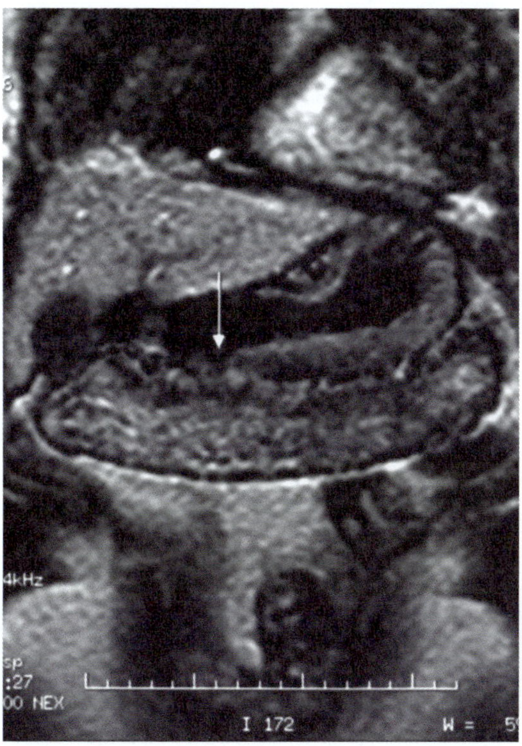

▼ **Fig. 95 g.**

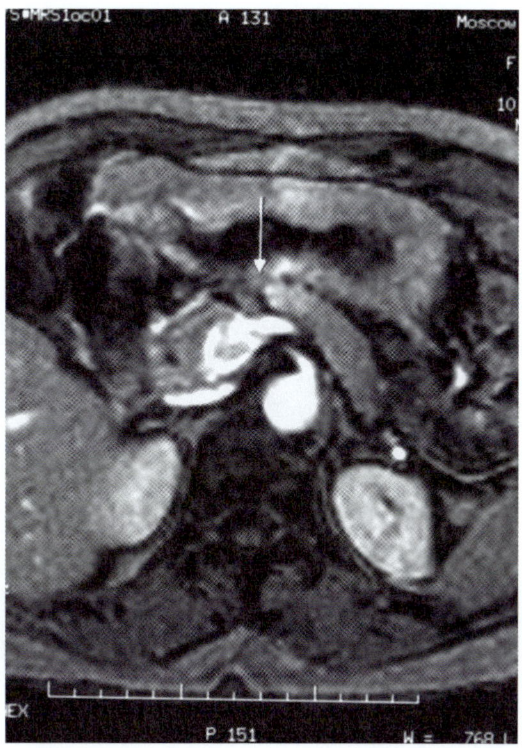

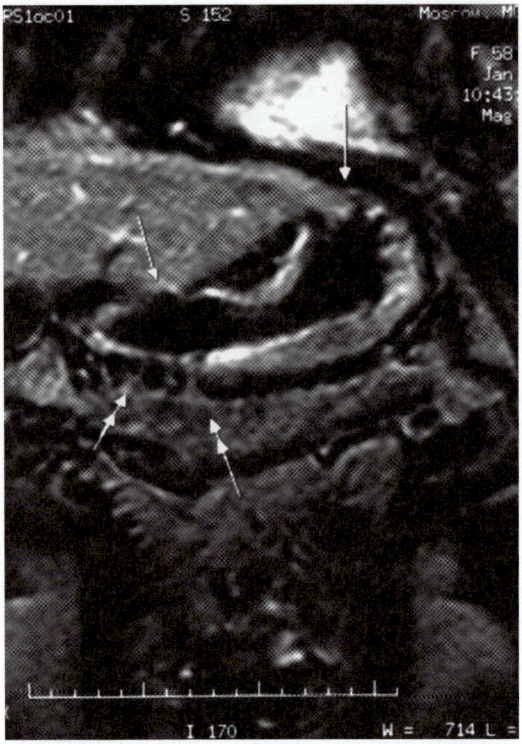

▲ Fig. 95 h.

▼ Fig. 95 i

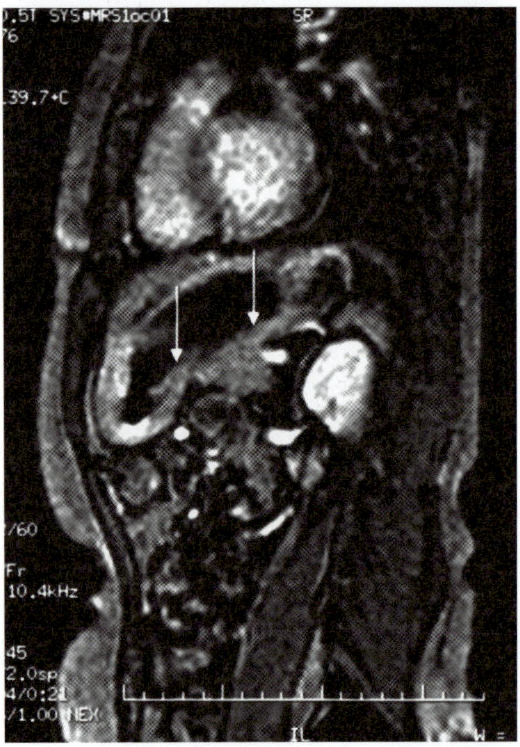

Fig. 95a–i. Female patient B., age 58. Diagnosis: gastric cancer. **a** Stomach roentgenogram (tight filling, vertical position, anterior projection): stomach cavity strongly decreased, the stomach is disfigured (rigid tube):, its contours are uneven over the entire length (arrows). **b** Stomach roentgenogram (tight filling, horizontal position, left posterior oblique projection): the stomach cavity markedly decreased, the stomach is disfigured (rigid tube), its contours are uneven (arrows). **c** Stomach roentgenogram (double contrast, horizontal position, anterior projection): failure to distend the stomach walls by double contrast because of their rigidity due to intramural infiltration (arrows). Conclusion: Infiltrative cancer of the stomach. In order to verify the extent of tumor spreading onto the neighboring anatomical structures, the patient was given MRI examination. **d** MR image (sagittal projection, T2 FSE): marked thickening of all walls due to infiltration extending from the subcardiac to the pyloric part (arrows); outer contours of the affected wall are indistinct, the outer contours are uneven. **e** MR image (coronary projection, FSPGR out of phase); the lower border of infiltration is distinctly visualized (arrow); the pyloric part is not changed. Irregular hypointense stripe at the level of the thickened wall of the stomach on the greater curvature, which does not exclude growth into the serous membrane. Intravenous contrast enhancement. **f** MR image (axial projection, FSPGR out of phase, with intravenous contrast enhancement – 20 ml Magnevist); marked accumulation of contrast medium in the thickened wall of the stomach; more vivid affection of the serous membrane and spread of infiltration to left lobe of the liver (arrow). **g** MR image (coronary projection, FSPGR out of phase, with intravenous contrast enhancement – 20 ml Magnevist); marked accumulation of contrast medium in the thickened wall of the stomach, more obvious growth into the serous membrane of the stomach and spread of infiltration onto the pancreas (arrow). **h** MR image (coronary projection, FSPGR out of phase, with intravenous contrast intensification – 20 ml Magnevist); marked accumulation of contrast medium in the thickened wall of the stomach; more vivid affection of the serous membrane and spread of infiltration to transverse colon and left lobe of the liver (arrows). **i** MR image (sagittal projection, FSPGR out of phase, with intravenous contrast enhancement – 20 ml Magnevist); marked accumulation of contrast medium in the thickened wall of the stomach; more vivid affection of the serous membrane and spread of infiltration to the pancreas (arrows). Conclusion: Infiltrative cancer of the stomach with invasion of left lobe of the liver, pancreas, and transverse colon.

Fig. 96a–g. Female patient V., age 36. Diagnosis: gastric cancer. **a** Stomach roentgenogram (tight filling, vertical position, anterior projection): the lesser curvature is pulled up, the contours are uneven; the angular notch is straightened, a flat niche in its projection (arrow). **b** Stomach roentgenogram (double contrast, horizontal position, right oblique projection): a depot of contrast medium on the lesser curvature (black arrow) with pronounced convergence of infiltrated folds; wall of lesser curvature is thickened and rigid due to intramural infiltration (white arrows). **c** Stomach roentgeno-

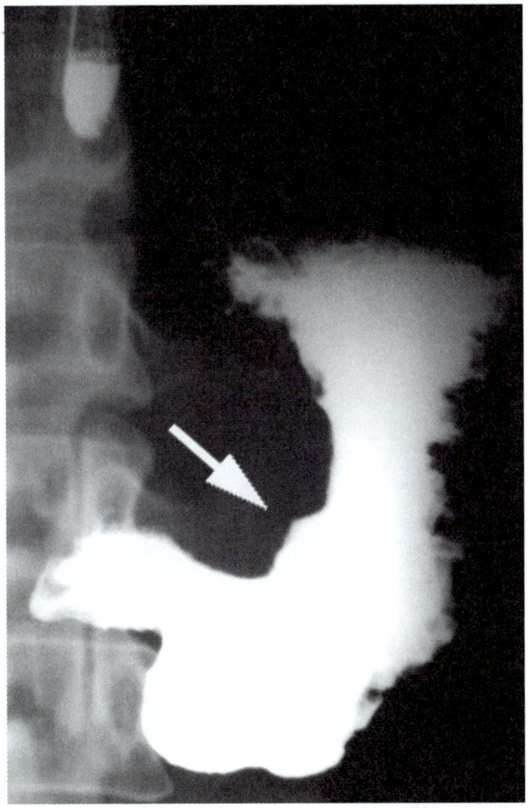

▲ **Fig. 96 a.**

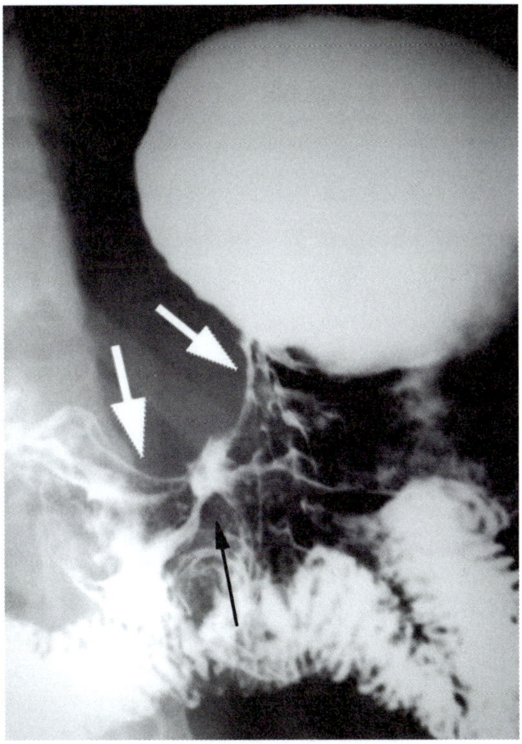

▲ **Fig. 96 b.** ▼ **Fig. 96 c.**

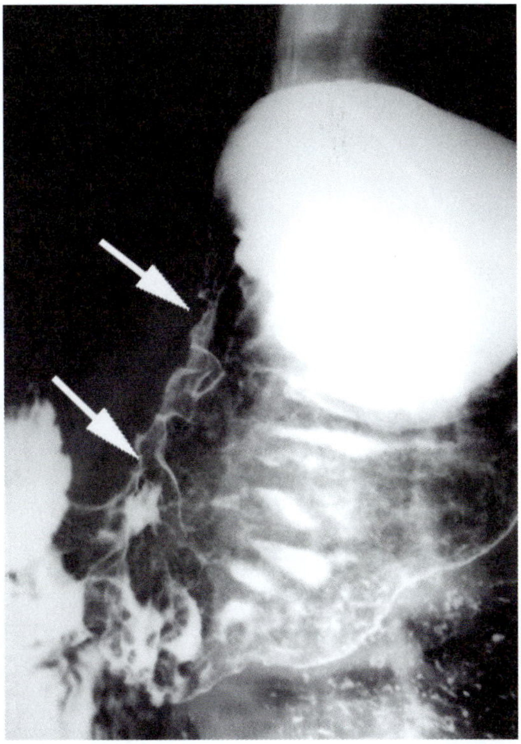

gram (double contrast, horizontal position, left half oblique projection): more distinctly visualized is thickened anterior wall closer to the lesser curvature due to intramural infiltration with convergence of the folds towards the involved part (arrows). In order to verify the spread of tumor, the patient underwent MRI. **d** MR image (coronary projection, position on the right side, T2 SSFSE): marked infiltration of the stomach walls in its lower half with marked deformation and circular narrowing of the lumen at this level. The cavity of the upper part is ectatic. **e** MR image (axial projection, FSPGR out of phase): infiltration spreads to upper parts of the stomach body by the lesser curvature. **f, g** MR images (coronary and axial projections, FSPGR out of phase): tumor infiltration spreads beyond boundaries of the stomach to form a single tumor conglomerate with enlarged lymph nodes of the lesser omentum and anterior and posterior pancreas; grows through the entire body and tail of the pancreas (arrows). Conclusion: Infiltrative-ulcerous cancer of the stomach with infiltration spreading to the pancreas and the lymph nodes of the abdominal cavity and the retroperitoneal space.

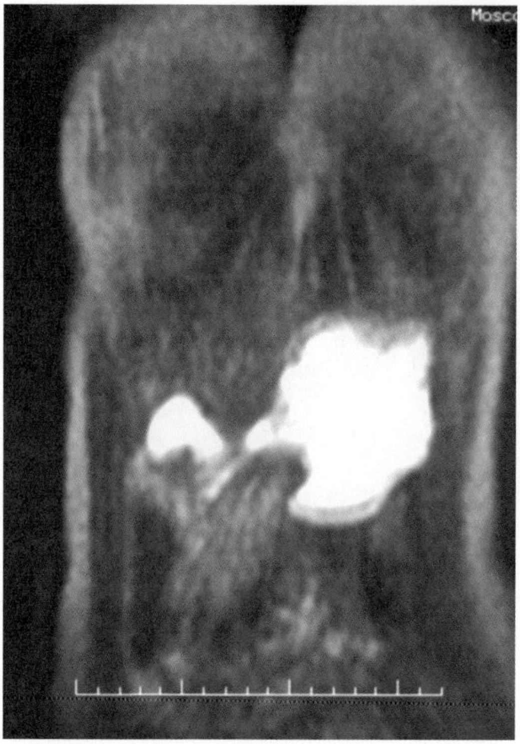

▲ **Fig. 96 d.**

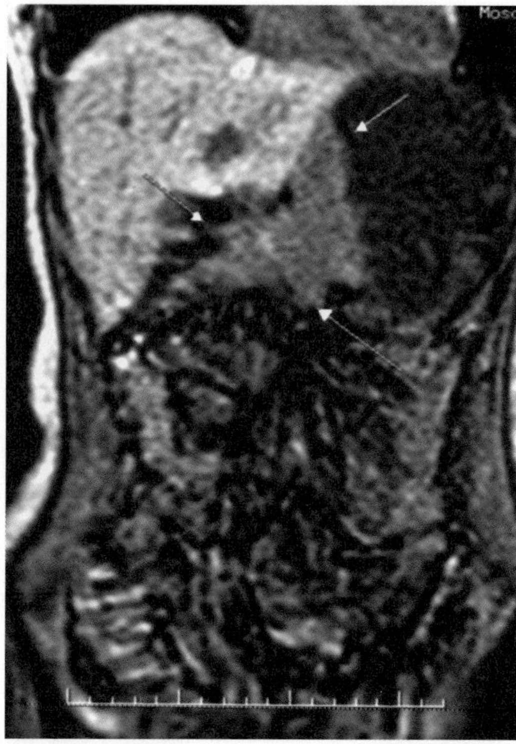

▲ **Fig. 96 f.**

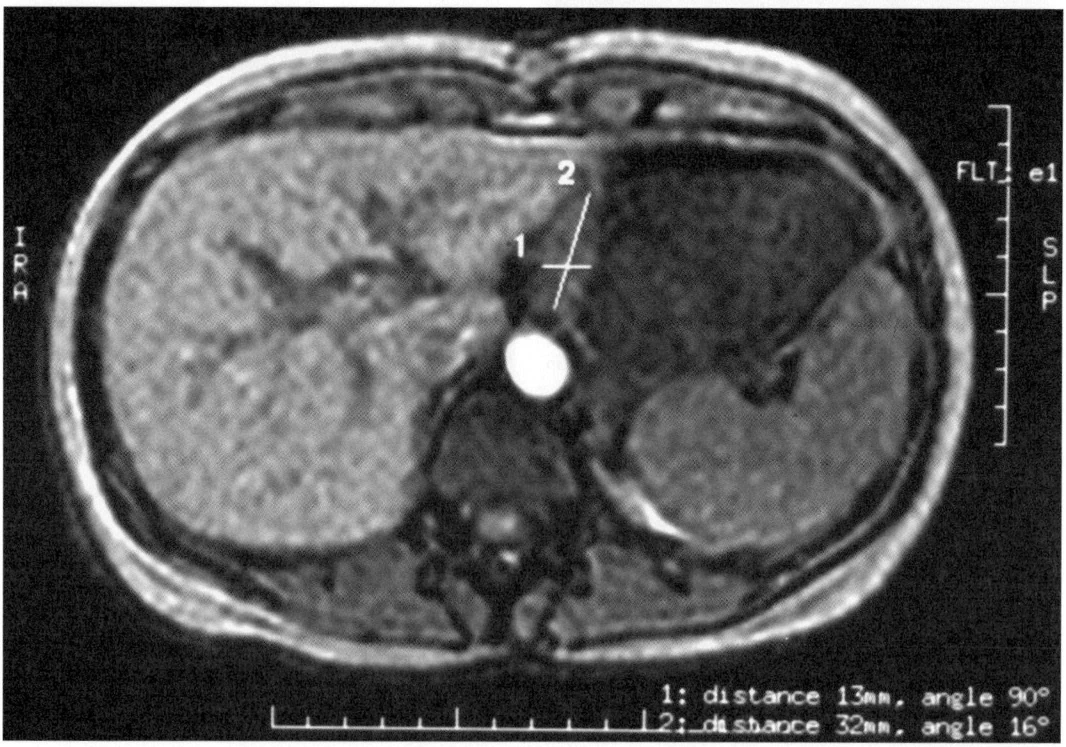

▼ **Fig. 96 e.**

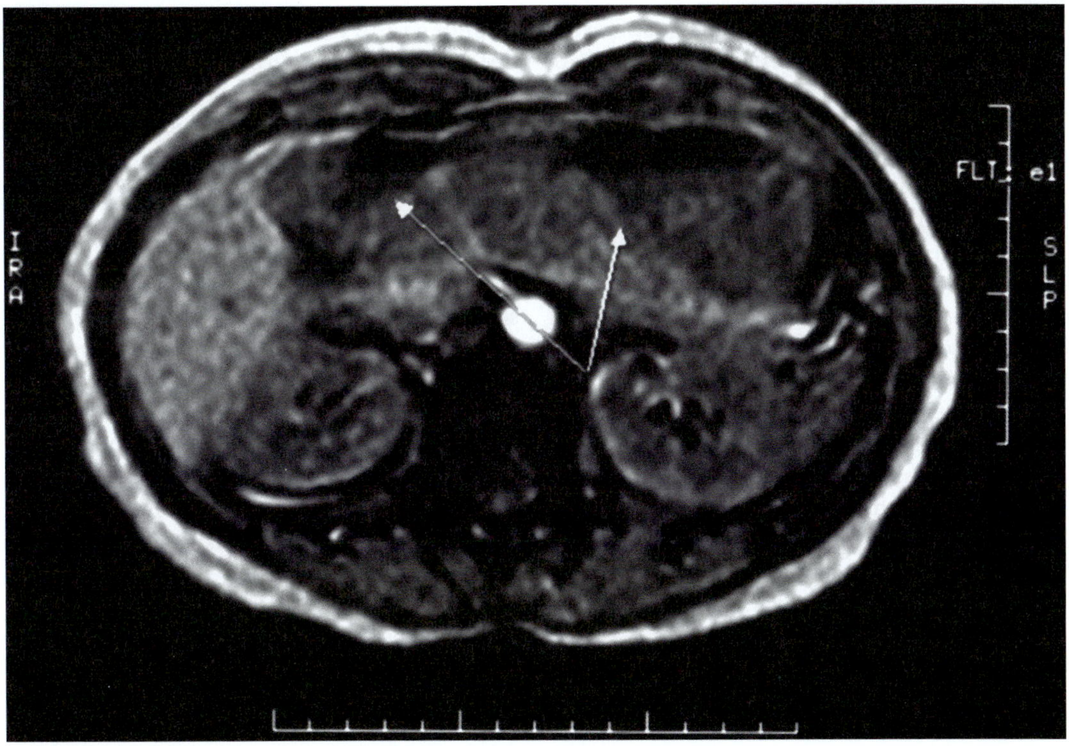

▲ Fig. 96 g.

As can be seen from this section on the MR signs of gastric cancer, this method falls within a stable scheme of radiological signs, although there are some specific MR signs. In our opinion, this is convincing proof of the necessity of using this method in some diagnostic situations. We are convinced that an orientation to both endoscopy and traditional radiology as basic landmarks makes it possible to use the potential of MRI in the diagnosis of stomach tumors to its maximum extent.

To conclude this section of our monograph let us emphasize some basic concepts. The condition of the stomach contours at the phase of its tight filling with barium sulfate suspension and thickening of the stomach wall in the region of its infiltration should be considered the main signs in the traditional X-ray of gastric cancer. For reliable detection of infiltration using these two signs, it is necessary to correct the entire method of conducting an X-ray examination of the stomach according to recommendations given in ▸ Chap. 4 and here.

Obligatory examination of a tightly filled stomach and the use of double-contrast radiology represent the optimal version of the traditional X-ray examination of the stomach for gastric cancer. The introduction into practical health-care systems of high-tech radiological methods markedly strengthens the role of radiological diagnosis of gastrointestinal pathologies, and gastric cancer in particular. Ultrasonography, computed tomography, and magnetic-resonance imaging used as additional methods of examination are an important contribution to the verification of blastomatous affection of the stomach and significantly enhance the role of radiological diagnosis on the whole.

Each of the methods that was introduced into radiological diagnosis during the last years of the twentieth century broadens the diagnostic potential of radiology in gastric cancer. Each of these methods has is own specific field of application in particular diagnostic situations. These include the estimation of the spread of tumor infiltration along the walls of the stomach and the adjacent anatomical structures, and some other aspects characterizing the anatomical feature of gastric cancer in each particular case.

It should be noted that the described signs of gastric cancer detectable with the use of these methods have one common base, depending on the same postulates that underlie the semiotics of traditional radio logy. Thus, these technologies are additional diagnostic methods, and their assessments should be based on findings of traditional radiology. Only so can their potentials be used to maximum effect. Each of these methods has its own specific features. Ultrasonography (when applied to cases of distal cancer and cancer of the lower half of the stomach body) can be used to determine sufficiently accurately the borders of tumor infiltration at the initial stage of its growth (3–4 cm). Computed tomography has the same advantages when used to examine the upper part of the stomach. MRI of the stomach has its own particular advantages.

Each of these methods makes its own specific contribution to cancer staging. They are especially helpful in cases where endoscopy and subsequent histological examination of bioptates fail to confirm the presence of tumor infiltration because of its most minute manifestations on the mucosal surface (intramural, diffuse – endophytic cancers). Thus, discovery of a small tumor infiltration by traditional radiology supplemented by double-contrast radiology may be confirmed by ultrasonography, computed tomography, or magnetic-resonance imaging. In some cases, the results of examinations by two of these techniques are sufficient to substantiate the necessity of a radical operation.

However, despite the clear advantages of these methods in the diagnosis of gastric cancer, they should be regarded only as additional techniques, whereas traditional radiology (an integral part of modern radiological diagnosis) and endoscopy remain the main methods for effective detection of gastric cancer.

Relationship Between Radiology and Endoscopy in the Diagnosis of Gastric Cancer

The relationship between X-ray and endoscopic examinations in the diagnosis of gastrointestinal pathologies have been intensively discussed ever since the invention of endoscopy and its introduction into practical medicine. During the first half of the twentieth century, the diagnosis of gastric cancer was the absolute prerogative of classical radiology, and by the 1930s, experience had accumulated in the treatment of gastric carcinoma. It then became clear that timely detection of such tumors is of primary importance. X-ray examinations became a significant aid in selecting therapeutic tactics, which was especially important in ulceration of the tumor. This stimulated surgeons to choose active strategies for treating ulcers located in the prepyloric part of the stomach. At the same time, advances in anesthesiology and surgery significantly broadened the scope of interventions, but the following soon emerged as the decisive prognostic factors include: stage of the tumor process, extent of invasion, and the presence of metastases. In that time it was difficult to detect minimally expressed metastatic processes, and physicians depended mainly on clinical symptoms.

The absence of efficient tools for the diagnosis of early gastric cancer was an obstacle to making needed changes in the traditional concept the disease. The demands of gastro-oncology for improvement of diagnostic means were realized in the modernization of X-ray equipment, making it possible to diagnose malignant tumors at their earlier stages (◘ Fig. 97).

In the middle of the 1950s, a new era opened in roentenogastroenterology: Japanese researchers developed the double-contrast technique. It was now possible not only to visualize the surface of barium-impregnated mucous membrane, but also to accurately judge the elasticity of the stomach wall by inflating the stomach with air, thus revealing tumor affections with sufficiently high accuracy.

The interest of physicians in roentgenology faded, however, with the invention of fiberoptic technology in 1958. Fibergastroscopy soon became very

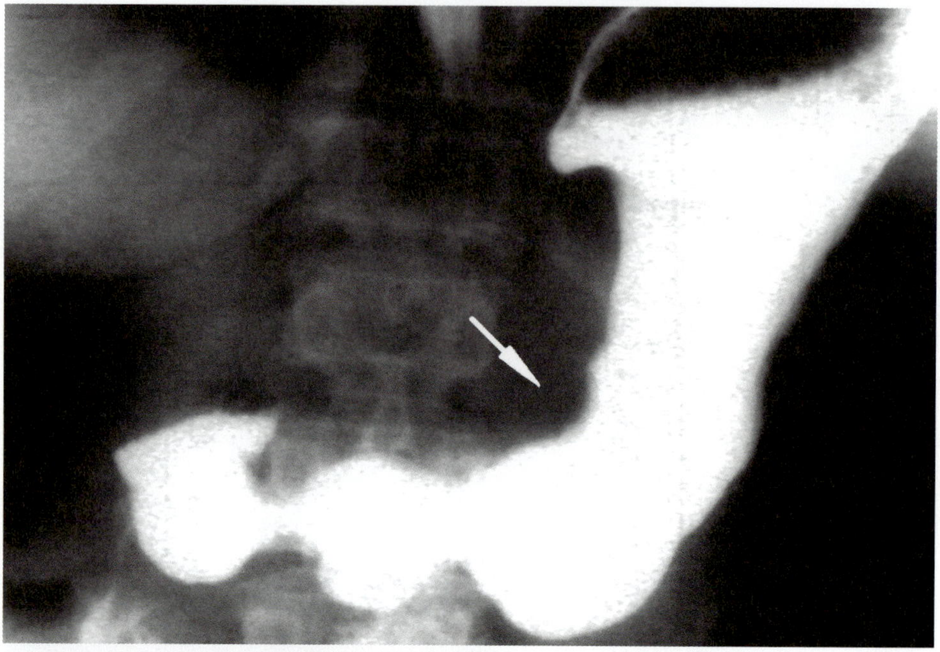

◂ Fig. 97 a.

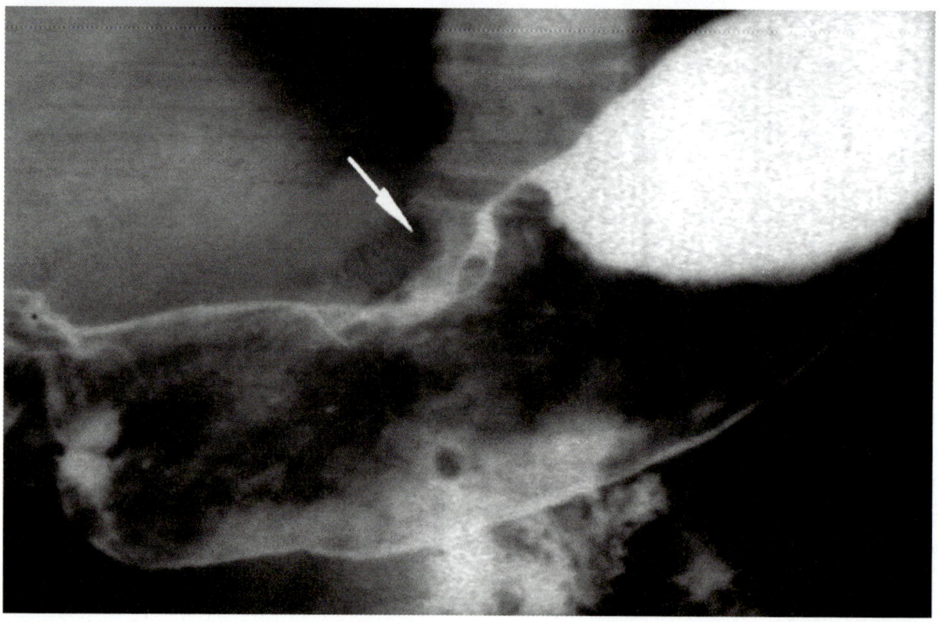

◂ Fig. 97 b.

Fig. 97a–e. Female patient I., age 61. Diagnosis: gastric cancer. **a** Stomach roentgenogram (tight filling, vertical position, anterior projection): the angular notch is straightened, a small infiltrated rigid platform is somewhat depressed into the stomach cavity with a characteristic serration (arrow). **b** Stomach roentgenogram (double contrast, horizontal position, anterior projection): thickened wall on the lesser curvature due to intramural infiltration prolapse into the cavity of an inflated stomach (arrow). Conclusion: Minor infiltrative cancer of the stomach cancer. **c** Endophotograph: a grayish site of the mucous membrane up to 1.5 cm in diameter with fine tuberosity is seen on the lesser curvature of the stomach body. Histological examination verified signet-ring cell carcinoma. **d** Macrospecimen of a resected stomach: a small portion of firm wall with folds of the mucous membrane converging toward it (arrowheads). **e** Fragment of a macrospecimen (strip): the stomach wall is thickened over a short length due to white intramural infiltration (arrows)

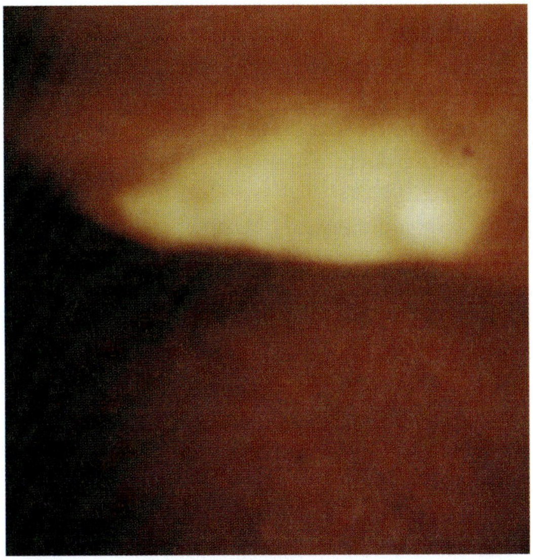

▲ Fig. 97 c.

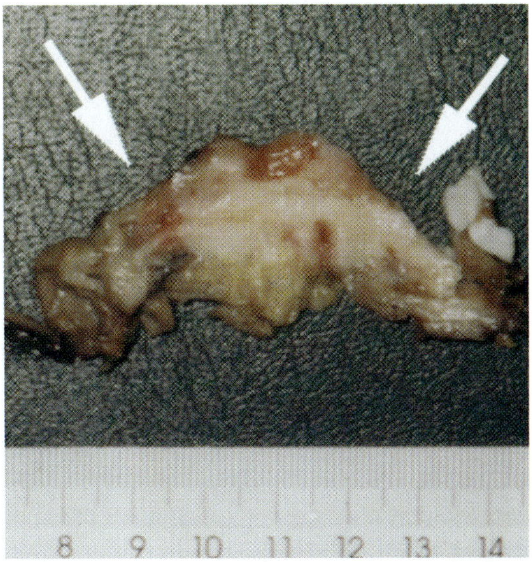

▲ Fig. 97 d.

▼ Fig. 97 e.

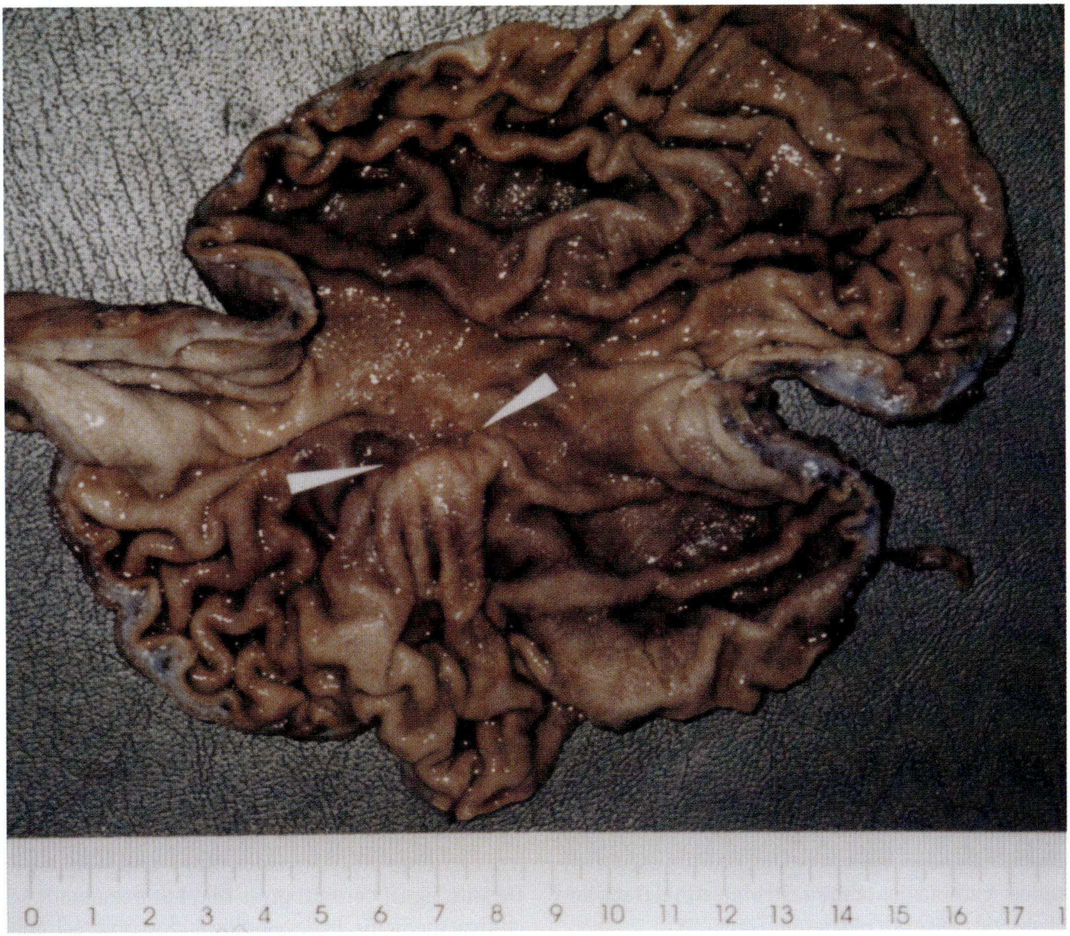

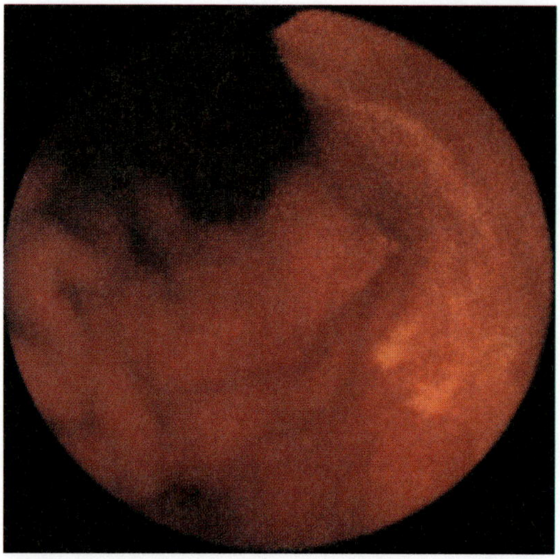

Fig. 98. Patient L., age 67. Diagnosis: gastric cancer. Endophotograph: a grayish site of the mucous membrane, 3 cm, on the posterior wall; tuberous surface; slightly depressed relative to the surrounding tissues. Histologically, adenocarcinoma.

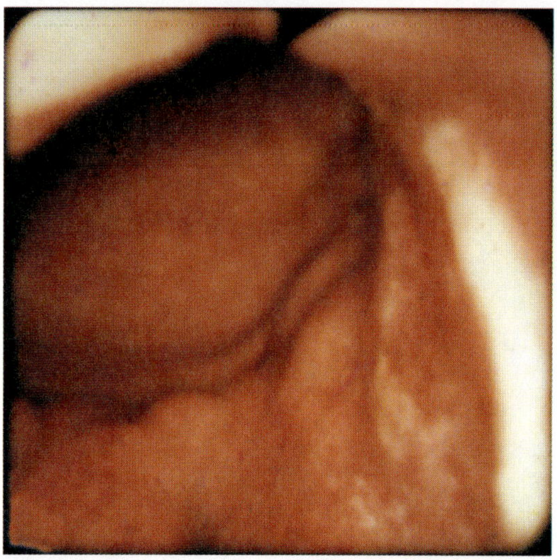

Fig. 99. Female patient K., age 54. Diagnosis: gastric cancer. Endophotograph: a portion of mucous membrane in the region of the lower third of the stomach on the greater curvature; uneven surface; slightly elevated over the surrounding tissues; color contrast between the infiltrated and visually intact tissues is absent. Histologically, adenocarcinoma with the signet-ring cell component.

popular, and a new era began in gastroenterology. Upgraded endoscopes were successfully used to diagnose pathologies of the gastrointestinal tract, and of gastric cancer in particular (Fig. 98).

Beginning in 1964, fibergastroscopes came in use. They were also used to take samples of tissues from the revealed foci of pathology. And since 1978, built-in photo and cinema cameras have been proposed for objective documentation of the endoscopic picture [201, 222, 232].

The introduction of fiberoptic endoscopes into clinical practice created the conditions for more accurate diagnosis of many diseases of the gastrointestinal tract. Adequate visualization of any part of the stomach and target biopsy have made this method especially highly effective (Fig. 99). It was quite natural that most clinicians showed a preference for endoscopy, believing that its efficacy was much higher than that of the traditional X-ray examination. Unfortunately, this incorrect view persists today. After almost half a century of the domination of endoscopy in the diagnosis of stomach pathologies, it has become clear that this error is fatal. The problem of early diagnosis of gastric cancer has not been resolved (Fig. 100).

Even now the importance of X-ray examinations is underestimated in oncology of the stomach (as well as in gastroenterology as a whole). Moreover, X-ray examinations are sometimes even refused. However significant the potentials of endoscopy, it cannot radically improve the early detection of gastric cancer. This is confirmed by the results of studies by S. Sjoblom et al. (1988), R. Ridolfi et al. (1998), and K. Newbold et al. (1989), who used fibergastroscopy as the only method of examination. The proportion of early diagnosed gastric cancers was only 3–7%, which indicates the only relative value of this approach.

At first, it seemed that visualization of the surface of the gastric mucosa and the possibility of taking tissue specimens for histological examinations made endoscopy an indispensable tool for differential diagnosis of peptic ulcer and primary ulcerative cancer of the stomach. Thus, endoscopy was given preference in the diagnostic algorithm. Without trying to diminish the importance of endoscopy, we must state, however, that timely diagnosis of dysplastic and metaplastic changes in the mucous membrane, particularly minor ulcerative cancer of the stomach, remains one of the most important problems in current gastroenterology and oncology. Despite significant progress that has been made in clinical medicine, in developing endoscopic technol-

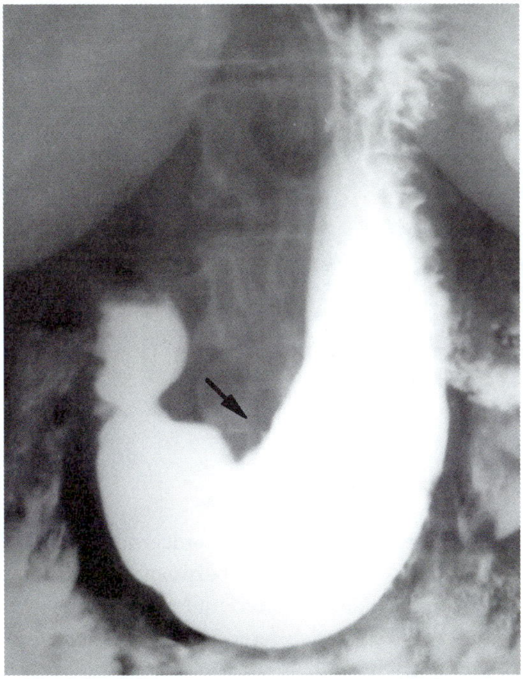

▲ **Fig. 100 a.**

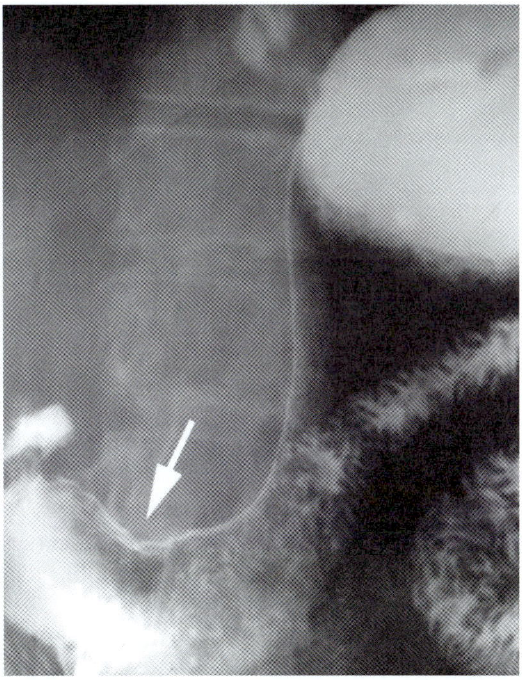

▲ **Fig. 100 b.**

▼ **Fig. 100 c.**

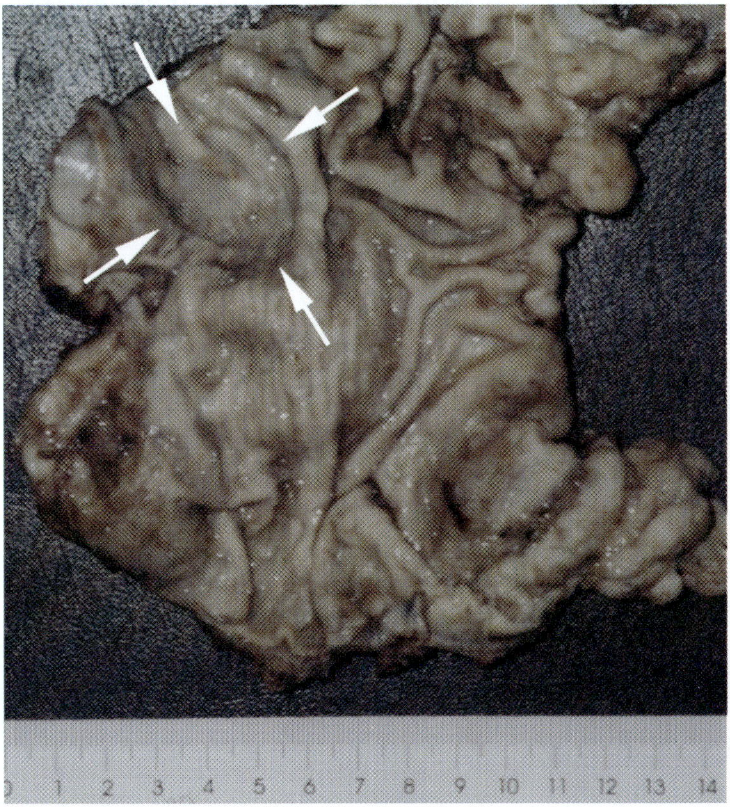

Fig. 100a–d. Female patient G., age 66. Diagnosis: gastric cancer. **a** Stomach roentgenogram (tight filling, vertical position, anterior projection): the angular notch is straightened, a rigid portion with a characteristic notch on the lesser curvature, slightly protruding into the cavity is seen (arrow). **b** Stomach roentgenogram (double contrast, horizontal position, anterior projection):wall of the antral part is thickened due to intramural infiltration (arrow). Conclusion: Minor infiltrative cancer of the antral part of the stomach. Endoscopy with subsequent histological examination of the bioptates failed to discover tumor cells. Based on reliable signs of blastomatous affection detected by traditional X-ray examination (double contrast) and despite the absence of histological confirmation, the patient was operated. **c** Macrospecimen of the resected stomach: the firm wall is covered with apparently intact mucous membrane (arrows). **d** Fragment of the macrospecimen (strip): the stomach wall is thickened due to tumor infiltration (arrows). Histologically, signet-ring cell carcinoma.

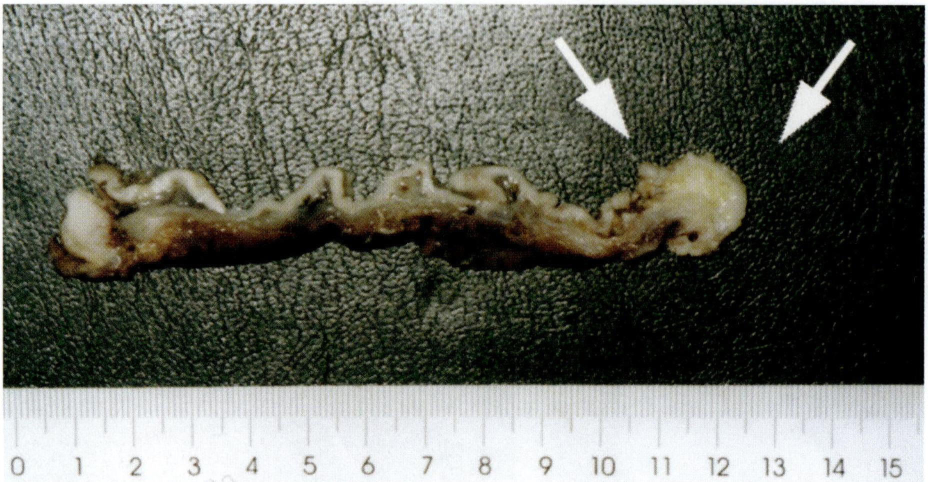

◀ **Fig. 100 d.**

ogy, and in improving methodology, the present situation with gastric cancer diagnosis remains discouraging (◘ Fig. 101) [16, 28].

According to some authors, by the time indications for operative treatment »chronic ulcer« have been established, cancer is diagnosed in 35–40% patients, and about 70% of all tumors of the stomach are discovered in patients with »ulcerous disease of the stomach.« Discrepancies between intravital and posthumous diagnoses account for 18% of the total number of dead who suffered from ulcer and cancer of the stomach [60].

We studied the problem of diagnosis of peptic disease in close cooperation with endoscopists and

▼ **Fig. 101 a.**

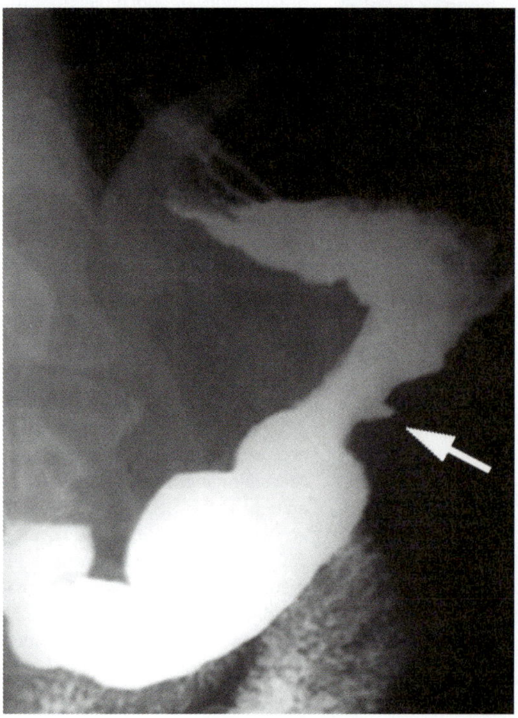

◘ **Fig. 101a–f.** Patient E., age 52. Diagnosis: gastric cancer. From anamnesis: complaints of epigastric discomfort and moderate pain for 2 months, rapid satiability after small meals. Endoscopy revealed an ulcer defect on the greater curvature of the stomach body. Histological examination failed to find tumor cells. After anti-ulcer therapy the patient felt subjective improvement, but repeated endoscopies did not confirm positive dynamics in the ulcer defect. X-ray examination was recommended. **a** Stomach roentgenogram (tight filling, vertical position, anterior projection): the stomach body is disfigured (rigid tube), an ulcer niche on the greater curvature not extending beyond the stomach contour (arrow). **b, c** Stomach roentgenograms (tight filling, vertical position, left quarter-oblique projection): stomach body is disfigured (rigid tube), a stable ulcer niche on the greater curvature not extending beyond the uneven and eroded contour of the greater curvature (arrows). **d** Stomach roentgenogram (double contrast, horizontal position, anterior projection): walls of the stomach body are thickened and rigid due to diffuse circular infiltration (arrows). Conclusion: Infiltrative-ulcerous cancer of the stomach body. Control endoscopy with subsequent histological examination of the bioptates revealed cells of signet-ring cell carcinoma. **e** Macrospecimen of the resected stomach: the wall is firm, ulceration of the mucosal surface with intramural infiltration of white color (arrows). **f** Fragment of the macrospecimen (strip): the stomach wall is thickened due to intramural infiltration of white color, which is seen over a significant distance from the ulcer crater (arrows).

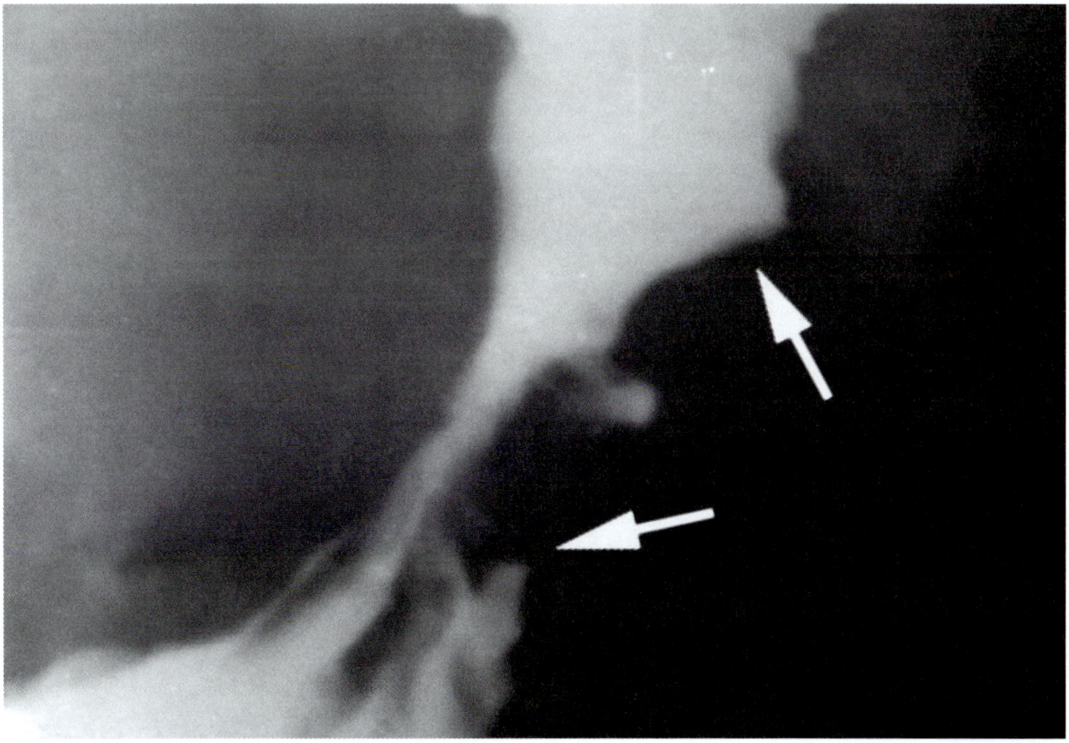

▲ Fig. 101 b.

▼ Fig. 101 c.

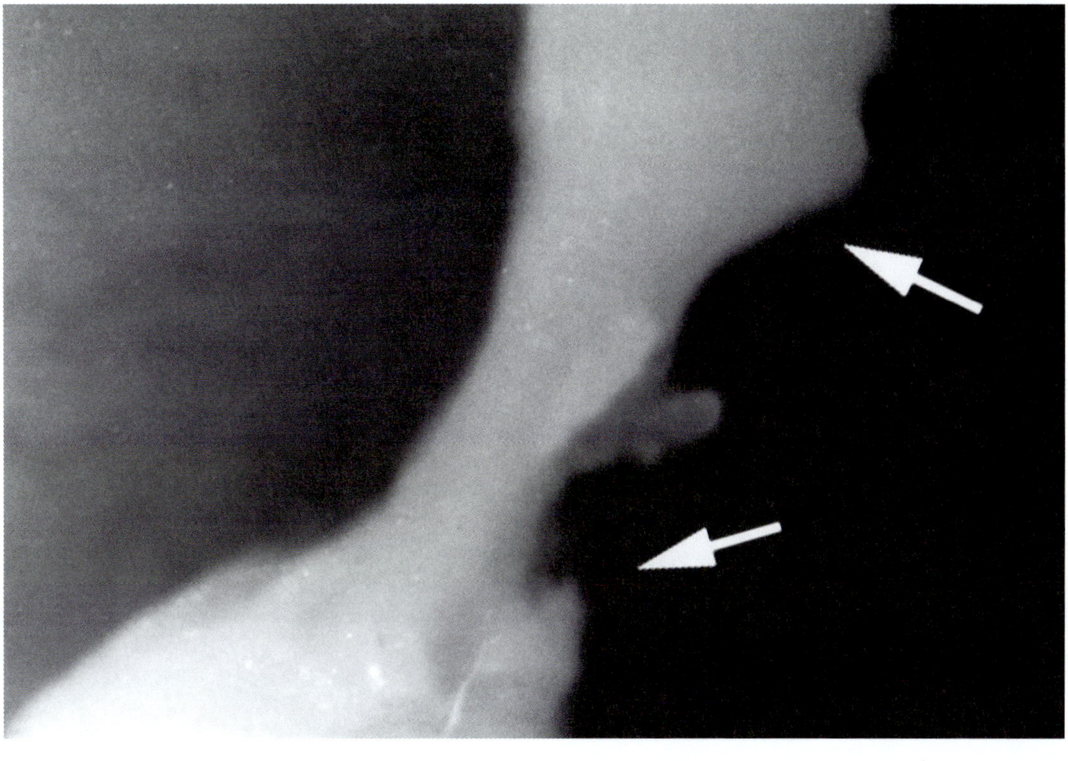

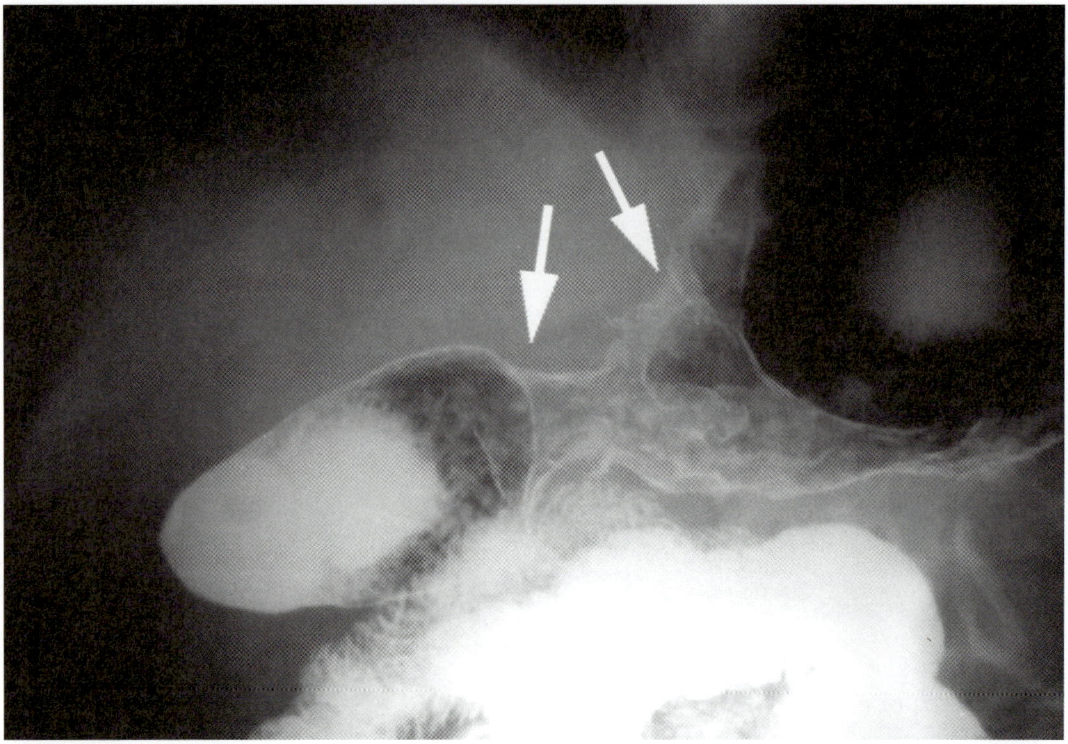

▲ Fig. 101 d.

▼ Fig. 101 e.

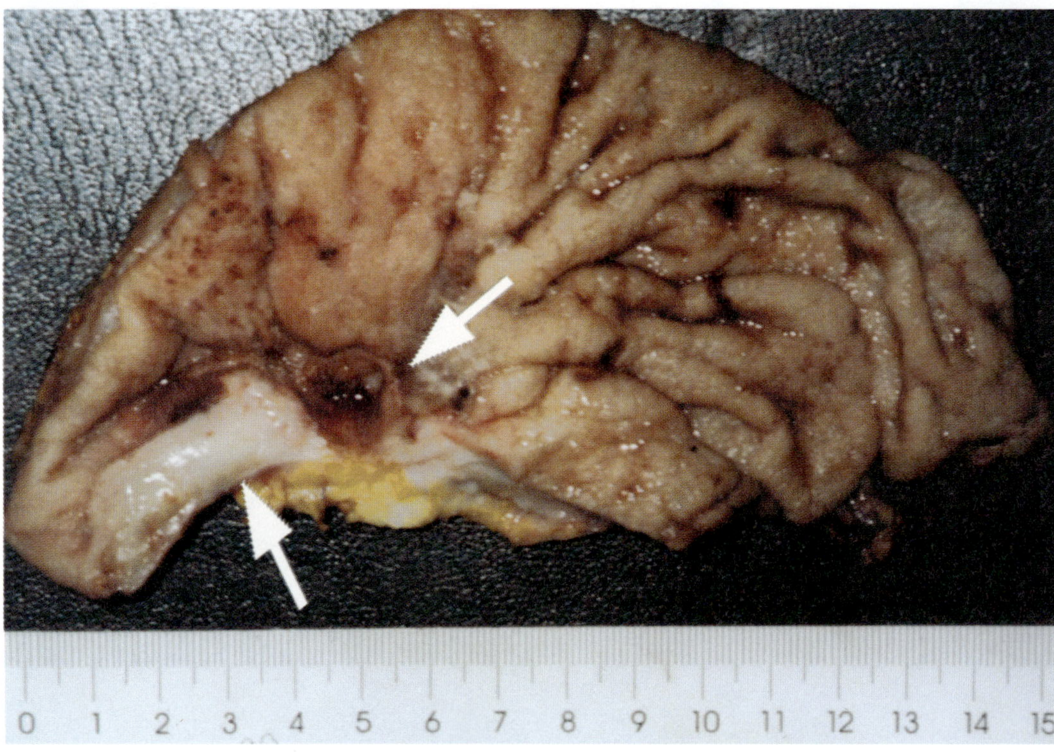

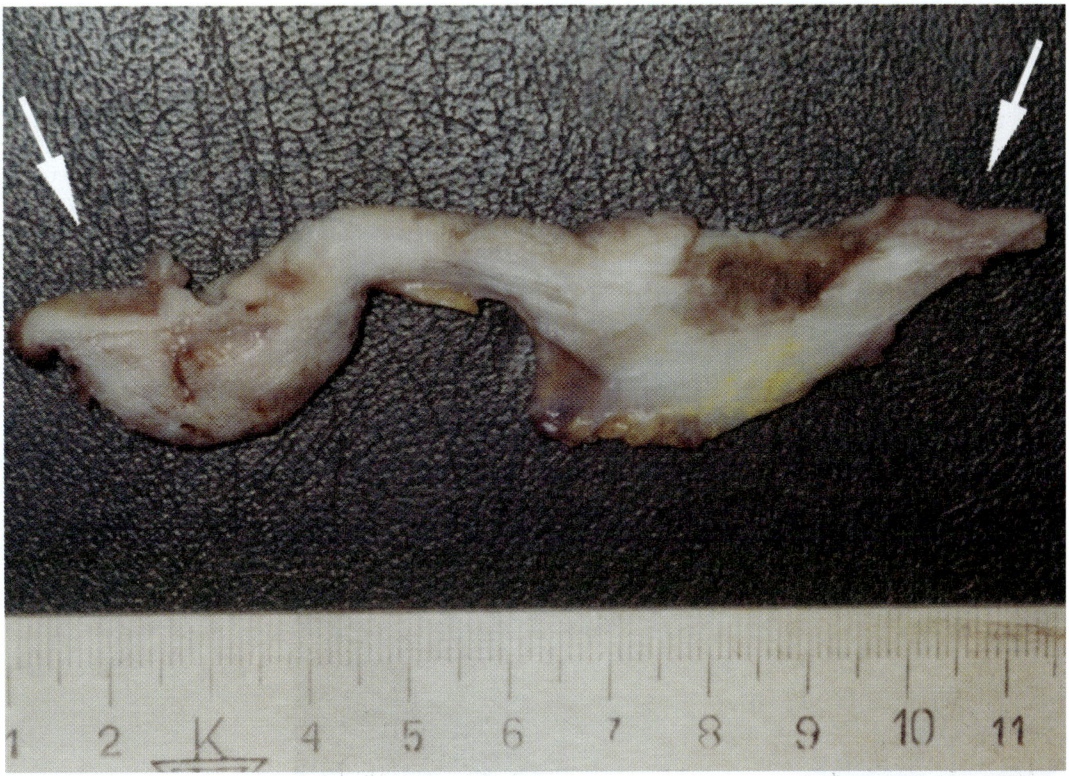

▲ Fig. 101 f.

▼ Fig. 102.

pathomorphologists for over 30 years to examine a great number of ulcer patients from the moment of primary establishment of the diagnosis to complete healing of the ulcer crater. A large number of these patients were observed from 1 to 3–5 years after cicatrization of the ulcer (◘ Fig. 102). Our experience gives us grounds to speak out on the problem.

The existing view of the absolute priority of endoscopy in the diagnosis of peptic ulcer and »primary ulcerous« cancer requires serious revision [32, 44, 51]. Some definitions that are often used in the medical literature should also be corrected.

First of all, the term »chronic ulcer«, which is often used in the literature, should be removed from the nomenclature. Only peptic ulcer may be »chronic«. Peptic ulcer is the manifestation of ulcerous disease. Ulceration of the stomach wall due to medication with non-steroid anti-inflammatory preparations has nothing to do with ulcerous disease. This is quite another nosological entity. The same holds for ulceration associated with cancer (◘ Fig. 103).

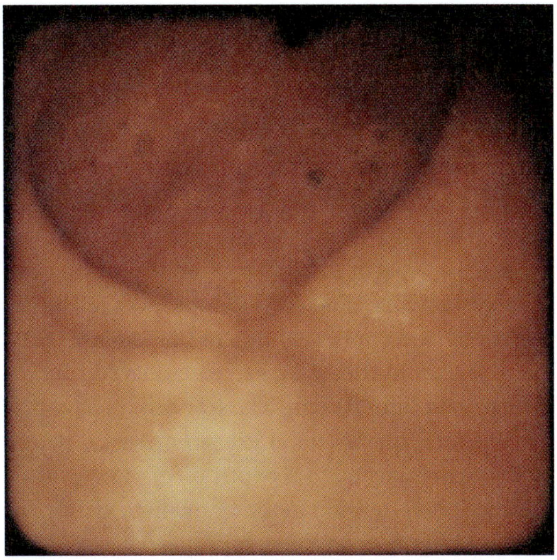

◘ **Fig. 102.** Patient O., age 40. Diagnosis: peptic ulcer in remission. Endophotograph: greater curvature of the antral part of the stomach is moderately disfigured due to transverse folds of the mucous membrane converging toward the funnel-shaped depression of the post-ulcer scar. The mucous membrane of the antral part is pale pink, smooth, and glassy.

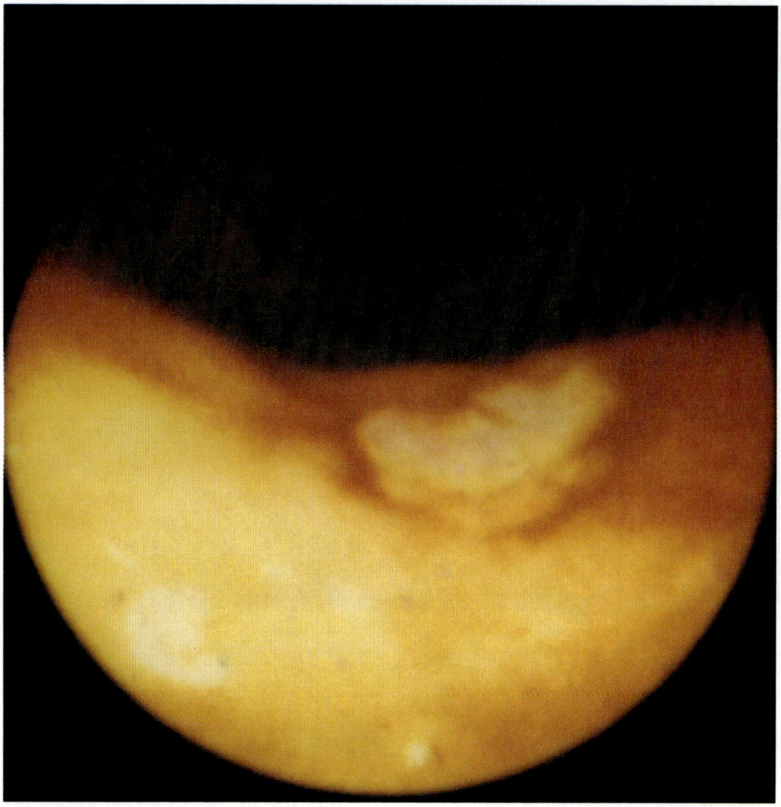

Fig. 103. Female patient A., age 50. Diagnosis: infiltrative cancer of the stomach body. Endophotograph: a flat ulcer of polygonal configuration, sized 0.7 x 0.3 cm, on the greater curvature of the upper third of the stomach body; even, sloping edges of pale-pink color, even floor lined with fibrin. Periulcerous mucous membrane is pale pink, smooth, and glassy. Histologically, adenocarcinoma with the signet-ring cell component.

Thus, ulcer can be only a symptom occurring in various pathologies, rather than a disease.

The results of our dynamic X-ray and endoscopic examinations of peptic ulcer patients show that the optimal time of ulcer niche healing is 1.5–2 months. In 85% of cases, the final form of ulcer healing is a post-ulcer scar giving a specific X-ray picture. In 3–5% of cases, the cured ulcer is not detectable with X-ray. In 8–10%, peptic ulcer can be exacerbated or complicated due to inadequate treatment. It should therefore be remembered that an ulcer proper cannot recur. The scar cannot have primary ulceration. Seasonal exacerbations of peptic ulcer are manifested by a peptic ulcer of new localization. It may develop in the immediate vicinity of the scar, but never on the scar proper.

Complications of peptic ulcer include only perforation, penetration, and bleeding. The concept of ulcer malignization is still a matter of dispute. Some insist that the absolute majority of ulcers are potentially malignant. Others reject the very idea of possible malignization. Most surgeons support the theory of malignization by the fact that 10–19% peptic ulcers become malignant. Based on our vast experience, and supported by current morphology concepts, we declare that this is impossible. We have not observed a single case of malignization of peptic ulcer. Reported cases of malignant transformation of peptic ulcer involved those in which ulcerous cancer was not diagnosed in due time. The frequency of such cases is 13.5–15% of all ulcers of the mucous membrane of the stomach. The literature data on ulcer malignization are nothing but a lame excuse for diagnostic error [28, 37, 51].

Such errors are directly connected with an excessive confidence in endoscopy and an underestimation of the potentials of current gastroroentgenology. The idea of ulcer malignization only discredits endoscopy, this valuable tool of examination, which, however, is unable to give full information in all cases, despite its indisputable role in the differential diagnosis of ulceration of gastric mucosa (Fig. 104) [28].

Current radiological methods can be used for the differential diagnosis of stomach ulcers. In the presence of relatively large (15 mm and over) ulcers, double-contrast radiology can reliably differentiate between malignant and benign ulcers. In cases of ulceration due to infiltrative-ulcerous cancer, the double-contrast method or inflation of the stomach with air alone (pneumogastrography) reveals the »ring« sign [44]. The X-ray picture in such cases shows a ridge of tumor infiltration around the ulcer crater against the background of air in the stomach cavity. No other ulcers of non-tumor origin, including the so-called callous ulcers, the frequency of which should also be revised, show the pattern of the infiltration ridge. We are absolutely sure that only »cartilaginous« firmness of the epithelial tumor can give a shadow on a roentgenogram showing the infiltration ridge. In cases of benign ulcers of the same size and localization, the X-ray image of a tightly filled stomach (double contrast) demonstrates a spot or drop. This can be explained by the fact that barium sulfate suspension is retained only in the ulcer crater, and it assumes irregular rounded shapes with distinct outlines, because the first ridge of infiltration, characteristic of blastomatous ulceration, is absent. Meanwhile, an inflammatory ridge, which is elastic, is distended on adequate inflation of the stomach [1, 58, 71, 182].

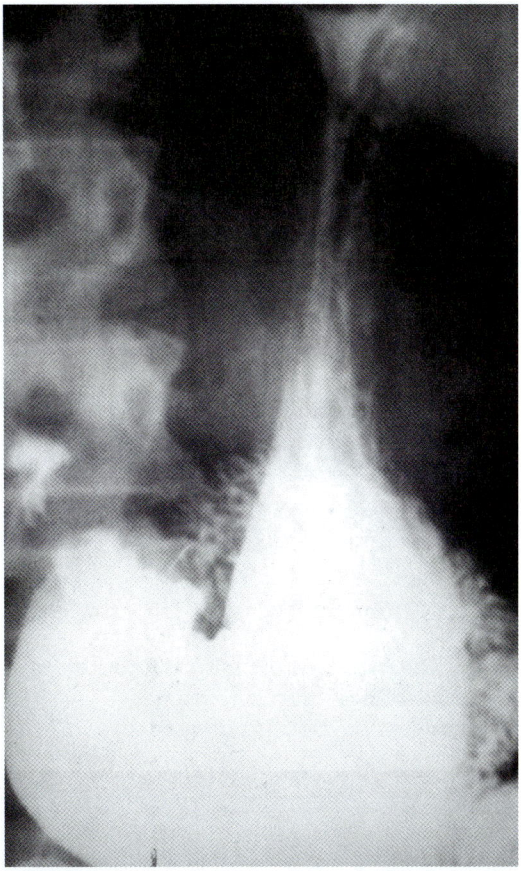

▲ **Fig. 104 a.**

▼ **Fig. 104 b.**

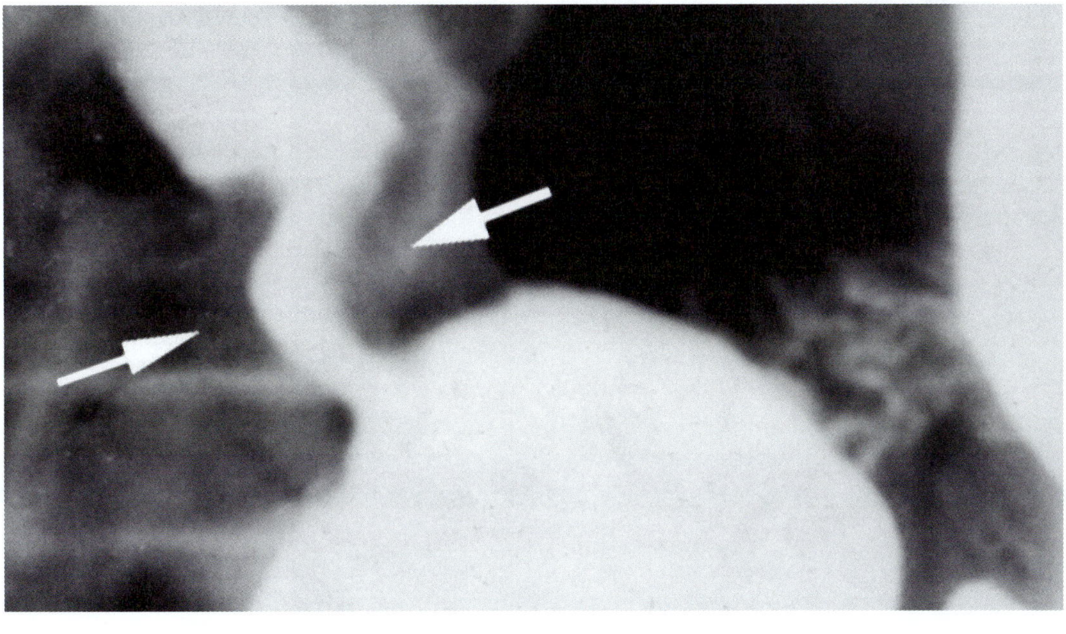

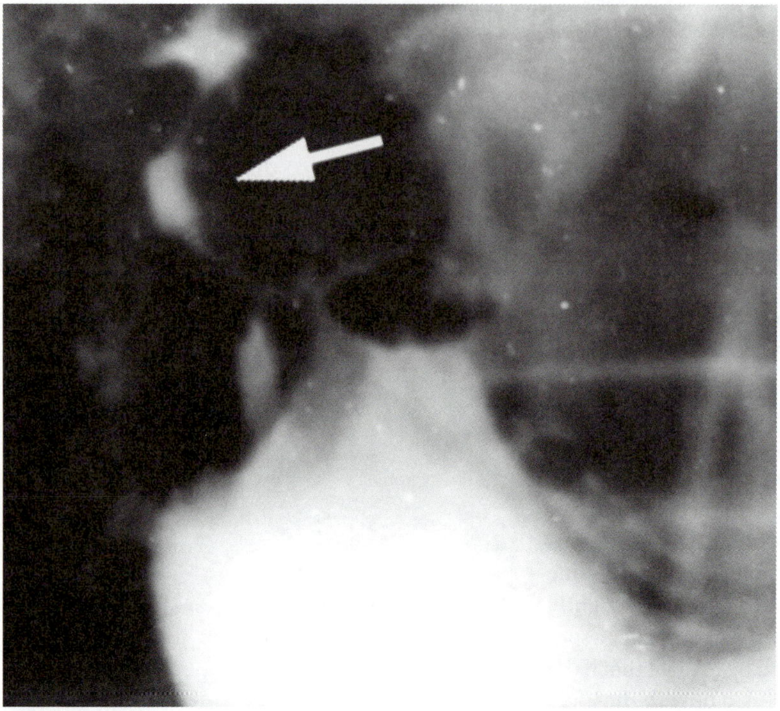

▲ **Fig. 104 c.**

▼ **Fig. 104 d.**

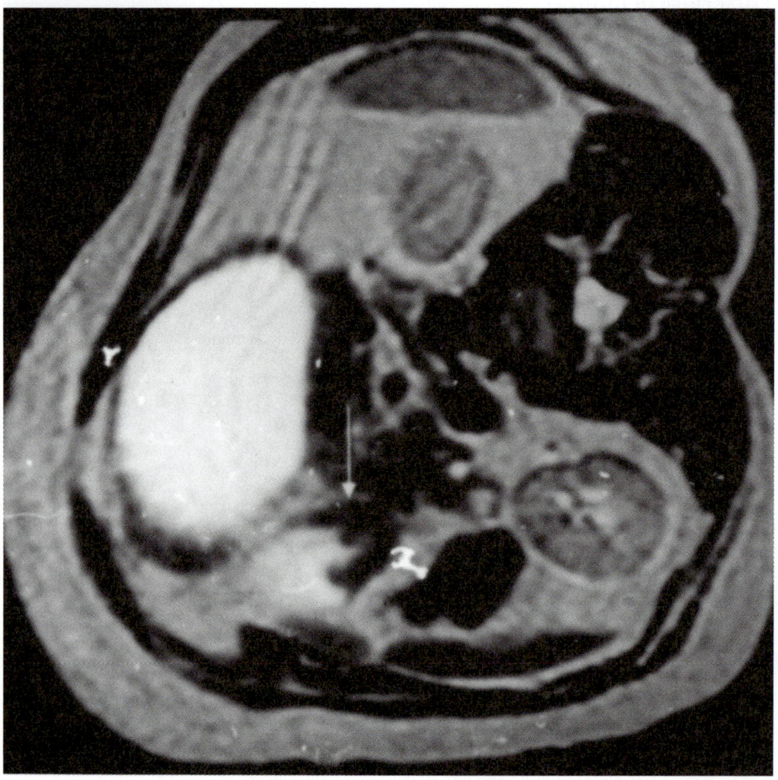

Fig. 104a–f. Patient H., age 49. Diagnosis: gastric cancer. From anamnesis: peptic ulcer for 6 years. Last complaints included marked epigastric pain. Loss of 8 kg. Endoscopy of the pyloric part of the stomach revealed rough cicatricial ulcerous deformation with an ulcer defect (8 x 3 cm) on the upper part of the posterior wall. Conclusion: Coarse cicatricial-ulcerous deformation of the pyloric part of the stomach with an ulcer. Histological examination of the bioptates failed to discover tumor cells. **a** Stomach roentgenogram (tight filling, vertical position, right quarter-oblique projection): the pyloric part of the stomach is unevenly narrowed, the sinus and the antral part are ectatic, evacuation is severely upset. **b** Stomach roentgenogram (tight filling, vertical position, anterior projection): the pyloric part of the stomach is strongly disfigured, the pylorus is elongated, its contours are uneven (arrows). **c** Stomach roentgenogram (tight filling, vertical position, anterior projection) after evacuation of the pyloric part: a depot of contrast medium in the disfigured pyloric part of the stomach (arrow). Conclusion: Roentgenologic picture of minor infiltrative-ulcerous cancer of the pyloric part of the stomach. In the absence of histological verification of gastric cancer, the patient was given MRI examination of the stomach. **d** MRI of the stomach (stomach cavity is filled with water, axial projection, position on the right side, T2 image): markedly thickened wall of the pyloric part of the stomach due to intramural infiltration. The inner contour of the affected wall is uneven, the outer contour is distinct with visualization of a thin hypointense stripe (arrow). The MR signal from the affected wall is heterogeneous and of low intensity. **e** MRI of the stomach

(stomach filled with water, axial projection, position on the right side, T2 image): circular constriction of the prepyloric part due to intramural infiltration over about 15 cm. The outer contour of the involved wall is distinct, signs of infiltration spread onto the pancreas head are absent. Distinct visualization of a hypo-intensive stripe between the affected stomach wall and the pancreas head (arrow). Conclusion: Initial signs of intramural blastomatous infiltration of the pyloric part of the stomach. Despite the absence of histological confirmation of the stomach tumor the patient was operated in view of radiological indications. **f** Fragment of a macrospecimen (strip): the wall of the pyloric part of the stomach is thick due to tumor infiltration of white color (arrows). Histologically, signet-ring cell carcinoma.

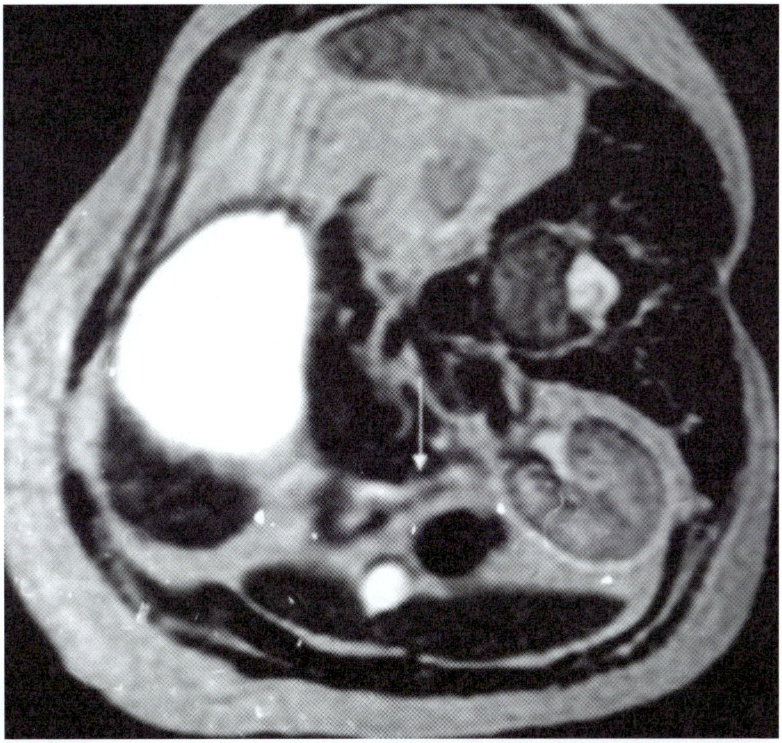

▲ **Fig. 104 e.**

▼ **Fig. 104 f.**

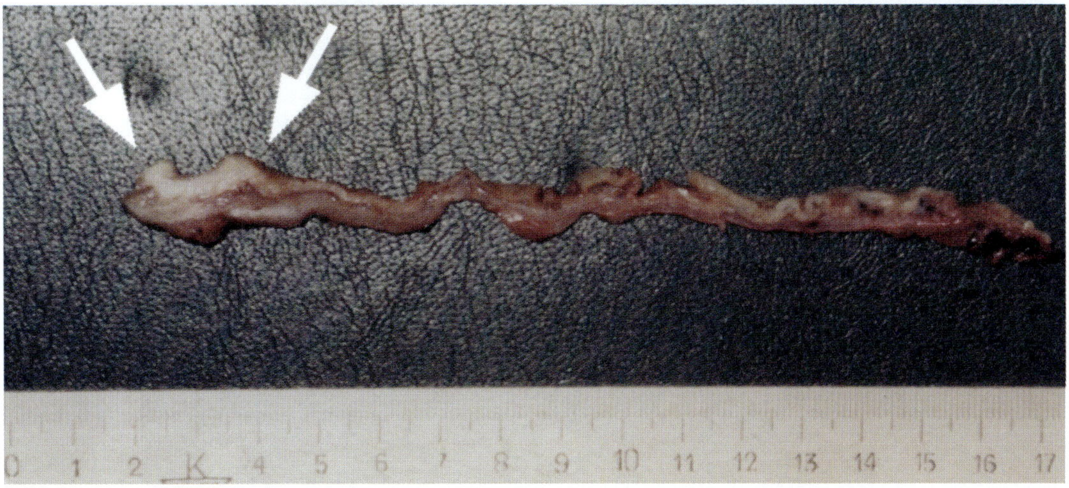

We were able to check the reliability of these two symptoms in dynamics in patients with peptic ulcer using control X-ray studies supplemented by the double-contrast method. In patients with ulcer of tumor origin, whose operation was postponed because of their refusal or the absence of histological confirmation of carcinoma, we observed enlargement of the ridge of infiltration around the ulcer. As the stomach filled with barium sulfate suspension, we observed enlargement of the ulcer crater. In control studies of patients with benign ulcers, the drop (spot), which is characteristic of peptic ulcer, diminished in size but preserved its shape and distinct contour. After 45 days, double-contrast radiology

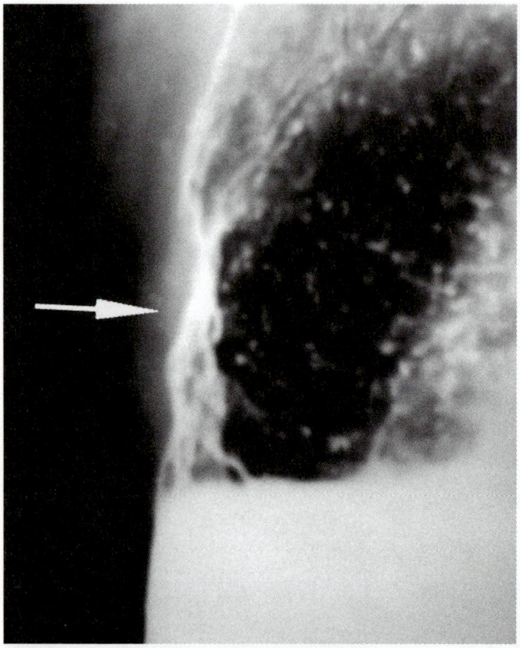

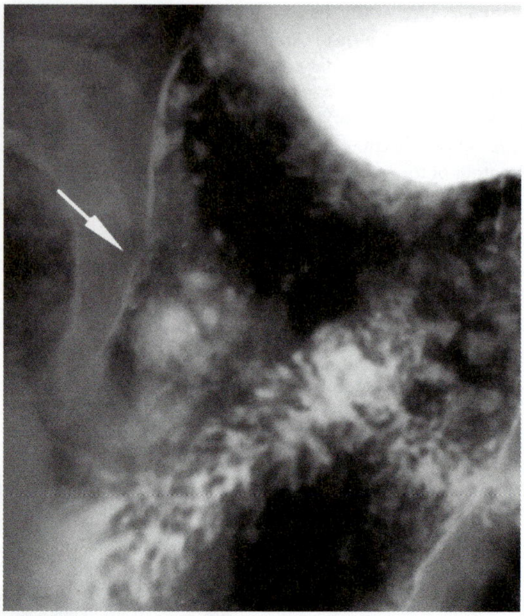

◀ Fig. 105 a.

▲ Fig. 105 b.

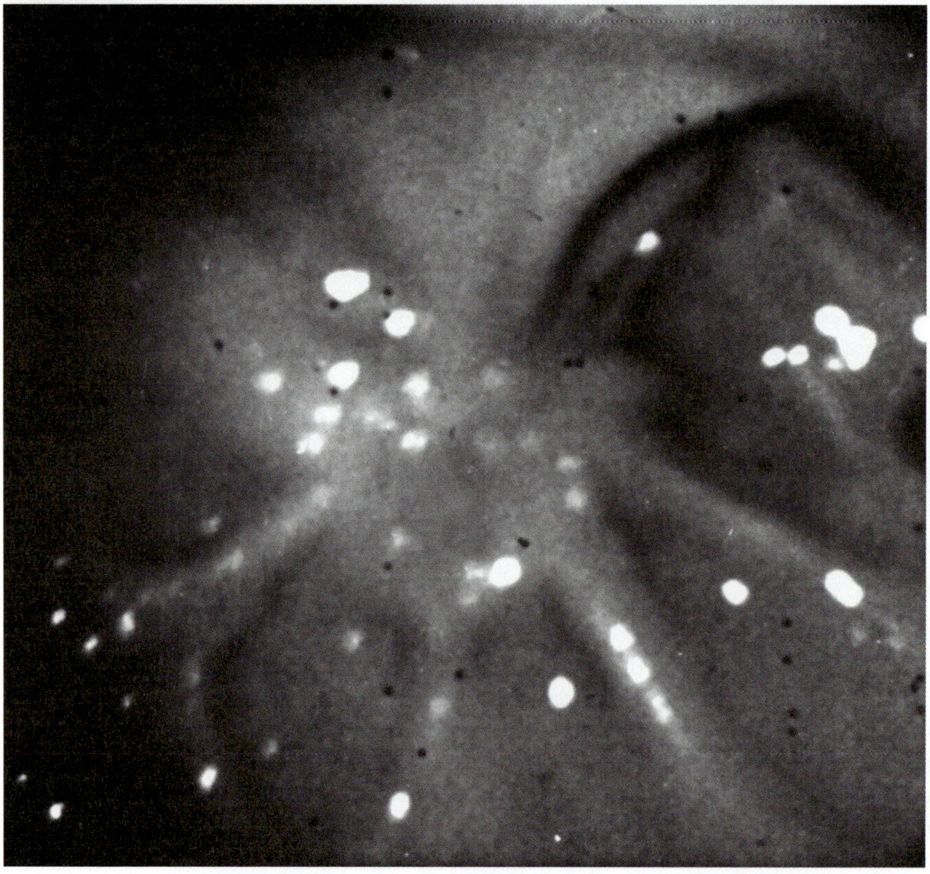

◀ Fig. 105 c.

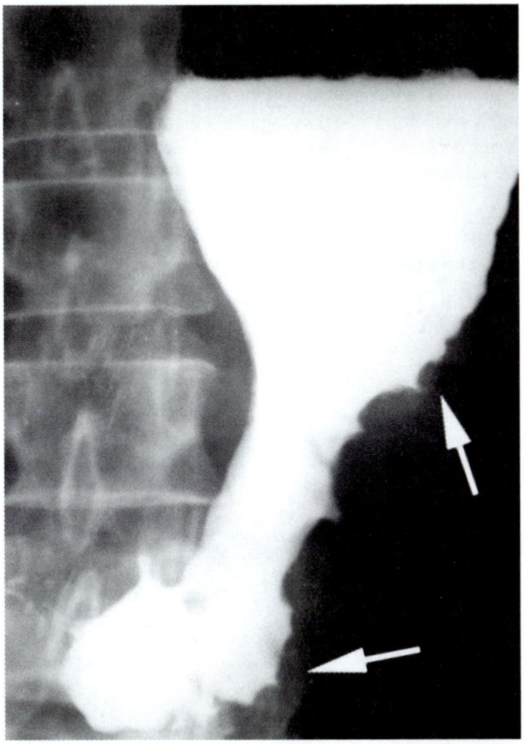

▲ Fig. 106 a. ▼ Fig. 106 b.

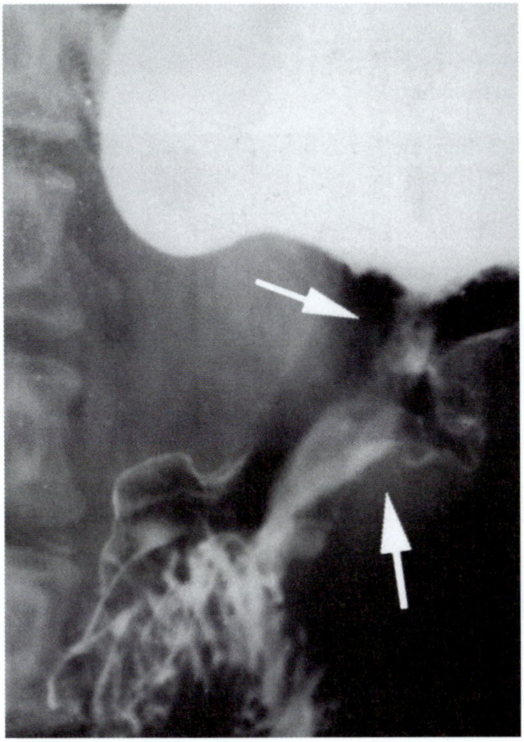

revealed post-ulcer scarring at the site of the former ulcer, which appeared as a small point with folds converging towards it. This is typical of a benign ulcer (◘ Fig. 105).

In expressing our view on the possible use of traditional radiology in the differential diagnosis of malignant and peptic ulcers on the stomach wall, we by no means want to belittle the benefits offered by endoscopy in verification of the nature of a stomach. We want only to present all the potentials of radiological diagnosis in gastroenterology to their full extent. While examining the stomach, the endoscopist pays special attention to the ulcer proper (its edges), whereas intramural infiltration, located mainly in the depth of the wall, is inaccessible to endoscopic visualization. (◘ Fig. 106) [32, 222].

◘ **Fig. 105a–c.** Patient D., age 52. Diagnosis: peptic ulcer in remission. Post-ulcer scar. Erosion of the mucosa. From anamnesis: peptic ulcer for many years with occasional seasonal exacerbations. Multiple X-ray and endoscopic examinations. At the present time the patient complains of intensifying epigastric pain after meals. **a, b** Stomach roentgenograms (double contrast): the anterior wall over a short length is slightly thickened (arrow). Small and large inclusions of barium sulfate suspension – erosions. Conclusion: Post-ulcerous scar. Erosion of the mucous membrane. **c** Endophotograph: sites of erosion of variable size are seen on the smooth and glassy surface of the mucous membrane. Histological examinations of bioptates taken during multiple endoscopies failed to reveal tumor cells. The patient was prescribed control X-ray and endoscopy.

◘ **Fig. 106a–e.** Patient K., age 58. Diagnosis: gastric cancer. From anamnesis: the patient has had peptic ulcer for many years. The last exacerbation persisted for 3 months. Epigastric pain, nausea, bitter taste in the mouth. Three endoscopies revealed an ulcer defect in the middle third of the stomach body on the posterior wall with folds converging towards the defect; positive dynamics – the ulcer size diminished from 2 to 0.3 cm. Instrumental palpation: the wall around the ulcer crater is elastic. Layers of proliferating epithelium against the background of inflammatory infiltration were determined histologically in bioptates taken during endoscopy. Findings of the third histological examination revealed signs of moderately active inflammation with epithelial dysplasia in one of the eight bioptates. Focal intestinal metaplasia and single mucus-containing cells of the proper mucous membrane. Helicobacter pylori of the 2nd degree. **a** Stomach roentgenogram (tight filling, vertical position, anterior projection): the stomach body is disfigured (rigid tube) with marked narrowing of the lumen. Uneven contours of the greater curvature (arrows). **b** Stomach roentgenogram (double contrast, horizontal position, anterior projection): pronounced deformation of the stomach body (rigid tube) with ulcerated infiltration on the posterior wall closer to greater curvature (arrows). In order to verify spread, the patient's stomach was examined by MRI. **c** MRI of the stomach (stomach cavity filled with water, sagittal projection, T2 image): 3 x 3 x 0.5 cm infiltration in the middle third of the stomach body on the posterior wall, closer to the greater curvature (arrow). Uneven contours. Ulcer to 0.5 cm in the central parts of the infiltration zone. **d** MRI of the stomach (stomach filled with water, coronary projection, T2 image): distinctly visualized infiltration of wall of the greater curvature (arrow). The inner contour of the involved wall is uneven, MR signal is heterogeneous and of moderate intensity. The outer contour is even, distinct, without signs of infiltration spreading beyond the limits of the stomach wall. Conclusion: Infiltrative-ulcerous cancer of the posterior wall of the stomach body. **e** Fragment of a macrospecimen (strip): submucous infiltration of white color over a short length (arrows) with minimal changes on the mucosal surface. Histologically, signet-ring cell carcinoma.

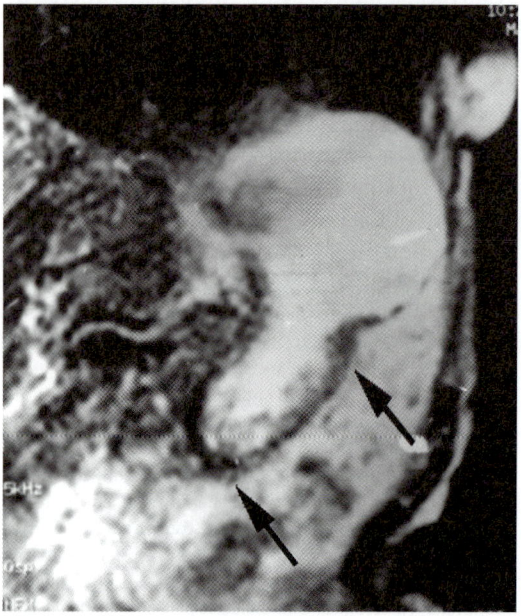

▲ **Fig. 106 c.**

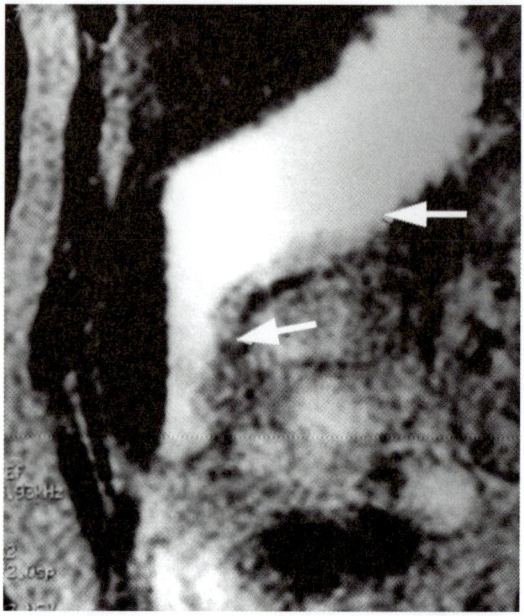

▲ **Fig. 106 d.**

▼ **Fig. 106 e.**

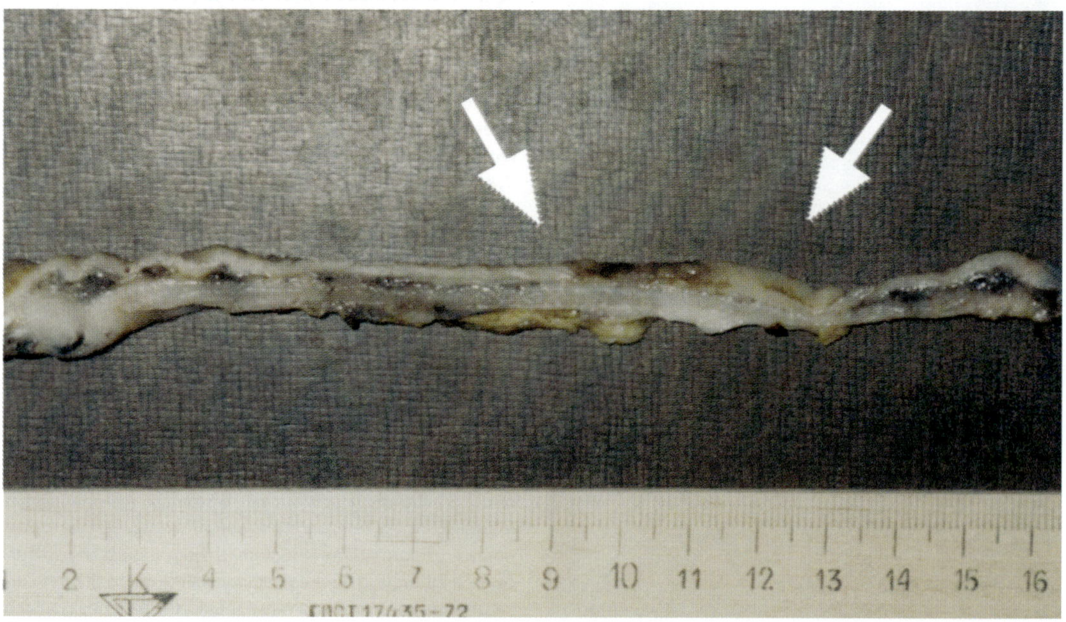

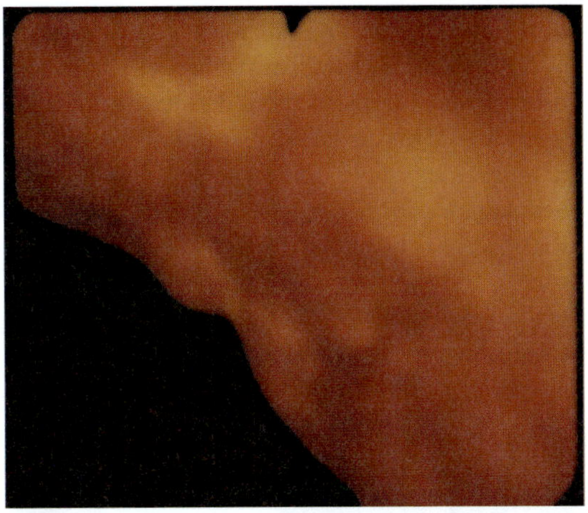

Fig. 107. Patient F., age 51. Diagnosis: peptic ulcer in remission. Endophotograph: post-ulcer scar on the mucous membrane of the lesser curvature of the stomach body.

Unfortunately, an increasing number of patients with endoscopically diagnosed peptic ulcer are treated today by laser, or »red light«, the therapeutic value of which is strongly doubted for peptic ulcer, without preliminary X-ray examination. Endoscopic control detects the absence of positive dynamics. Using the double-contrast technique, it was possible in some cases to reveal signs of intramural tumors with marginal ulceration. Multiple bioptates were examined for signs of tumor; the results were negative. The low informative value of endoscopic biopsy is explained by the fact that diffuse cancer normally originates in the deep parts of the mucous membrane, whereas biopsied material usually includes elements of reactively changed columnar epithelium. The material taken from the floor of the ulcer crater also has no informative value, because it includes mostly fibrin and necrotic detritus. In other words, we are talking about infiltrative-ulcerous cancer of the stomach with atypical course, and the endoscopist who experiences difficulties in diagnosing cancer has to resort to radiological diagnosis. Unfortunately, this happens only after the course of physiotherapy has been given [48].

Thus, it is necessary to revise and correct the approach to the use of X-ray and endoscopic examinations in the diagnosis of gastric cancer, particularly its ulcerative forms, and in dynamic observations of patients with peptic ulcer. The diagnostic scheme is as follows:

1. Primary diagnosis – roentgenological and endoscopic (with biopsy)
2. First control examination following treatment after 3–4 weeks – X-ray alone
3. Second control examination, usually the last, 6–7 weeks after the start of treatment – roentgenological and endoscopic (with biopsy)

As can be seen from this scheme, the endoscopic examination is conducted at the stage of primary diagnosis and on healing of the ulcer crater; tissue specimens are taken for histological examinations in both cases (Fig. 107). Traditional radiology is involved at the stage of primary diagnosis (together with endoscopy) and in dynamic monitoring of treatment (without endoscopy). Radiology and endoscopy with histological examination of bioptates are used only for the final evaluation. We stress again the importance of a complex approach to the diagnosis of gastrointestinal diseases. The diagnostic algorithm we propose precludes diagnostic errors that are possible in the period of clinical examination.

Confirmation of our position on the relationship between radiology and endoscopy in the diagnosis of gastric cancer can be found in some publications [60, 171, 185]. Each method separately cannot point to the diagnosis, especially in cases of infiltrative and infiltrative-ulcerous cancer of the stomach.

Studies carried out in recent years show that there may be significant discrepancies in the results of histological examination of materials taken during biopsy and following radical surgery. In cases where cancer of the stomach cannot be verified prior to the operation these can be as great as 17–33% [59].

Morphological studies aimed searching for cancer cells cannot meet the current requirements either. The absence of cancer cells in bioptates does not rule out the presence of gastric cancer.

Examination of lymphoid infiltrate helps to establish the diagnosis and prognosis of tumors of various localizations. In morphological diagnosis, valuable information is supplied by determining the quantity of intraepithelial mononuclear leukocytes, especially those with histological signs of activation, which are characteristic of adenocarcinoma. In severe dysplasia (currently regarded as neoplasia) of gastric epithelium, a content of activated intraepithelial leukocytes exceeding 6/1000 epitheliocytes is a bad prognostic sign. Quantitative determination of tumor markers in human blood serum at a sensitivity of 73% and specificity of 89% cannot always accurately answer whether or not blastomatous affection is present [12, 77].

Permanent comparison of radiological and endoscopic findings during the past 30 years, with subsequent verification by histological examination of tissue specimens or by clinicoroentgenological observation of patients who did not have surgery for various reasons, leads us to conclude that there is a need for revision of the role of endoscopy in the diagnosis of not only ulcerative forms of gastric cancer, but even more of diffusely spreading carcinomas.

This is connected with the limited potentials of endoscopy in view of changes in the morphogenesis of tumor affections. Thus, despite the rapid development of endoscopy with biopsy and subsequent histological examination of the bioptates, diagnosis of early cancer (which is decisive for complete cure) remains very low at 3–7%. The low rate of radical operative interventions for gastric cancer and the low postoperative 5-year survival have remained unchanged for 40 years, and this is explained by the late diagnosis [40, 86]. The significantly high percentage of untimely diagnosis pertains to endophytic cancers. This anatomical variant of cancer, especially with predominantly submucous spread of the tumor, is the most difficult to diagnose. Researchers are therefore trying to find new ways to diagnose diffuse gastric cancer (chromatogastroscopy, loop biopsy in fibergastroscopy, improved double-contrast technologies, measuring thickness of the stomach wall using ultrasonography, computed tomography, magnetic-resonance imaging, endoscopic ultrasonography, etc.).

In cases of predominantly submucous growth, cancer infiltration can be accompanied for a long time by only insignificant changes in the mucous membrane and mild disorders in the structure of the stomach wall. Here, the importance of endoscopy decreases significantly. Atypical cells, in such cases, occur in small complexes surrounded by powerful growths of connective tissue (which are sometimes mistaken for a curable ulcerous defect of the mucous membrane). This creates significant difficulties for the morphological verification of the disease. It also explains the former, incorrect interpretation of linitis plastica as being the result of an inflammatory process. Today, linitis plastica is regarded as one of the most malignant forms of gastric cancer, in which tumor grows mostly in the submucous coat over a long period of time (Fig. 108) [28, 34, 53].

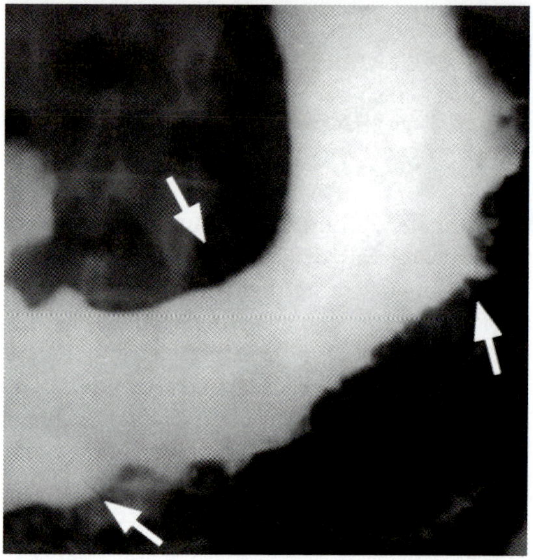

▲ Fig. 108 a.

▼ Fig. 108 b.

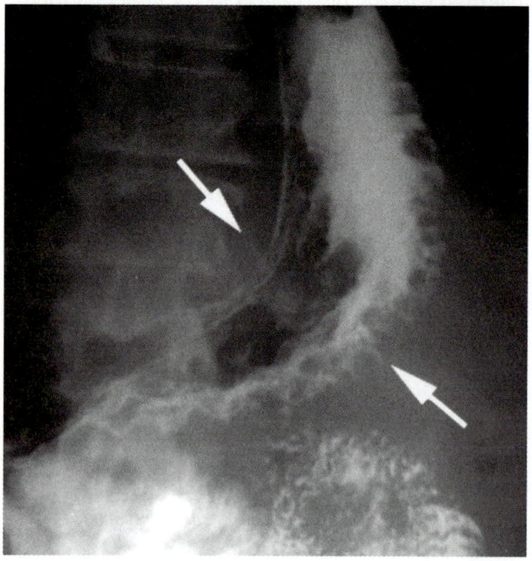

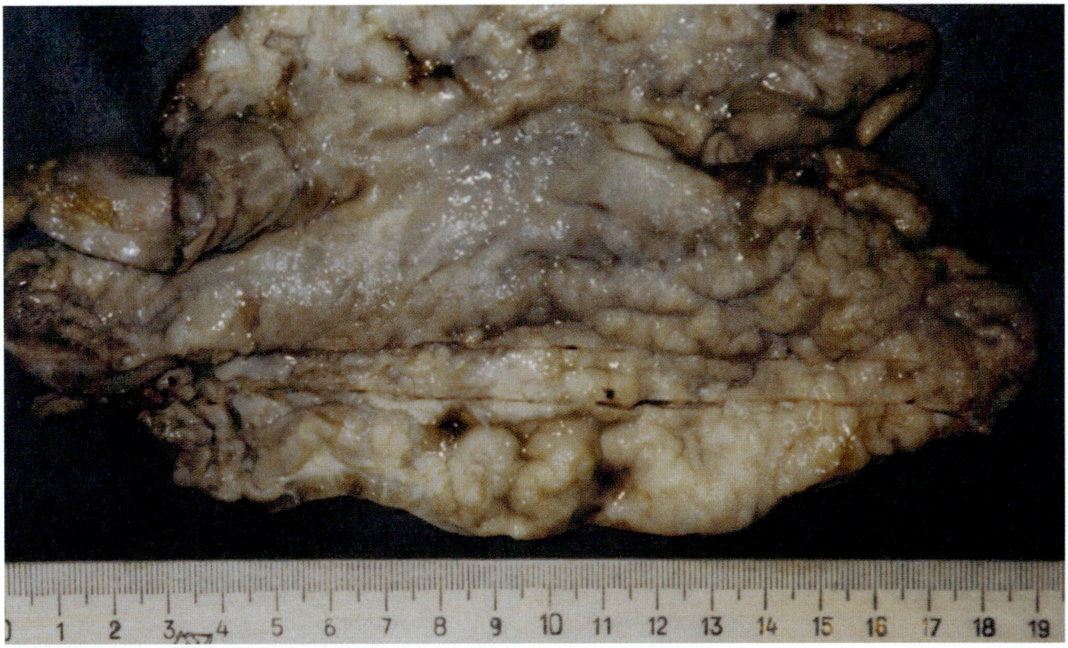

▲ Fig. 108 c.

▼ Fig. 108 d.

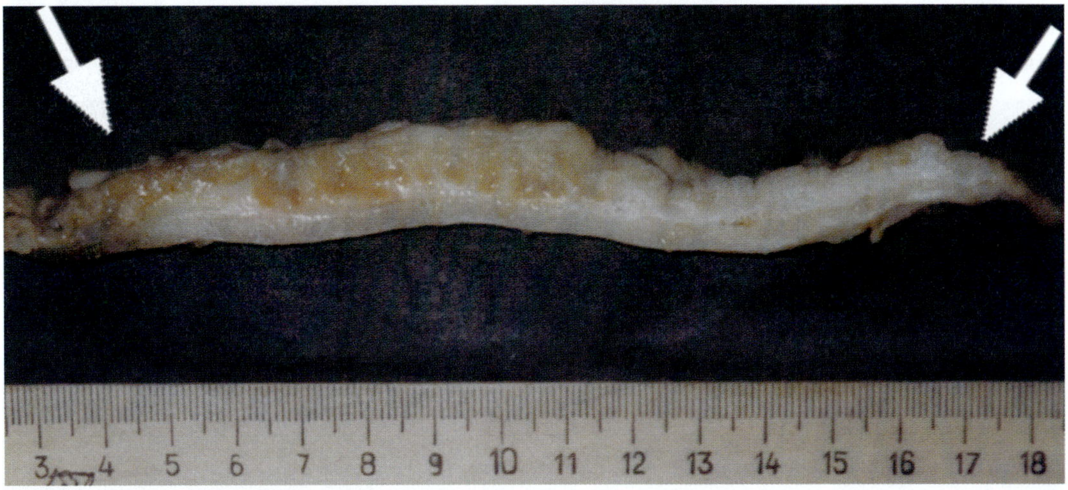

◘ **Fig. 108a–d.** Female patient Zh., age 63. Diagnosis: gastric cancer. **a** Stomach roentgenogram (tight filling, vertical position, anterior projection): stomach cavity decreased, lesser curvature shortened and depressed, walls of the sinus are uneven (arrows). **b** Stomach roentgenogram (double contrast, horizontal position, anterior projection): the walls are rigid and thickened due to circular intramural infiltration (arrows). Conclusion: Infiltrative cancer of the stomach. **c** Macrospecimen of a resected stomach: the wall is firm over the entire length due to intramural infiltration. **d** Fragment of the macrospecimen (strip): the wall is thickened, white tumor tissue infiltrating the stomach wall is seen (arrows). Histologically, signet-ring cell carcinoma.

The endoscopic picture depends largely on localization of the tumor. In cases where the tumor is found mainly on the lesser curvature of the stomach body or in the antral part, slightly elevated sites of infiltration with indistinct margins are also revealed, firm (to instrumental palpation) and sometimes covered with a grayish coat (◘ Fig. 109). Small flat ulcers in the center of the »infiltrate« are not infrequent.

If the affected region is limited largely to the greater curvature of the stomach, markedly thick-

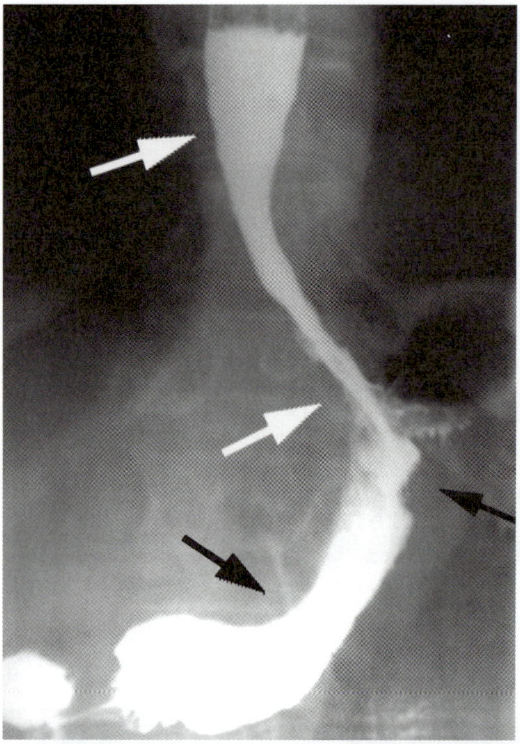

▲ Fig. 109 a.

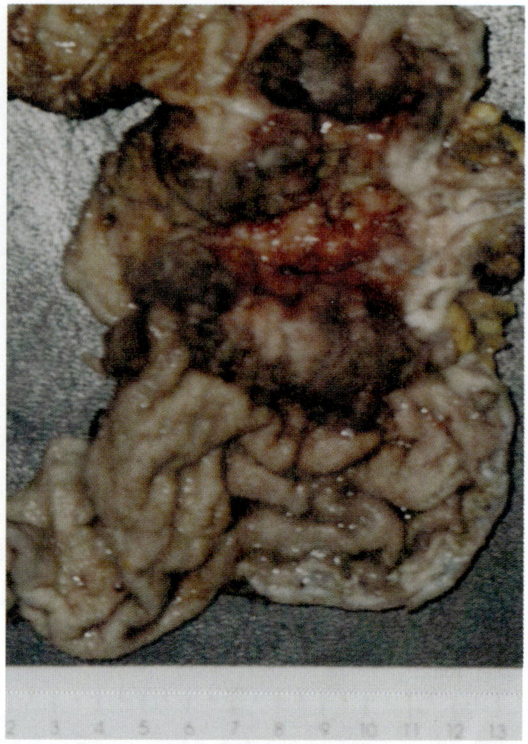

▲ Fig. 109 c.

▼ Fig. 109 b.

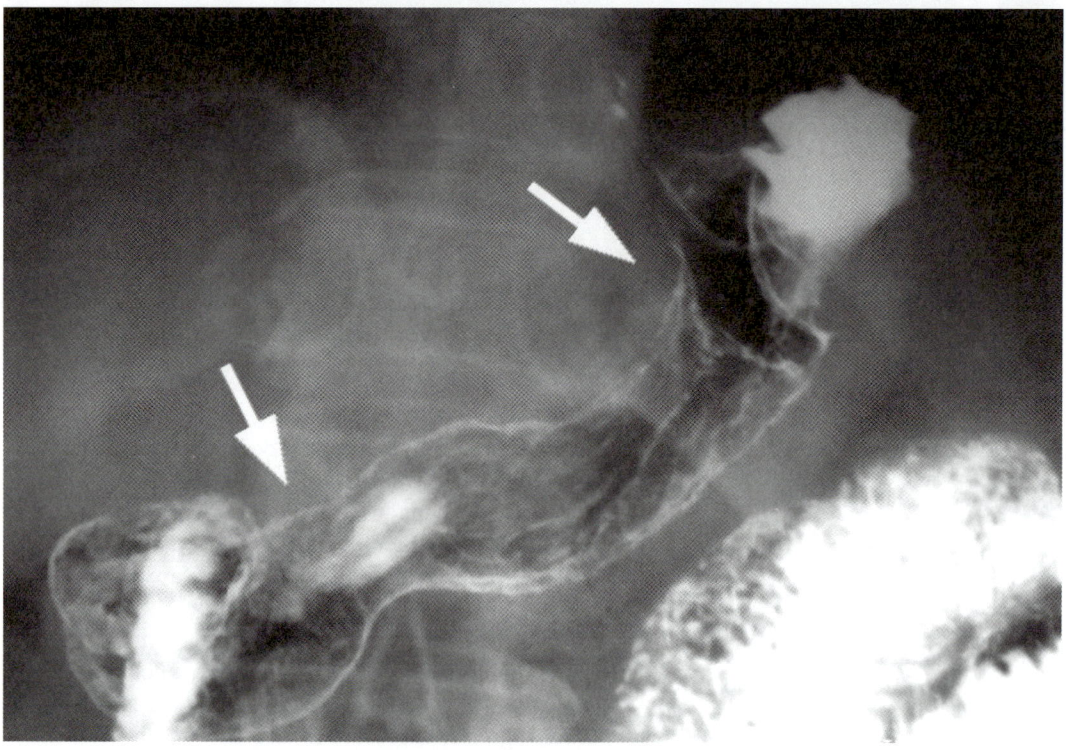

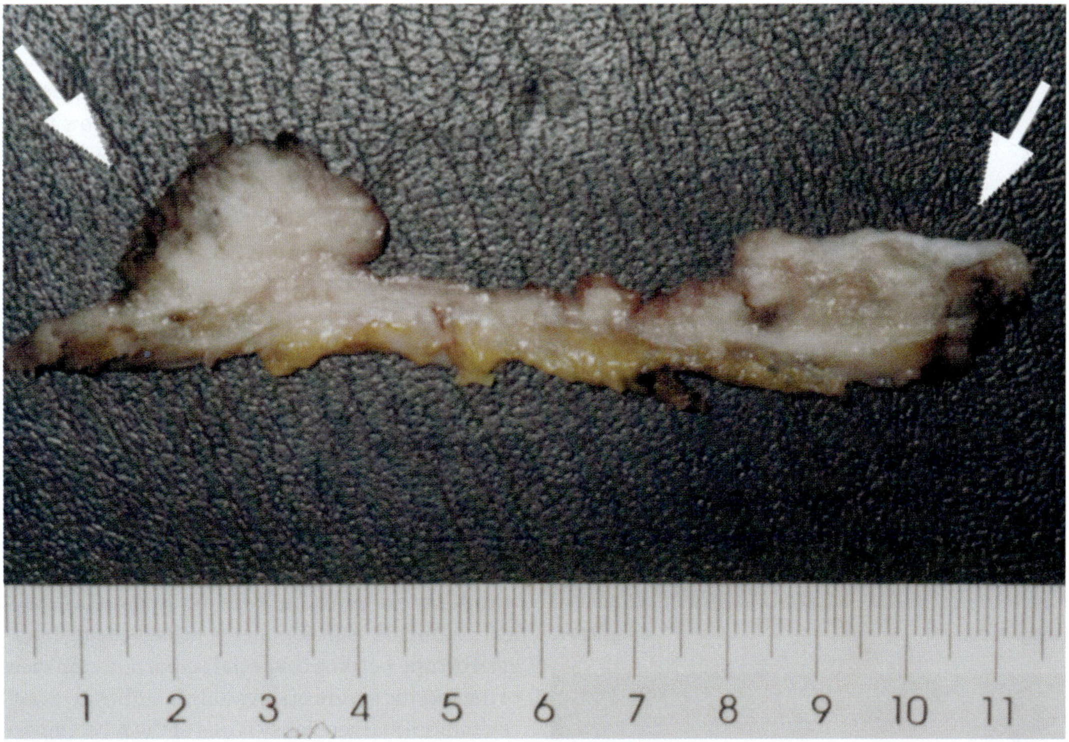

▲ **Fig. 109 d.**

■ **Fig. 109a–d.** Patient E., age 55. Diagnosis: gastric cancer. **a** Stomach roentgenogram (tight filling, vertical position, anterior projection) at the moment of contrast medium passage through the gastroesophageal junction: the lower third of the esophagus is irregularly narrowed, the contours are uneven (white arrows); the stomach cavity is markedly decreased, the stomach is disfigured (rigid tube), its contours are uneven (black arrows). **b** Stomach roentgenogram (double contrast, horizontal position, anterior projection): the cavity is decreased significantly, the walls are rigid due to diffuse circular intramural infiltration (arrows). Conclusion: Infiltrative cancer of the stomach with invasion of the esophagus. **c** Macrospecimen of the resected stomach: the inner surface of the stomach is occasionally covered with a grayish coat, the wall is firm over the entire length due to tumor infiltration which invades the esophagus. **d** Fragment of the macrospecimen (strip): wall is thickened, white tumor tissue is seen over entire length, which infiltrates the stomach wall (arrows). Histologically, adenocarcinoma with the signet-ring cell component.

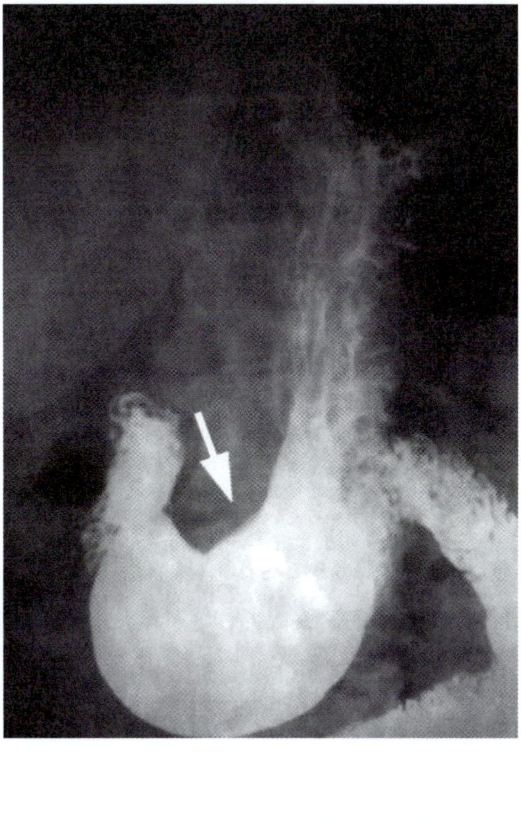

► **Fig. 110 a.**

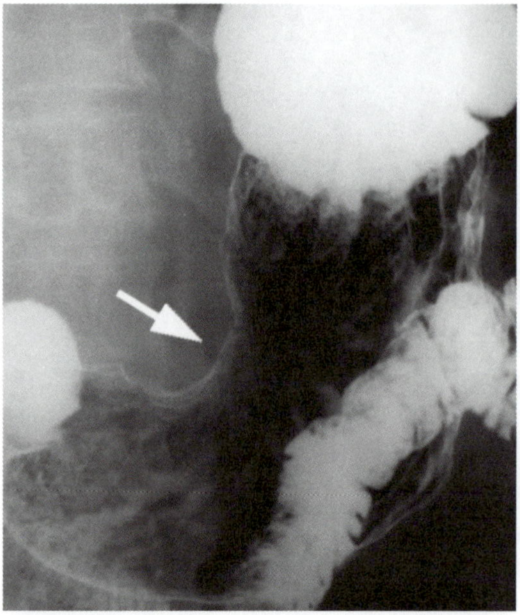

▲ **Fig. 110 b.** ▼ **Fig. 110 c.**

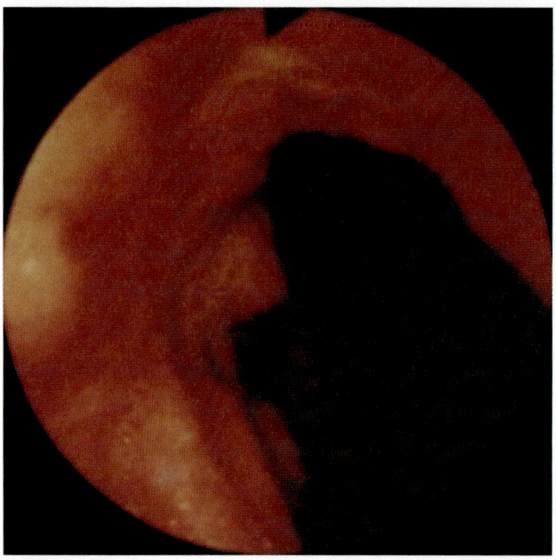

Fig. 110a–c. Female patient S., age 64. Diagnosis: gastric cancer. **a** Stomach roentgenogram (tight filling, vertical position, anterior projection): the angular notch is straightened, the lesser curvature is depressed (arrow). **b** Stomach roentgenogram (double contrast, horizontal position, anterior projection): the wall of the notch is thickened due to intramural infiltration (arrow); the folds converge toward the involved site of the wall. Conclusion: Infiltrative cancer of the angular notch. **c** Endophotograph: mucous membrane is grayish pink, dull, with uneven surface; occasional scarlet papillary growths with a fibrin coat can be seen on the anterior wall and the lesser curvature of the stomach body. Stomach lumen is disfigured and narrowed. Histologically, adenocarcinoma with the signet-ring cell component

ened infiltrated rigid folds (sometimes eroded) do not stretch after intensive inflation of the stomach with air. In some cases, changes on the mucous membrane amount to only a small, shallow ulcer that looks benign, but during surgery, the infiltration can be seen to spread to the submucous and muscular coats. Regardless of the location of tumors, they have one property in common. Obvious changes on the surface of the mucous membrane must be visualized by endoscopy (Fig. 110). If the changes show only slightly on the surface of the mucous membrane, and the growth is mainly in the submucous coat, endoscopic examination proves ineffective.

In most cases, the changes revealed by endoscopy must be differentiated from various hyperplasias of the mucous membrane and post-ulcer deformities of the stomach, which are known to interfere with X-ray examination. Here, findings of histological examination of bioptates obtained during fibergastroscopy become of special importance. In view of the specific nature of spreading in infiltrative cancer, multiple target biopsy is one of the most important requirements. At least five to seven specimens of tissues should be taken from the parts of the stomach wall which are in question based on X-ray examination and endoscopy. Target endoscopy of the mucous membrane is reasonable only when it is based on the findings of a preliminary roentgenological examination, which suggests that a particular part of the stomach should be visualized endoscopically (Fig. 111) [241, 259].

In explaining the reasons for the inappropriate use of endoscopy in Russia, most authors indicate a lack of adequate attention on the part of the endoscopist. As an example, they cite the results of gastric cancer control in Japan, where endoscopy is widely used for diagnostic purposes. In our opinion, however, the reason for late diagnosis of gastric cancer may not be connected with the endoscopists' lack of attention. In order to understand the inability of endoscopy alone to reveal gastric cancer, it suffices to compare the results of gastric cancer diagnosis (a) by stages, (b) by the 5-year survival, and (c) by the death rates in USA and Japan, where high-quality endoscopy is available everywhere. An analysis of published data shows that in Japan, where endoscopy is preceded by an X-ray examination, the results

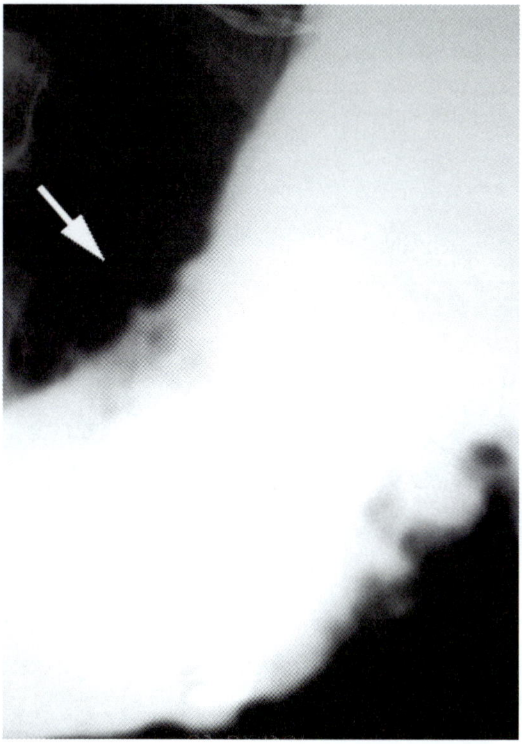

▲ **Fig. 111 a.**

are better by several orders of magnitude than in the USA, where endoscopy alone is normally used.

X-ray examination of the stomach prior to endoscopic inspection ensures qualitative performance in two stages [24]:

1. Chromogastroscopy, i.e., intravital staining of the stomach mucosa during endoscopic examination
2. Endoscopic resection of the stomach mucosa from the area of pathological change, which was revealed preliminarily by X-ray or fibergastroscopy

The following two methods are mainly used to stain gastric mucosa: a 0.5% methylene blue solution (the dye method) or a 0.2% solution of indigo carmine (the contrast method). Both are based on visual contrast between the pathologically changed tissues and intact surrounding tissues. The method of staining with methylene blue is based on the active absorption of the stain in the foci of intestinal metaplasia and dysplasia of the gastric epithelium (stain diffusion through the membrane of malignant tumor cells). The method employing indigo carmine, which does not stain the cells of the stomach mucosa, is based on distribution of the stain over the surface of the mucous membrane, giving a contrast image of its relief and pathologically changed parts.

Thus, target chromogastroscopy helps to visualize in detail pathological changes in the mucous membrane of the stomach, to locate them and determine their size, to verify changes in the relief and structure of the mucosal surface, and to take the necessary tissue specimens. However, as we have already said, target biopsy is unable to solve the diagnostic problem in all cases, especially in detecting early forms of infiltrative cancer of the stomach by examining a small number of specimens. Very often it is unable to establish a correct diagnosis of early gastric cancer or to estimate the extent of tumor invasion. A much larger fragment is often needed for a reliable conclusion.

Endoscopic resection of the mucous membrane from the suspected region can provide such large specimens. At present, the following two methods are most popular and widely used in clinical practice:

1. A standard loop excision
2. Aspiration of a specimen using a distal cap

Appropriately conducted endoscopy based on preliminary X-ray findings has far greater diagnostic value and a lower probability of possible complications during the procedure.

The reason for unsatisfactory diagnosis of gastric cancer should be sought in quite a different field. In infiltrative tumor growth the gastroscopic picture is far less conspicuous; this impedes not only verification of the nature of affection, but also visualization of its manifestations. In addition, there is the strong tendency toward an increasing proportion of endophytic new growths in the overall picture of gastric cancer and the decreasing number (or almost complete lack) of roentgenological examinations. Thus the absolute majority of tumors are revealed only in their far advanced stages, despite the expanding network of endoscopic units.

Unfortunately, the results of microscopic examination of specimens taken during target endosco-

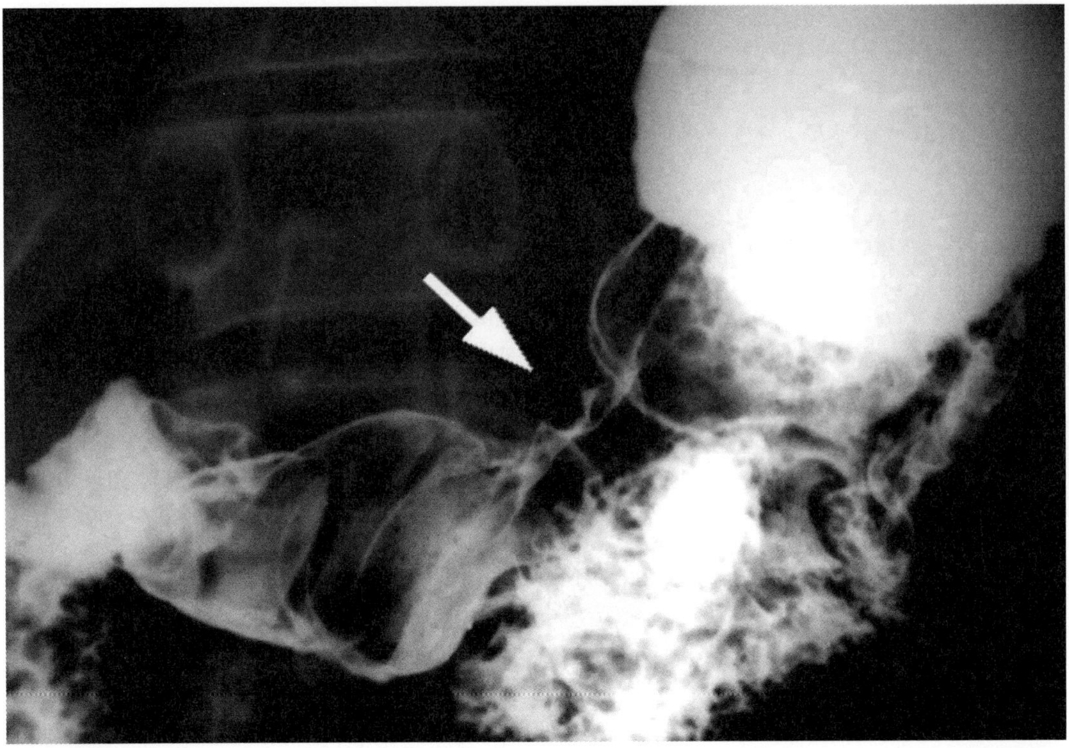

▲ Fig. 111 b.

▼ Fig. 111 c.

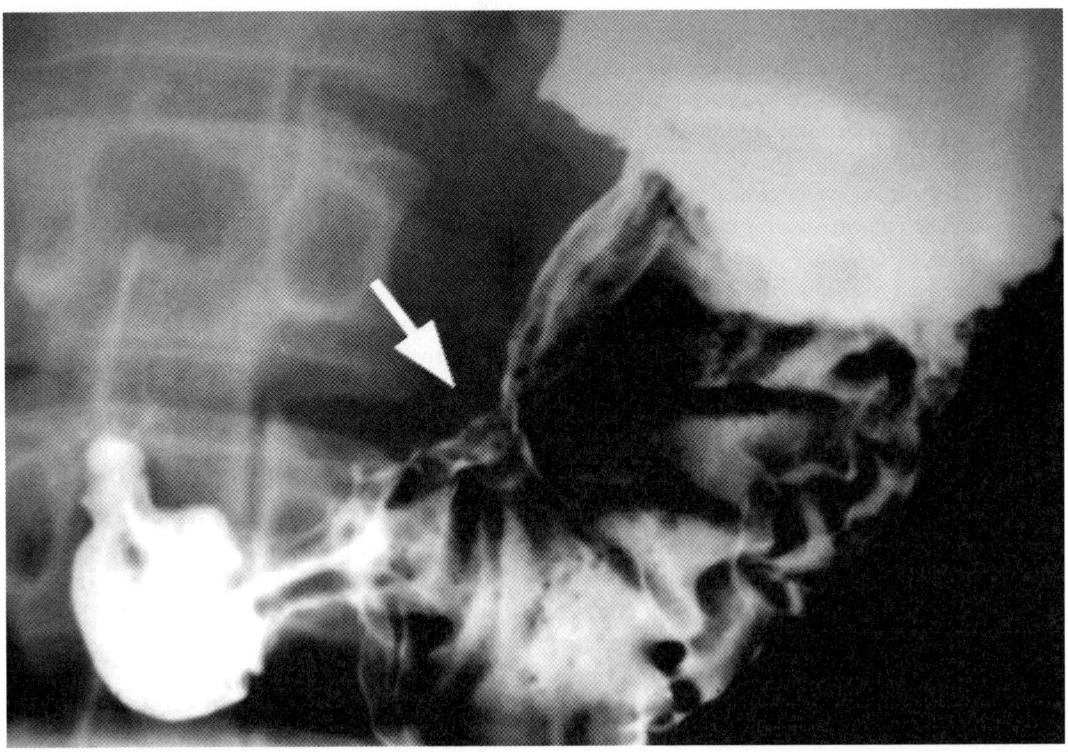

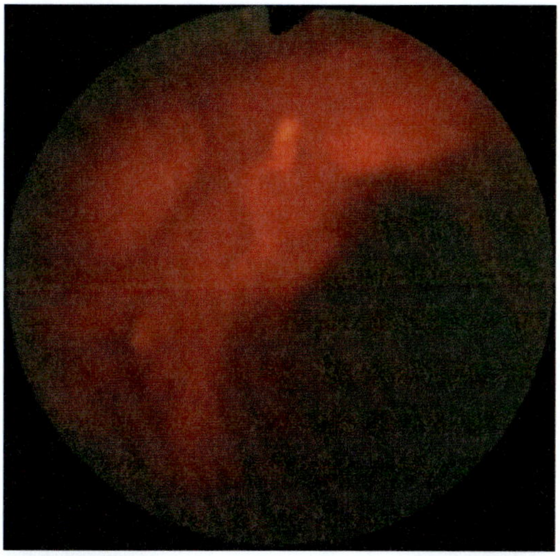

▲ **Fig. 111 d.**

Fig. 111a–d. Patient I., age 48. Diagnosis: gastric cancer. **a** Target stomach roentgenogram (tight filling, vertical position, anterior projection): the angular notch is straightened, its contour is uneven (arrow). **b** Stomach roentgenogram (double contrast, horizontal position, anterior projection): the contour is uneven, the wall is rigid, folds converge toward the affected part of the angular notch (arrow). **c** Stomach roentgenogram (double contrast, horizontal position, right half-oblique projection): with the optimal projection during roentgenotelescopy thickened wall of the notch due to intramural infiltration is visualized (arrow) with converging folds. Conclusion: Infiltrative cancer of the angular notch. **d** Endophotograph: a portion of mucous membrane with a diameter of about 3 cm, slightly elevated over the surrounding tissues is seen in the lower third of the stomach body at the border of the anterior wall and the lesser curvature; some mucosal folds converging toward the affected site do not straighten on inflation of the stomach with air. The mucous membrane in this region is scarlet, rough, with two eccentrically placed flat ulcers to 0.3 cm in diameter. Histologically, adenocarcinoma with the signet-ring cell component.

py often turn out to be of low informative value. Errors in morphological verification of the nature of infiltrative tumors of the stomach are connected to a great extent with their structure. There is a strikingly large proportion of diffuse forms of tumors compared with other histological versions of malignant new growths of gastric mucosa. According to some authors, scirrhous cancers alone account for 41–65% of all gastric carcinomas [97, 131,156, 157, 174]. The microscopic picture of this type of new growth is characterized by the presence of a marked fibroplastic component. It appears as the spread of connective tissue, which surrounds occasional cancer cells or their small aggregations with strong ridges. This explains the serious difficulties we face while establishing the character of a pathology. According to M. Kanter et al. (1985) and Evans et al. (1986), up to one fourth of all diagnostic errors are due to incorrect interpretation of the revealed changes. The complexity of identifying tumor infiltration is confirmed indirectly by the old and persistent concept of the inflammatory genesis of linitis plastica – a form of diffuse cancer.

While discussing the reason for decreasing effectiveness of histological and cytological studies in revealing the endophytic form of gastric cancer, it is necessary to note such factors as the incorrect choice of the site for taking tissue specimens, technical difficulties in conducting biopsy, and the predominantly submucous spread of the process.

According to data in the literature, the best way to avoid mistakes in selecting the site for taking tissue specimens is to take many samples. The accuracy of morphological diagnosis increases from 70% to 98% if the number of bioptates increases from one to six or seven [201, 224].

It is more difficult to get around another cause of incorrect verification of the nature of pathology: mostly submucous spread of the tumor. In such cases, in addition to correct selection of the site for biopsy, it is necessary to take a tissue specimen from the submucous coat. However, the small (0.2 x 0.2 cm) branches of biopsy forceps can take only specimens of the mucous membrane. The situation is even more aggravated by the fact that even »sophisticated« methods of biopsy, such as loop biopsy, needle aspiration biopsy, artificial electro-ulceration with subsequent taking of the material from the ulcer using common forceps, or using »gigantic« forceps, are effective in not more than 50% of cases (Kaneki et al. 1983, Iishu et al. 1986, Graham et al. 1989, Levin et al. 1990). The results of our observations are more optimistic: Using »gigantic« forceps of our own design enhanced the efficacy of biopsy to 65–70% [37, 222].

In our opinion, standardization of the method could improve endoscopic identification of infiltrative tumors. Experience with radiological diagnosis of gastrointestinal pathologies, malignant tumors included, shows that using standardized programs (other conditions being the same) increases the efficacy of examinations. Nevertheless, an obliterated and atypical visual picture, characteristic mostly of the early stages of gastric cancer or of later stages of the disease with submucous spread of the tumor, may significantly decrease the efficacy of fibergastroscopy (■ Fig. 112).

The accumulated experience indicates that an examination done in compliance with all current requirements can give us highly accurate information on the nature of the disease, and in some situations can outline the extent of spread. This is because even at the very early stages of cancer there may be a marked tendency to mostly submucous spread of tumor infiltration, giving a specific X-ray picture of uneven contours (with tight filling), wall thickening, and local decrease of elasticity (with double contrast). Traditional X-ray examination with filming gives the endoscopist additional information on the nature of the revealed changes and also on the best site for target biopsy using the relevant methods and appropriate tools.

Our vast experience in diagnosing the pathology in question indicates that many errors and difficulties in identifying minor forms of cancer may be avoided by using a complex of the traditional radiological and endoscopic examinations. Mutual exchange of information obtained by either of the methods increases the efficacy of early detection of infiltrative new growths with correct interpretation of the obtained results. Opposition to any of these methods can only harm the patient.

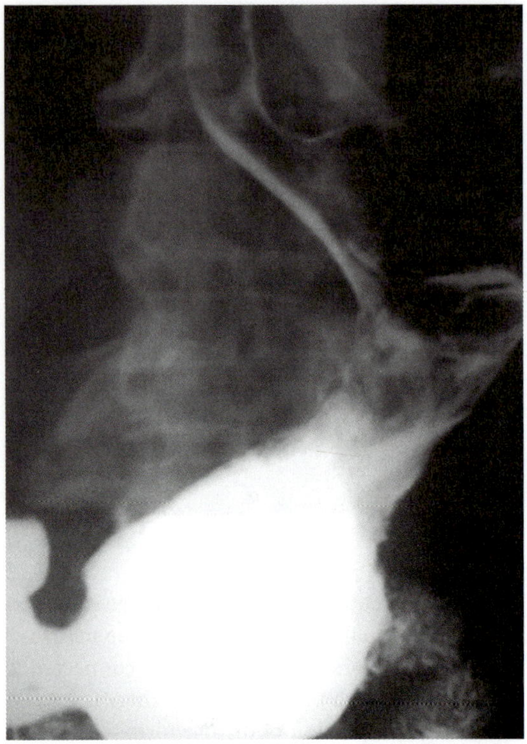

▲ **Fig. 112 a.**

▼ **Fig. 112 b.**

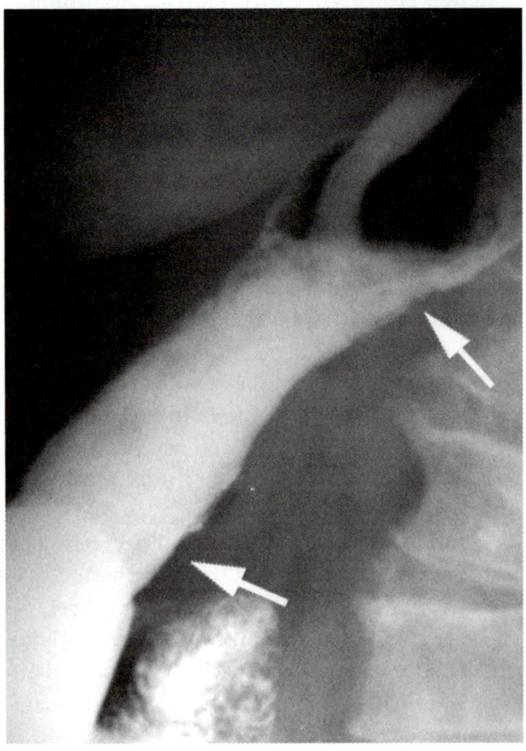

■ **Fig. 112a–d.** Female patient M., age 68. Diagnosis: gastric cancer. **a** Stomach roentgenogram (tight filling, vertical position, anterior projection): stomach body is disfigured (rigid tube), gastroesophageal junction is wide open. **b** Stomach roentgenogram (tight filling, vertical position, left lateral projection): stomach body is disfigured (rigid tube), uneven contours of the posterior wall of the body (arrows). **c, d** Stomach roentgenograms (double contrast, horizontal position, left oblique projection, lateral projection): stomach cavity is decreased, walls of the stomach body and its upper part are thickened and rigid due to diffuse circular intramural infiltration (arrows). Conclusion: Infiltrative cancer of the stomach body with invasion of the esophagus. The patient was operated. Histologically, signet-ring cell carcinoma.

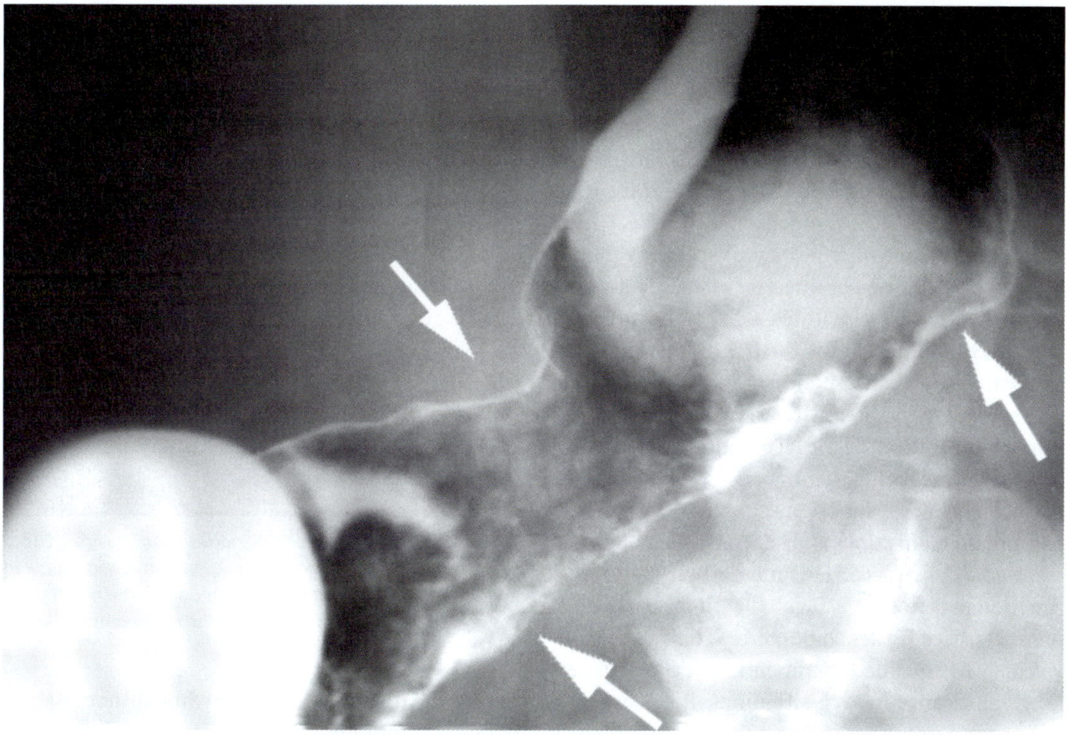

▲ Fig. 112 c.

▼ Fig. 112 d.

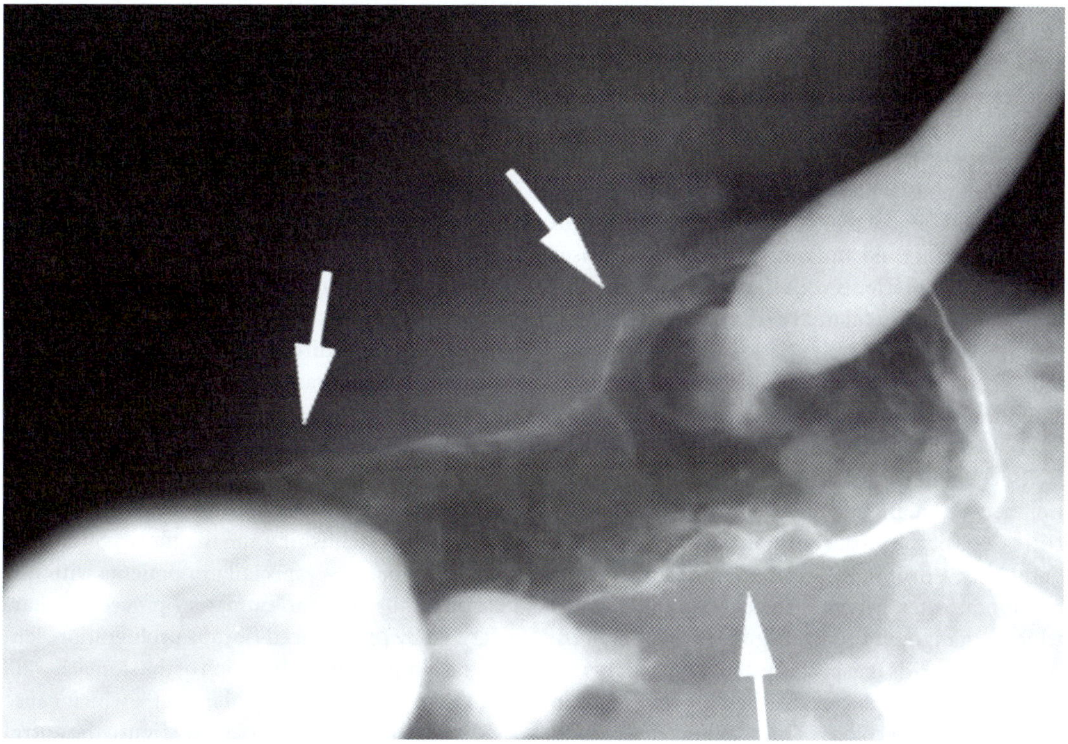

No less complicated is endoscopic identification of the nature of so-called organic stenosis of the pyloric part of the stomach. In the presence of exacerbation of the primary disease, endoscopy of ulcer-caused stenosis detects some features of malignancy: hyperemia, edema of the mucous membrane, vulnerability to physical contacts, and the like. Or the tumor tends to mostly submucous spread. Valuable information can be obtained by instrumental palpation, which can estimate elasticity of the wall. Possible revival of peristalsis during fibergastroscopy in a patient with exacerbation of peptic ulcer, which is described in the literature, is, in our opinion, unimportant for the differential diagnosis. There is another incorrect belief that in cancer, even at its early stage, the motor function is absent. Peristalsis in blastomatous affections is absent only when the muscular coat is involved. This means that motor dysfunction may not be associated with the early stage of cancer, because it is characteristic only of deep invasion. The so-called therapeutic test acquires certain significance in such situations. It consists in a 2- to 3-week course of intensive anti-inflammatory therapy with subsequent radiological and endoscopic examinations. If the condition stems from an ulcer, the dynamics will be distinctly positive: edema and hyperemia of the mucous membrane will subside, peristalsis will be restored, etc. The pyloric function is restored in some cases as a result of the formerly existing functional spasm, which was mistaken for stenosis. Radiological examination is reasonable and effective in such situations. Although the presence of fluid and mucus, and in some cases food masses, interferes with the examination, skillful use of the classical method and double contrast help to verify the characteristic signs of blastomatous affection, on the basis of which one can conduct a differential diagnosis [55].

Data on the pathogenesis of gastric cancer that have accumulated to date indicate a close connection between malignant affection and chronic gastritis – one of the most common varieties of gastric pathology. Chronic inflammation of the mucous membrane often becomes the background against which a malignant tumor originates and develops. Atrophic gastritis is especially dangerous in this respect, and it is emphasized as being a risk factor in current gastro-oncology. This explains to a certain degree the difficulties we face while differentiating between symptoms preceding cancer and signs that characterize tumor infiltration. It should be remembered that, in their early stages, neither gastric cancer nor chronic gastritis have pathognomonic signs. In advanced cancers, which are characterized by disintegration of tumor, metastases, and invasion of the neighboring anatomical structures, there appear subjective signs and changes that are detectable by instrumental examinations and leave no doubt as to the true nature of the pathology.

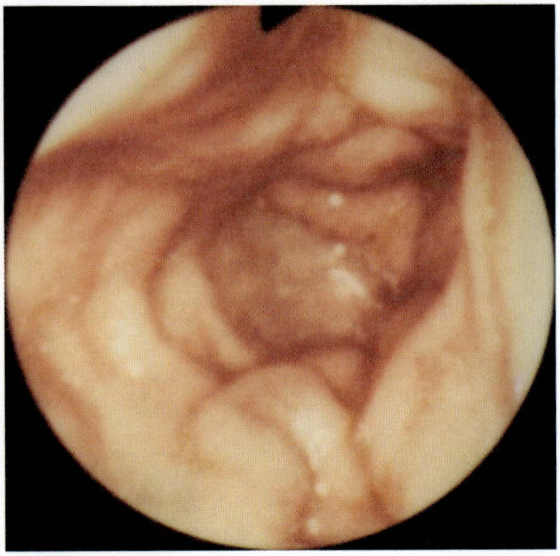

Fig. 113. Patient G., age 41. Diagnosis: antral gastritis. Endophotograph: the antral part is strongly disfigured and narrowed due to rough transverse folds, which do not straighten completely after insufflation of air. The mucous membrane is pale pink, smooth, and glassy.

Based on such situations, clinicians concluded that it is possible to differentiate clinically between gastritis and gastric cancer. This, in turn, explains why the patient is directed to an endoscopist without a preliminary traditional X-ray examination of the stomach. Experience shows that this approach lengthens the diagnostic search significantly. By giving the patient an X-ray examination with subsequent endoscopy we have considerably shortened the time for establishing the diagnosis. Situations sometimes occur – especially in patients with diffuse intramuscular inflammatory processes, characterized by pronounced fibrous proliferation, leuko- and lymphocytic infiltration of the stomach wall, and thickening of its muscular coat – which cause rigidity of the wall, narrow and disfigure the antral part of the stomach, and cause disorders in peristalsis. Endoscopic examination alone is not enough to establish an accurate diagnosis, even if this is chronic gastritis, the most common pathology.

The symptoms described were the basis for the concept of »rigid antral gastritis«. Contrarily, we think it more reasonable to use the term »diffuse interstitial gastritis«, which demonstrates the connections between meta- and anaplastic processes in the stomach wall. Moreover, rigidity proper sometimes becomes a subjective factor in conclusions made by an endoscopist. Difficulties arising during the examination of such patients may be ruled out by the skilled performance of endoscopy. At the same time, the final conclusion as to the nature of the disease can only be reached by morphological examination of bioptates (Fig. 113). Sometimes repeated endoscopy is required after a course of anti-inflammatory therapy, because a single examination cannot always diagnose these pathologies.

Difficulties in verifying the character of the pathology arise in Ménétrier's disease. Differential diagnosis and exclusion of a possible tumor require fibergastroscopy and biopsy. In order to verify the diagnosis morphologically, bioptates must contain tissues taken from the submucous coat, because the process often begins in the epithelium of the glandular floor of the mucous membrane (Fig. 114).

Ménétrier's disease manifests endoscopically as hyperemia and edema of the mucous membrane and severe thickening of the folds, which are sometimes covered with polypoid growths. It is important to study the functional symptoms for a differential diagnosis. Stretching of the folds and distinct reduction of their caliber (which are detectable by endoscopy) leave practically no doubt as to the inflammatory nature of hyperplasia of the mucous membrane. The benign character of changes is also confirmed by the preservation of a certain elasticity of the walls, which is detectable by X-ray examination at the phase of double contrast, as well as by instrumental palpation during endoscopy. Disfiguring and narrowing of the stomach lumen in the gigantic-fold type of endophytic cancer do not disappear even during inflation of the stomach with air; wall rigidity also remains stable at the double-contrast phase during the X-ray examination. Locations of erosion and submucous bleeding in the involved zone are also important for the differential diagnosis. In Ménétrier's disease, erosions are usually few and are located on the fold apices, but in infiltrative cancer these changes are multiple and more often located between the folds.

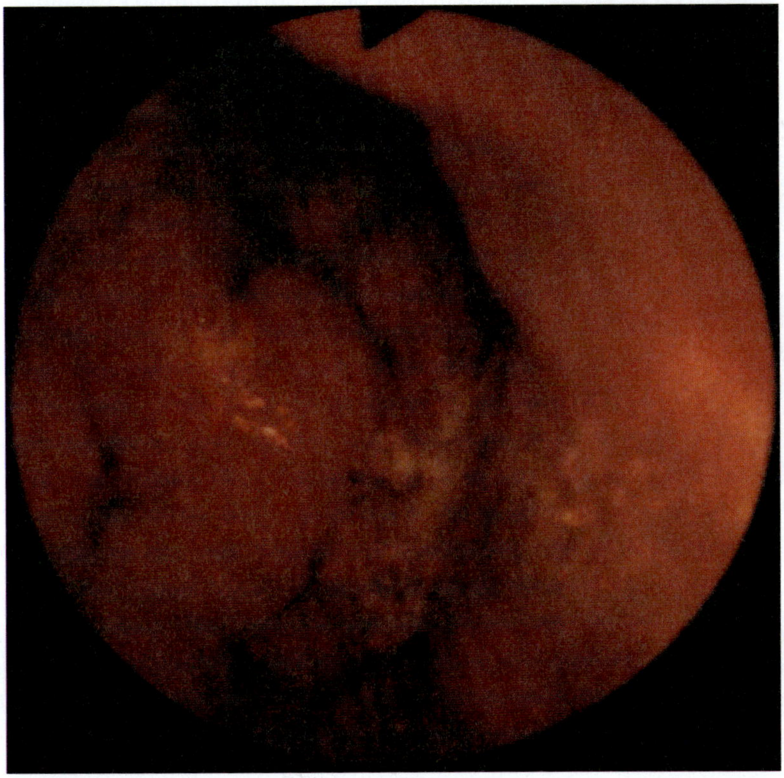

Fig. 114. Patient L., age 56. Diagnosis: Ménétrier's disease. Endophotograph: very thick and closely spaced sinuous folds in the stomach body on the greater curvature, which do not straighten after stomach inflation with air. The mucous membrane is hyperemic and edematous; occasional sites with fibrin deposits

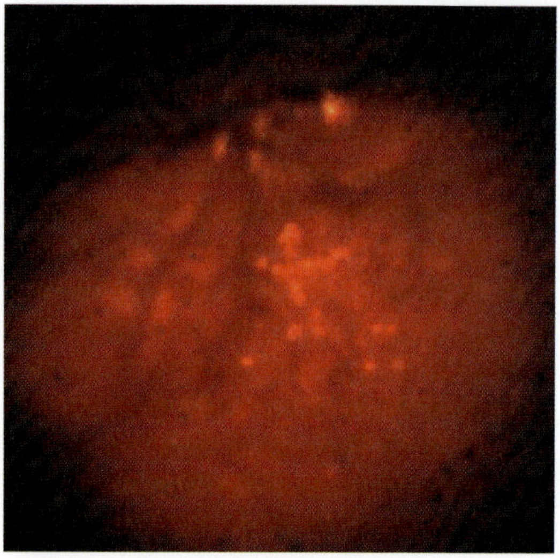

Fig. 115. Patient V., age 62. Diagnosis: infiltrative cancer concurrent with atrophy of the gastric mucosa. Endophotograph: against the background of marked vascular injection in the submucous coat, seen is a dull portion of the mucous membrane lacking vascular pattern, with punctate submucous hemorrhages and rough surface. Histologically, adenocarcinoma.

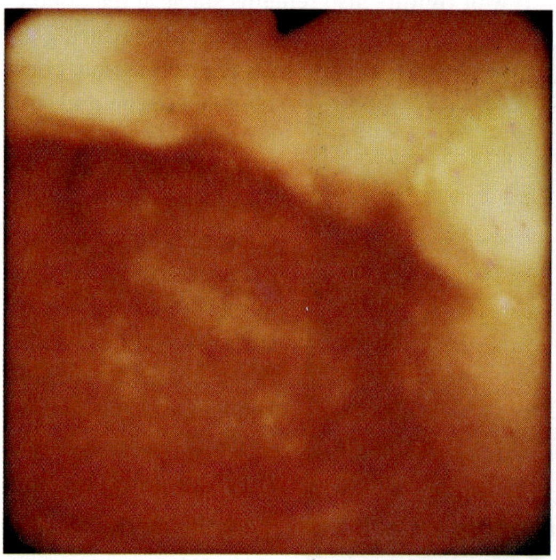

Fig. 116. Female patient O., age 43. Diagnosis: superficial gastritis. Endophotograph: the mucous membrane of the stomach is pink, smooth, and glassy, with foci of hyperemia.

It should be noted that in some cases, endoscopic signs of the tumor are difficult to distinguish from visual signs of atrophic and superficial forms of gastritis (Fig. 115), but thorough and purposeful examination and interpretation of the revealed changes can give grounds to suspect cancer even in cases where the differential diagnosis is difficult. Thus, in the endoscopic picture resembling atrophic gastritis (smooth relief of the mucous membrane, its whitish shade, absence of folds), the tumor character is evidenced by the focal nature of affection, by the color contrast between the »frosted« infiltrated wall and surrounding scarlet intact tissues, and by the absence of a vascular pattern in the tumor zone.

Endoscopic signs that are common to both superficial gastritis and diffuse cancer include smooth relief in the involved zone, its uniform elevation, hyperemia, edema, and easy vulnerability on physical contact. The differential diagnosis in such cases is based mostly on inflammatory changes in the mucous membrane which are less pronounced in gastritis than in cancer, but this parameter is so relative and subjective that, in our opinion, it cannot be regarded as convincing (Fig. 116). In addition, the limited nature of affection, the local character of the changes, their homogeneity, and the rigidity of tissues are the distinguishing signs of tumor in such cases (Fig. 117). A correct diagnosis can be established in most cases with a preliminary traditional roentgenological examination. Moreover, the complex approach, including radiological diagnosis and endoscopy, with subsequent histological examination of the tissue specimens obtrained, guarantees a correct diagnosis.

Thus, establishing the diagnosis of gastric cancer, especially in its early stages, requires rational use of all modern methods of examination (radiological, endoscopic, morphological). The initial and very important stage includes the use of the traditional X-ray examination based on the study of stomach contours and also on information obtained by double-contrast radiology. Using the complex of methods of radiological diagnosis (ultrasonography, CT, MRI) in difficult diagnostic cases requiring verification broadens the possibilities for correct assessment of the radiologically revealed changes and helps to carry out purposeful and adequate endoscopy with the taking of tissue specimens for histological examination. With due account to the specific character of the spread of infiltrative cancers, which presents the greatest difficulties for their identification, much effort should be directed at increasing the efficacy of endoscopic diagnosis, by conduct-

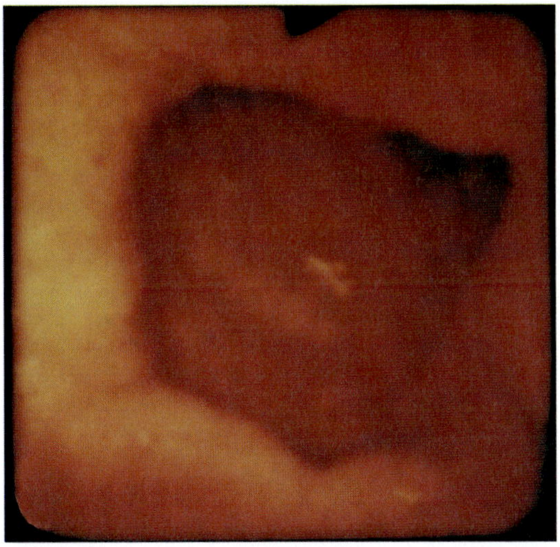

Fig. 117. Patient D., age 60. Diagnosis: gastric cancer. Endophotograph: the lumen of the stomach is hyperemic and narrowed due to circular intramural infiltration. Histologically, signet-ring cell carcinoma.

ing multiple target biopsies and also by improving methods for taking tissue specimens from deeper parts of the mucous and submucous coats. New potentials for timely detection of minor endophytic gastric cancer, which is usually characterized by meager and atypical clinical signs (or to be more accurate, by their absence) may be realized by conducting control X-ray examinations of persons belonging to the so-called risk groups (e.g., patients with chronic inflammatory diseases of the stomach).

The problem of diagnosing diffuse cancer is the problem of diagnosing gastric cancer on the whole, because infiltrative tumors account for the discouraging statistics of advanced cancer in modern gastro-oncology. The problem of early diagnosis and adequate treatment can only be solved with due consideration of all available signs in radiological and endoscopic studies of tumor infiltration. The new technologies of radiological diagnosis, such as ultrasonography, computed tomography, and magnetic-resonance imaging, provide additional help in particular situations.

Some Correction of Current Views on Cancer Location in Various Parts of the Stomach

According to the modern concept, the main sites of cancer localization in the stomach are believed to be its distal part, the posterior wall, and the lesser curvature. However, a large proportion of tumors originate on the greater curvature and the anterior wall of the stomach wall [28, 29, 33, 129]. This fact has not been given wide recognition owing to the old belief that these parts of the stomach are rare sites of primary cancer lesions. Therefore, we think it necessary to propose amendments to the existing structure of radiological examination of the stomach affected by tumor, based on our own experience. Our concept of the localization of gastric cancer is supported by A. Marzcell et al. (1989) and V. Eckardt et al. (1990), who point to the increasing incidence of carcinomas localized primarily on the anterior wall and the greater curvature of the stomach. P. Percivale et al. (1989) and J. Breaux et al. (1990) reported that cancer of the greater curvature occurs in 12.9% and cancer of the anterior wall in 8–10% of cases [99, 117]. This should stimulate a revision of the existing semiotic and methodological concepts in the diagnosis of gastric cancer. The orientation must be the search for endophytic tumors, particularly in the upper part of the stomach, where infiltrative cancer is especially frequent [31, 33, 35, 39]. Thus, we want to describe some signs of cancer in its early stages in those parts of the stomach which are unduly neglected by the modern cancer investigation protocols.

Cancer of the Cardiac Part

The diagnosis of tumors of the cardiac part of the stomach is associated primarily with the anatomical properties of this region. These include: pronounced relief, permanently changing zone of the functioning cardia, and the specific distribution of muscle fibers in this part of the stomach wall. Compression and palpation are impossible here.

It is necessary to note that the traditional method of detecting tumors of the upper part of the stomach does not meet the requirements of modern gastro-oncology. The opinion is still held that dysphagia is the most specific symptom of cancer of the upper part of the stomach. Meanwhile, practical experience shows that this symptom appears, as a rule, at those stages of the disease when radical surgery is already impracticable or has little effect (Fig. 118) [9, 18, 155].

In order to increase the efficacy of practical radiology in revealing cancer of the upper part of the stomach, it seems reasonable to divide this type of cancer into five groups according to the type of tumor:

1. Tumors of the cardia. Depending on the initial localization, this group should be subdivided into the following:
   a. Cancer of the cardia proper
   b. Supracardiac cancer
   c. Subcardiac cancer
   d. Precardiac cancer
   e. Retrocardiac cancer
2. Tumors of the anterior wall of the upper part of the stomach
3. Tumors of the posterior wall of the upper part of the stomach
4. Tumors of the stomach fundus
5. Tumors of the greater curvature of the upper part of the stomach

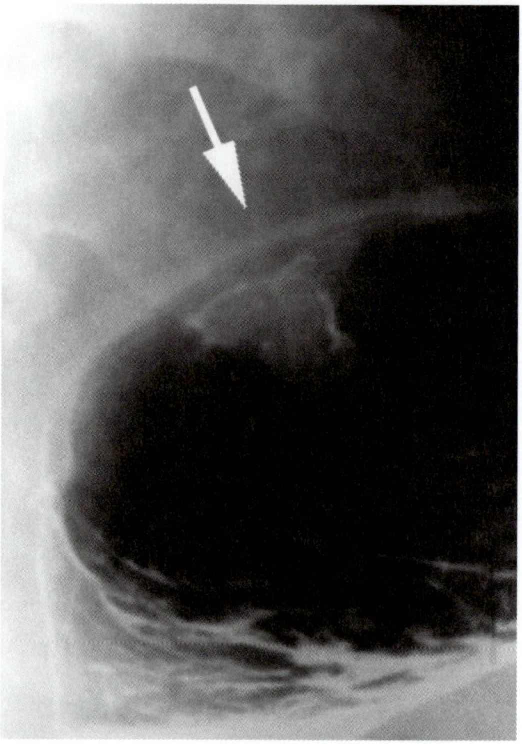

▲ **Fig. 118 a.** ▼ **Fig. 118 b.**

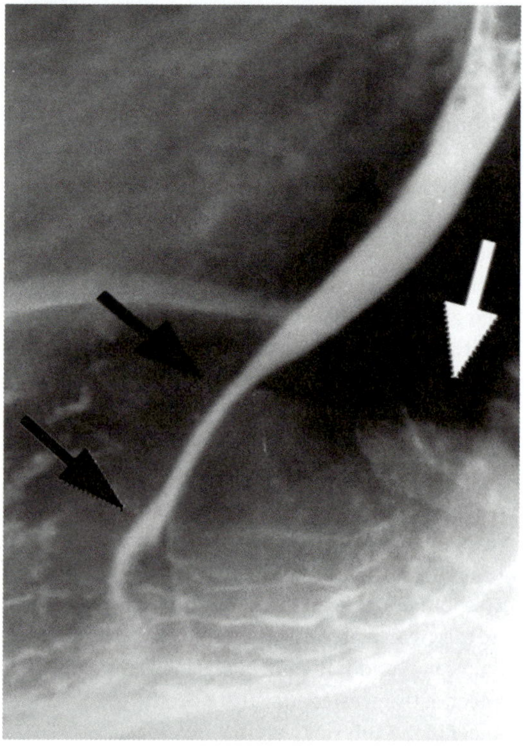

Fig. 118 a–f. Female patient E., age 67. Diagnosis: gastric cancer. **a** Roentgenogram of the upper part of the stomach (double contrast, vertical position, anterior projection): wall of the fundus is thickened due to intramural infiltration (arrow). **b** Roentgenogram of the upper part of the stomach (double contrast, vertical position, left lateral projection) at the moment of contrast medium passage through the gastroesophageal junction: the abdominal segment of the esophagus is unevenly narrowed (black arrows) due to spreading infiltration (white arrow). **c** Roentgenograms of the upper part of the stomach (double contrast, horizontal position, left posterior oblique projection): more distinctly visualized is thickening of the fundus walls due to intramural infiltration (black arrows); atypical relief of the cardiac rosette (white arrows). Conclusion: Infiltrative cancer of the upper part of the stomach with invasion of the esophagus. In order to estimate spread of infiltration onto the neighboring organs and tissues, the patient was examined by computed tomography. **d, e, f** Computed tomograms (tight filling with E-Z-CAT DRY, supine position): the wall of the fundus is thickened due to intramural infiltration spreading to the left crus of the diaphragm and the spleen (arrows). Endoscopic examination proved to be infeasible due to markedly narrowed esophagus.

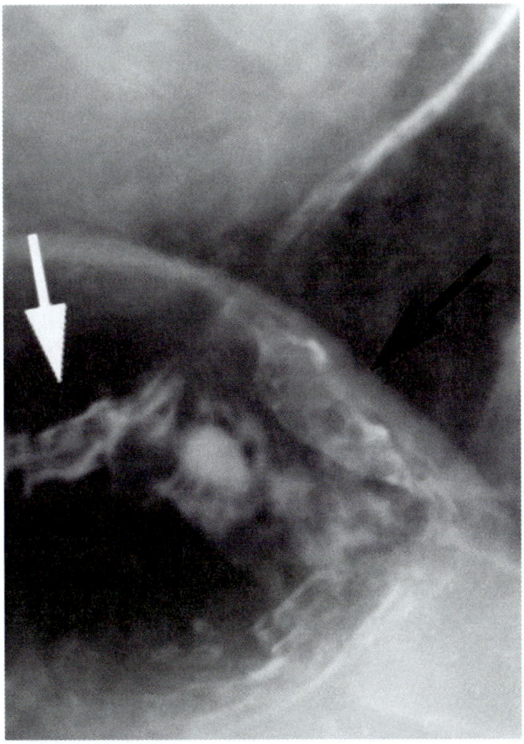

▲ Fig. 118 c.

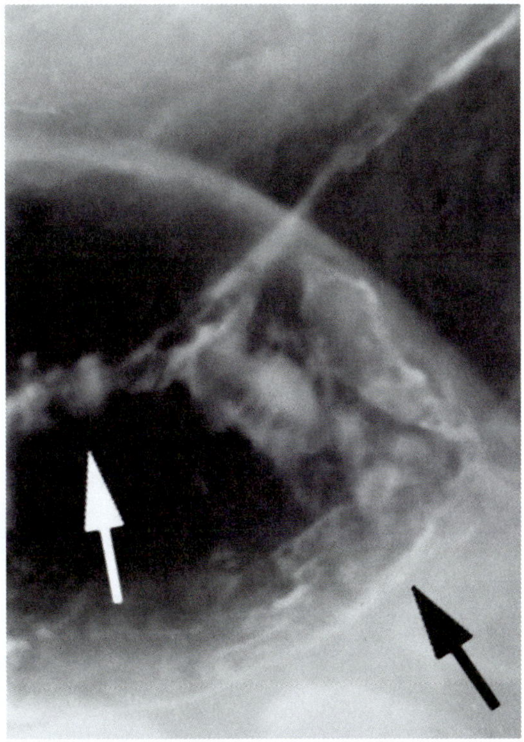

▲ Fig. 118 c.

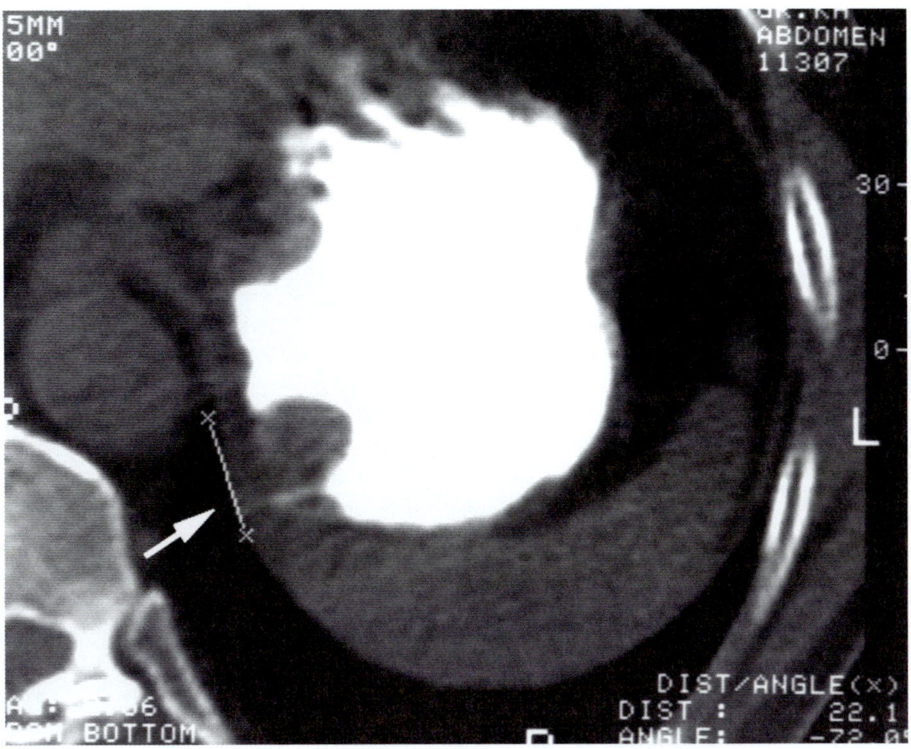

◀ Fig. 118 d.

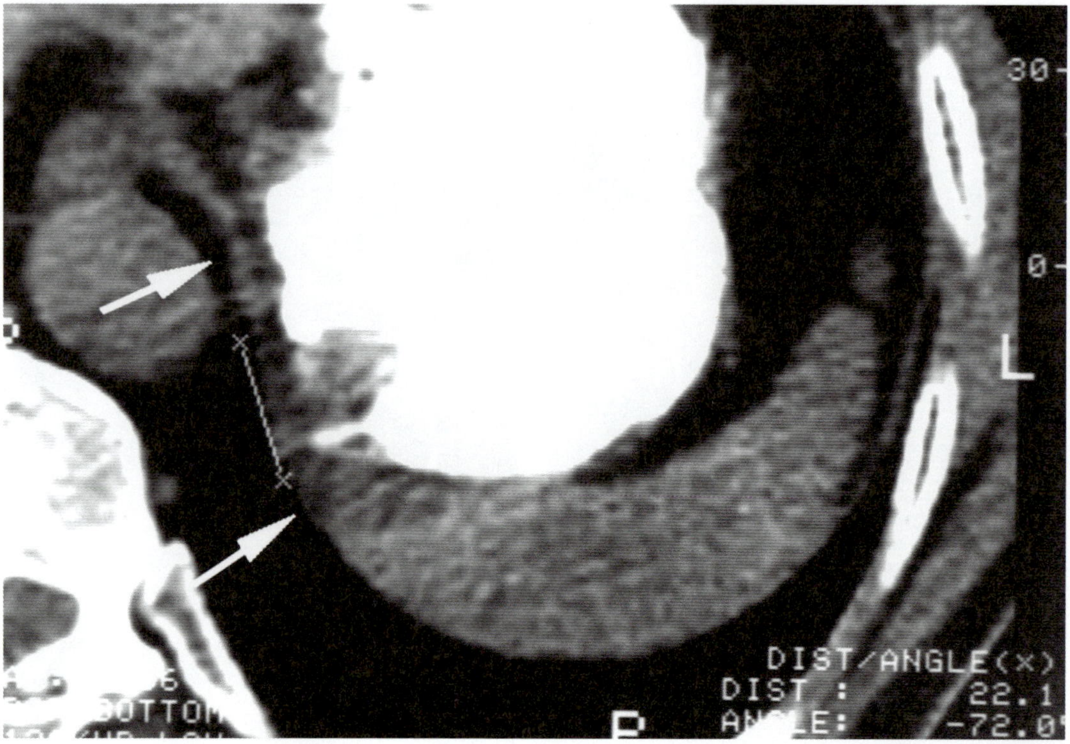

▲ Fig. 118 e.

▼ Fig. 118 f.

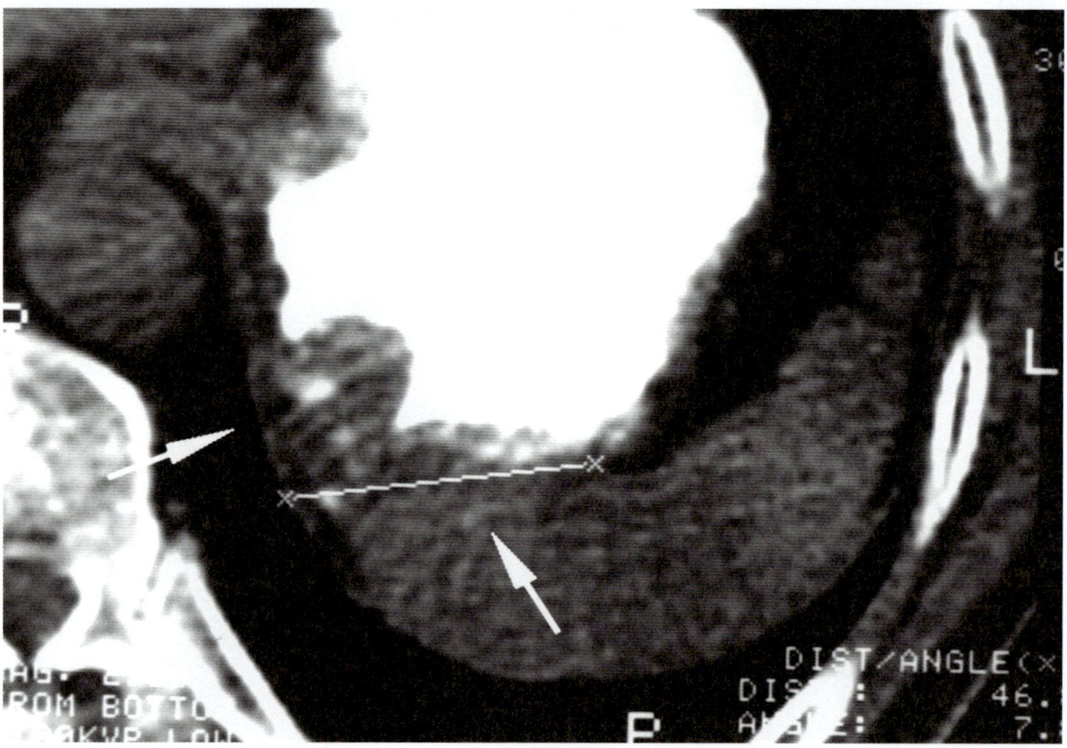

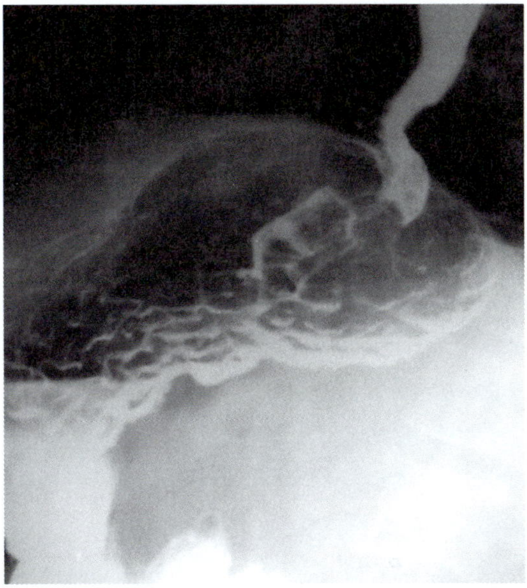

▲ **Fig. 119 a.**

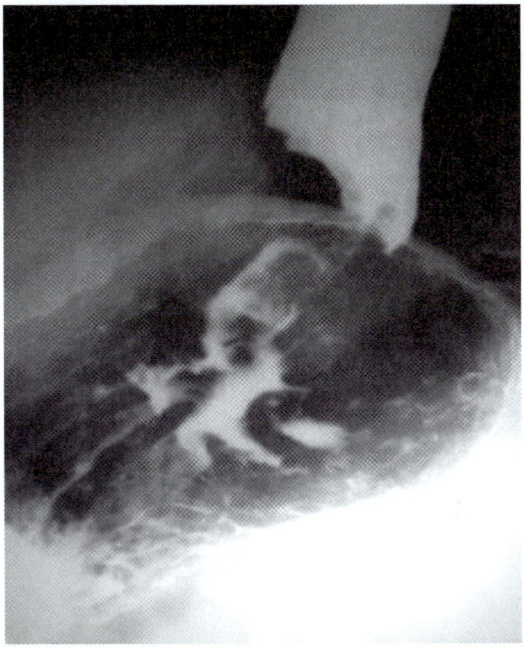

▼ **Fig. 119 b.**

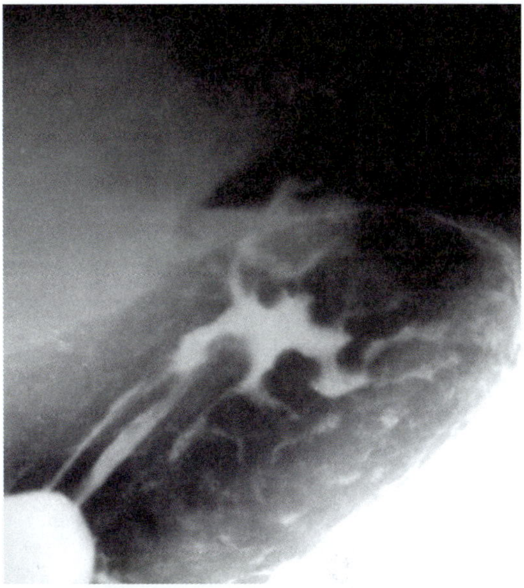

▲ **Fig. 119 c.**

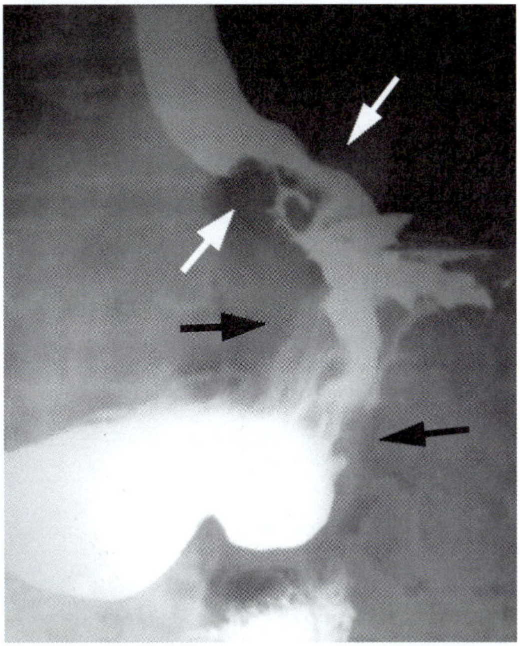

▼ **Fig. 120 a.**

Fig. 119 a–c. Patient D., age 58. Diagnosis: gastric cancer. **a** Stomach roentgenogram (tight filling, vertical position, left lateral projection) at the moment of contrast medium passage through the gastroesophageal junction: the abdominal segment of the esophagus is unevenly narrowed, its contours are uneven and eroded, the walls are rigid. **b** Roentgenogram of the upper part of the stomach (double contrast, horizontal position, left posterior oblique projection) at the moment of contrast medium passage through the gastroesophageal junction: mucosal folds terminate near the cardia; the contours of the abdominal segment of the esophagus are uneven and eroded. **c** Roentgenogram of the upper part of the stomach (double contrast, horizontal position, left posterior oblique projection): atypical relief of the cardiac rosette (cardioesophageal junction); termination of mucosal folds is distinctly visualized. Conclusion: Infiltrative cancer of the upper part of the stomach with invasion of the esophagus. Histologically, signet-ring cell carcinoma.

Fig. 120 a–e. Patient I., age 62. Diagnosis: gastric cancer. **a** Stomach roentgenogram (tight filling, vertical position, anterior projection) at the moment of contrast medium passage through the gastroesophageal junction: uneven narrowing of the abdominal segment of the esophagus (white arrows), uneven and eroded contours of the body and the upper part of the stomach (black arrows). **b** Stomach roentgenogram (double contrast, horizontal position, left lateral projection): atypical relief of the cardiac rosette (cardioesophageal junction), the walls are rigid and thickened due to diffuse circular intramural infiltration (arrows). **c, d** Roentgenograms of the upper part of the stomach (double contrast, horizontal position, left lateral projection) at the moment of contrast medium passage through the gastroesophageal junction: uneven narrowing of the abdominal segment of the esophagus, uneven contours (arrow). Conclusion: Infiltrative cancer of the upper part of the stomach with invasion of the abdominal segment of the esophagus. **e** Endophotograph: the cardiac part is greatly narrowed due to spread of tumor which embraces the stomach walls circularly. Histological examination of the bioptates verified signet-ring cell carcinoma.

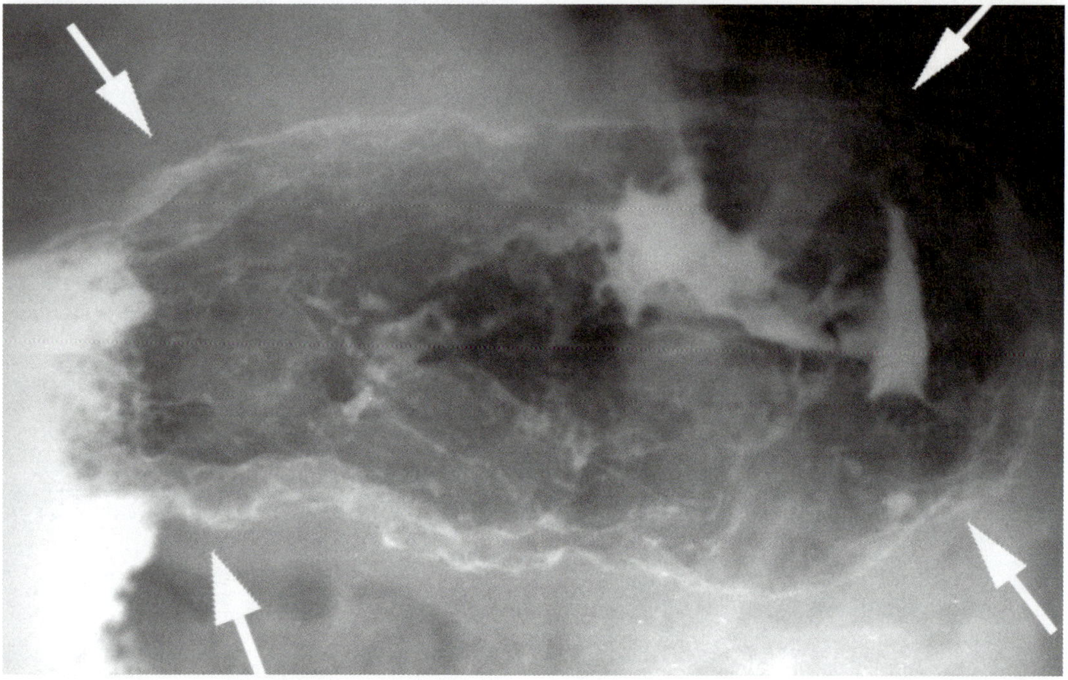

▲ **Fig. 120 b.**

▼ **Fig. 120 c.**

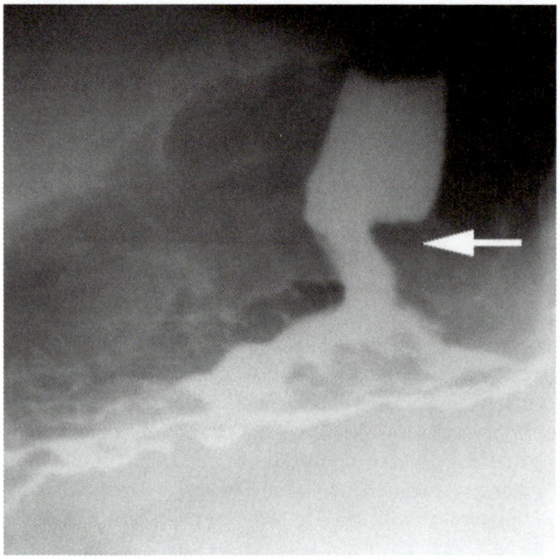

▼ **Fig. 120 d.**

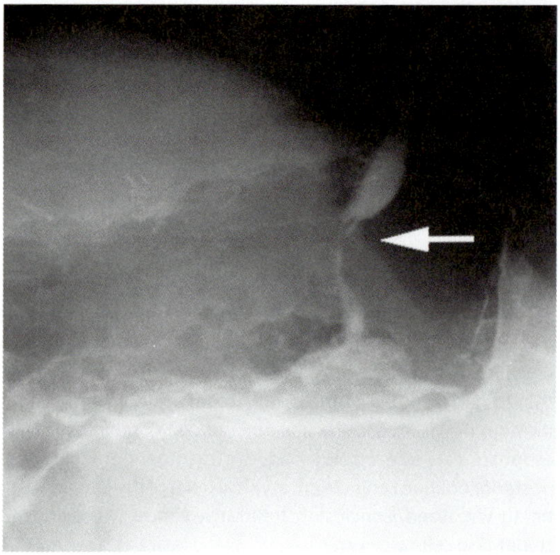

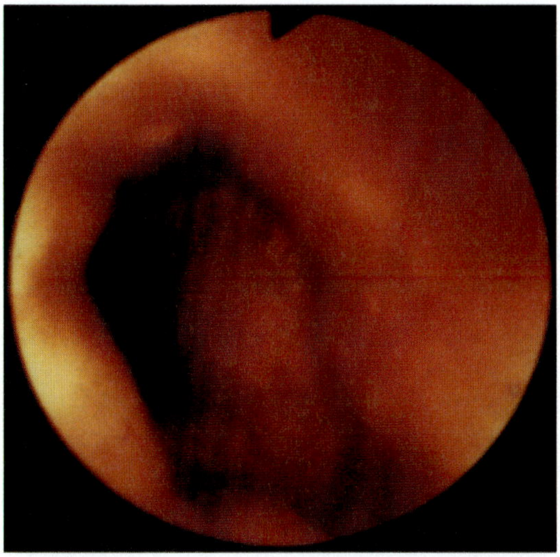

▲ Fig. 120 e.

Localization of the tumor within the boundaries of a given part of the stomach is the basic factor influencing the onset, the character, and terms of development of clinical symptoms. Thus, a tumor originating in the immediate vicinity of the cardiac sphincter relatively soon invades the abdominal segment of the esophagus to cause dysphagia (◘ Fig. 119). With a tumor located at a distance from the cardia, e.g., on the posterior wall or the greater curvature, this symptom occurs much later or not at all (◘ Fig. 120). But the initial site of the tumor does not determine the development of this or that clinical symptom exclusively. It also has a significant effect on the formation of radiological signs. Every experienced radiologist knows that there is a great difference between the traditional X-ray picture of cancer of the cardia and that presented by cancer of the posterior wall of the upper part of the stomach and the stomach fundus (◘ Figs. 121 and 122). Secondary changes characterizing further progress of the tumor differ as well. In some cases, these are invasion of the esophagus, in others the diaphragm, and in still others the splenic hilus, the pancreas, etc. [63, 82, 147, 151].

Thus, tumors originating in various locations of the upper part of the stomach can differ in at least three aspects:

1. Clinical symptoms
2. Signs of blastomatous affection detectable by radiological methods
3. Complications associated with further growth of the tumor

Our experience and the data in the literature show that the traditional X-ray examination, based on the classical method of the first gulp and examination of the mucous membrane relief against the background of the air bubble, can diagnose proximal gastric cancer in 75–92% of cases [31, 38, 42, 52]. But these are generally advanced forms of cancer, in which diagnosis does not lead to cure. Although there are publications regarding early cancer of this part of the stomach, diagnosis of this tumor remains very complicated, and in some cases infeasible.

◘ **Fig. 121 a–c.** Female patient B., age 69. Diagnosis: gastric cancer. **a** Stomach roentgenogram (tight filling, vertical position, anterior projection): organic changes are not detectable. **b** Stomach roentgenogram (double contrast, vertical position, left lateral projection): the specific radiating pattern of the cardiac rosette is absent (arrows). **c** Stomach roentgenogram (double contrast, vertical position, left lateral projection): atypical relief of the cardiac rosette (arrows). Conclusion: Infiltrative cancer of the cardiac part of the stomach. The patient was operated. Histologically, signet-ring cell carcinoma.

▼ **Fig. 121 a.**

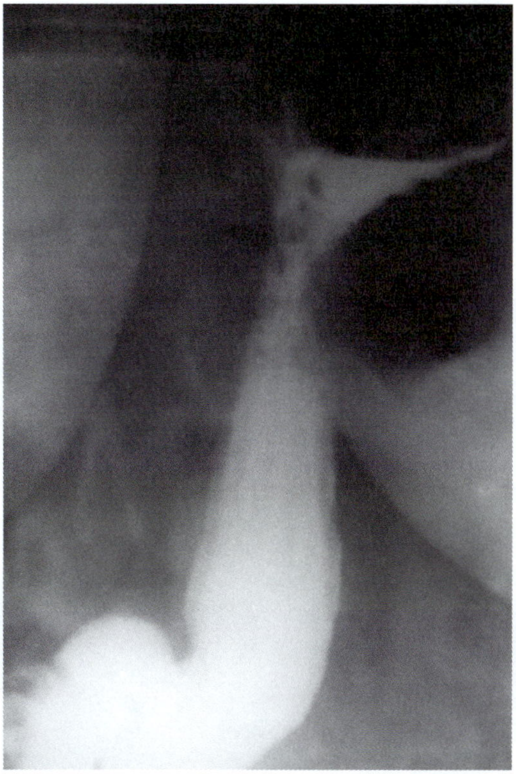

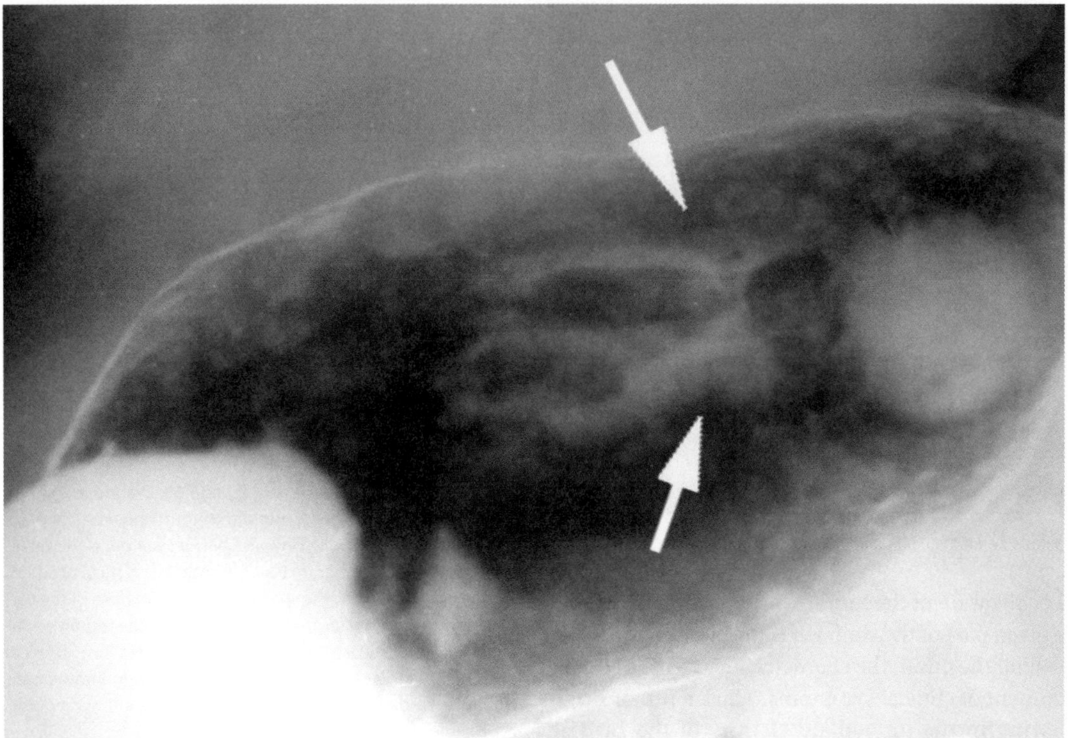

▲ Fig. 121 b.

▼ Fig. 121 c.

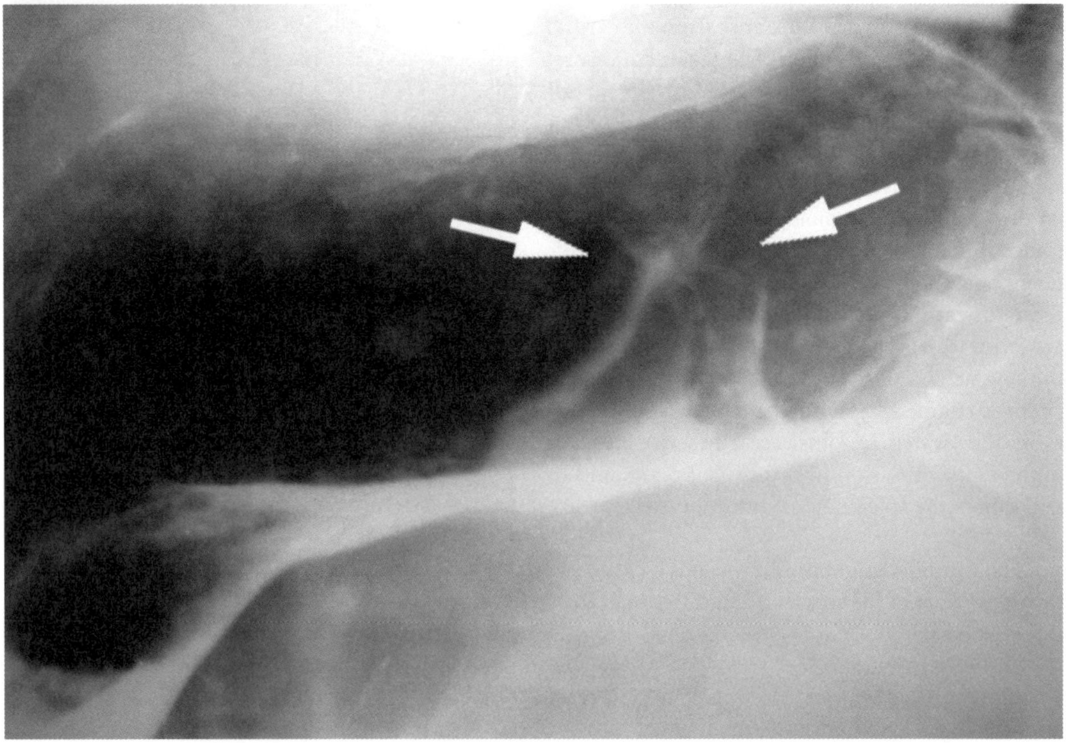

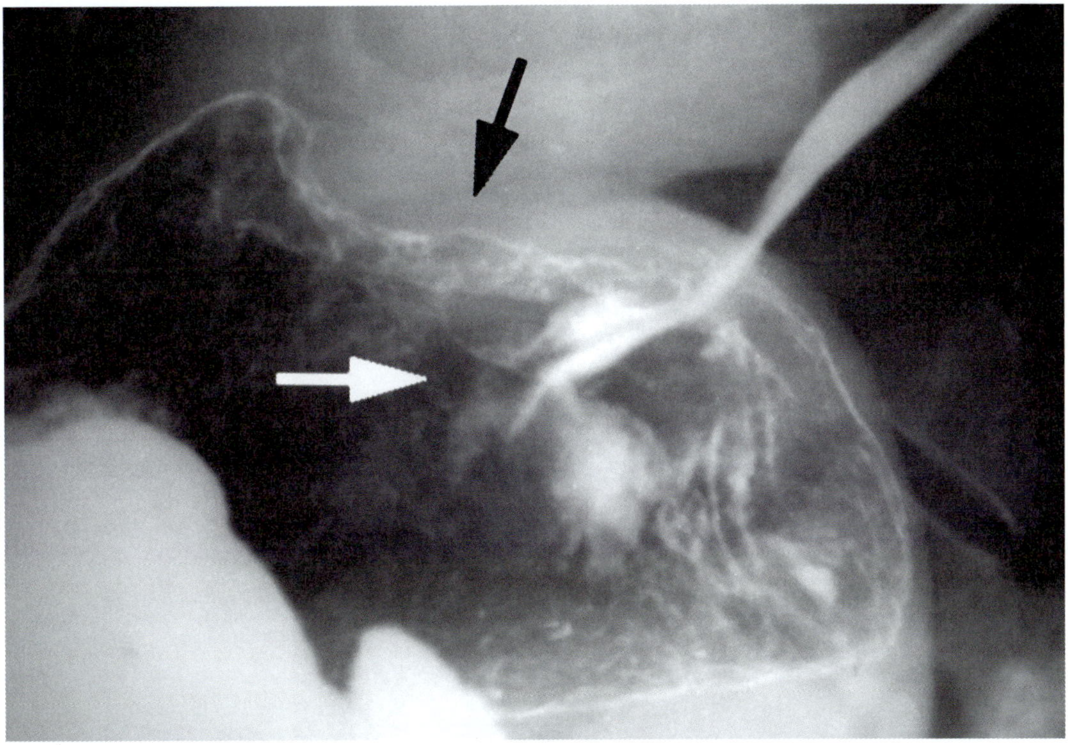

▲ **Fig. 122 a.**

▼ **Fig. 122 b.**

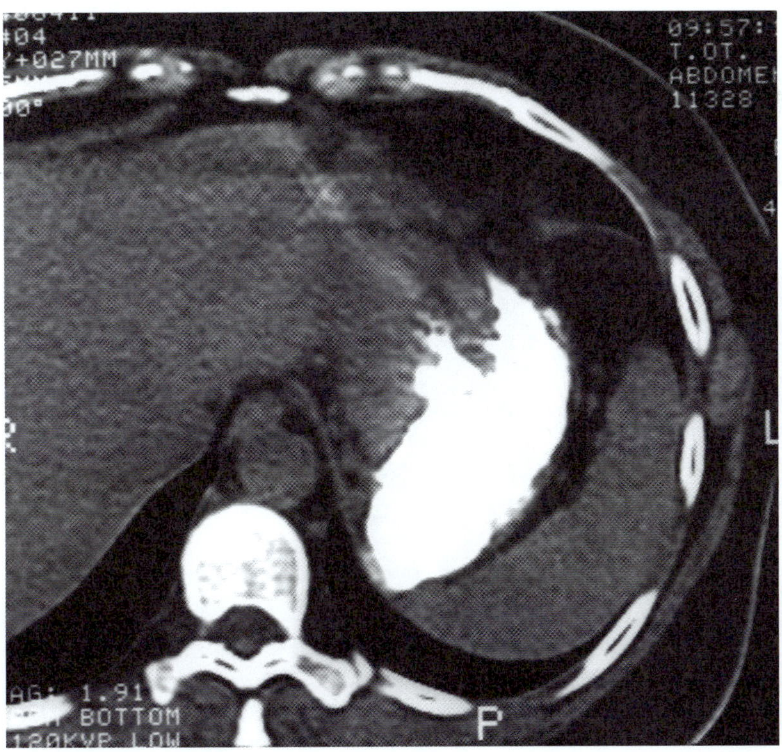

Fig. 122 a–g. Female patient K., age 55. Diagnosis: gastric cancer. **a** Stomach roentgenogram (double contrast, horizontal position, left lateral projection): the upper part of the stomach is disfigured, the anterior wall is thickened and rigid due to intramural infiltration (black arrow), atypical relief of the cardiac rosette (white arrow), the esophagus patency unimpaired. In order to verify the spread of infiltration onto the esophagus, the patient was examined by computed tomography. **b, c** Computed tomograms of the stomach (tight filling with E-Z-CAT DRY, supine position, the level of the stomach fundus): walls are thickened due to intramural infiltration. **d, e** Computed tomograms of the stomach (tight filling with E-Z-CAT DRY, supine position, the level of the cardiac and subcardiac parts): infiltration spreads to the abdominal segment of the esophagus (white arrow), the exophytic tumor component is visualized (black arrow). Conclusion: Cancer of upper part of the stomach with invasion of the esophagus, mixed type of growth. **f** Macrospecimen of a resected stomach: the exophytic component in the upper part (arrows) with the changed surrounding relief; infiltration spreads to the esophagus. **g** Fragment of the macrospecimen (strip): stomach wall is thickened due to intramural infiltration component of white color (arrows). Histologically, adenocarcinoma with the signet-ring cell component.

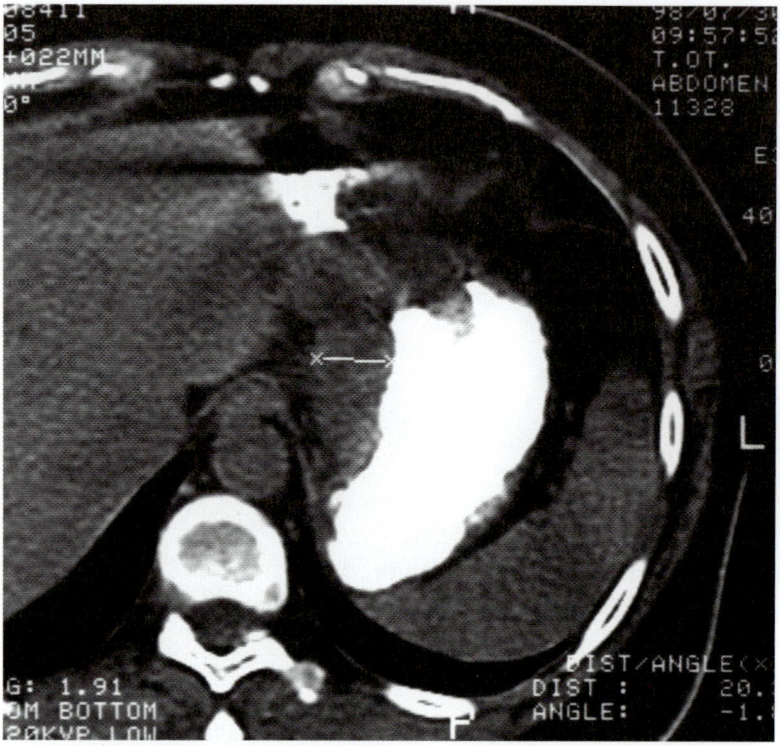

◂ **Fig. 122 c.**

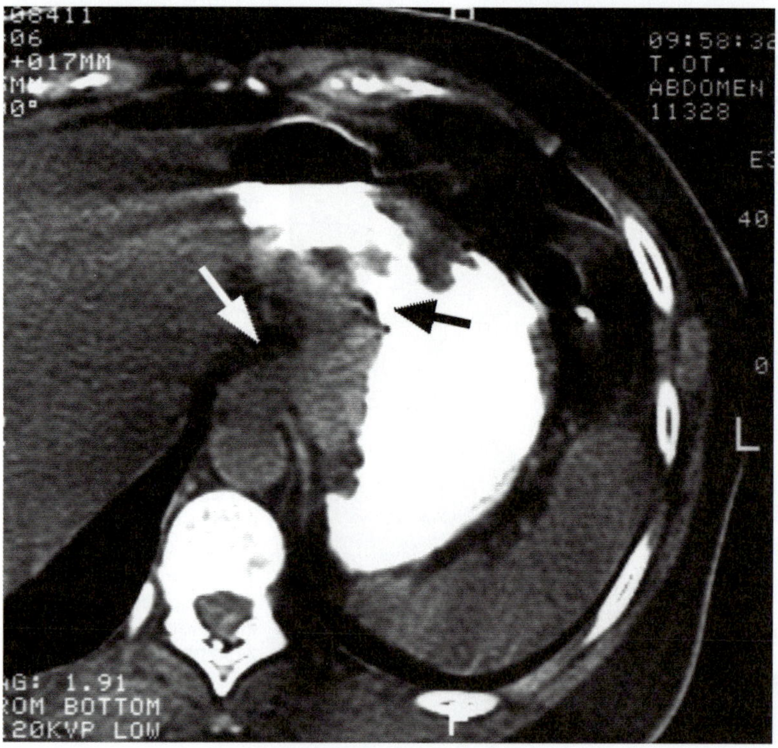

◂ **Fig. 122 d.**

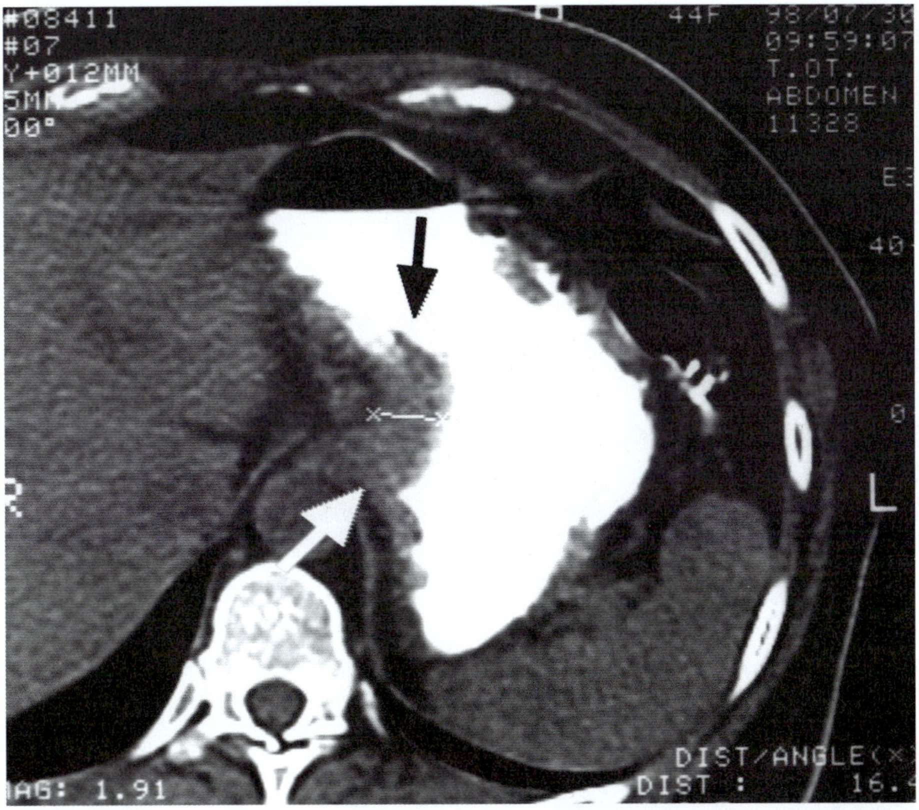

◀ Fig. 122 e.

▼ Fig. 122 f.

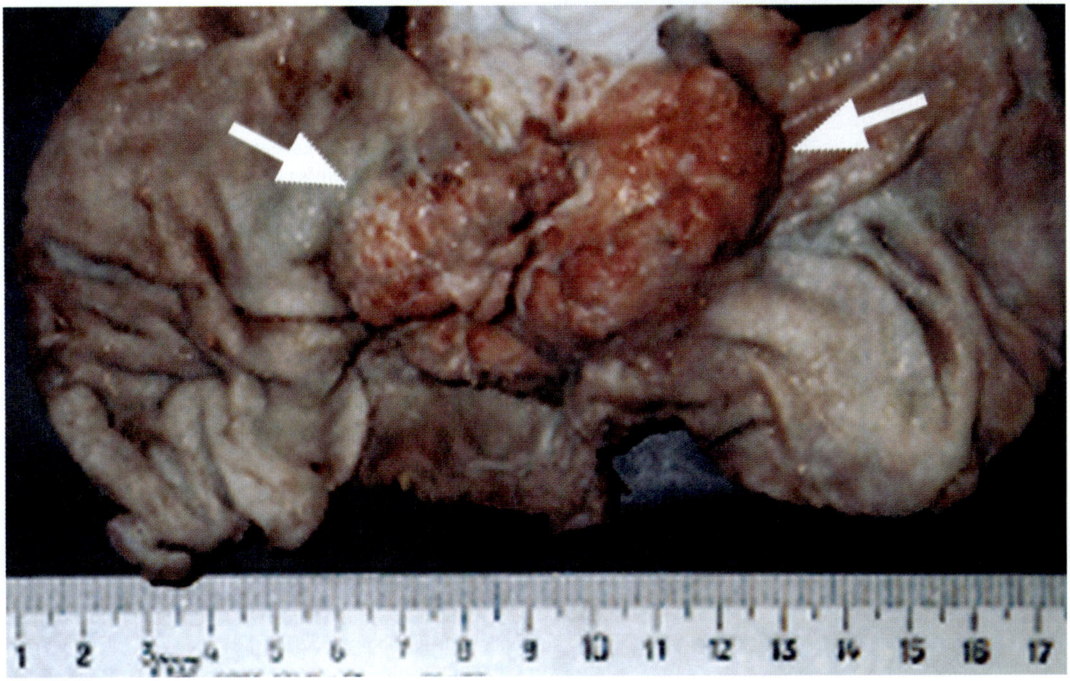

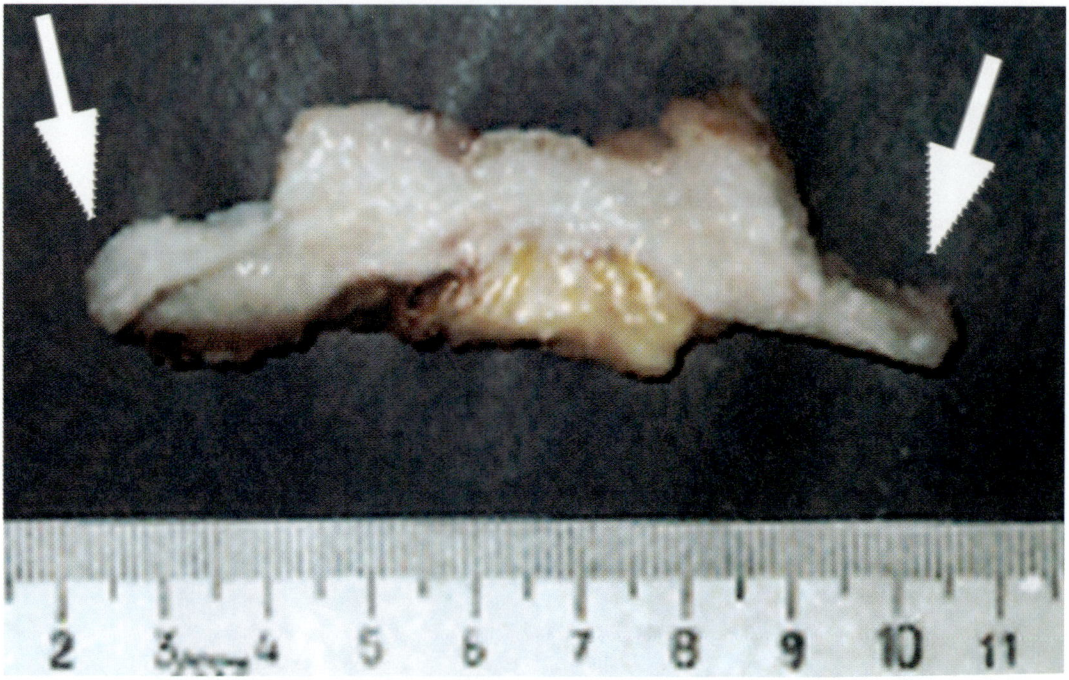

▲ **Fig. 122 g.**

▼ **Fig. 123 a.**

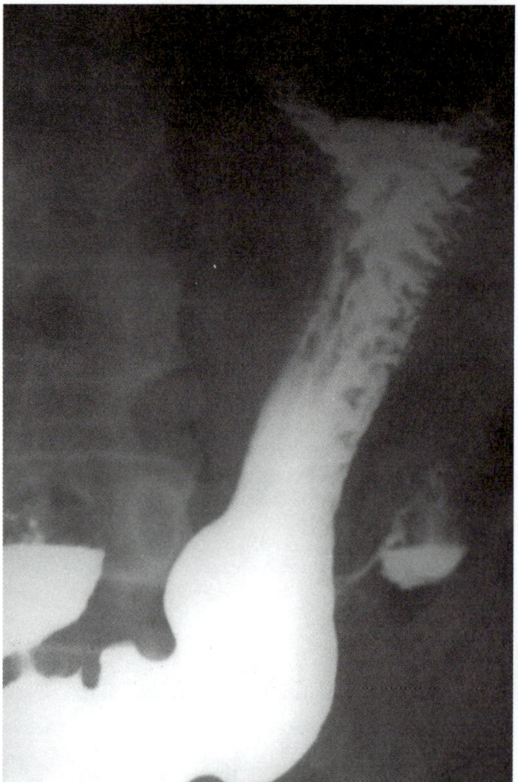

Fig. 123 a, b. Patient S., age 38. Diagnosis: gastric cancer. **a** Stomach roentgenogram (tight filling, vertical position, anterior projection): organic changes are not detected. **b** Stomach roentgenogram (double contrast, horizontal position, left posterior oblique projection): stomach contour depressed on the anterior wall of upper part of the stomach, the wall at this level is rigid, the folds terminate near the infiltration (arrows). Conclusion: Infiltrative cancer of the anterior wall of the upper part of the stomach. The patient was operated. Histologically, non-differentiated cancer.

Fig. 124 a–e. Female patient A., age 70. Diagnosis: gastric cancer. **a** Stomach roentgenogram (tight filling, vertical position, anterior projection): walls of the subcardiac part are thickened due to intramural infiltration (arrows). **b** Roentgenogram of the stomach and the lower third of the esophagus (tight filling, vertical position, anterior projection) at the moment of contrast medium passage through the gastroesophageal junction: uneven narrowing of the abdominal segment of the esophagus, its contours are uneven (arrow). **c, d** Stomach roentgenograms (double contrast, horizontal position, left lateral projection): atypical relief of the cardiac rosette (white arrows), anterior wall is thickened due to intramural infiltration (black arrows). **e** Roentgenogram of the stomach and the lower third of the esophagus (double contrast, horizontal position, left lateral projection) at the moment of contrast medium passage through the gastroesophageal junction: abdominal segment of the esophagus is unevenly narrowed, its contour uneven and eroded (arrow). Conclusion: Infiltrative cancer of the upper part of the stomach with invasion of the esophagus. The patient was operated. Histologically, adenocarcinoma with the signet-ring cell component.

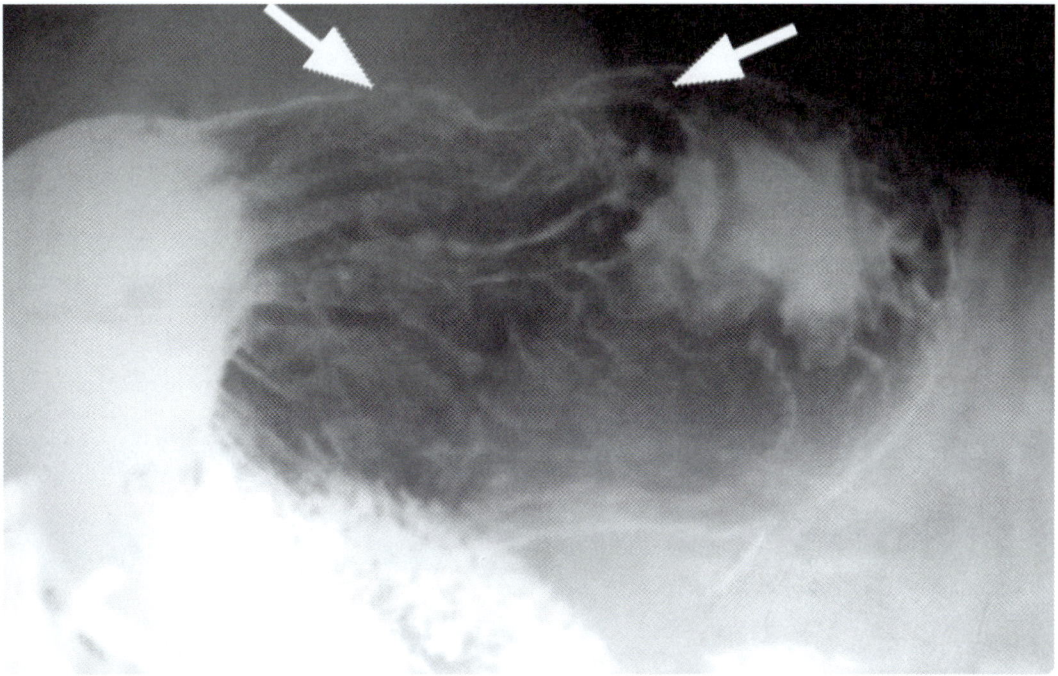

▲ **Fig. 123 b.**

▼ **Fig. 124 a.**

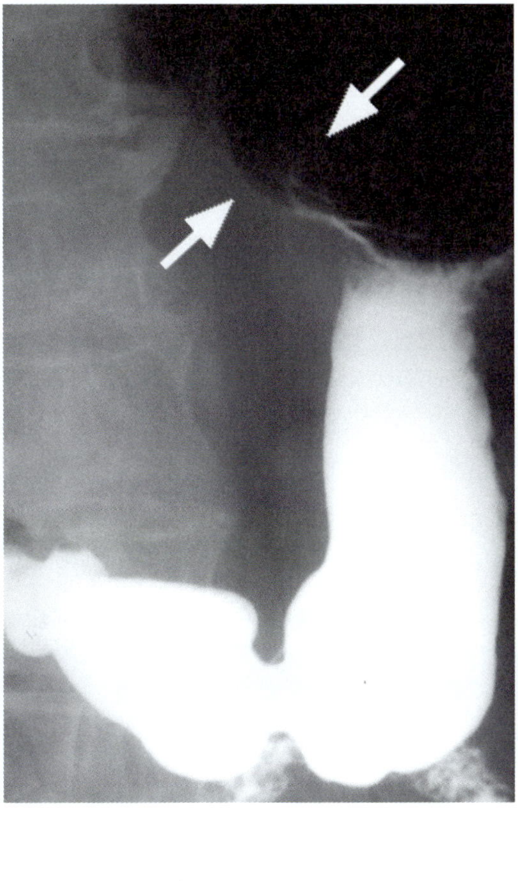

▼ **Fig. 124 b.**

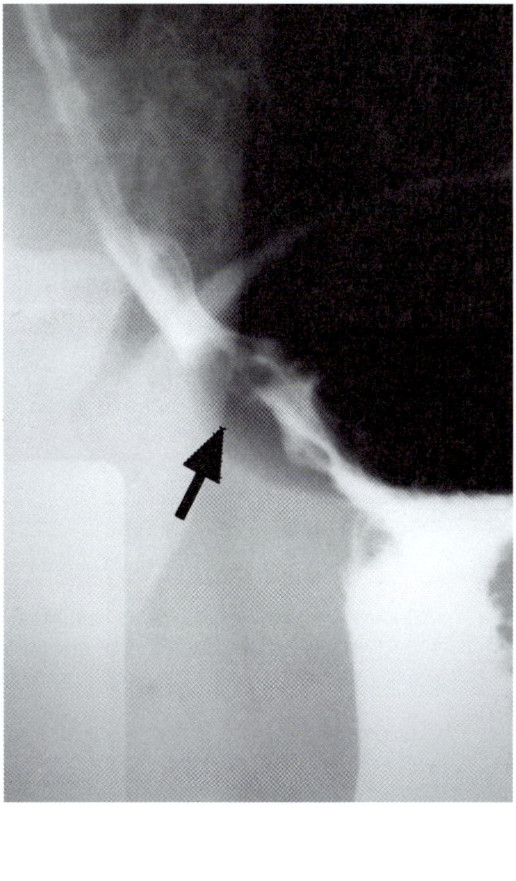

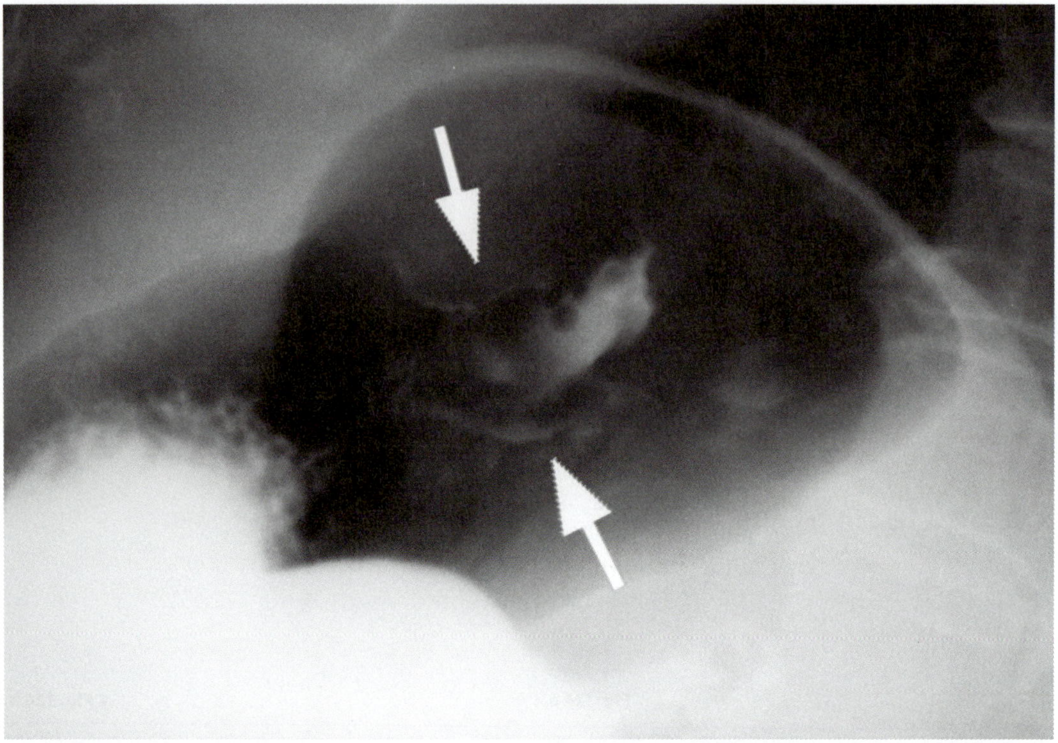

▲ Fig. 124 c.

▼ Fig. 124 d.

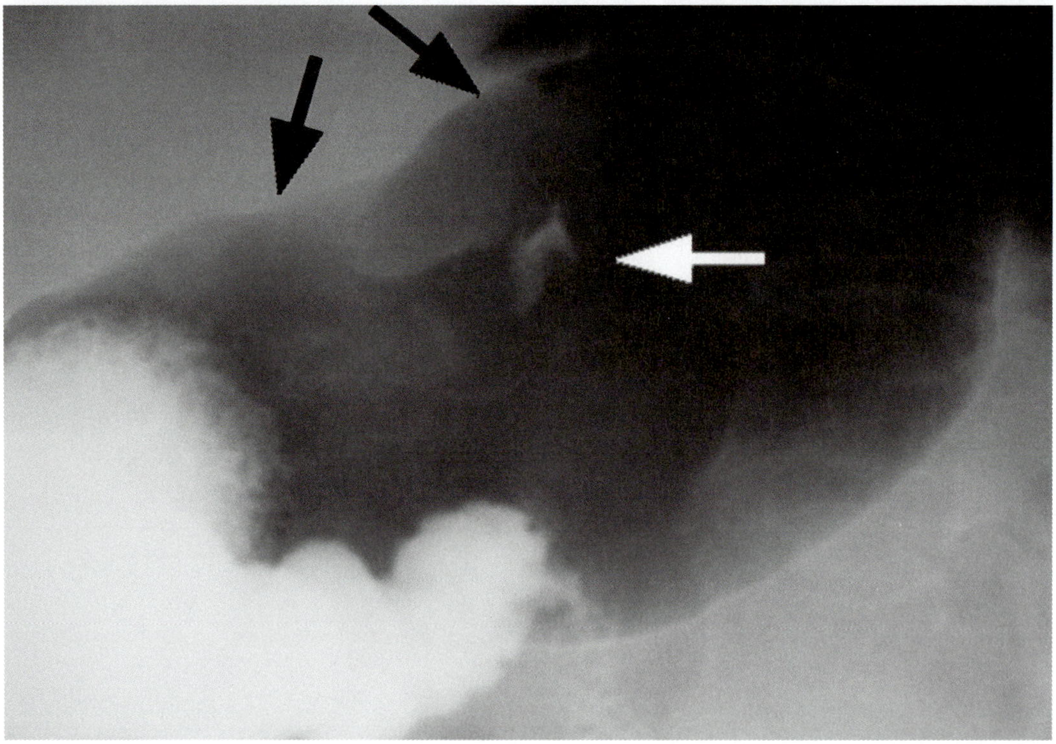

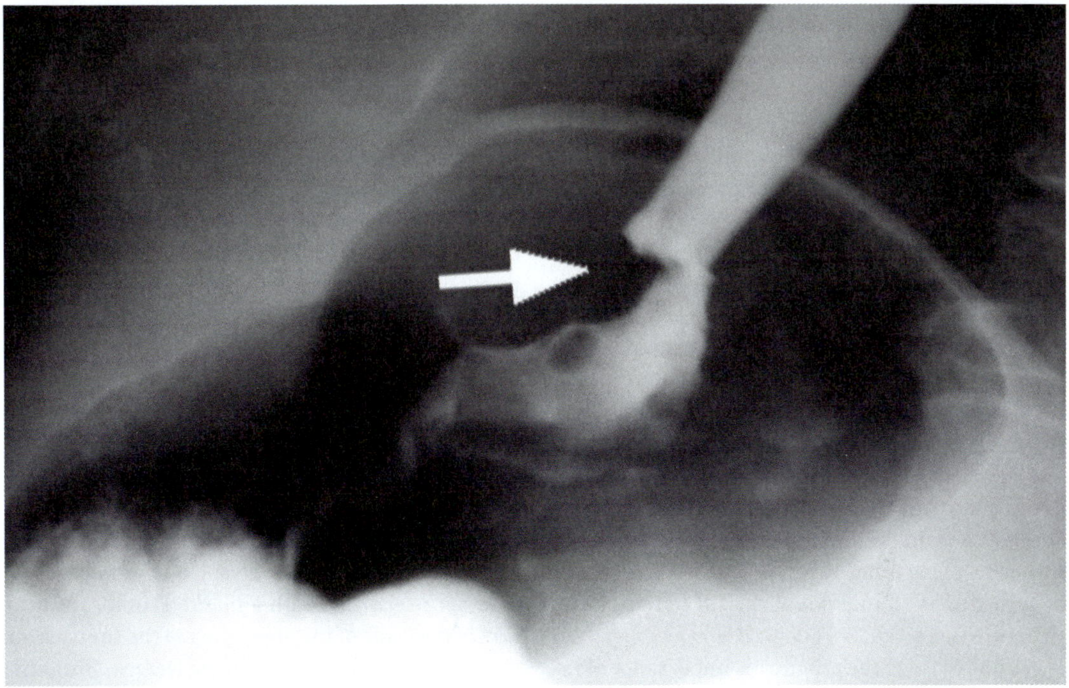

▲ **Fig. 124 e.**

M. Mori, Y. Adachi, and K. Nakamura et al. (1987) report that early cancers of the upper part of the stomach account for only 1% among similar tumors in other localizations (◘ Fig. 123). Sometimes, proximal cancer is diagnosed in cases where more than two walls of the upper part of the stomach are involved e.g., posterior wall and cardia; fundus and cardia; greater curvature and cardia; anterior wall and cardia (◘ Fig. 124). Affection of only one wall is revealed in comparatively rare cases, this usually being the anterior wall of the upper part of the stomach. The reasons for this disappointing result are found in the absence of clinical signs in the early stages of the process and in the complicated anatomical structure of this region, the visualization of which requires special approaches. The main problem is the presence of the so-called blind zones for both traditional X-ray examination and endoscopy. In other words, cancer of the upper part of the stomach may run an asymptomatic course for a long time. Known clinical, radiological and endoscopic signs are sometimes insufficient to establish the diagnosis of cancer at the stage when adequate treatment may cure the patient.

Another specific feature is the anatomic-functional formation known as the cardioesophageal rosette (junction). Its normal functional and anatomical structure is characterized by the convergence of esophageal folds straight into the cardiac folds. For this reason, owing to the only slightly marked submucous coat of the interfold space, the folds remain impregnated with barium sulfate suspension in adequately performed double-contrast radiology. Their imaging differs depending on individual variations, as was described in ► Chap. 5.

We meet with certain difficulties while conducting a differential diagnosis of the early signs of cancer of the cardia and rosette imaging. The difficulties are especially serious in the absence of sufficient clinical gastroesophageal symptoms. These difficulties are even more aggravated in endoscopic evaluation of the early manifestation of the tumor, again because of the close vicinity of the cardioesophageal junction and meager signs of tumor on the surface of the gastric mucosa. In such situations we are assisted by CT or MRI of the stomach. These methods give us additional information on the limited thickening of the wall, and at this level we are looking for the signs characteristic of the initial changes in the esophagus. This, after all, helps us to verify the diagnosis (see ▸ Fig. 83). Unfortunately, in the absence of these techniques, we have to resort to dynamic observation of the patient using traditional roentgenology and endoscopy. Our experience shows that after several months, sometimes after a year, endoscopy and biopsy confirm our initial diagnosis, and the patient can undergo surgery. But in some cases, this turns out to be »normal« imaging of the cardioesophageal junction. On the one hand, such cases serve to confirm the need to abandon the existing concept that only histological verification is an indication for surgery. In the absence of information supplied by CT and MRI, which confirm pathology in such patients, we are guided by the dynamic observations. In the absence of signs of tumor for a sufficiently long time (up to a year), this picture may be regarded as an individual variant of the rosette structure (see ▸ Fig. 50b) [35, 47, 226].

With regard to the prognostic importance of radiological and endoscopic signs, it is necessary to point out that most of the signs described are characteristic of advanced tumors. The affected cardia, which the classical roentgenologists compared to a rigid tube, a thickened infiltrated fundus, an additional shadow of the tumor against the background of the air bubble – all indicate cancer at a far advanced stage and the futility of attempts to help the patient. The signs of tumor spreading to the esophagus have the same significance.

Here it is necessary to discuss some specific properties of the neoplastic process at this localization. Retrospective analysis of the available clinical and X-ray signs of cancer of the upper part of the stomach shows that this cancer grows for a relatively long time without causing such discomfort to the patient that he seeks medical aid. Despite the large size of the tumor, the clinical picture (unmotivated weakness, low capacity for work, poor appetite, gastric discomfort, unexplained loss of weight, depression) may be so inconspicuous that only long-standing symptoms may cause the patient to visit his doctor. Again, dysphagia must be regarded as a late clinical symptom resulting from the spread of tumor infiltration to the abdominal segment of the esophagus. Some authors state that early dysphagia may develop owing to the concurrent esophageal spasm, but we have always found infiltration of the esophagus in patients with dysphagia, using radiological examination of the esophagus and the stomach (traditional X-ray plus double contrast, CT, MRI) in combination with endoscopy and biopsy. We observed dysphagia developing at various stages of the disease. The extent of affection and the severity of changes in the lower third of the esophagus and the upper part of the stomach did not always agree with the time of onset and severity of dysphagia. We have observed cases of proximal cancer of the stomach and invasion of the esophagus in which it was very difficult to establish the primary affection of the stomach and impossible to visualize the cardia endoscopically. The first symptoms of dysphagia appeared at least 1–1.5 months before endoscopic examination revealed a typical picture of cancer. The reverse was also possible: Dysphagia was absent altogether in patients with a marked tumor infiltration of the walls of the upper part of the stomach, or the first symptoms of dysphagia were so insignificant that it was possible to establish its onset only from anamnestic data going back several months before the patient complained. This means that analysis of clinical symptoms can suggest the initial location of the tumor in a particular upper portion of the stomach prior to surgery and morphological study of the resected material: In the former case, we have the tumor of the cardia with rapid involvement of the esophagus, and in the latter the tumor originated at a relatively long distance from the cardiac rosette (see ▸ Figs. 51 and 87). On this aspect, we agree with S. Kholdin (1952) and W. Sweet (1976), who indicated that cancer of the lower parts of the esophagus was closely connected with blastomatous infiltration of the stomach wall. The prevalence of tumors in the lower third of the esophagus is actually due to overlooking cancer of the cardia; isolated affection of the abdominal and other lower segments of the esophagus is a very rare occurrence. In other words, discovery of blastomatous affection of the lower third of the esophagus must lead the radiological diagnostician and endoscopist to perform a thorough examination of the stomach despite the difficulties arising from severely impaired patency. In our opinion, the pressing task of current radiological diagnosis consists not in simply detecting the signs characteristic of affection of the cardioesophageal junction and abdominal segment of the esophagus (»elongation« of the esophagus, splashing of the barium sulfate suspension, wall thickening, etc.); these signs may be specific but they have no positive prognostic potential. Rather, it consists in revealing signs of the presence of operable new growths, which might be a valuable supplement to endoscopic findings. Although endoscopy with lateral lenses is very effective, inspection of this part of the stomach remains difficult. The X-ray examination also meets with some insoluble problems. This points up how serious the problem is. It is especially difficult to reveal pathology in patients with so-called cascade stomach. This is often the result of cancer of the posterior wall of the upper third of the stomach body and the cardia, or of a tumor, the size of which does not exceed that of the cardiac zone. Detection of such new growths requires the entire available set of X-ray methods, including double contrast in addition to tight filling.

Concerning blastomatous affection of the upper part of the stomach, it is necessary to note the possible diagnostic use of the air bubble, which is always present in the stomach. We mean the so-called symptom of air redistribution or an elongated air bubble. Epstein and Wasch (1944) were the first to indicate that the changed shapes of the air bubble in the stomach might be used for diagnostic purposes. However, we do not think that this phenomenon can be regarded as pathognomonic for endophytic cancer of the stomach, because this also occurs during the cicatrization of large benign ulcers owing to the formation of fibrous tissue. Air can also be redistributed in the stomach under pressure exerted on it from various formations and space-occupying processes (enlarged left lobe of the liver, cyst, tumor extending from the neighboring organ, and the like). Despite the low specificity of this sign, its presence discovered during examination of the patient with gastric symptoms narrows down the range of pathologies which might be considered in the given case. The sign is simple. to detect. It is necessary only to examine the abdominal cavity attentively before the patient ingests barium sulfate suspension and to evaluate the suspected part of the stomach with orientation to the obligatory presence of the air bubble under the left arch of the diaphragm. In contrast to its normal position in the stomach fundus, the air bubble in such situations has a »tail« in the stomach body, and the amount of air is much greater than that in the normal air bubble.

Other signs of pathology of the upper parts of the stomach manifested by changes in the air bubble, which are of secondary importance as regards their prognostic value, are an additional shadow, which is characteristic of exophytic new growths, and also a significantly increased stomach–diaphragm distance due to tumor infiltration in the stomach fundus, which is not displaced during deep breathing due to its growth into the adjacent organs. The air redistribution sign is of greater importance than the described changes because it occurs in patients with relatively small and operable carcinomas.

▼ **Fig. 128 a.**

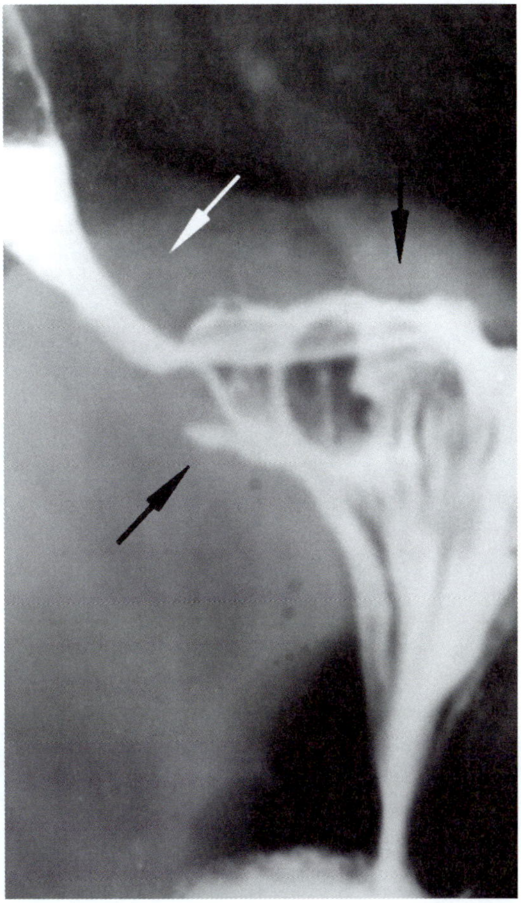

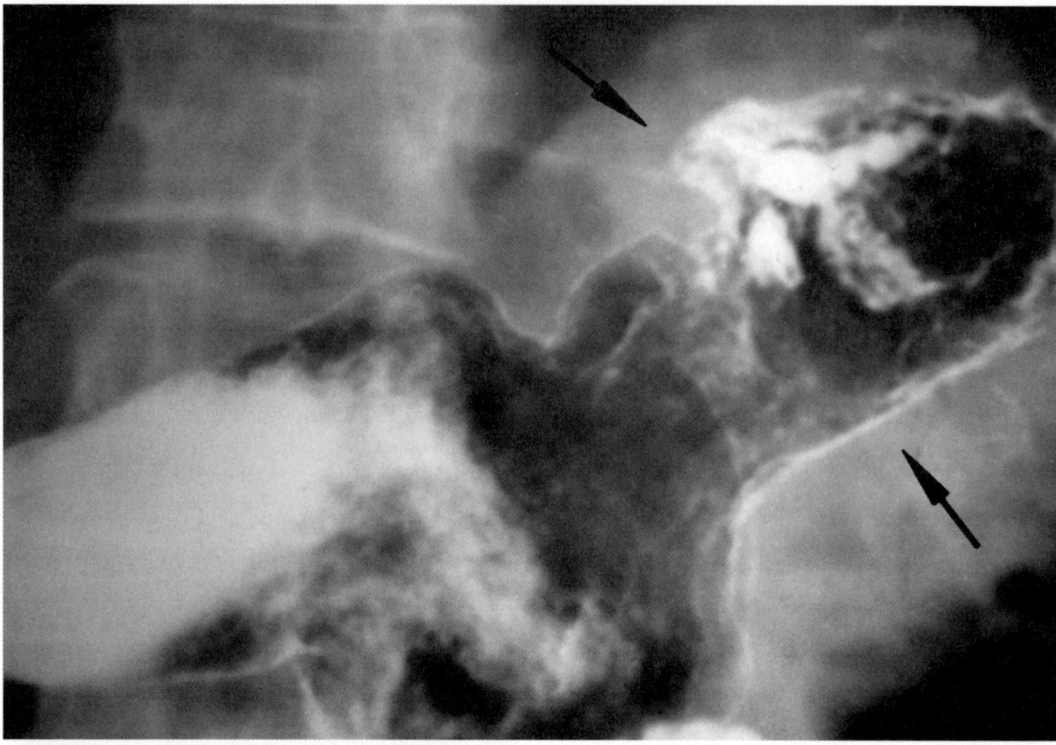

▲ **Fig. 128 b.**

▼ **Fig. 128 c.**

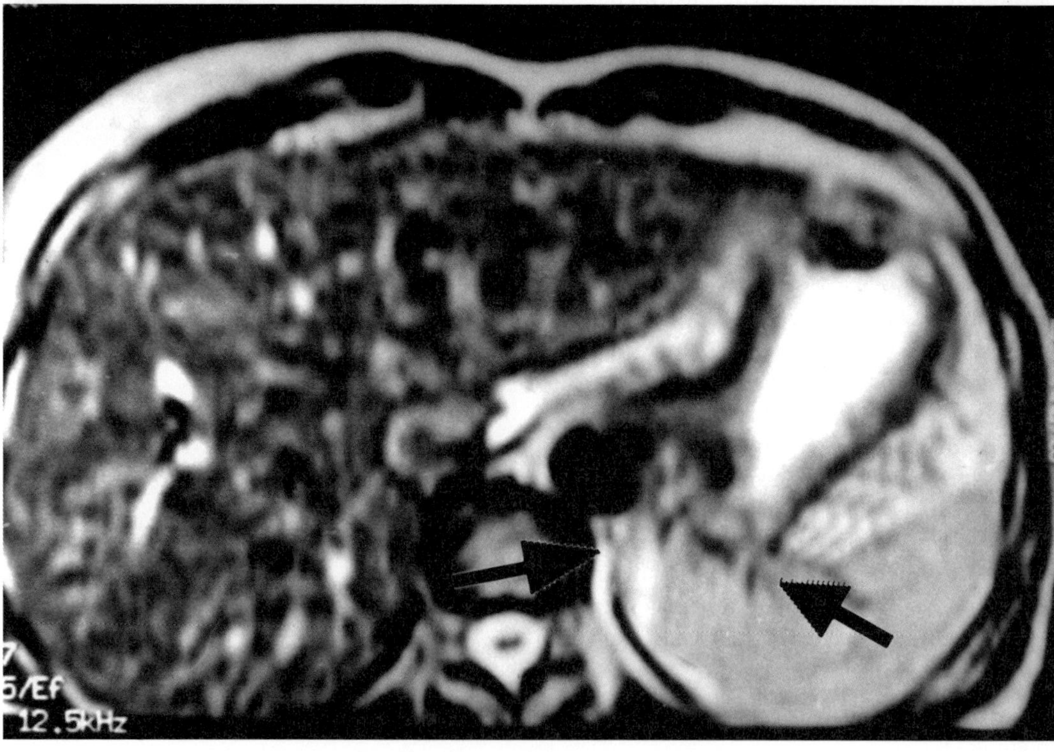

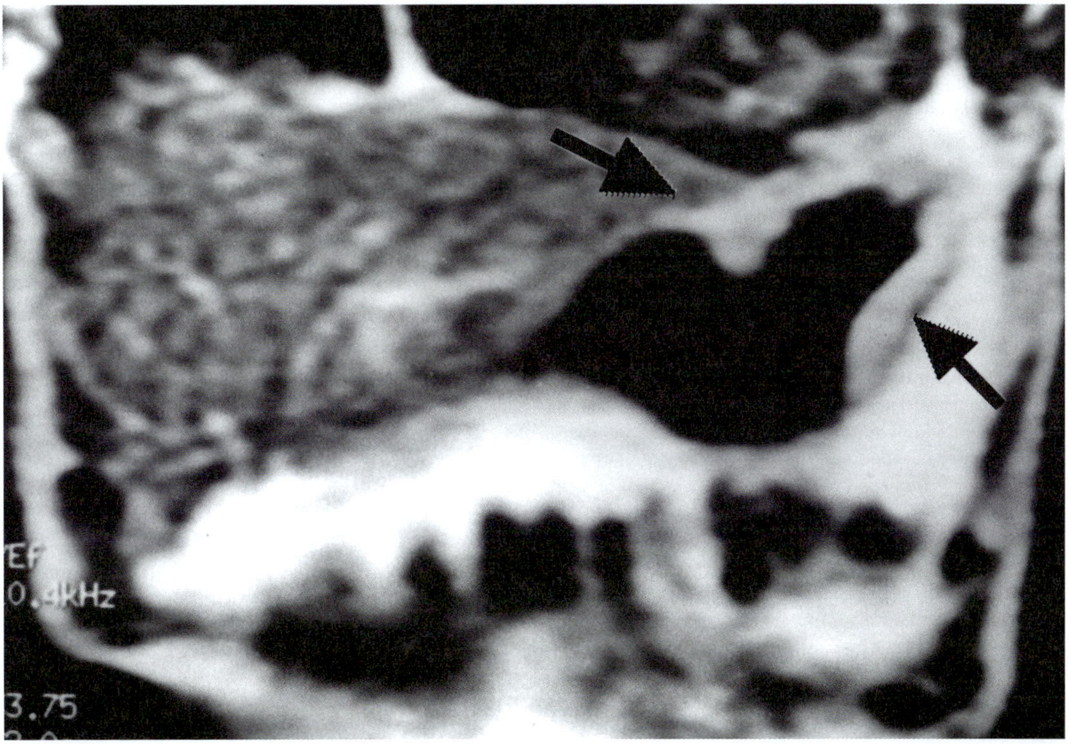

▲ **Fig. 128 d.**

▼ **Fig. 128 e.**

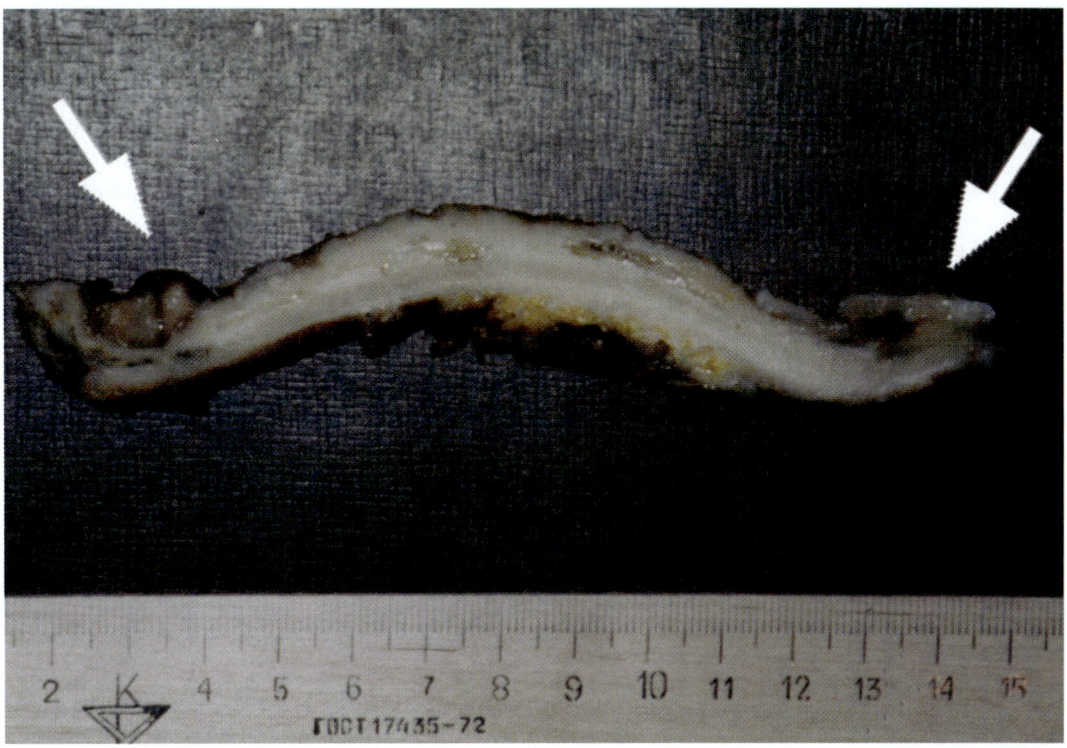

Fig. 128 a–e. Female patient V., age 53. Diagnosis: gastric cancer. **a** Stomach roentgenogram (tight filling, vertical position, anterior projection): contour of the cardiac part and the fundus is uneven (black arrows), the abdominal segment of the esophagus is circularly narrowed, with a small suprastenotic dilatation (white arrow). **b** Stomach roentgenogram (double contrast, horizontal position, left posterior oblique projection): walls of the upper part are thickened and rigid due to intramural infiltration (arrows). Conclusion: Infiltrative cancer of the upper part of the stomach with invasion of the esophagus. In order to verify the infiltration spread, the patient was examined by MRI. **c** MRI (axial projection, level of upper part of the stomach, T2 image): walls of the fundus are thickened unevenly due to intramural infiltration. Infiltration spreads onto the abdominal segment of the esophagus with strongly narrowed lumen, and also onto the left crus of the diaphragm and the medial edge of the spleen (arrows). **d** MRI (coronary projection, level of upper part of the stomach, T2 image): uneven thickening of the fundus walls with infiltration spread to the upper two thirds of the stomach body (arrows). Conclusion: Infiltrative cancer of the body and the upper part of the stomach with invasion of the abdominal segment of the esophagus, the left crus of the diaphragm, and the medial edge of the spleen. **e** Fragment of a macrospecimen (strip): the wall of the stomach is thickened due to intramural infiltration of white color (arrows). Histologically, signet-ring cell carcinoma.

Fig. 129 a–c. Patient V., age 43. Diagnosis: cancer of the lower third of the esophagus with invasion of the cardiac part of the stomach. Complaints of dysphagia, vomiting after meals, which continued for 3 months. Weight loss, 10 kg. **a** Roentgenograms of lower third of the esophagus (tight filling, vertical position, anterior projection) at the moment of contrast medium passage through the gastroesophageal junction: the lower third of the esophagus is unevenly circularly narrowed; uneven contours. A depot of contrast medium in the supradiaphragmatic segment (arrow). **b** Roentgenogram of lower third of the esophagus (tight filling, vertical position, left lateral projection) at the moment of contrast medium passage through the gastroesophageal junction: an ulcer niche with eroded contours on the anterior wall of the supradiaphragmatic segment of the esophagus (arrow), atypical relief of the cardioesophageal junction. **c** Roentgenogram of upper part of the stomach (double contrast, vertical position, anterior projection): thickened wall of the cardia due to tumor infiltration is seen against the background of the air bubble with the stretched folds of the proximal part of the stomach (arrow). Conclusion: Infiltrative cancer of the cardiac part of the stomach with involvement of the esophagus. Ulceration of the anterior wall of the supradiaphragmatic segment of the esophagus. The patient was operated. Histologically, squamous cell cancer. Such cases are relatively rare. As a rule, cancer occurs in the stomach with subsequent spread to the esophagus. Nevertheless, traditional X-ray examination with double contrast reveals affection of the cardiac part of the stomach. This is another confirmation of our point of view that radiological methods of examination should be used again in gastroenterology.

Double-contrast radiology has the greatest potential in the traditional X-ray examination of the upper parts of the stomach. Only this method can demonstrate wall thickening and loss of elasticity at the initial stages of the malignant process. Thick and rough folds add to the double-contrast imaging, and this suggests malignancy. At the same time, it should be noted in this connection that it is possible to study contours of the upper part of the stomach using some manipulations such as changing the patient's position from vertical to tilted, or from horizontal to vertical, which helps to estimate the condition of the walls in cascade stomach.

During recent decades, there has been a distinct tendency toward an increasing occurrence of tumors in the upper part of the stomach. This is the point of particular concern to specialists, because cardioesophageal cancer has the worst prognosis when compared with tumors of all other localizations (Fig. 128).

It has become commonplace that when discussing new growths in this localization we usually mean advanced cases. The main reason for oncological neglect is that the patients present late for medical attention, i.e., they do not visit the doctor until the dysphagia dominates the clinical picture, indicating the spread of the process onto the esophagus. The difficulty of diagnosing proximal cancer is due (in addition to the late clinical manifestations) to the fact that the prevalence of endophytic forms over exophytic forms is not taken into consideration. The radiological semiotics of cancer of the upper part of the stomach continues to be based on the old signs of exophytic new growth (additional shadow, splashing of barium sulfate suspension, etc.).

Another problem has become the subject of special concern for gastroenterologists in recent years. This is the so-called specialized columnar epithelium, or Barrett's esophagus (Barrett epithelium; the lower part of the esophagus is lined with cylindrical epithelium; gastrointestinal metaplasia). Barrett's esophagus is an acquired disease in which squamous epithelium of the esophagus is replaced by cylindrical epithelium, owing to the prolonged attack on the mucous membrane by gastric contents; it is regarded as a complication of gastroesophageal reflux alongside with ulcers and peptic strictures of the esophagus. The British surgeon

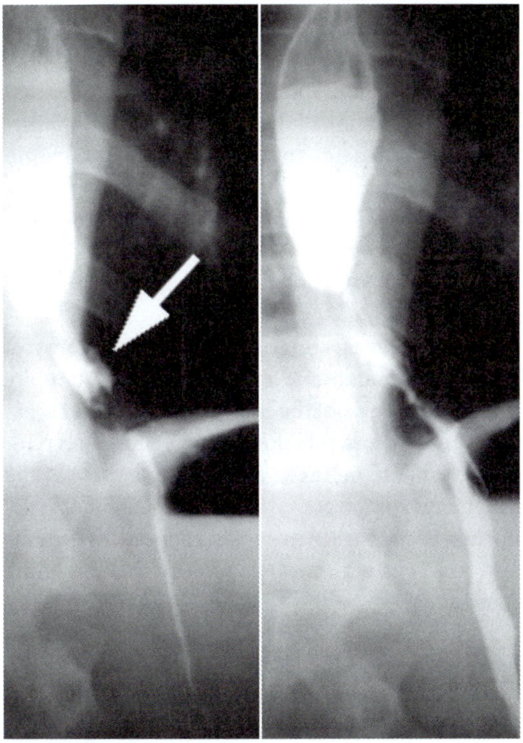

▲ **Fig. 129 a.**

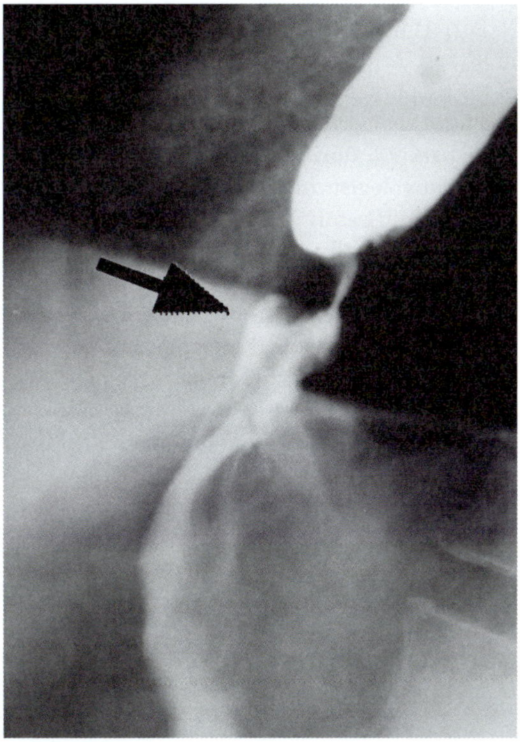

▲ **Fig. 129 b.**

▼ **Fig. 129 c.**

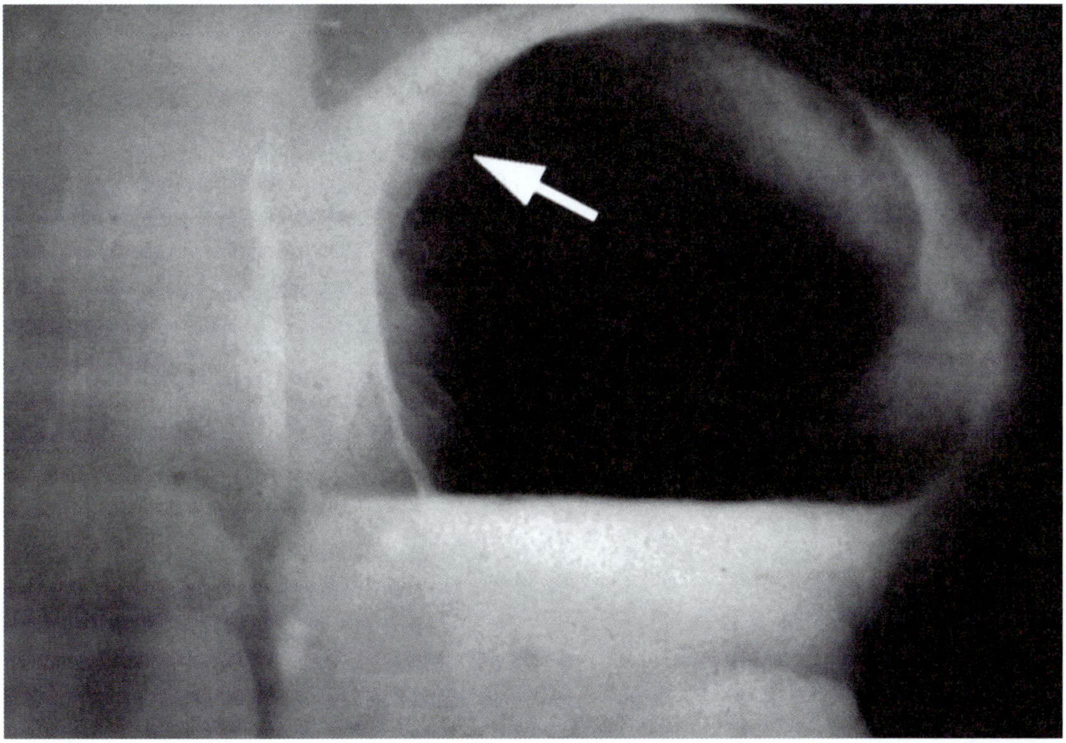

N. Barrett was the first to describe the syndrome in 1950; it includes hernia of the esophageal hilus of the diaphragm, peptic ulcer of the esophagus, and focal changes in the mucous membrane of its distal part [93]. During recent years, the interest of gastroenterologists in Barrett's esophagus has increased significantly. This is explained by the epidemic spread of this pathology worldwide (beginning in the 1980s) and by the considerably increasing occurrence of proximal cancer of the stomach. Gastrointestinal metaplasia is regarded by the gastroenterological community as a precancerous condition, because the incidence of adenocarcinoma in such patients is 30 times higher than in the population as a whole.

Histological examination of columnar epithelium, which results from metaplasia and replaces multi-layered squamous epithelium, differentiates between the following three types of cells in accordance with Barrett's classification:

1. Fundal
2. Cardiac or transitional
3. Specialized intestinal

7

Columnar epithelium of the stomach is practically identical to epithelium of the fundus and the cardia, whereas the specialized cylindrical epithelium has the properties of gastric and intestinal epithelium: The cells have cilia on their surfaces and crypts containing mucus-forming goblet-shaped, and entero-endocrine cells. Combinations of various forms of metaplasia of the esophageal epithelium are also possible, but the absorbing capacity of these cells is insufficient, as distinct from true enterocytes. Therefore, intestinal-type metaplasia is regarded as incomplete. Esophageal metaplasia may extend to a distance of 3–15 cm from the line of transition of the gastric epithelium to the esophageal epithelium.

Endoscopically, the following two types of Barrett's esophagus are distinguished:

1. A short segment of the Barrett esophagus – metaplasia extends for less than 3 cm
2. A long segment of the Barrett esophagus – metaplasia extends for more than 3 cm

There are some factors predisposing to development of Barrett's esophagus. Thus, hernia of the esophageal hiatus of the diaphragm occurs in 75–80% cases, and dysfunction of the lower esophageal sphincter develops in 19–20% patients. There are no pathognomonic symptoms of Barrett's esophagus, and its clinical symptoms do not differ from those of the gastroesophageal reflux, but it should be noted that about 95% of patients experience heartburn.

At the present time, endoscopy with biopsy of the mucous membrane is commonly used for diagnostic purposes, but the endoscopic signs are sometimes meager and therefore, between four and 15 bioptates should be taken from various parts of the esophagus spaced at 1–2 cm. On esophagoscopy, the portion of cylindrical metaplasia appears hyperemic and contrasts with the pale pink epithelium of the esophagus.

Since patients with Barrett's esophagus are highly predisposed to adenocarcinoma, it is necessary to note again that roentgenology should be returned to the field of gastroenterology as soon as possible. The lower segments of the esophagus of patients with X-ray signs of reflux esophagitis will then be examined by the endoscopist more thoroughly. The necessary number of tissue specimens will be taken to facilitate the diagnosis of blastomatous processes at the earlier stages (◘ Fig. 129).

Thus, from the current standpoints of epidemiology and morphology of gastric cancer, tumors of the upper part of the stomach have become the pressing problem of gastro-oncology in the twenty-first century.

Cancer of the Antral and Pyloric Parts

Blastomatous affection of the distal part of the stomach occurs quite frequently. Although its incidence tends to decrease, it is necessary to note that this concerns only exophytic tumors and in a small number of countries, where to human health has a high priority. The most prevalent cancers are infiltrative tumors, the occurrence of which remains at about the same level (◘ Fig. 130).

Pyloric cancers are a special problem in the detection of distal tumors. They occur less frequently

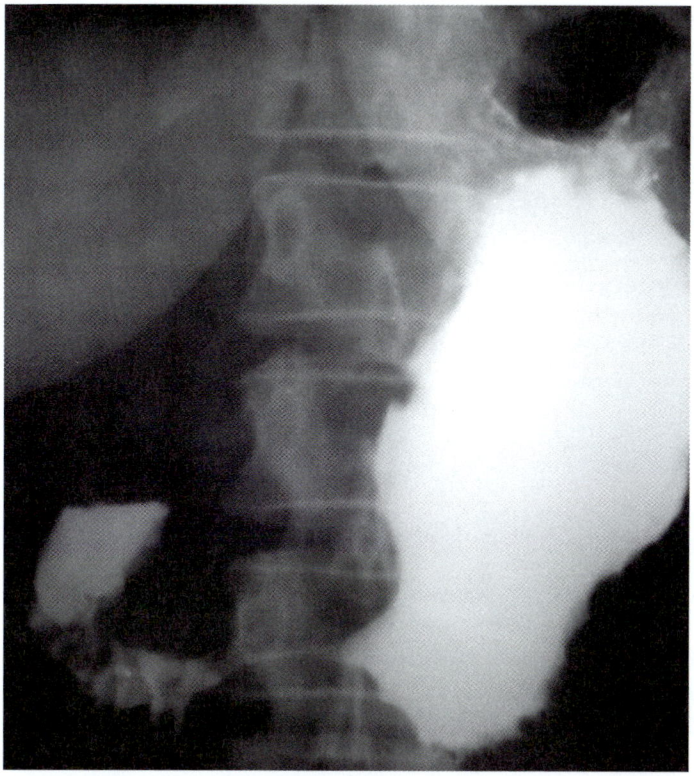

Fig. 130 a–c. Female patient U., age 62. Diagnosis: gastric cancer. **a** Stomach roentgenogram (tight filling, vertical position, anterior projection): cavity of the distal part is decreased, the distal part is disfigured (rigid tube), its contours are uneven, the walls are rigid. **b, c** Stomach roentgenograms (double contrast, horizontal position, anterior projection): circular infiltration of the distal part of the stomach, markedly rigid walls, thickened wall of the lesser and the greater curvatures of the stomach body due to infiltration spreading in the proximal direction (arrows). Conclusion: Infiltrative cancer of the distal part of the stomach with invasion of the stomach body. The patient was operated. Histologically, signet-ring cell carcinoma.

◂ **Fig. 130 a.**

▾ **Fig. 130 b.**

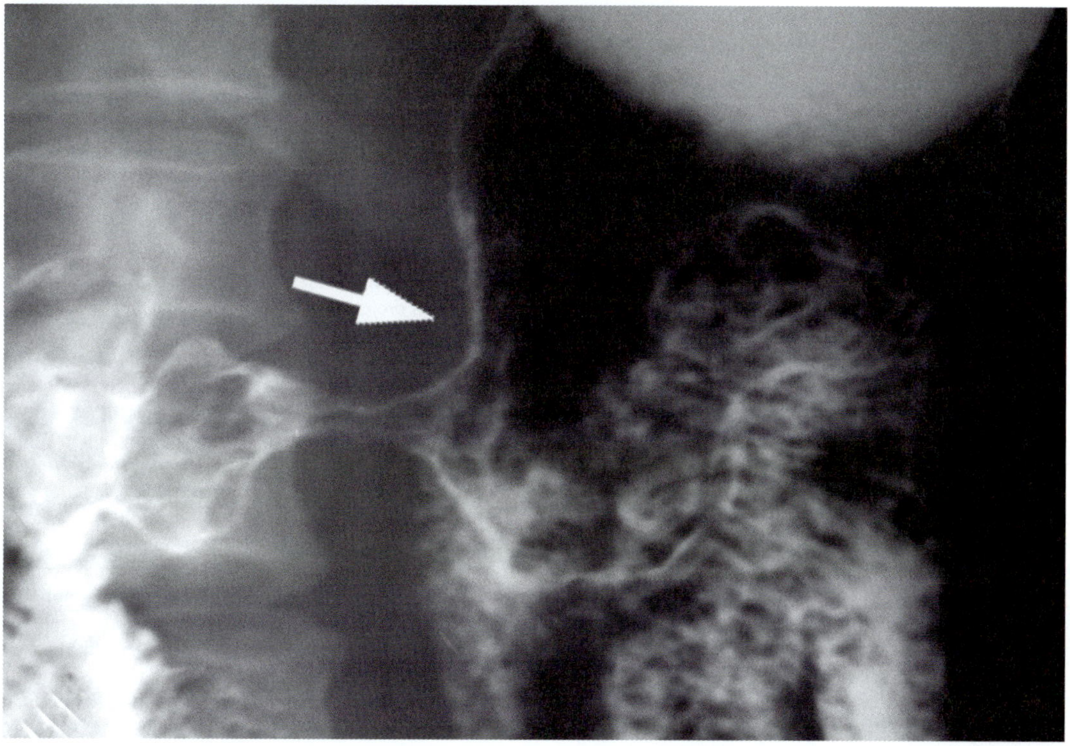

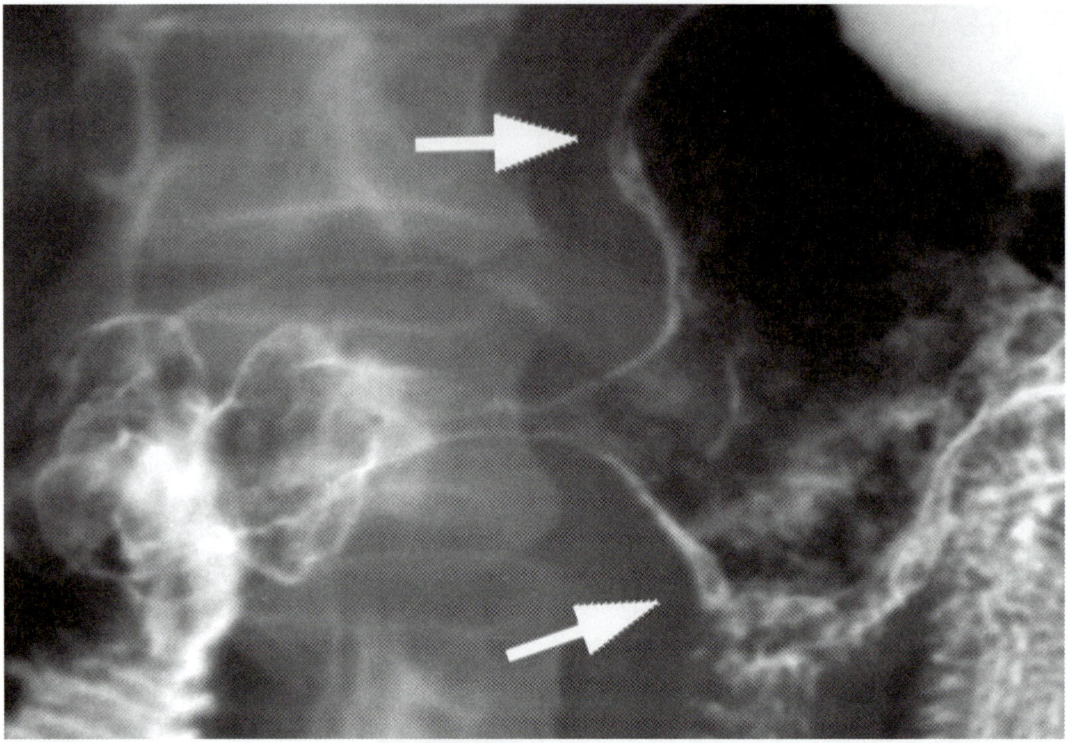

▲ **Fig. 130 c.**

▼ **Fig. 131 a.**

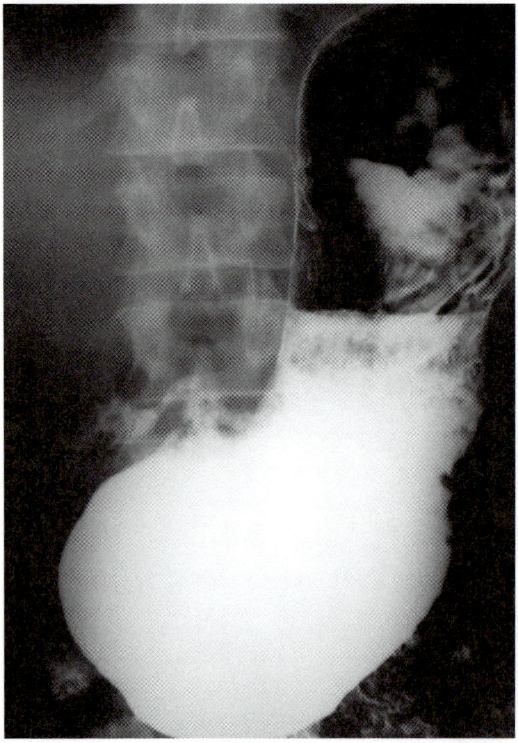

Fig. 131 a, b. Patient I., age 57. Diagnosis: gastric cancer. **a** Stomach roentgenogram (tight filling, vertical position, anterior projection): the pyloric part is narrowed, the lesser curvature of the distal part is very short, the sinus sags, the evacuating function of the pylorus is upset. **b** Stomach roentgenogram (double contrast, horizontal position, anterior projection): marked convergence of the folds in the direction of the thickened portion of the wall of the lesser curvature in the pyloric part (arrow). Conclusion: Infiltrative cancer of the pyloric part of the stomach. The patient was operated. Histologically, signet-ring cell carcinoma.

Fig. 132 a–e. Female patient G., age 63. Diagnosis: gastric cancer. **a** Stomach roentgenogram – (tight filling, vertical position, anterior projection): cavity of the distal part and the lower third of the stomach body is decreased, the lesser curvature is short and depressed, its contours and contours of the greater curvature are uneven (arrows). **b, c** Stomach roentgenograms (tight filling, vertical position, anterior projection): the cavity is diminished, evacuation is accelerated. Uneven contours, rigid walls, the angular notch straightened (arrow). **d** Stomach roentgenogram (double contrast, horizontal position, anterior projection): the walls of the distal part and the body of the stomach are thickened and rigid due to circular intramural infiltration. Conclusion: Infiltrative cancer of the distal part of the stomach with invasion of the stomach body. **e** Endophotograph: the stomach lumen is disfigured, narrowed, the mucous membrane is grayish pink, dull, with uneven surface, readily injured on contact, the folds in this region are completely smoothed down. Histological examination of the bioptates verified signet-ring cell carcinoma of the stomach.

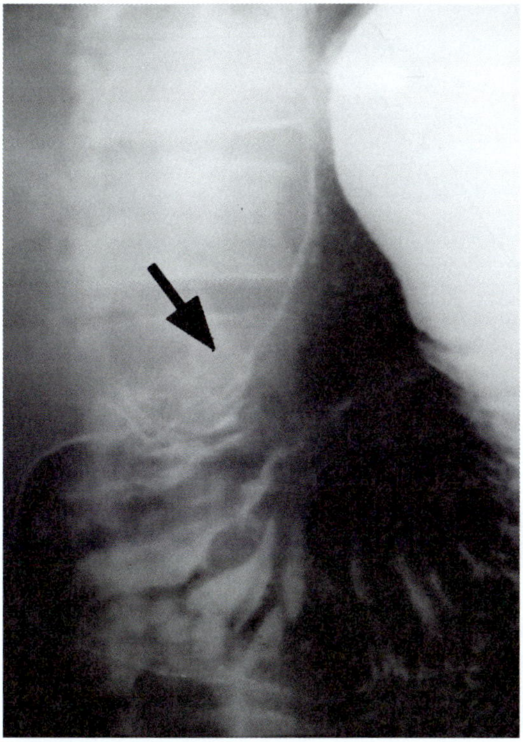

▲ **Fig. 131 b.**

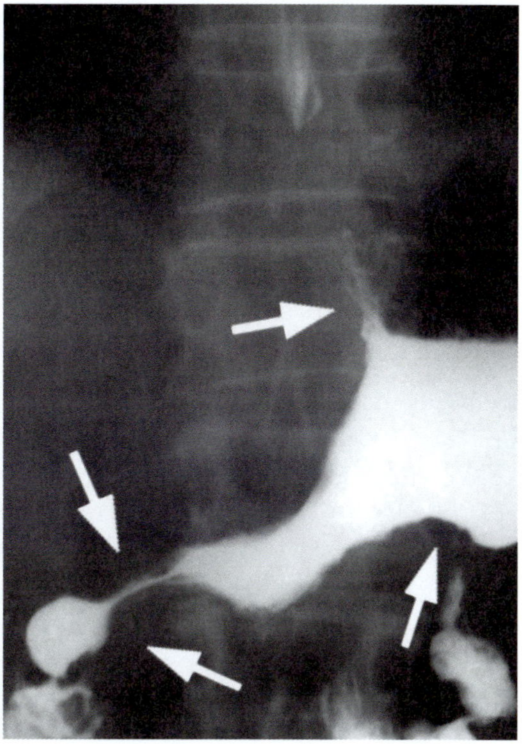

▲ **Fig. 132 a.**

▼ **Fig. 132 b.**

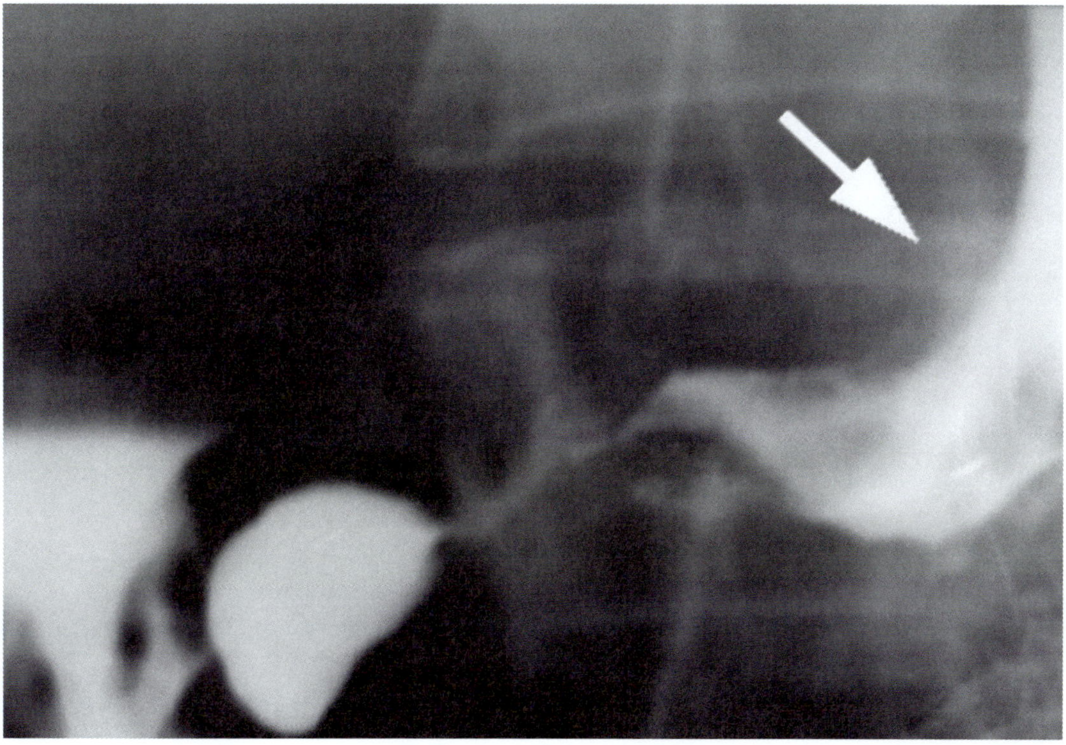

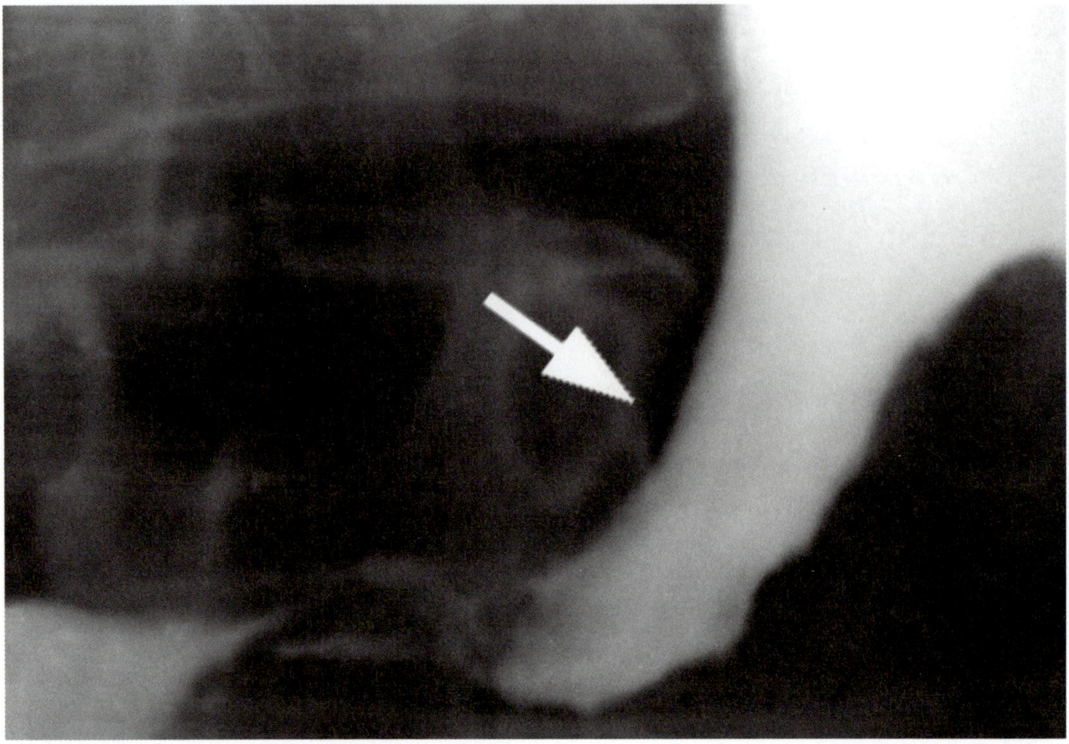

▲ Fig. 131 c.

▼ Fig. 132 d.

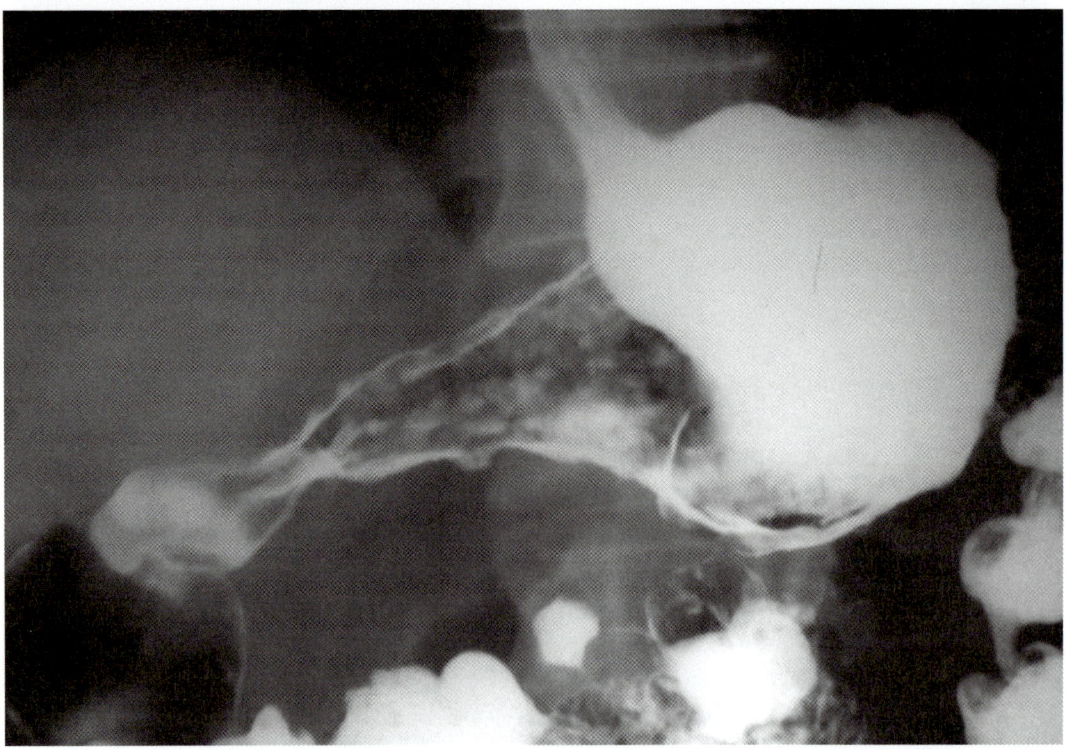

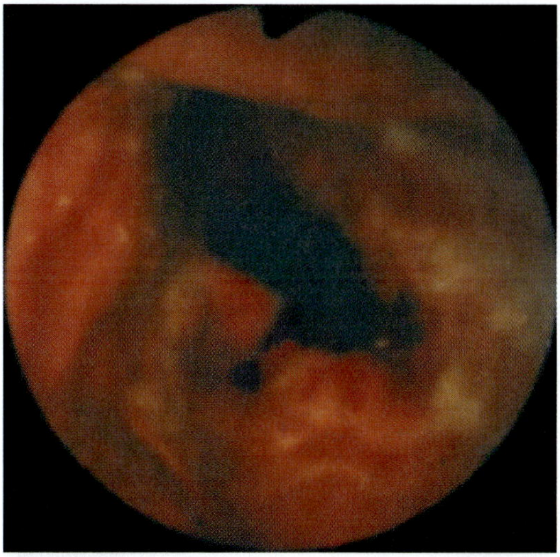

▲ **Fig. 132 e.**

than antral cancers. According to some authors, they account for 4–16% of all gastric carcinomas. Nevertheless, it would be reasonable to discuss them as one group because of their common clinical manifestations [185, 223]. Because of their location in the pylorus, even relatively small tumors manifest by obstructive symptoms at the early stages of their growth (■ Fig. 131). As distinct from stenosis, the pylorus may develop incompetence due to infiltration, and the patients experience constant hunger while losing weight (■ Fig. 132). Practical experience shows that early clinical symptoms induce the patient to seek medical aid, but X-ray and endoscopic examinations sometimes prove ineffective for timely detection of the tumor in this zone; the anatomy of the pylorus is the most difficult for radiological examination and endoscopy. In addition, distal cancers must be differentiated from stenoses of the pyloroduodenal region. The diagnosis of ulcerous stenosis with obliterated or indistinct clinical signs is often established in patients with this localization of cancer (■ Fig. 133). As the infiltrative forms of tumor growth predominate in this part, the diagnosis is even more difficult due to the specific anatomical and functional properties of this part of the stomach and the absence of marked symptoms of organic affection, interpreted in most situations to be the result of the inflammatory process. But patients often go to the doctor when their tumor is already easily palpable (■ Fig. 134) [42]. Conspicuous manifestations of pyloroduodenal pathologies resulted in rapid accumulation of clinical data, the importance of which is difficult to overestimate even today. As knowledge of the nature of obstruction of the pyloric part grew, two aspects emerged. First, the necessity of selecting the proper degree of operative intervention implies preoperative establishment of the cause and the spread of the pathological process (■ Fig. 135) [66]. Second, research into the role of cancers of the linitis plastica type influenced the present situation as regards identification of the nature of pyloric stenosis (■ Fig. 136). The basic concepts of this research remain unchanged today. In current publications we meet the same point of view on the onset of the primary focus of infiltration in the prepyloric part and on tumor spreading in the proximal direction. As regards ulcers of the pyloric part, most researchers agree that they are usually malignant [10].

▼ **Fig. 133 a.**

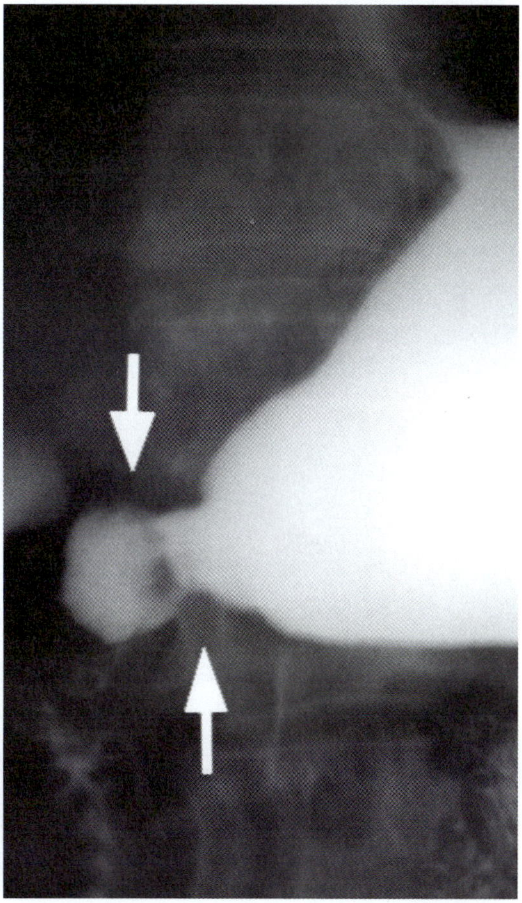

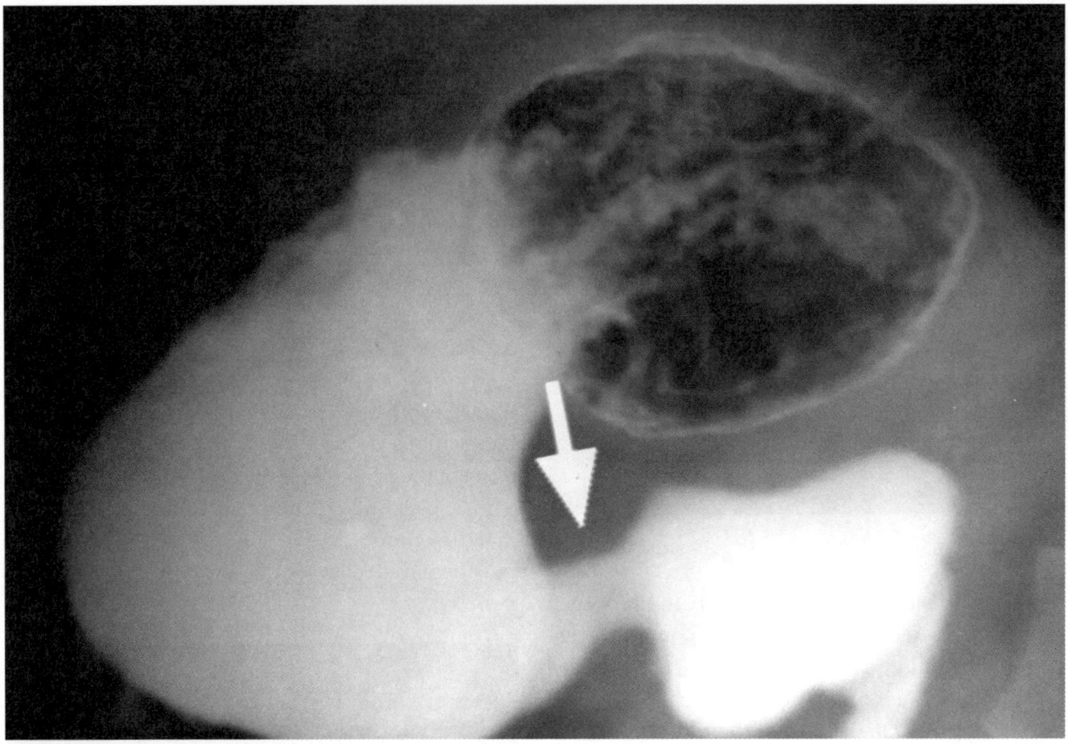

▲ Fig. 133 b.

▼ Fig. 133 c.

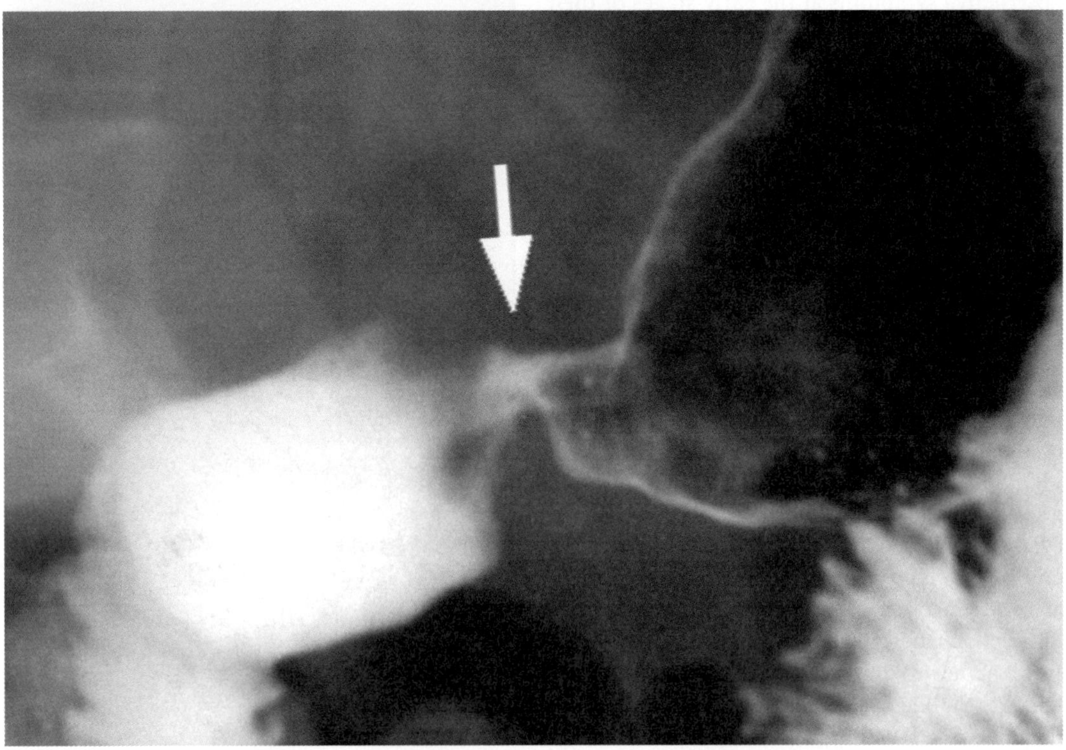

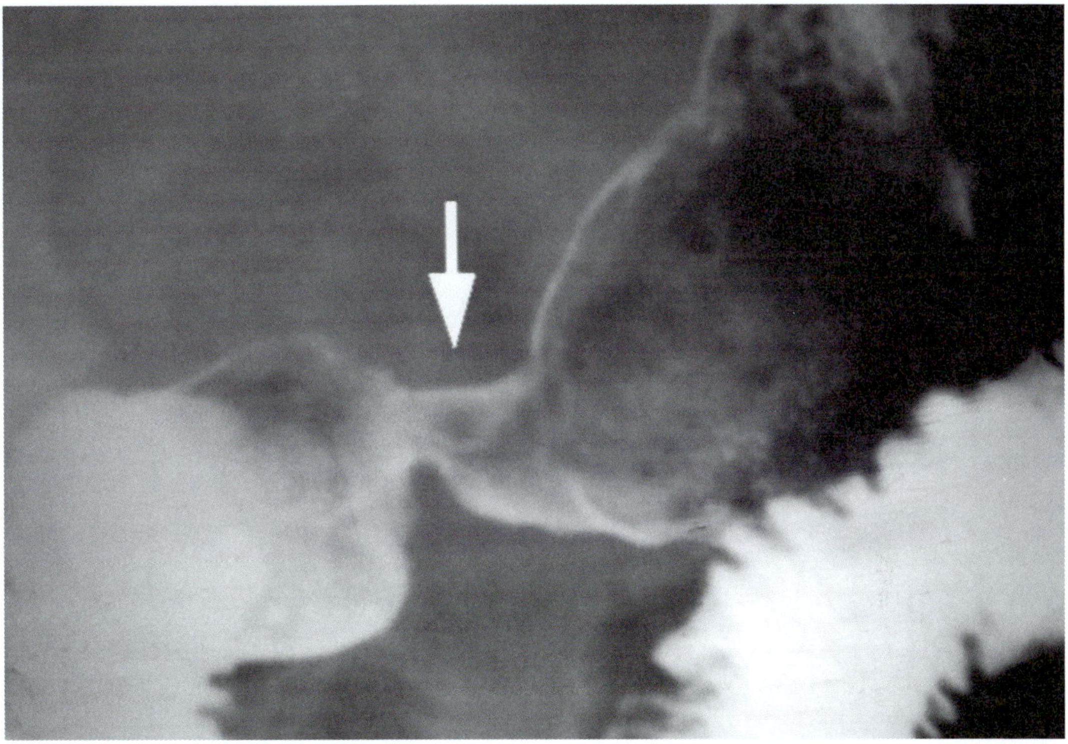

▲ Fig. 133 d.

▼ Fig. 133 e.

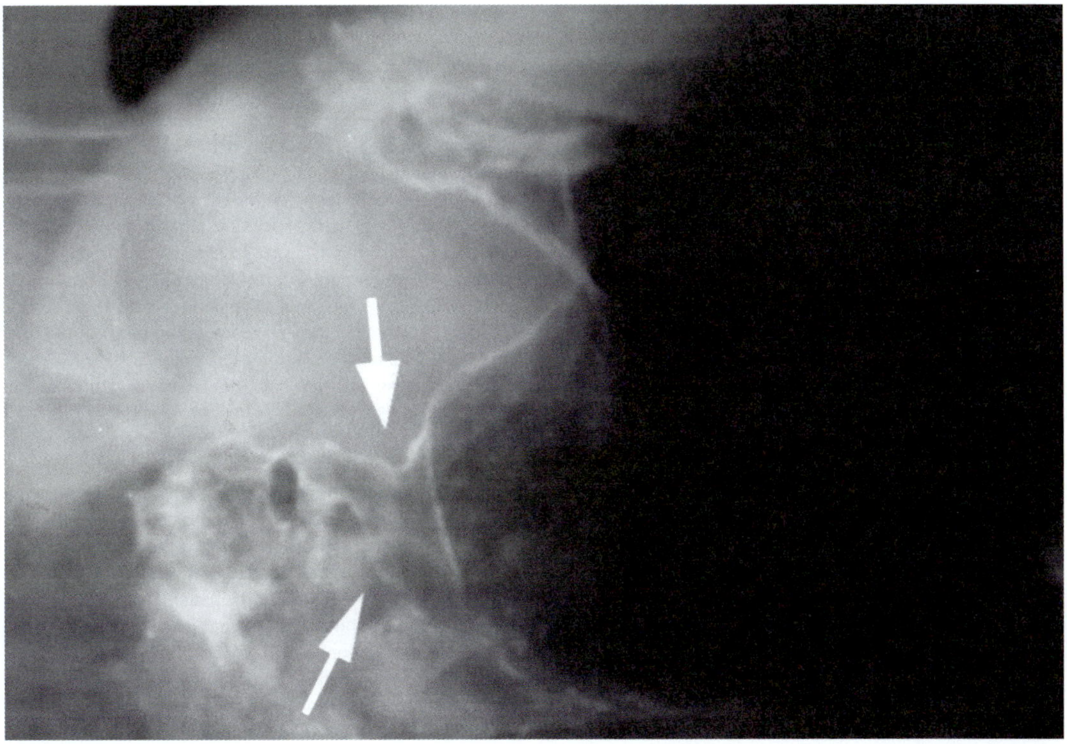

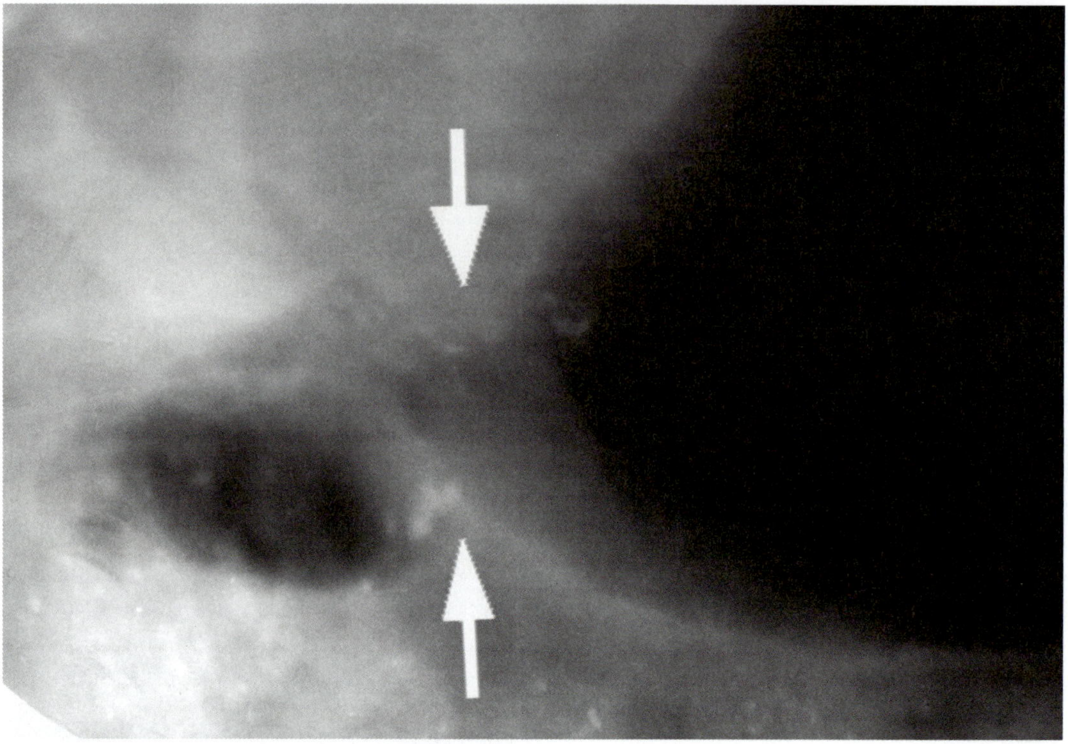

▲ Fig. 133 f.

▼ Fig. 134 a.

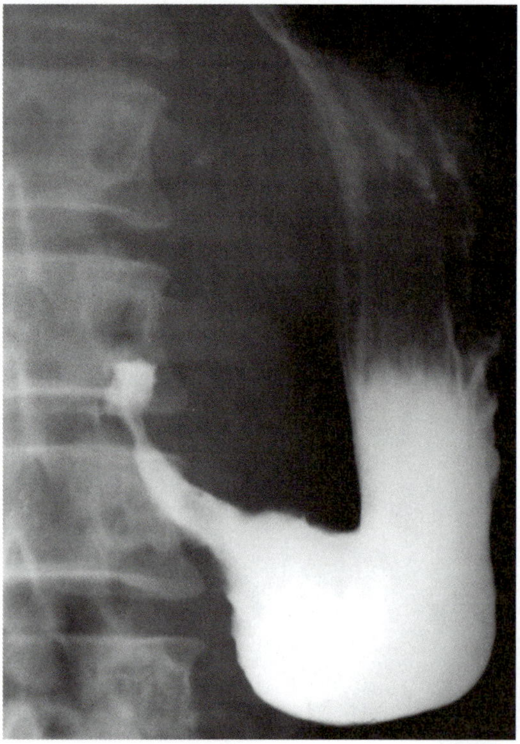

Fig. 133 a–e. Patient L., age 65. Diagnosis: gastric cancer. Complaints of occasional vomiting, usually in the second half of the day. The feeling of overfilled stomach after meals. Anamnestic data: endoscopy conducted about 2 months earlier revealed a small ulcer in the pyloric part of the stomach. Histological examination of bioptates failed to find tumor cells. Control endoscopies did not reveal positive dynamics. X-ray examination of the stomach was recommended. **a** Stomach roentgenogram (tight filling, vertical position, anterior projection): the pyloric part is disfigured, narrowed, the walls are rigid (arrows). **b** Stomach roentgenogram (tight filling, horizontal position, left posterior oblique projection): the pyloric part is disfigured (rigid tube) (arrow). **c, d** Stomach roentgenograms (double contrast, horizontal position, anterior projection): the pyloric part is disfigured, the walls are rigid, the lesser curvature has the shapes of a rigid platform with a depot of contrast medium (arrow). **e, f** Stomach roentgenograms (double contrast, horizontal position, anterior projection) after additional ingestion of a gas-producing mixture and practically complete evacuation of the barium sulfate suspension: the walls of the pyloric part of the stomach are thickened and rigid due to circular intramural infiltration (arrows). Conclusion: Infiltrative-ulcerous cancer of the pyloric part of the stomach. The patient was operated. Histologically, signet-ring cell carcinoma.

Fig. 134 a–c. Patient K, age 46. Diagnosis: gastric cancer. **a** Stomach roentgenogram (tight filling, vertical position, anterior projection): the pyloric part and the distal half of the antral part are narrow, evacuation function of the pylorus is upset, the

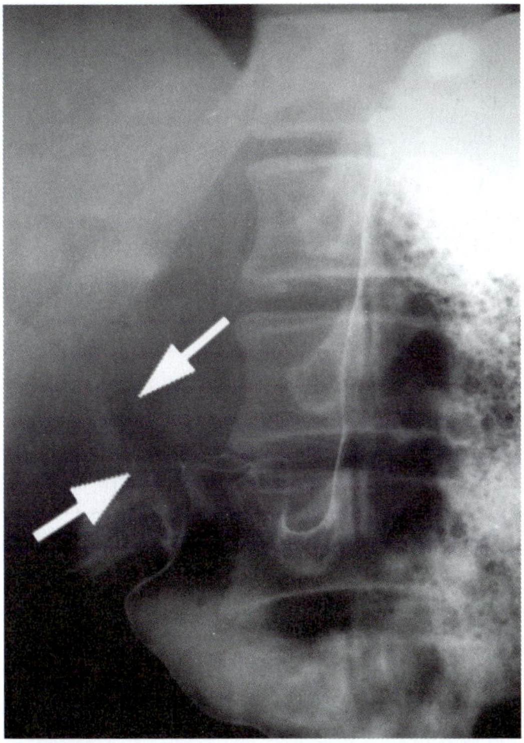

▲ **Fig. 134 b.**

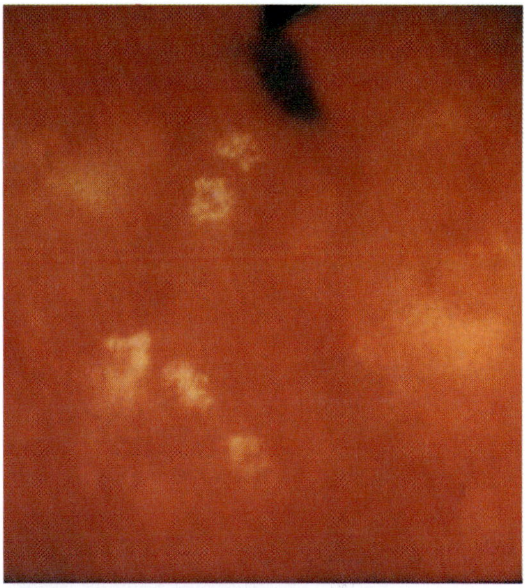

▲ **Fig. 134 c.**

walls are rigid. **b** Stomach roentgenogram (double contrast, horizontal position, anterior projection): the pyloric part and the distal half of the antral part are narrowed, the walls are thickened and rigid due to circular intramural infiltration (arrows). Conclusion: Infiltrative cancer of the pyloric part of the stomach with invasion of the antral part of the stomach. **c** Endophotograph: the pyloric part of the stomach is very narrow and disfigured, the mucous membrane is spotted: grayish pink spots against the background of hyperemia; the surface is smooth and glassy. Histological examination of the bioptates verified signet-ring cell carcinoma.

Fig. 135 a–c. Patient S., age 59. Diagnosis: gastric cancer. **a** Stomach roentgenogram (tight filling, vertical position, anterior projection): antral part of the stomach is disfigured (hourglass), the angular notch is straightened, contours are uneven (arrows). **b** Stomach roentgenogram (double contrast, horizontal position, anterior projection): walls of the antral part, the sinus, and the stomach body are thickened and rigid due to diffuse circular intramural infiltration (arrows). Conclusion: Infiltrative cancer of the antral part of the stomach with involvement of the stomach body. **c** Endophotograph: the antral part of the stomach is strongly disfigured and narrowed. The mucous membrane is scarlet, infiltrated, with uneven surface. Ulceration with tuberous firm margins and flat uneven floor covered with necrotic mass is seen on the greater curvature. Histological examination of bioptates verified signet-ring cell carcinoma.

▼ **Fig. 135 a.**

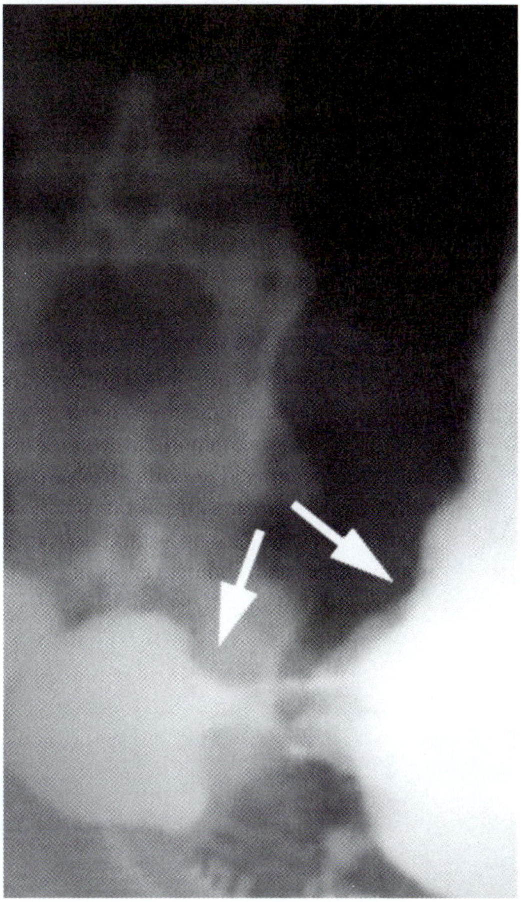

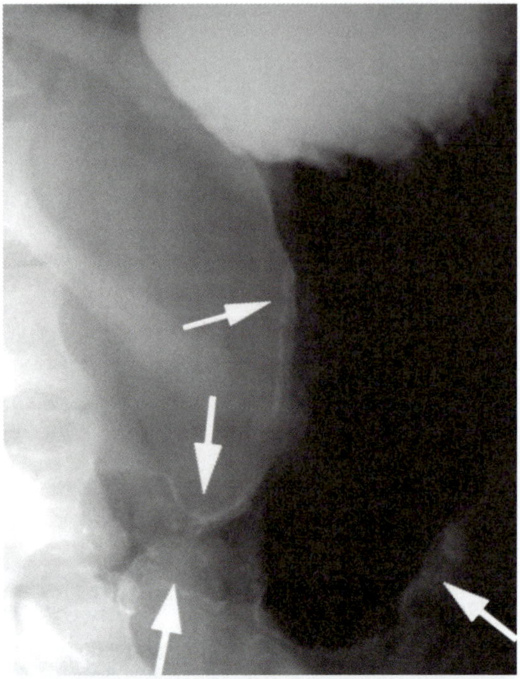

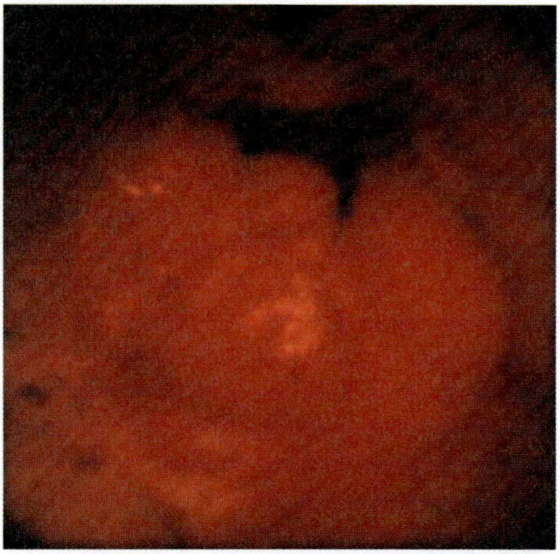

▲ Fig. 135 c.

◄ Fig. 134 b.

▼ Fig. 136 a.

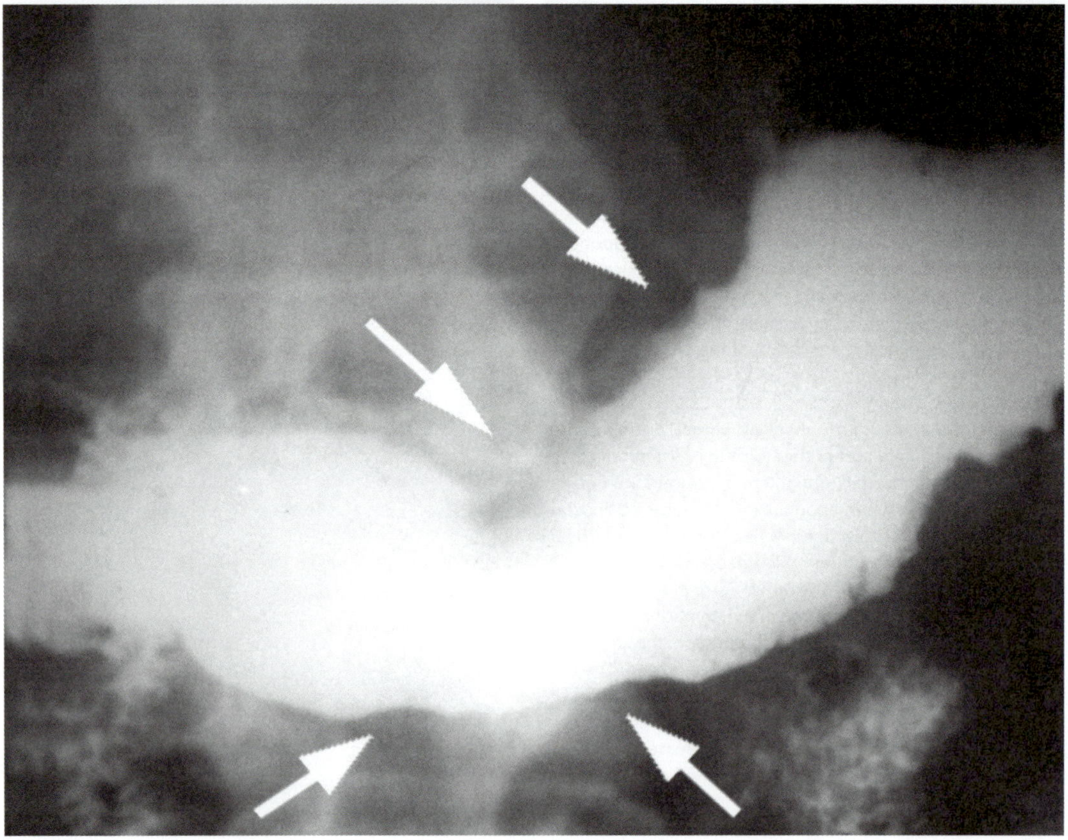

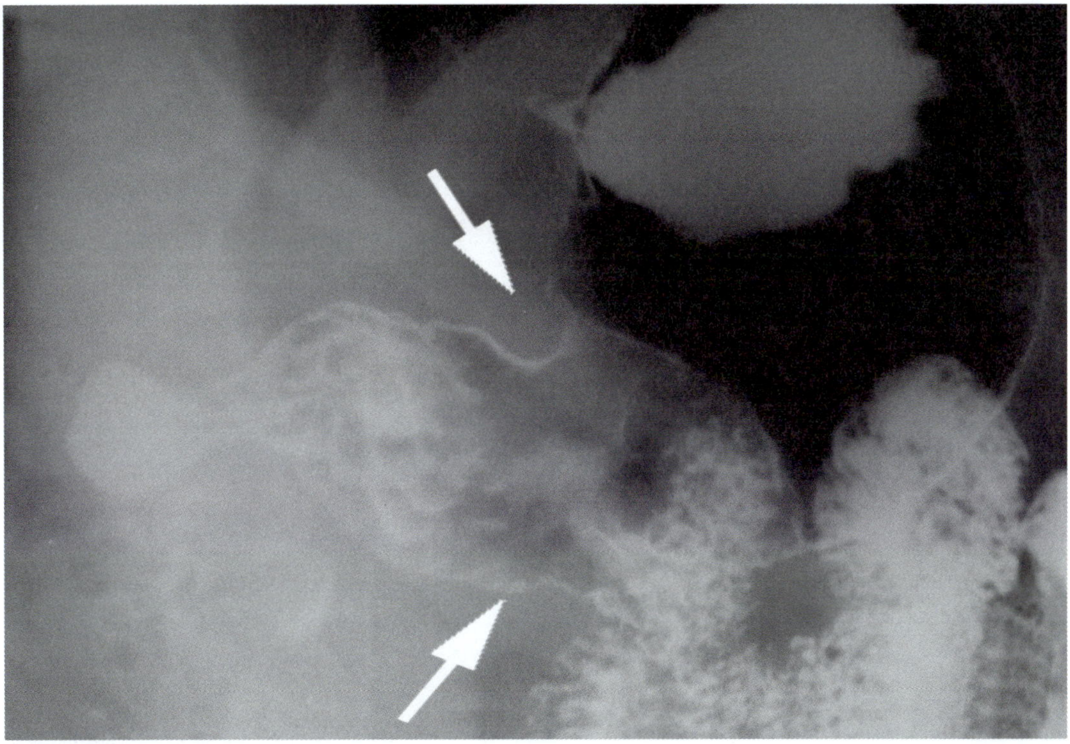

▲ **Fig. 136 b.**

▼ **Fig. 137 a.**

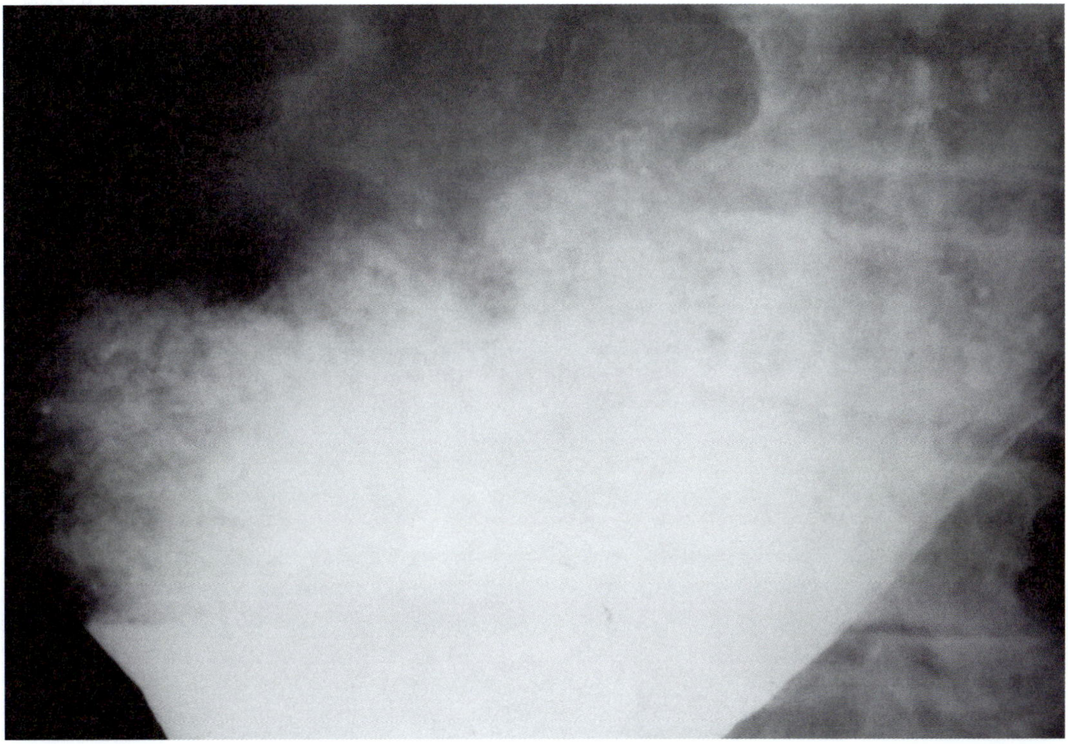

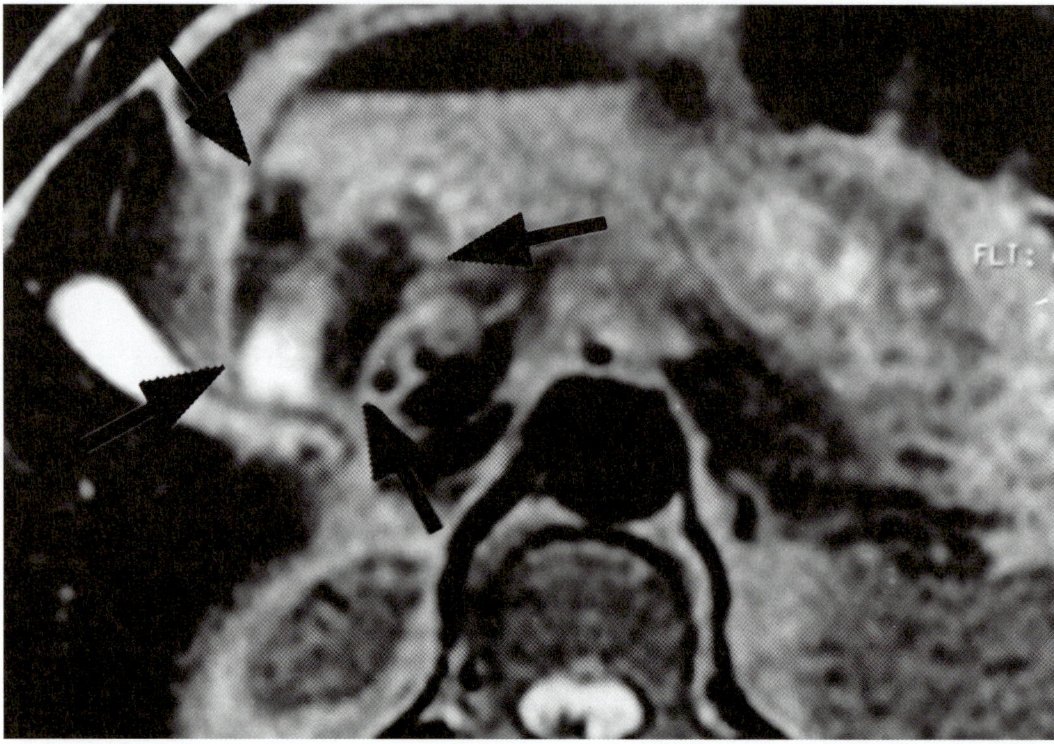

▲ Fig. 137 b.

▼ Fig. 137 c.

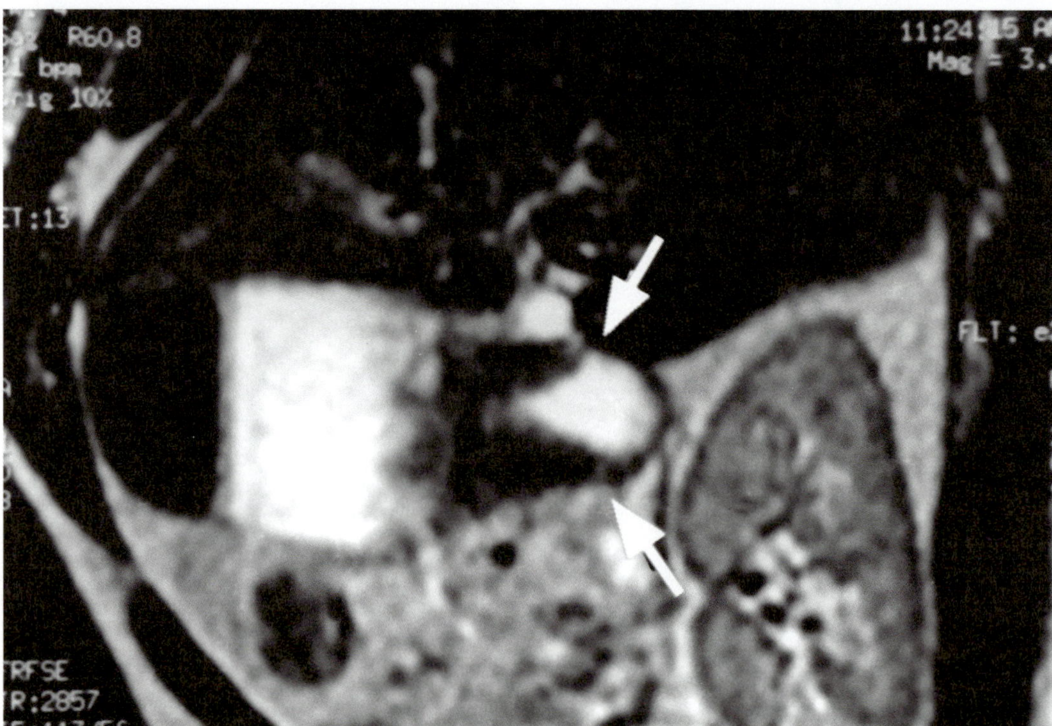

Fig. 136 a, b. Patient M., age 68. Diagnosis: gastric cancer. **a** Stomach roentgenogram (tight filling, vertical position, anterior projection): uneven contours of the distal part and the body of the stomach; straightened angular notch (arrows). **b** Stomach roentgenogram (double contrast, horizontal position, anterior projection): the walls of the distal part and the body of the stomach are thickened and rigid due to diffuse circular intramural infiltration (arrows). Conclusion: Infiltrative cancer of the distal part of the stomach with spread onto the stomach body. The patient was operated. Histologically, adenocarcinoma with the signet-ring cell component.

Fig. 137 a–c. Patient K., age 61. Diagnosis: gastric cancer. **a** Stomach roentgenogram (tight filling, vertical position, anterior projection): the cavity is strongly ectatic, the fasting stomach contains much fluid and mucus; pronounced evacuation disorder. In the absence in the patient's anamnesis of gastroduodenal ulcer, the X-ray picture is more likely to be interpreted as a tumor affection of the pyloric part of the stomach. In order to verify etiology of the so-called stenosis of the pyloric part of the stomach, endoscopy with multiple biopsy was recommended. Endoscopy revealed severely narrowed upper part of the stomach. Histological examination of the bioptates failed to find tumor cells. The patient was examined by MRI. **b** MR image of the stomach (axial projection, level of the pyloric part of the stomach, T2 image): the pyloric part of the stomach is circularly narrowed due to intramural infiltration of its walls for a length of about 45 mm with the maximum wall thickness to 20 mm; the inner outline of the narrowed part is uneven and blurred, the outer sufficiently distinct. Signs of involvement of the perigastric cellular tissue are absent (arrows). **c** MR image of the stomach (sagittal projection, level of the pyloric part of the stomach, T2 image): more distinct is the lower border of the intramural infiltration (arrows). Conclusion: Infiltrative cancer of the pyloric part of the stomach. The patient was operated. Histologically, non-differentiated cancer. As seen from this example, MRI of the stomach proved to be the method by which it was possible to verify the nature of the so-called stenosis of the pyloric part of the stomach before operation and to confirm findings of the traditional roentgenological examination. Endoscopy failed to verify the nature of the so-called stenosis.

Fig. 138 a, b. Female patient Sh., age 58. Diagnosis: gastric cancer. **a** Stomach roentgenogram (tight filling, vertical position, anterior projection): the cavity is decreased, the angular notch is straightened, the lesser curvature is shortened and depressed (arrows); **b** Stomach roentgenogram (double contrast, horizontal position, anterior projection): walls of the distal part and body of the stomach are thickened and rigid due to circular intramural infiltration (arrows). Conclusion: Infiltrative cancer of the distal part and the body of the stomach. The patient was operated. Histologically – signet-ring cell carcinoma.

The need for early diagnosis of gastric cancer stimulated oncologists to make a more thorough study of pyloric cancers. Simultaneously, they evaluated the potentials of X-ray methods, which were directed at the functional symptoms (disordered evacuation, residues of barium sulfate suspension within a defined lapse of time, etc.) because of the insignificant number of determinable morphological signs of organic affection. But in our studies of cancer and ulcer stenosis we arrived at the conclusion that the current semiotics of such affections, based mostly on signs of far-advanced cancers, cannot adequately lead to an early diagnosis, nor can it differentiate the two conditions (Fig. 137). The pyloroduodenal zone can be the site of localization of rarer diseases, such as tuberculosis, syphilis, rigid antral gastritis, or erosive gastritis. In addition, difficulties can arise in the presence of perigastric commissures and depressions in the so-called hypertrophic pylorostenosis, secondary changes in the gastroduodenal junction in patients with benign or malignant affection of the hepato-pancreatic-duodenal zone. Unfortunately, we must admit that at present, these conditions are identified only during surgery, because it is sometimes impossible to verify the diagnosis using available technical facilities.

The main reason for this unsatisfactory situation is that these tumors are mostly endophytic, and not adequately covered by roentgenological and endoscopic semiotics (Fig. 138). This is a difficult problem. Stomach deformations, which occur in

▼ Fig. 138 a.

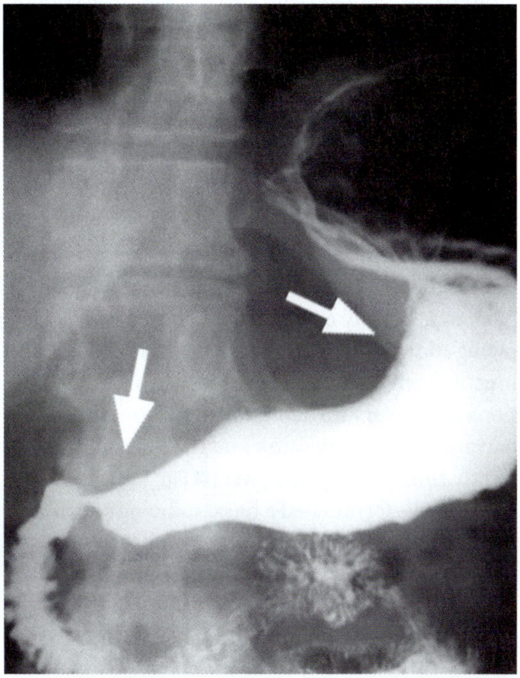

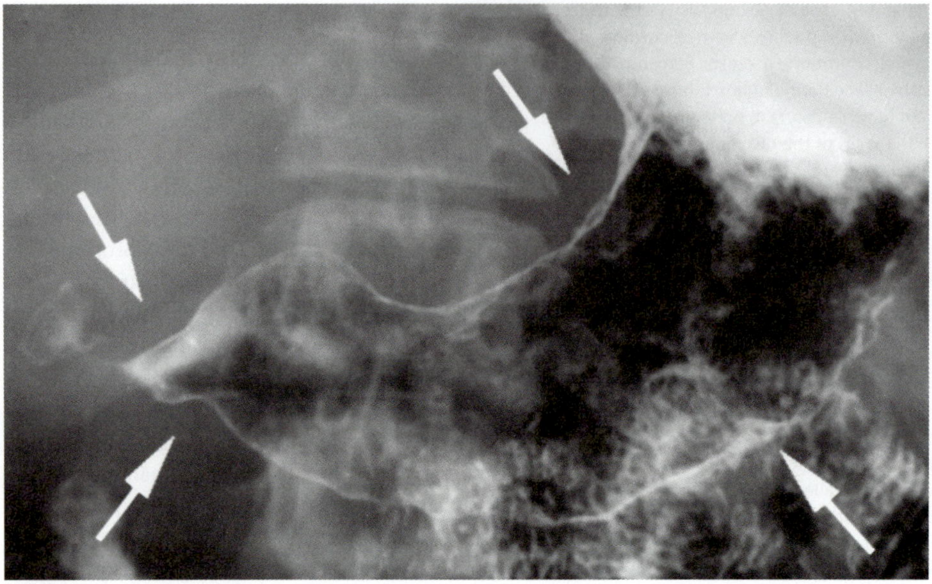

◂ **Fig. 138 b.**

such situations, can interfere with endoscopy (which is used by most oncologists) and biopsy. The limited potentials of fibergastroscopy, which gives a rather non-specific picture as regards differential diagnosis, and insufficient knowledge of radiological diagnosis (in some cases, sheer ignorance of it), makes clinicians take unusual measures such as laparotomy, or frequent and futile attempts to obtain histological confirmation by examining bioptates taken during endoscopy. M.S. Levin et al. (1990) provide a good illustration of such a situation: A patient was operated on only when the diagnosis was established after the fifth attempt to obtain a positive result of endoscopic biopsy, 18 months after the patient's first visit [184].

Serious difficulties arise during a traditional X-ray examination, because so-called stenosis of the pylorus is usually accompanied by stomach ectasia owing to the presence of food residues, liquid, and mucus. Early diagnosis of tumors in such localizations is also very difficult due to the greatly diluted barium sulfate suspension and the infeasibility of it tightly filling the pyloric part (◘ Fig. 139).

We have formulated a basic radiology semiotics for the pathology under discussion based on signs of infiltrative growth, which can be present even in cases with insignificant affection of the stomach wall. The current traditional orientation toward the signs of diffuse tumor is the main reason for an unfavorable prognosis, even when the diagnosis is successful. This is true for both roentgenological and endoscopic examinations [48, 55].

The recent tendency to decline radiological diagnosis leads to dramatic results. The widely used fibergastroscopy often fails to establish the true cause of the patient's deteriorated condition and only states the presence of ulceration and erosion, or even finds »intact« mucous membrane in this part of the stomach. Common biopsy proves useless in cases with submucous tumors, which do not manifest on the surface of the mucous membrane.

In such cases, X-ray findings acquire major importance in the diagnostic algorithm. But due to the small size of the tumor, the traditional techniques do not always supply sufficient information. Determination of thickness and elasticity of the walls using double-contrast radiology becomes especially important here. If the tumor is small, it is impossible to detect the presence of the well-known signs such as concentric narrowing or rigidity of walls of the antral part of the stomach, which suggest the spread of malignancy not only to the pyloric part but also to the neighboring structures. The situation becomes even more serious in the presence of concurrent peptic ulcers, which, together with erosive gastritis, mask submucous tumors and lead to an incorrect radiological and endoscopic diagnosis (◘ Fig. 140).

Fig. 139 a–f. Female patient P., age 71. Diagnosis: gastric cancer. **a** Stomach roentgenogram (tight filling, vertical position, anterior projection): the stomach contains much fluid, mucus, and food residue; the evacuation function of the pylorus is upset. **b** Stomach roentgenogram (tight filling, vertical position, anterior projection) after ingestion of an additional portion of contrast medium: the pyloric part is unevenly narrowed, its walls are rigid, vigorous peristaltic activity of the intact parts of the stomach is seen. **c, d** Stomach roentgenograms (tight filling, vertical position, anterior projection): pyloric part is unevenly narrowed due to circular infiltration of its walls (arrow); the evacuation function of the pylorus is upset. **e** Stomach roentgenogram (double contrast, horizontal position, anterior projection): walls of the pyloric part are thickened and rigid due to circular intramural infiltration (arrow). Conclusion: Infiltrative cancer of the pyloric part of the stomach. **f** Endophotograph: pyloric part of the stomach is disfigured, greatly narrowed (resembling a sleeve), the mucous membrane in this region is grayish pink, tuberous, with a fibrin coat; the pylorus is not differentiated. Histological examination of the bioptates taken during endoscopy verified signet-ring cell carcinoma.

Fig. 140 a–d. Patient K., age 53. Diagnosis: gastric cancer. **a, b** Stomach roentgenograms (tight filling, vertical position, anterior projection): pyloric part is unevenly narrowed due to circular infiltration of its walls; the evacuation function of the pylorus is normal. **c** Stomach roentgenogram (double contrast, horizontal position, anterior projection): walls of the pyloric part are thickened and rigid due to circular intramural infiltration. Conclusion: Infiltrative cancer of the pyloric part of the stomach. **d** Endophotograph: pyloric part of the stomach is disfigured, narrowed like a sleeve, the mucous membrane is hyperemic, with rough surface and a fibrin coat. Histological examination of the bioptates taken during endoscopy verified non-differentiated cancer.

▼ **Fig. 139 a.**

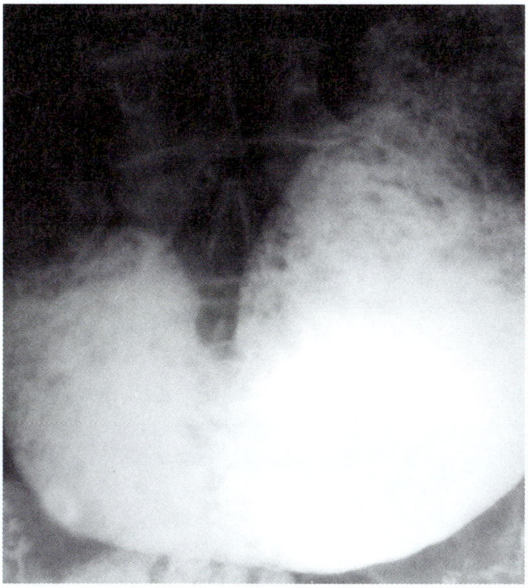

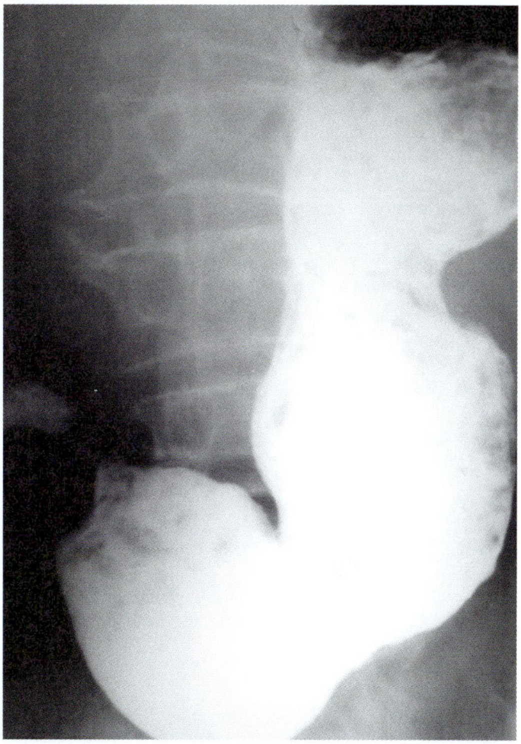

▲ **Fig. 139 b.**

▼ **Fig. 139 c.**

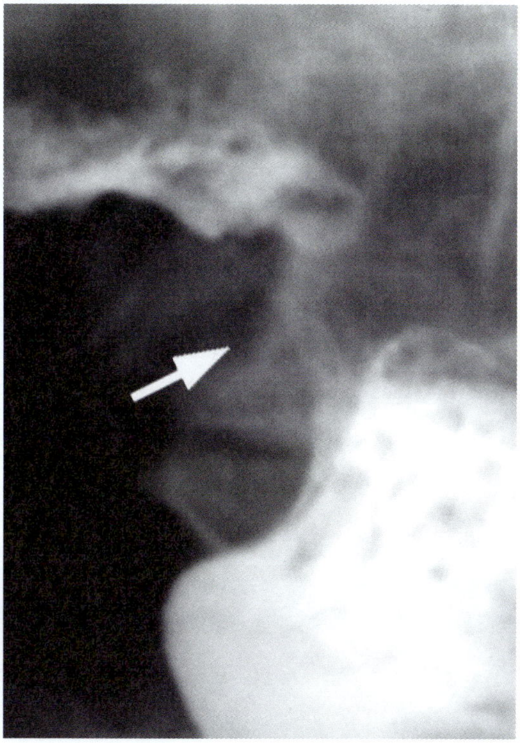

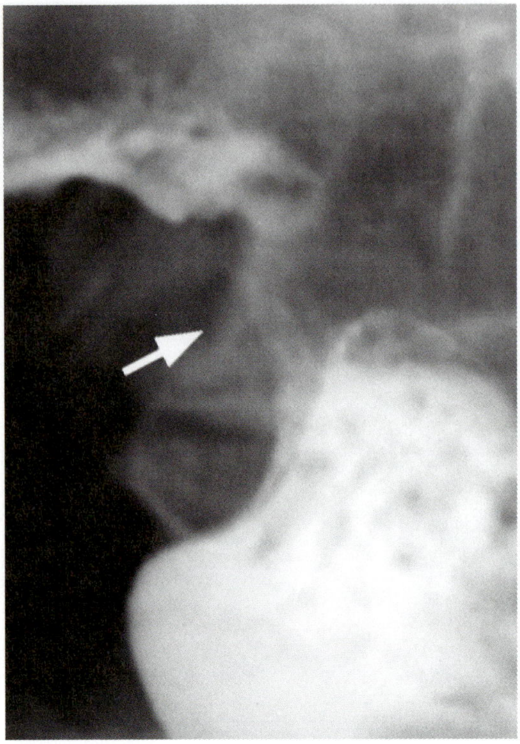

◄ Fig. 139 d.

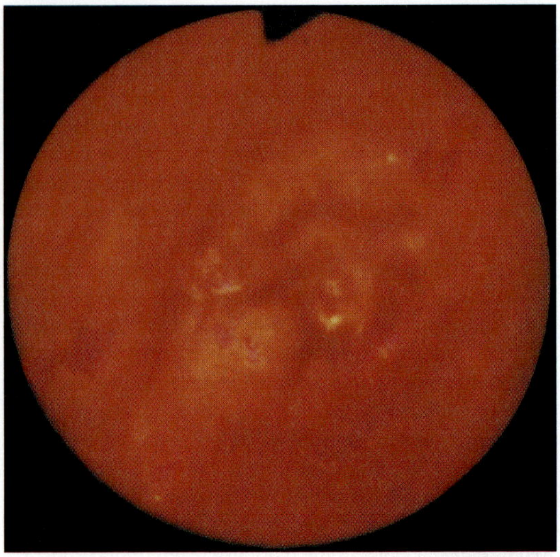

▲ Fig. 139 f.

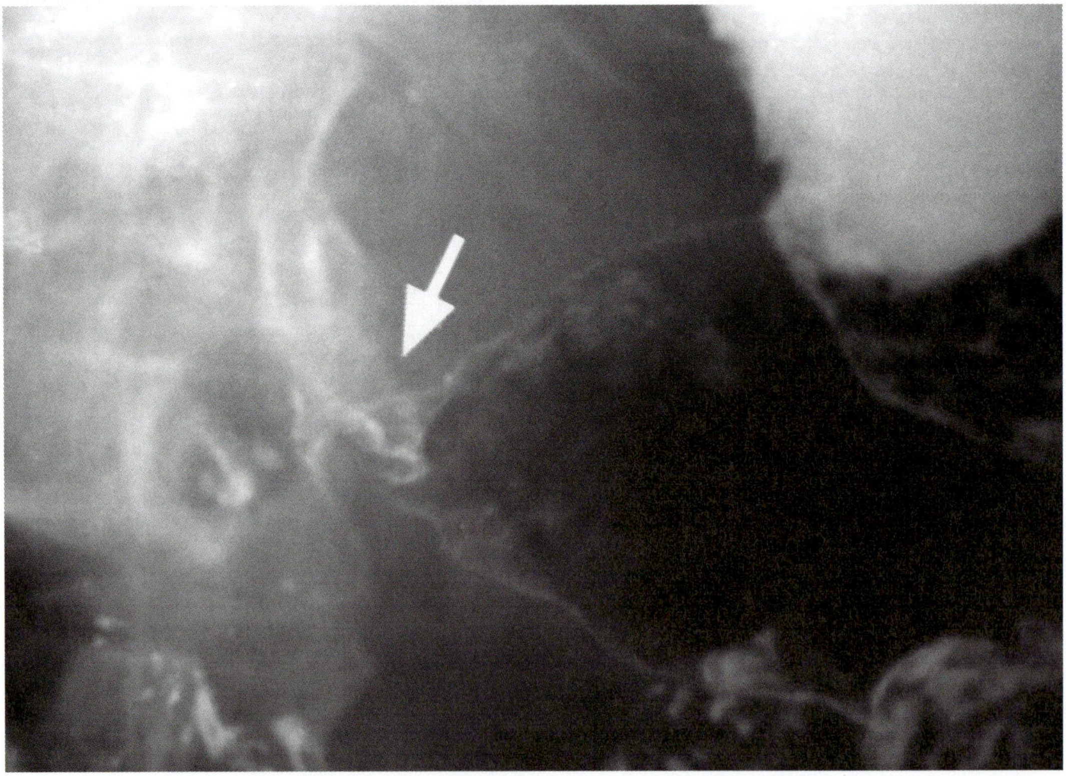

▼ Fig. 139 e.

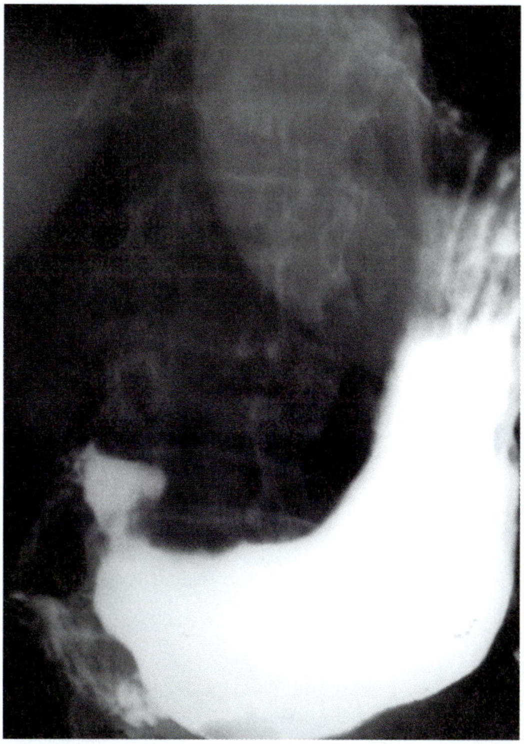

▲ Fig. 140 a.

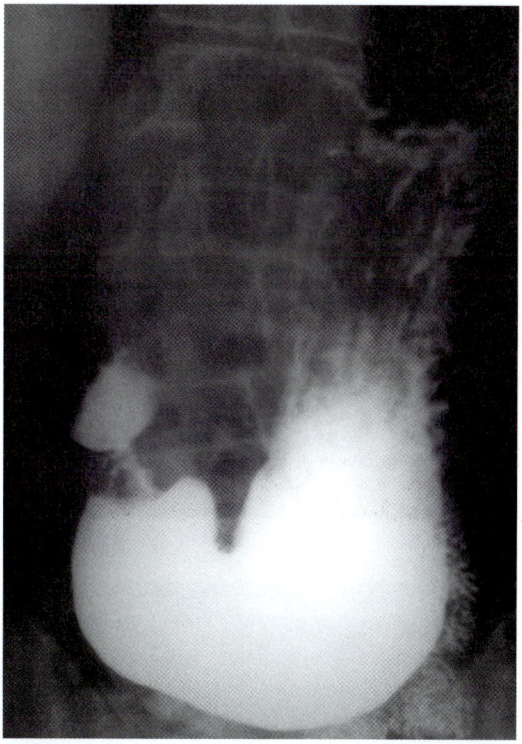

▲ Fig. 140 b.

▼ Fig. 140 c.

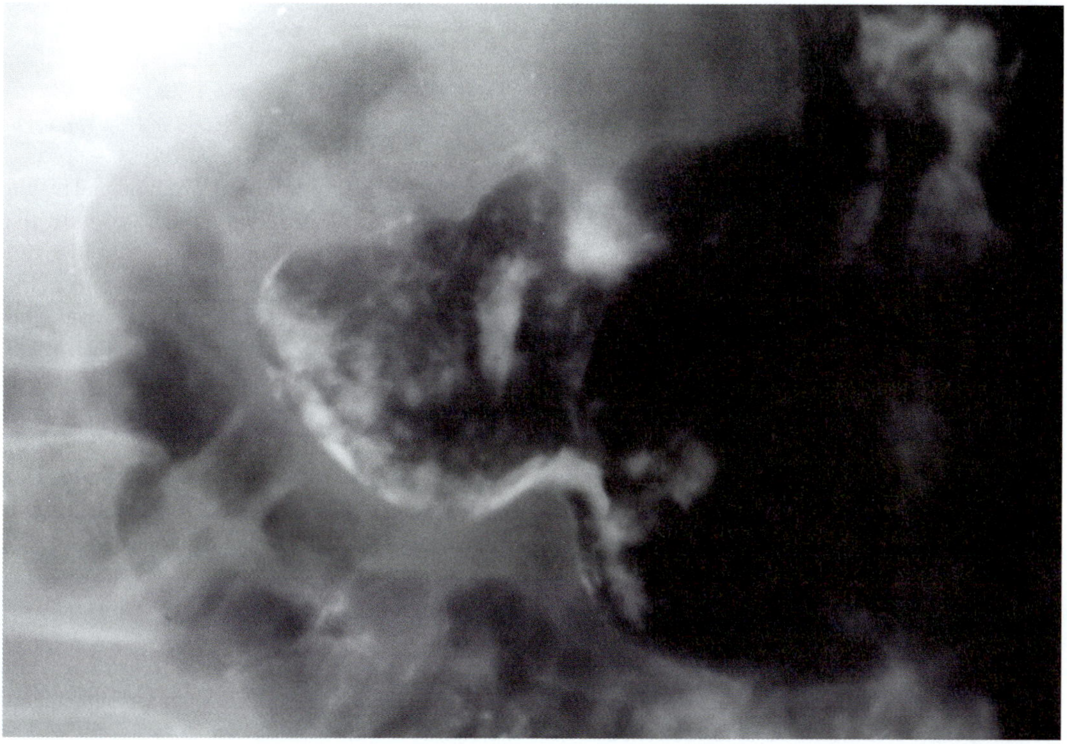

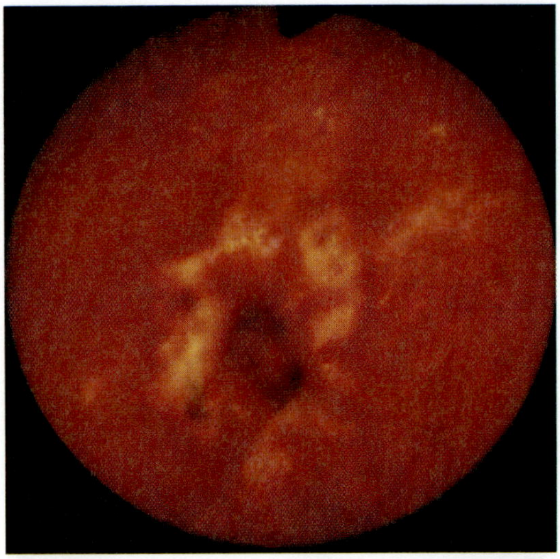

▲ Fig. 140 d.

▼ Fig. 141 a.

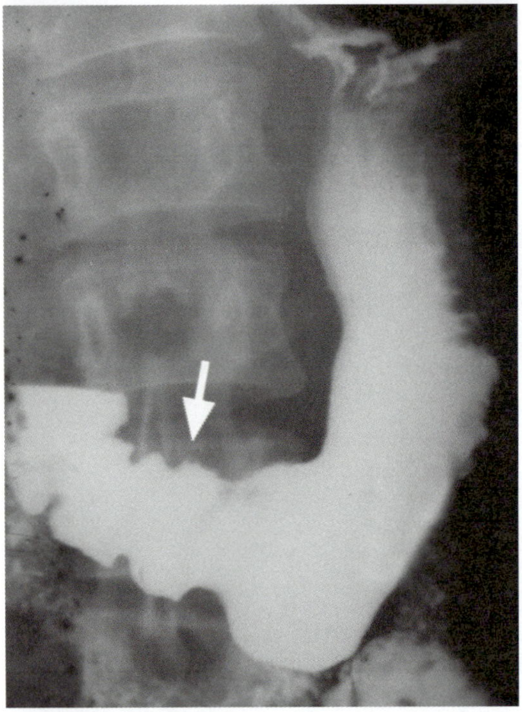

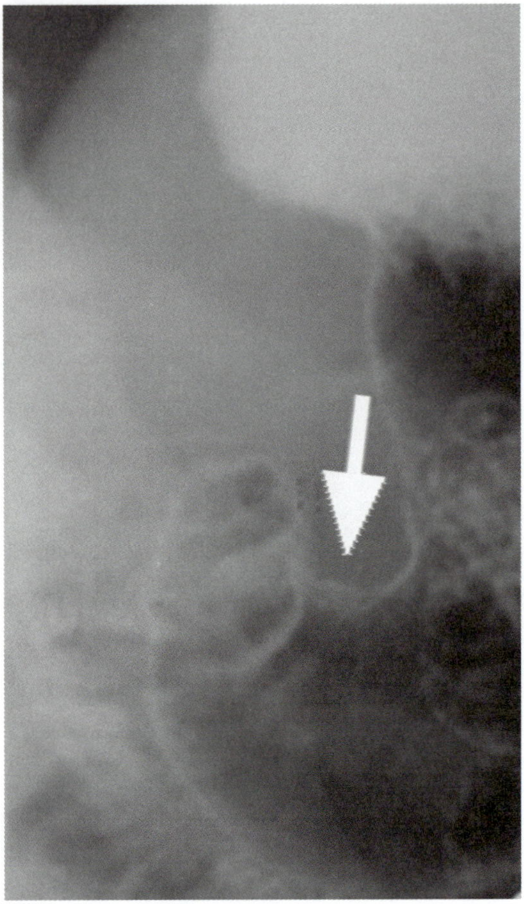

▲ Fig. 141 b.

Nevertheless, modern radiological diagnosis is able to solve these difficulties, which only appear to be unsurpassable obstacles to a correct and early diagnosis of cancer of the prepyloric part of the stomach. Here we stress again that good visualization of the morphological substrate can be obtained only with certain specific techniques of examination. One of these is target imaging of the pyloroduodenal region in the vertical and horizontal positions with the maximum possible tight filling. This technique can be used to estimate the contours, the elasticity of the wall, its rigidity, the extent of the involved area, and the presence of ulcers. At the same time, during examination in the vertical position, tight filling of the pylorus is often difficult in the presence of liquid, mucus, and food residues. Therefore, radiography in the vertical position should preferably be done after the patient is raised from the horizontal position, which is optimal for filling this region.

The double-contrast investigation plays an important role in the diagnosis of distal cancer. It can give the image of the tumor in its true size because the tumor becomes »trimmed« with the intact wall of the stomach as it is inflated with air. Imaging of the stomach wall with double-contrast radiology

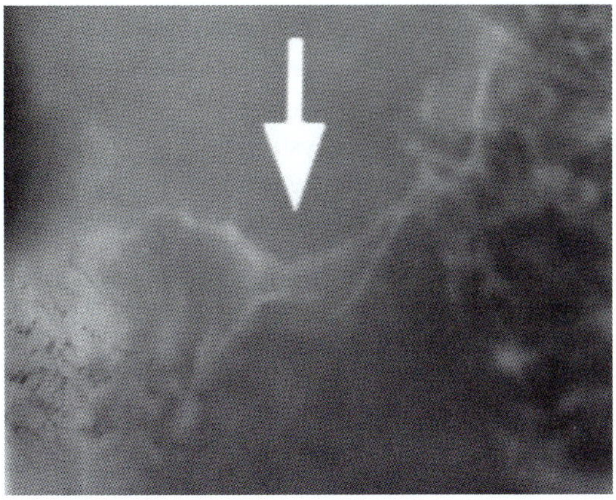

▲ Fig. 141 c.

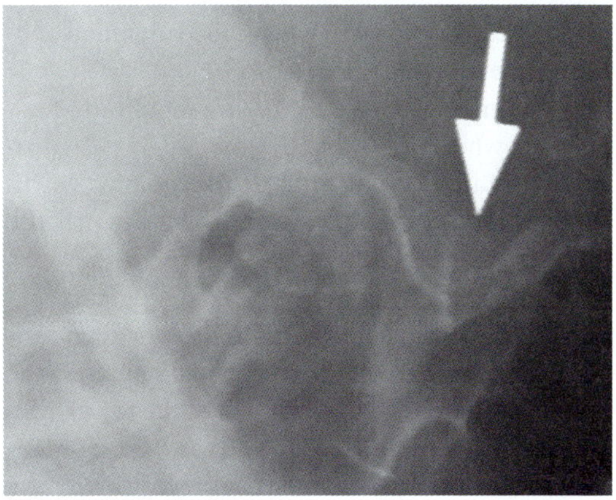

▲ Fig. 141 c.

Fig. 141 a–c. Patient V., age 58. Diagnosis: gastric cancer. **a** Stomach roentgenogram (tight filling, vertical position, anterior projection): uneven contour of lesser curvature of the antral part (arrow). **b** Stomach roentgenogram (double contrast, horizontal position, right oblique projection): wall of the lesser curvature of the antral part is thickened and rigid due to intramural infiltration (arrow). **c** Stomach roentgenograms (double contrast, horizontal position, right oblique projection): the walls of the prepyloric part are thickened and rigid over a length of about 2 cm due to intramural infiltration (arrows). Conclusion: Initial infiltrative cancer of the distal part of the stomach. The patient was operated. Histologically, adenocarcinoma with the signet-ring cell component.

makes it possible to differentiate between benign stenosis and malignant tumor. In patients with cancer, as distinct from cicatricial-ulcerous stenosis, the thickness of the walls in the distal part of the stomach greatly exceeds normal thickness. Concerning these signs of the blastomatous process, we must point out that one particular sign should not be considered separately from others. Clinical manifestations must also be taken into consideration in such situations.

While discussing pathologies of the pylorus, we would like to dwell on the spread of tumor in the distal direction, i.e., to the bulb and the post-bulbar part of the duodenum. The classical concept of the infiltrative process of the linitis plastica type suggests a casuistic possibility of total affection of the gastrointestinal tract: Spread of the process in the distal direction is connected largely with blastomatous lymphangitis.

To summarize what has been said about distal gastric cancer, we should like to note once again some points in radiological diagnosis of the so-called pylorostenosis. Not infrequently, while planning a stomach resection for ulcer of the pyloroduodenal zone accompanied by severe evacuation dysfunction of the pylorus, the clinician still doubts the correctness of his decision because of the serious difficulties in preoperative establishment of the pathology. Serious deformational changes occurring with stenosis of the zone in question create special conditions for the traditional X-ray and endoscopic examinations. They considerably reduce the informative value of endoscopy, which is regarded as the final preoperative method of establishing the diagnosis. In such situations, the main responsibility should be shifted to radiological diagnosis, because much experience has been gained with it in revealing diffuse cancers, the prevailing oncological pathology in this zone [45, 73].

The entire systematized radiological semiotics of infiltrative cancers of the stomach is most closely connected with a special complex of methodological techniques aimed at the maximum imaging of intramural tumor process. This optimism is based on the possibility of currently used pneumographic and traditional components of gastroenterology to reveal thickening of the wall and its elasticity, which, in addition to evaluating the condition of the mucous membrane, effectively reveals tumor infiltration in this part of the stomach, which is the most difficult to access for an accurate diagnosis (Fig. 141). It follows, therefore, that, considering the importance of the final interpretation of the evacuation dysfunction of the pylorus, one must entertain the possibility of radiological diagnosis of the so-called organic stenosis of the pyloroduodenal region [55].

It is time to revise the existing set of radiological signs which are still used not only by gastroenterologists and surgeons, but also by radiological diagnosticians, who choose not to deal with the diagnosis of early gastric cancer because they lack faith in the potentials of modern radiological diagnosis. This pertains first of all to the so-called residues of barium sulfate suspension that remain in the stomach for 24 h after the start of the X-ray examination. This must not be regarded as a sign of organic stenosis of the pyloroduodenal region. We have often observed cases in which primary examination of the stomach revealed all the signs believed to suggest organic stenosis of the pyloroduodenal region: boat-shaped ectatic stomach, which is found below the pectineal line, and significant residue of contrast medium after 24 h. Three to four weeks after conservative treatment, the stomach of such patients assumed a normal shape, while contrast medium was evacuated from the stomach even earlier (◘ Fig. 142). There are two aspects of major importance regarding the so-called organic stenosis of the stomach. The radiologist has to understand the cause of this stenosis (to be more exact, stable evacuation dysfunction of the pyloroduodenal region), whether it be a tumor with localization in the pylorus or the prepyloric part of the stomach, or a non-tumor pathology. This question can be answered with a traditional X-ray examination based on the polypositional principle, with tight filling of the stomach by a large amount of contrast medium, double contrast, and sometimes with air alone. If a small tumor is diagnosed, which causes stenosis owing to its specific location, the problem requires no further investigation. If a gastric tumor is ruled out, however, it is necessary to estimate very carefully the degree to which organic and functional components are involved. In any case, great care must be taken in interpreting the results of the examination. Of course, much depends on the clinical status of the patient. We have already expressed our negative attitude about the various pharmacological tests which are used to obtain more reliable information in these and other difficult differential-diagnosis situations. According to our data, this only adds to the difficulties of diagnosis, by masking the true picture. Our principle is a completely physiological X-ray examination of the stomach. Furthermore, pharmacological tests do not differentiate between functional disorder of evacuation and organic dysfunction. Only repeated X-ray examinations after one or several courses of treatment can lead to the final diagnosis. This is especially true for patients with gastroduodenal peptic ulcer, in whom stable evacuation dysfunction is due to edema and marked antral gastritis, symptoms that are relieved by prolonged adequate treatment. This position is confirmed by special studies conducted in Italy: Anti-Helicobacter therapy resulted in complete cure in 20 of 22 patients with diagnosed stenosis. In 17 patients signs of stenosis disappeared completely after 2 months and in three patients after 6 months. In other words, there was no actual organic stenosis, but rather a functional spasm of the pylorus in the presence of inflammatory changes. This confirms the important role of inflammatory and functional components of the »stenosis« picture, which is considered to be classical, and stresses the necessity of dynamic observation of such patients, including follow-up observation. With regard to evacuation dysfunction of the pyloroduodenal region, it is necessary to note that radiological diagnosis has obvious advantages over endoscopy for verifying the cause of so-called stenosis of this part of the stomach due to its specific anatomo-functional properties. In addition to data reported by the Italian researchers, our own observations of such patients confirm the need for substantial correction of the accepted set of signs characterizing so-called organic stenosis of the stomach.

◘ **Fig. 142 a–d.** Female patient Ya., age 54. Functional spasm of the pylorus. **a** Stomach roentgenogram (tight filling, vertical position, anterior projection): the antral part and the sinus of the stomach are ectatic, the stomach walls are even, evacuation function of the pylorus is disordered. **b** Stomach roentgenogram (tight filling, vertical position, anterior projection) in 24 h: residue of barium sulfate suspension is seen in the stomach cavity. Repeated endoscopy with biopsies failed to detect tumor cells. In the absence of signs of blastomatous affection, as evidenced by the main two instrumental methods, the patient was given conservative treatment. The same patient observed 3 weeks later. **c** Stomach roentgenogram (tight filling, vertical position, anterior projection): organic changes are not detectable, stomach contours are even, timely evacuation. **d** Stomach roentgenogram (tight filling, vertical position, anterior projection) in 24 h: the stomach is free of barium sulfate suspension, which is evenly distributed in the large intestine.

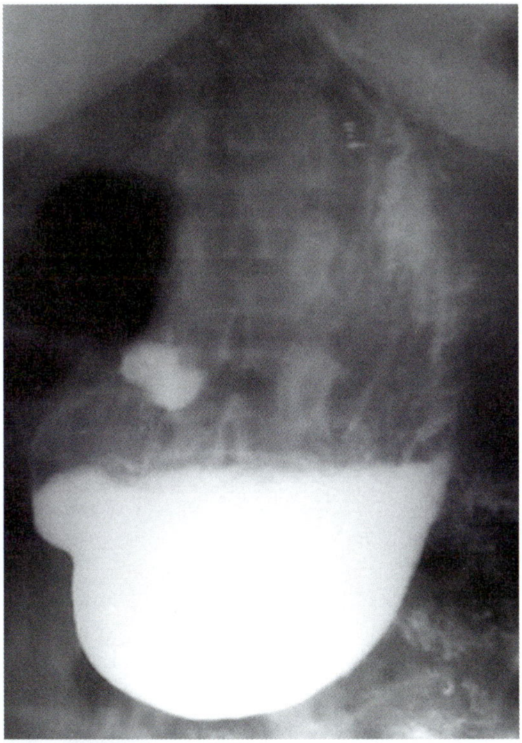

▲ Fig. 142 a.

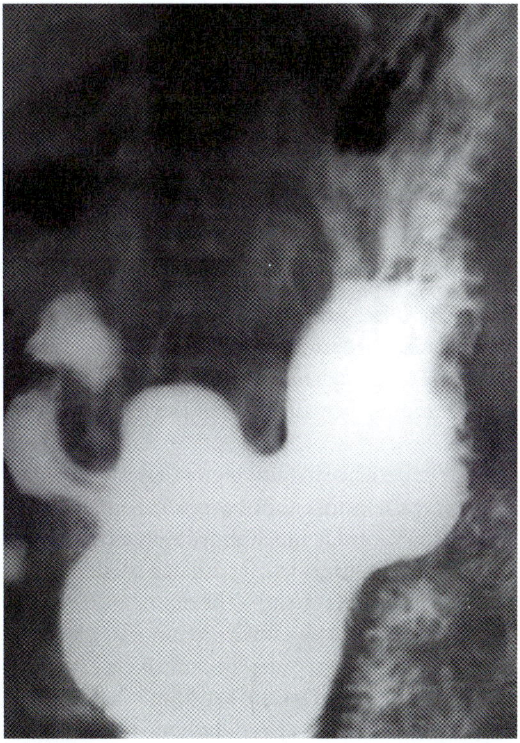

▲ Fig. 142 c.

▼ Fig. 142 b.

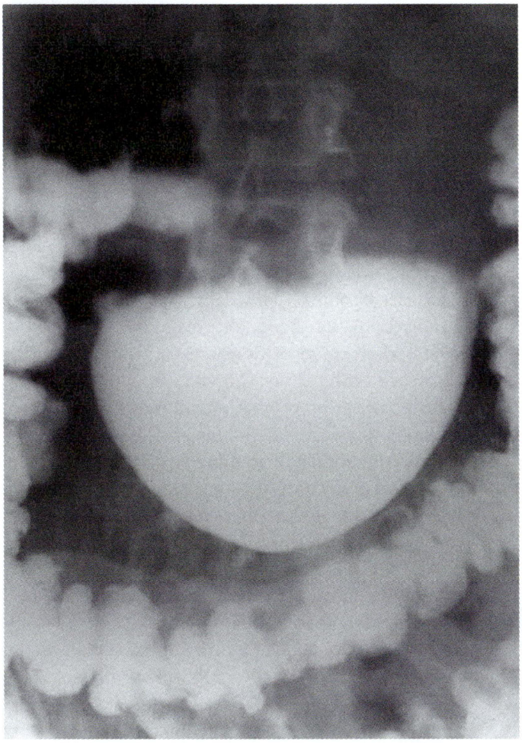

▼ Fig. 142 d.

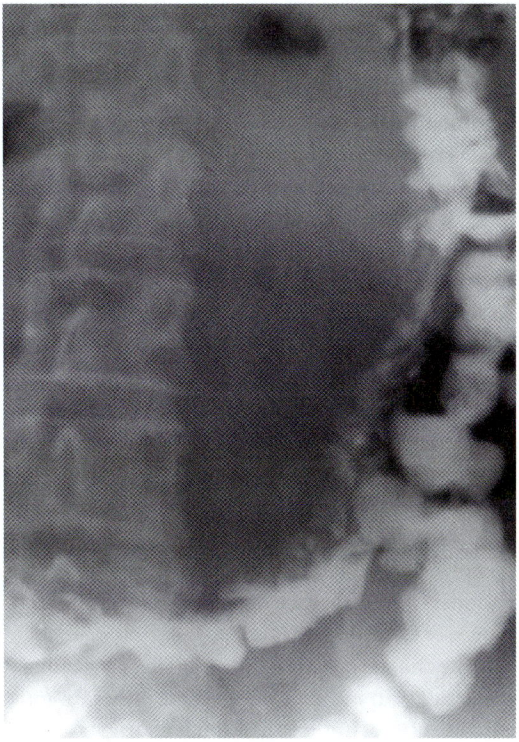

Cancer of the Greater Curvature

Until recently, the greater curvature was believed to be a rare localization of gastric cancer. For this reason, the literature contains only few reports on studies of tumors of the greater curvature. According to some authors, primary blastomatous affection of the greater curvature occurs in 1–3%, and they did not regard this pathology as an independent localization form. Other authors indicate a higher incidence of cancer of this localization (7.3–8.9%), but the results of screening demonstrate a much higher percentage of primary affection of the greater curvature.

Our experience in radiological diagnosis of gastric cancer shows that its primary localization on the greater curvature is much more frequent than reported by the authors who estimated it as 12.9% [41, 46, 99]. For several reasons – the main one being the absence of endoscopic confirmation – we observed patients with primary affection of the greater curvature for a year and longer. We found that the final stage of these tumors was endophytic fibrous carcinoma type infiltration of all walls of the stomach. This led us to conclude that a considerable portion of diffuse intramural cancers originate on the greater curvature. Thus, we think it necessary to discuss the diagnosis of tumors located on the greater curvature in more detail (◘ Fig. 143) [31, 34].

Owing to the specific anatomo-functional properties of the greater curvature, additional approaches to detecting the early signs of tumor are necessary. These approaches are not included in the existing standard methodology for reasons discussed in previous chapters. The standard methodology regards affections of the greater curvature in general, and tumors in particular, as a rarity. Most cancers originating on the greater curvature are not detected for the following two reasons: (a) the presence of pronounced mucosal folds, extending in a dorsal-ventral direction on the greater curvature, which respond to inflammatory disease and often do not stretch during X-ray and endoscopic examinations; (b) the absence of special additional techniques of examination [41].

The clinical picture of blastomatous affection of the greater curvature is not specific either. In most cases, cancer of this localization is characterized by an asymptomatic course, although some patients may complain of dull pain unassociated with meals and continuing for the greater part of the day. Other clinical symptoms, including loss of body weight, do not develop in all patients, and if they do, it is at later stages of the disease.

▼ **Fig. 143 a.**

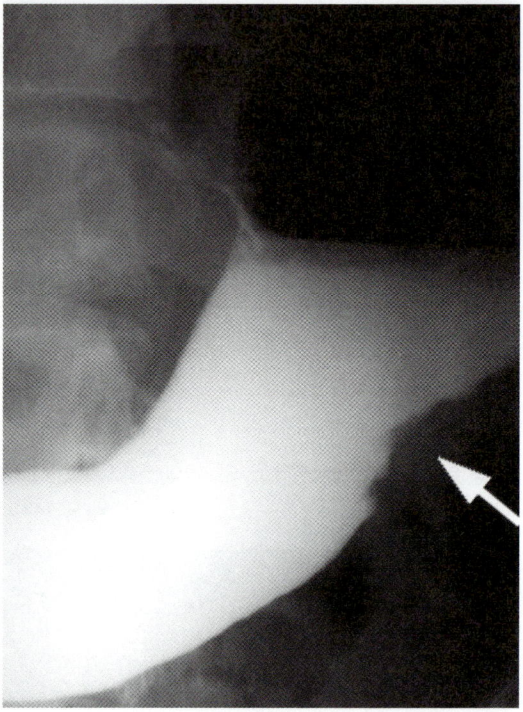

◘ **Fig. 143 a–e.** Patient I., age 55. Diagnosis: gastric cancer. **a** Stomach roentgenogram (tight filling, vertical position, anterior projection): uneven contour of the greater curvature (arrow). **b** Stomach roentgenogram (tight filling, vertical position, anterior projection), dosed compression: more distinctly visualized is the eroded contour of the greater curvature of the stomach body (arrows). **c** Stomach roentgenogram (tight filling, vertical position, anterior projection), dosed compression: intensified compression reveals a depot of contrast medium (arrow). **d** Stomach roentgenogram (double contrast, horizontal position, anterior projection): the wall of the greater curvature is thickened due to intramural infiltration; visualized at the center is a small rounded light image corresponding to an ulcer crater (arrow). Conclusion: Infiltrative-ulcerous cancer of the greater curvature of the stomach body. **e** Endophotograph: visualized in the region of the stomach sinus is a portion of mucous membrane, to 3 cm in diameter, which is slightly elevated over the surrounding tissues; the surface is rough, of grayish pink color, with flat linear ulceration at the center. Histological examination of the bioptates verified non-differentiated cancer.

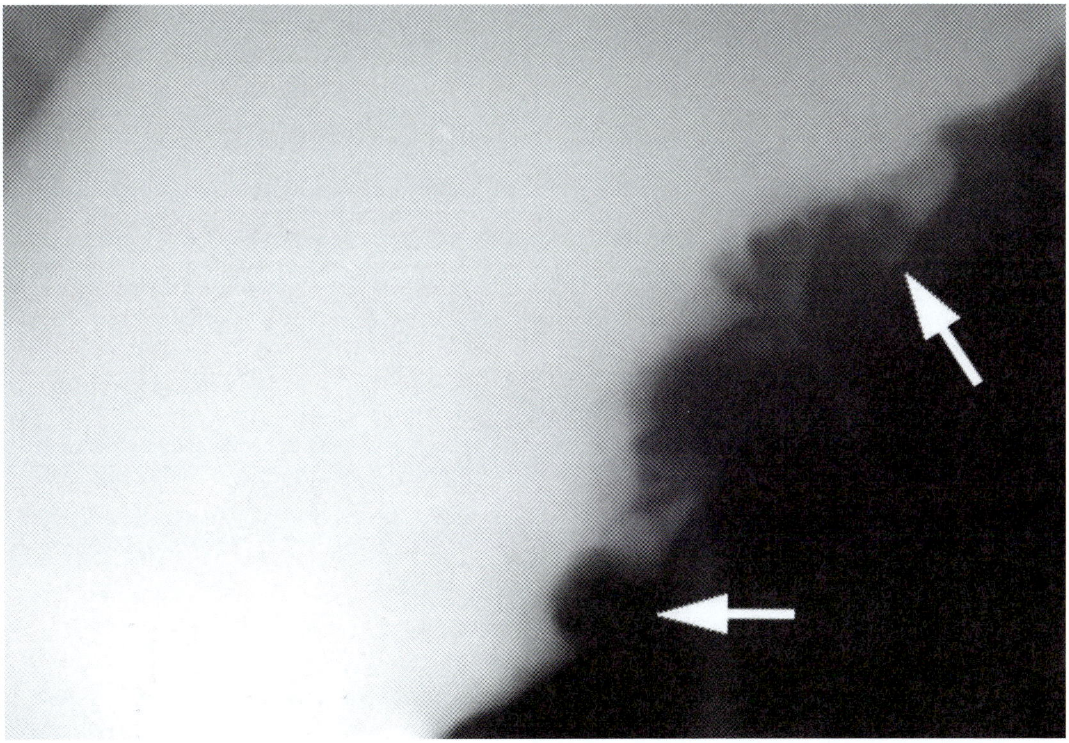

▲ **Fig. 143 b.**

▼ **Fig. 143 c.**

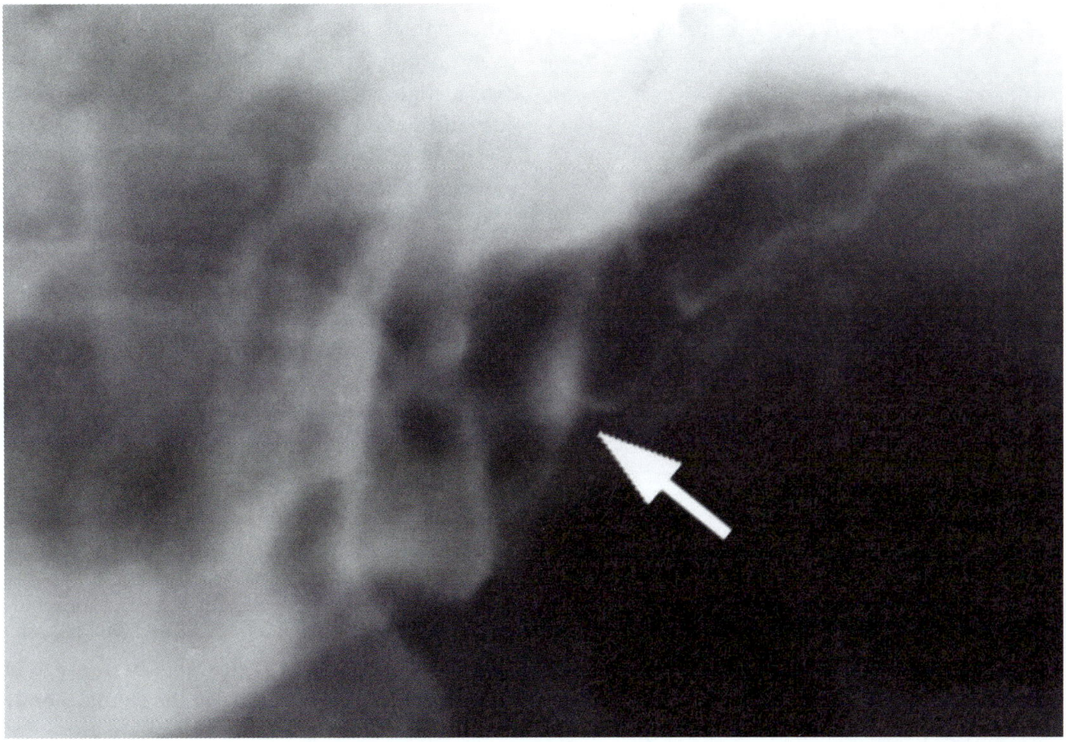

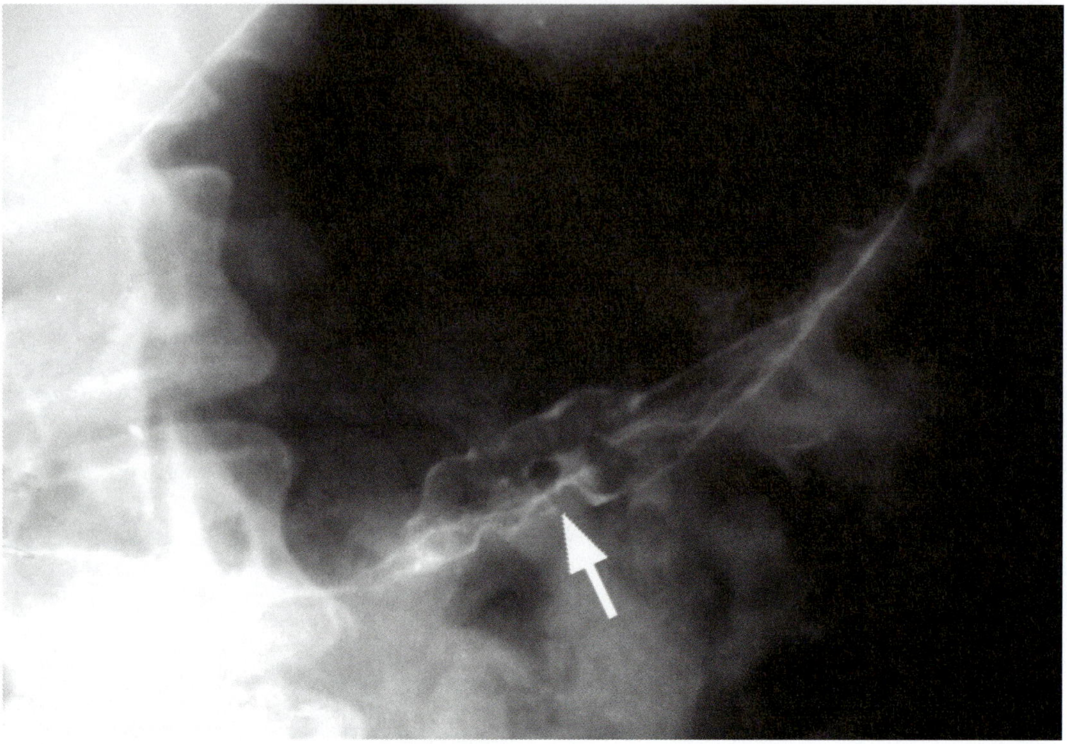

▲ Fig. 143 d. ▼ Fig. 143 e.

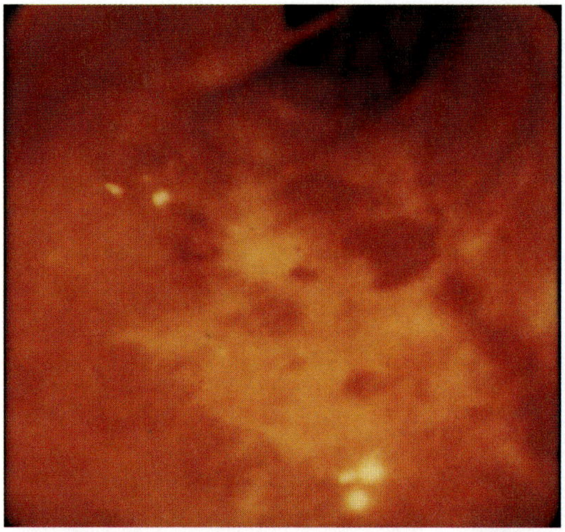

Malignant tumors of the linitis plastica and scirrhous type are usually characterized by the absence of a pronounced clinical picture. Even more difficult is clinical diagnosis of primary lesions in the »dumb« zone of the greater curvature of the stomach, in its upper third, where, according to H. Fukotomi and T. Sakita (1984), infiltration of the wall may be of significant thickness whereas its function may be relatively normal. At the same time, these authors indicate a high incidence of cancer of the greater curvature of the lower third of the stomach body. The number of tumors at this site exceeds that of tumors on the lesser curvature, the anterior wall, and posterior wall taken together. In our observations, this part of the stomach was affected in 57.6% of all cancer cases, the primary location of which was the greater curvature, and as a rule, additional methodological efforts were necessary for thorough study. As we have already noted, blastomatous infiltration often spreads to the higher parts, and eventually results in the classical linitis plastica type diffuse affection of the stomach. The necessity of improving the diagnosis of tumors of the greater curvature becomes even more apparent if we remember that the results of surgery for cancer of this localization are somewhat better compared with cancers of other localizations. This was true in cases of early detected infiltrative tumors, a considerable percentage of which were located primarily in the stomach body in the region of the greater curvature. In our opinion, the solution here is to screen risk groups for gastric cancer (some authors call them asymptomatic subjects) [8, 57, 73].

Unfortunately, in spite of numerous publications stressing the importance of a complex use of radiological methods in combination with fibergastroscopy (with biopsy) to detect cancer of the greater curvature, many clinicians continue to depend on endoscopy alone. Meanwhile, practical experience shows that routine endoscopy with the traditional technique of taking tissue specimens, has less informative value in such cancers than in those at other locations. The mucosal relief of the greater curvature is so rich that it is very difficult to reveal minor changes in this part of the stomach, the more so if the submucous coat is involved.

The X-ray examination aimed at early diagnosis of new growths in this part of the stomach consists in a thorough study of a series of target X-rays imaging not only the mucosal relief but also the contour of the greater curvature during tighter filling of the stomach with barium sulfate suspension. The study at the phase of tight filling is mandatory. To this end, the patient has to ingest an additional portion of barium sulfate suspension (Fig. 144) [36, 41, 54].

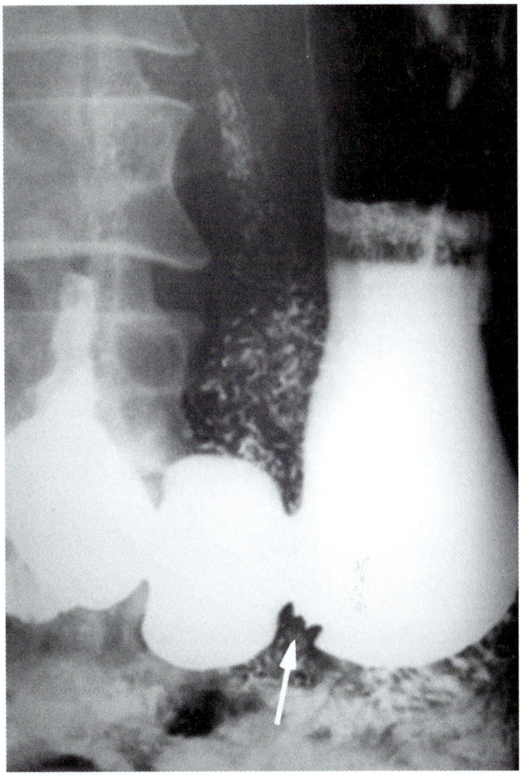

▲ **Fig. 144 a.** ▼ **Fig. 144 b.**

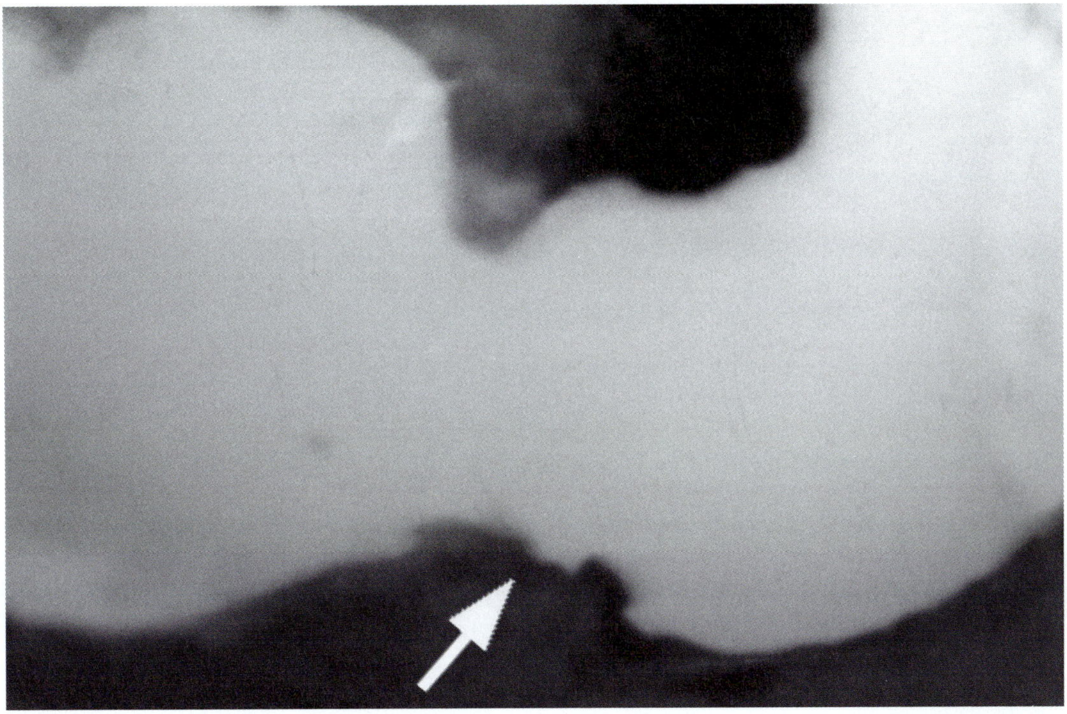

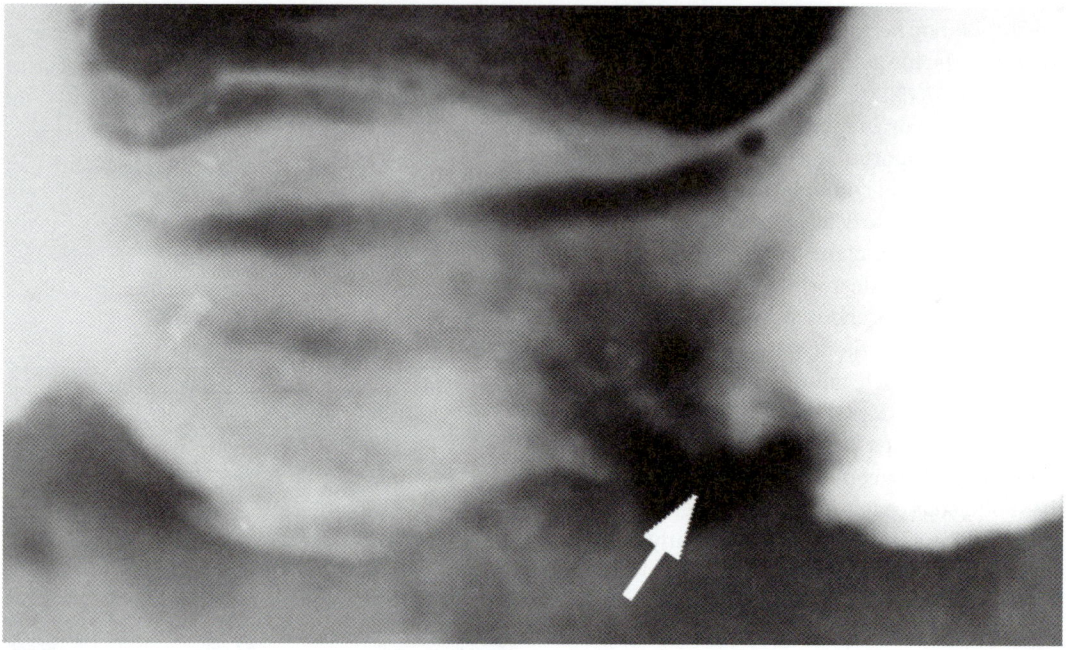

▲ Fig. 144 c.

▼ Fig. 144 d.

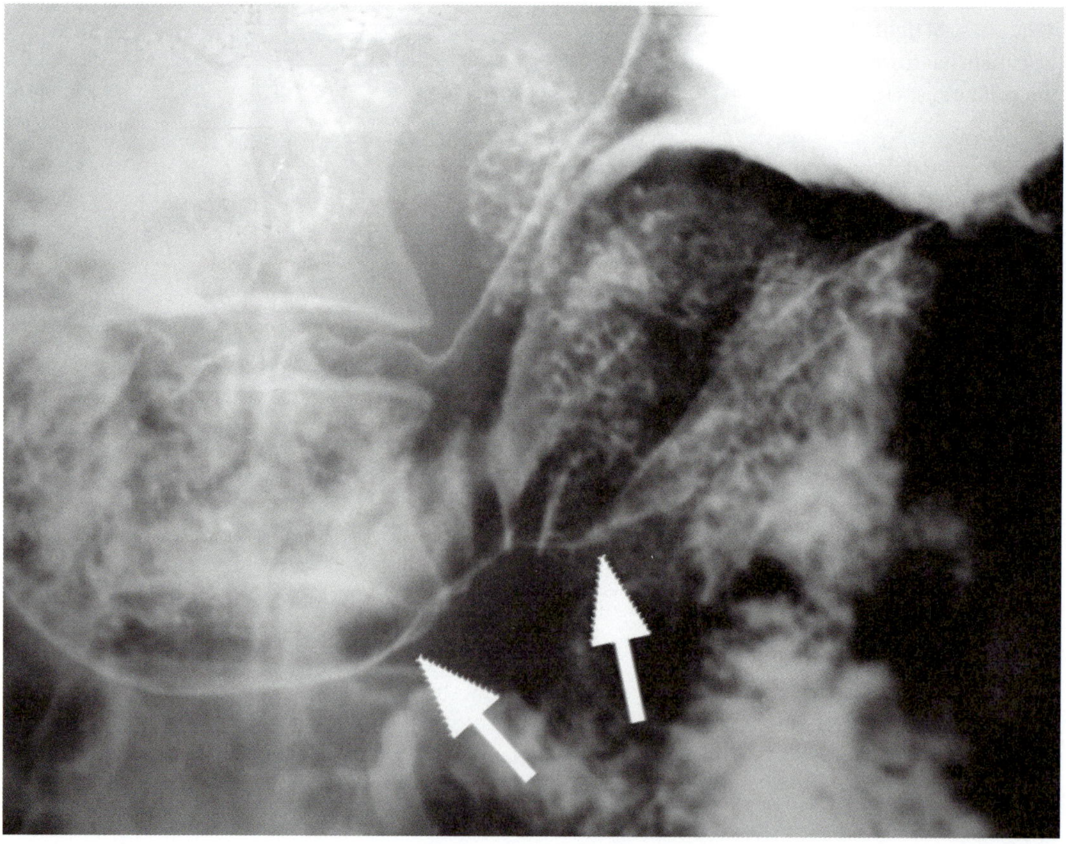

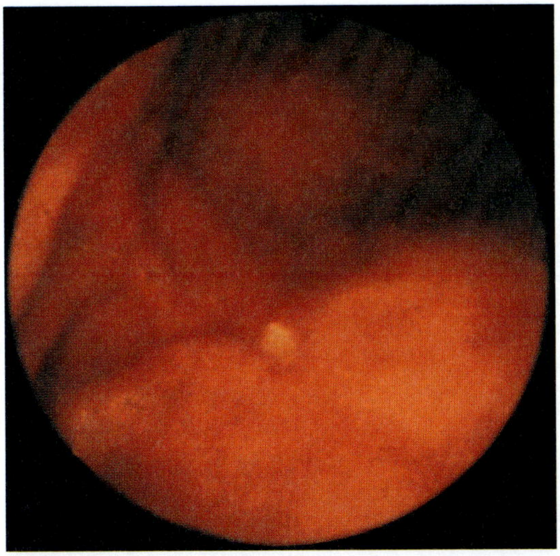

▲ **Fig. 144 e.**

Fig. 144 a–g. Female patient V., age 48. Diagnosis: gastric cancer. **a** Stomach roentgenogram (tight filling, vertical position, anterior projection): on the greater curvature in the proximal portion of the antral part visualized is a small portion of an uneven contour, which is slightly depressed into the stomach cavity (arrow); peristalsis is seen over the entire length. **b, c** Stomach roentgenograms (tight filling, vertical position, anterior projection), dosed compression: a site of infiltration with a centrally located niche of irregular rounded shape within confinements of the stomach contours (corresponding to the revealed changes) is seen (arrows). **d** Stomach roentgenogram (double contrast, horizontal position, anterior projection): a portion of infiltrated wall is seen on the greater curvature of the proximal part of the antral part with folds converging towards infiltration (arrows). Conclusion: Infiltrative-ulcerous cancer of the greater curvature of the antral part of the stomach. **e** Endophotograph: a portion of the mucous membrane of grayish pink color, with a rough surface, slightly elevated over the surrounding tissues is seen in the sinus of the stomach on its greater curvature; folds of mucous membrane converge toward the margins of this portion; ulceration sized 0.4 x 0.3 x 0.1 cm is seen at the center of infiltration; its margins are scarlet, the floor is covered with a fibrin coat. Histological examinations of the bioptates verified non-differentiated cancer. **f** Macrospecimen of the resected stomach: the wall of the greater curvature is firm; a portion of the intramural infiltration with folds converging towards it is visualized (arrows). **g** Fragment of the macrospecimen (strip): the stomach wall is thickened due to intramural infiltration (arrows).

▼ **Fig. 144 f.**

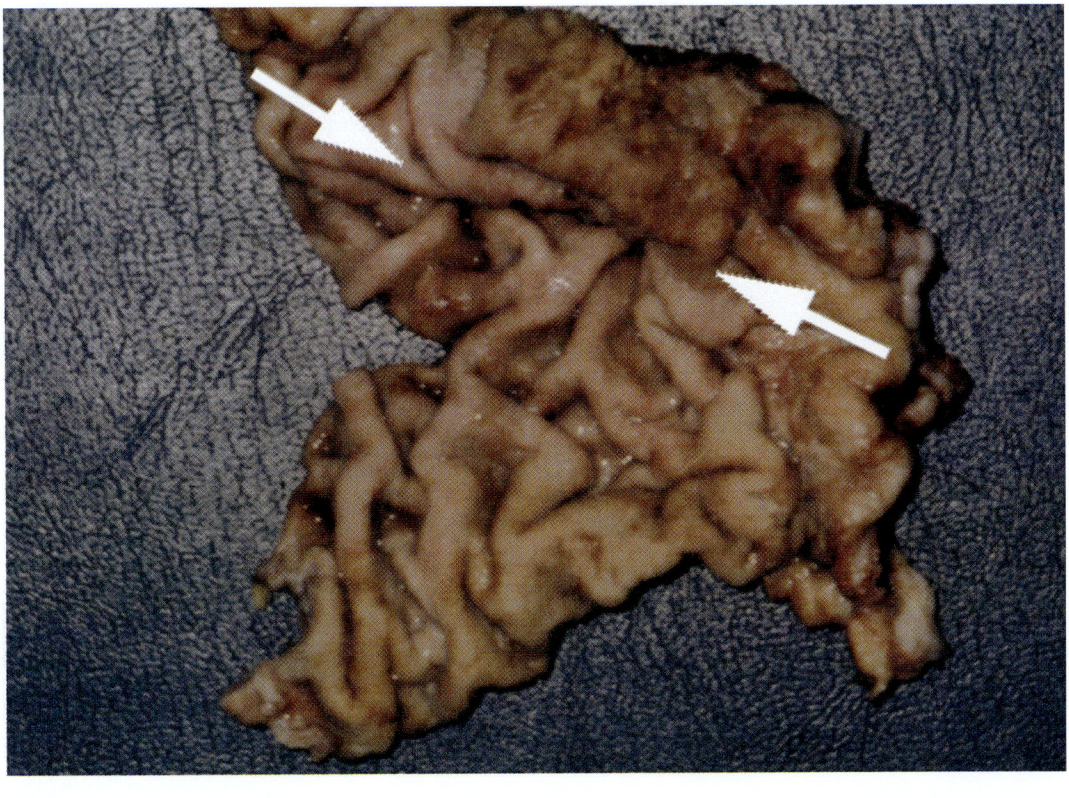

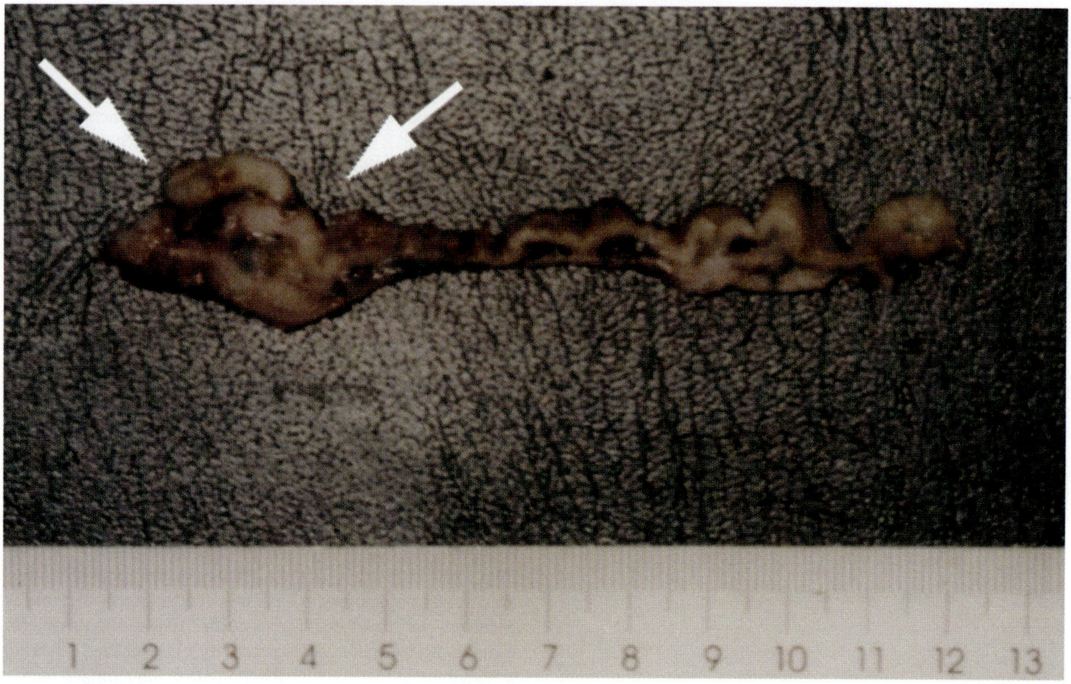

▲ **Fig. 144 g.**

▼ **Fig. 145 a.**

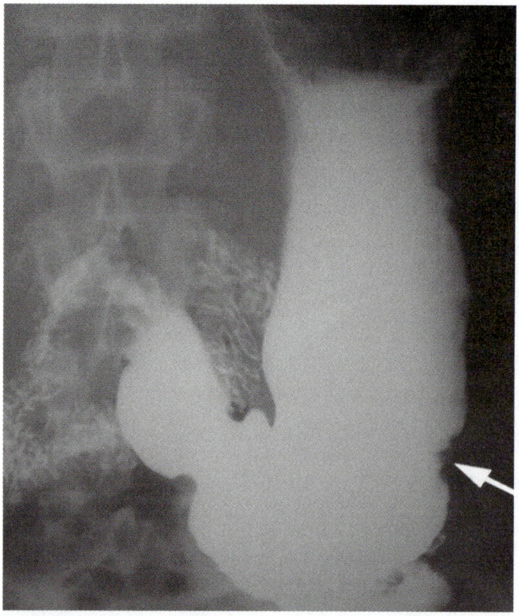

▼ **Fig. 145 b.**

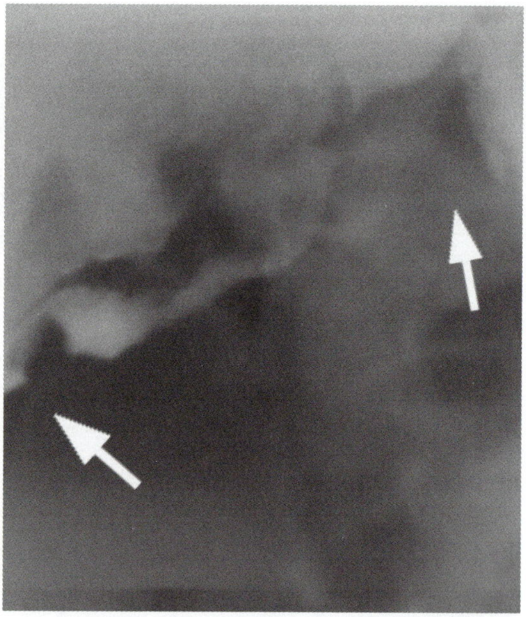

Fig. 145 a–d. Patient A., age 61. Diagnosis: gastric cancer. **a** Stomach roentgenogram (tight filling, vertical position, right anterior quarter-oblique projection): uneven contour of the greater curvature of the sinus (arrow). **b, c** Stomach roentgenograms (tight filling, vertical position, left half-oblique projection), dosed compression: folds converge toward the infiltration on the greater curvature (arrows). **d** Stomach roentgenogram (double contrast, horizontal position, anterior projection): a portion of infiltrated wall on the greater curvature of the sinus with thickened folds converging toward this portion (arrow). Conclusion: Infiltrative cancer of the greater curvature of the stomach sinus. The patient was operated. Histologically, signet-ring cell carcinoma.

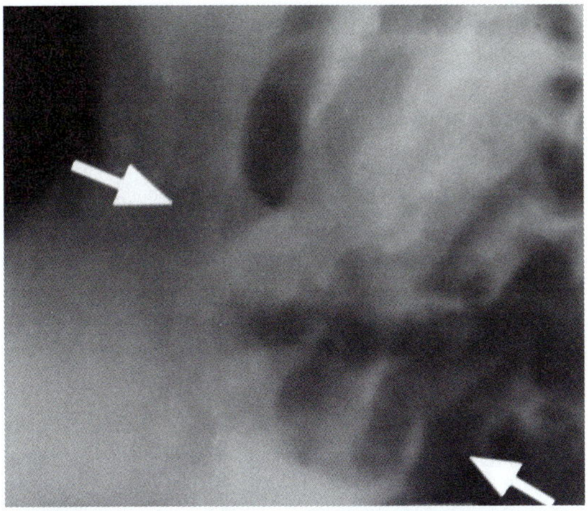

▲ Fig. 145 c. ▼ Fig. 145 d.

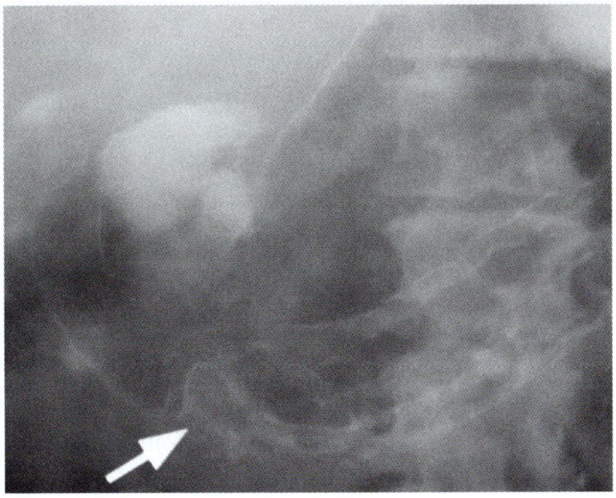

The double-contrast investigation is of special importance. It helps to assess not only the condition of the mucous membrane but also the stomach wall thickness. The method is universal, because in addition to visualizing organic changes it also helps to detect functional disorders, which are manifested by decreasing elasticity of the infiltrated stomach wall. Quantitative information obtained by this method exceeds the findings of any other modification of classical methods of examination without double contrast. Neither the presence of peristaltic activity nor the absence of deformation of the relief can today confirm the absence of endophytic gastric cancer. Diffuse cancers of the greater curvature are the main difficulty in classical roentgenology; at the same time, this is a field where the informative value of X-ray studies is not worse than that of fibergastroscopy (◘ Fig. 145).

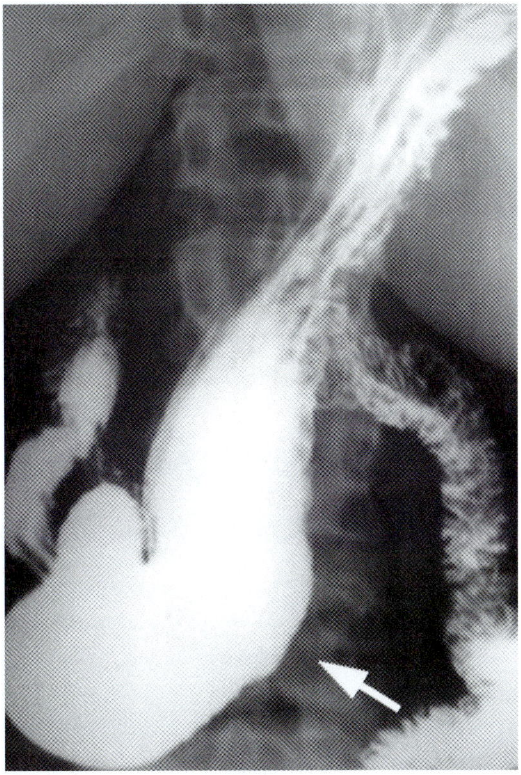

▲ **Fig. 146 a.**

◘ **Fig. 146 a–g.** Female patient Ch., age 42. Diagnosis: gastric cancer. **a** Stomach roentgenogram (tight filling, vertical position, left anterior quarter-oblique projection): uneven contours of greater curvature on lower third of stomach body (arrow). **b, c, d, e** Stomach roentgenograms (tight filling, vertical position, left half-oblique projection), dosed compression: visualized at different degrees of compression is a depot of contrast medium with infiltration ridge and folds converging toward it (terminating at the periphery) on the greater curvature in lower third of stomach body (arrows). Conclusion: Infiltrative-ulcerous cancer of the greater curvature of the lower third of the stomach body. Endoscopy with subsequent histological examination of bioptates failed to reveal tumor affection. The patient was examined by MRI of the stomach. **f** MR image of the stomach (coronary projection in conditions of tight filling of the stomach cavity with water, T2 SSFSE): uneven contour of the greater curvature in the lower third of the stomach body (arrow). **g** MR image (coronary projection, tight filling of the stomach with water, FSPGR out of phase): uneven contour of the greater curvature in the lower third of the stomach body. The wall is thickened over a distance of 28 mm, heterogeneous MR signal (arrows). The serous membrane is seen at all levels, including the site of wall thickening. Conclusion: Infiltrative-ulcerous cancer of the greater curvature in the lower third of the stomach body without involvement of the serous coat of the stomach wall. The patient was operated. Histologically, non-differentiated cancer.

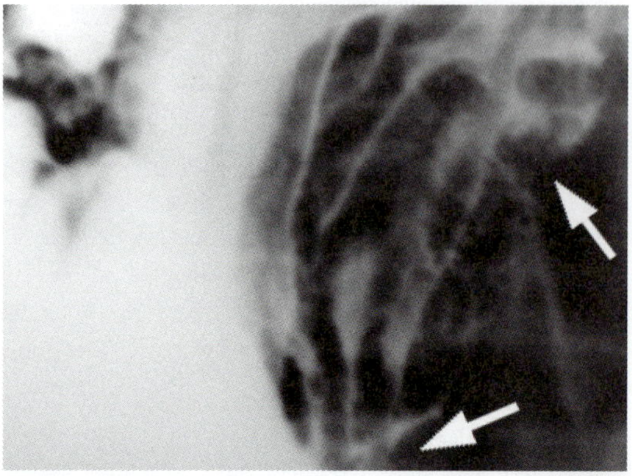

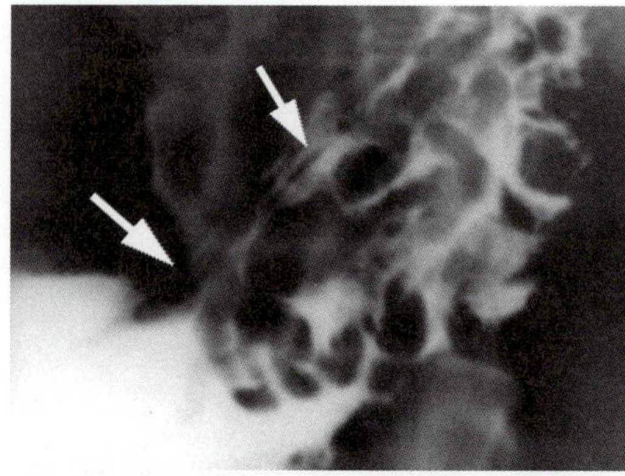

▲ Fig. 146 b. ▼ Fig. 146 c. ▲ Fig. 146 d. ▼ Fig. 146 e.

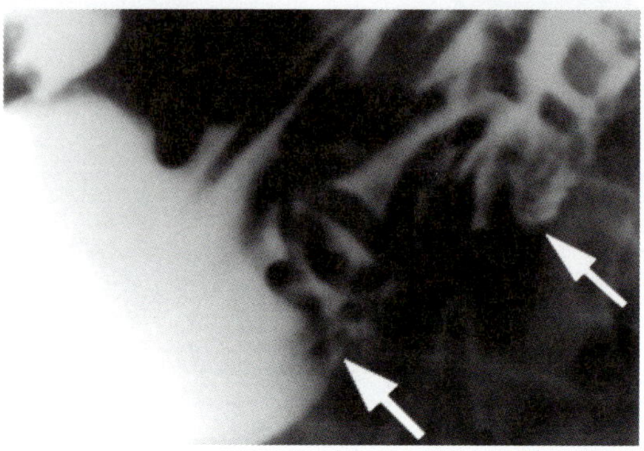

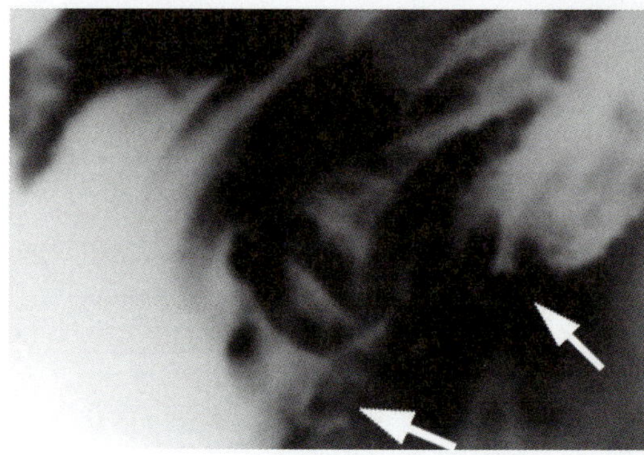

In some of our observations, the double-contrast investigation proved to be the only effective tool to diagnose cancer of the greater curvature at its initial stage. Another field of application of this method is target endoscopy, during which tissue specimens are taken from the zone where X-ray examination has suspected the presence of a tumor. Bioptates are taken using instruments (aspiration, needle, »hot« biopsy, etc.) specially designed for taking tissue specimens from the submucous coat. But G. Caletti et al. (1989) indicate that these methods often prove ineffective. Verification of the site for taking tissue specimens by staining the mucous membrane of the stomach affected by superficially growing tumor, which is effective in 95–97% of cases, becomes infeasible with submucous spread of the tumor [24]. X-ray findings become decisive in such cases.

Close cooperation between a radiological diagnostician and an endoscopist is the guarantee of successful detection of gastric cancer. Japanese researchers united radiology and endoscopy in a single program for examination of risk groups for gastric cancer, based on standardized semiotics, methodology, and surgical treatment, to attain unprecedented success in diagnosis and treatment.

Ulcerated tumors occur mostly on the greater curvature. Although they are possible to diagnose at present, they nevertheless remain a serious problem in gastroentero-ocology. Difficulties that arise in revealing tumor substrate on the greater curvature add to the problems of differentiating between benign and malignant ulcerations. Additional problems arise with signs which are not characteristic of typical cancer ulcers. Either they are difficult to identify or they resemble common peptic ulcer. X-ray examinations in such cases revealed depression on the contour and a niche (as distinct from blastomatous ulceration of the lesser curvature, which extends beyond the limits of the stomach contour in rare cases). The ridge of infiltrated tissue is more pronounced; the folds may converge not toward the ulcerated site but toward the infiltration ridge (■ Fig. 146) [46].

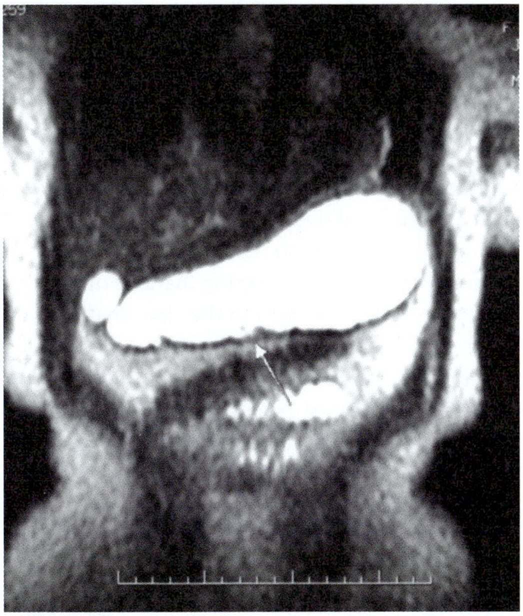

▲ **Fig. 146 f.** ▼ **Fig. 146 g.**

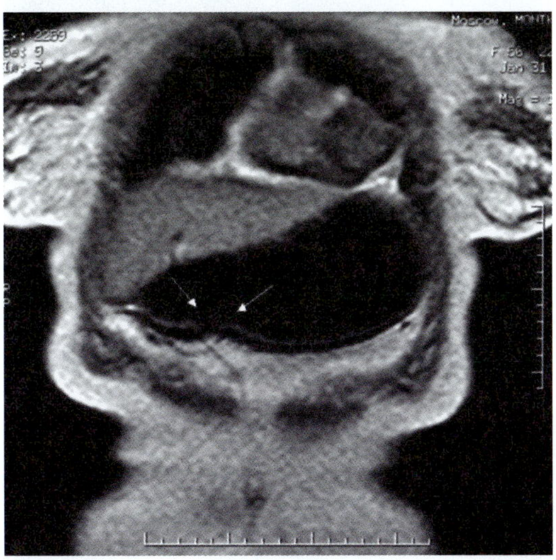

Specific ulceration of the greater curvature and differential diagnosis became the subject of concern of oncologists early in the twentieth century, at the dawn of roentgenology. Holmes and Hempton (1932) concluded from their observations that all ulcers of this localization require surgery. Smith and Jordan (1948) strengthened the opinion that ulcers on the greater curvature are malignant in 60% cases. Bourdeau et al. (1951) and McClone and Robertson (1953) revealed malignant ulceration of the greater curvature in 49–56% of all ulcers of the stomach. This concern of the specialists was shared by radiologists.

In the 1950s and 1960s, many publications dealt with the problem of X-ray diagnosis of malignant and benign ulcers of the greater curvature. They all reflected the inability of classical radiology, based on the traditional method of tight filling, to establish definite criteria for differential diagnosis of these conditions. Signs of malignant ulcers (convergence of mucosal folds toward the ulcer, their termination at the infiltration ridge, location of the niche within the confinements of the stomach contours, etc.), which are more characteristic of pathologies of the lesser curvature, are often useless in conditions affecting the anatomical and functional properties of the greater curvature.

We want to explain our opinion on infiltrative cancer of the greater curvature based on the results of studies using traditional methods and the double-contrast technique with obligatory endoscopy as an additional tool of examining the abdominal cavity and the stomach (in recent years we have also used ultrasonogrpaphy, CT, or MRI). Our experience shows that a methodologically correct examination can reveal some signs that are quite specific for infiltrative-ulcerous cancer. The most important of these, which help to establish the radiological diagnosis, are the following: irregular shapes of the ulcer crater with overhanging and eroded contours, walls thickened to various degrees and to various lengths, upset peristalsis, and elasticity of the stomach walls.

We want to note again that with discovery of any ulcer of the stomach, and especially on its greater curvature, the main objective of the radiological diagnostician is to rule out blastomatous infiltration. Even with dynamic observation during treatment of the patient, in cases where endoscopic signs of ulceration disappear, only the stability of intramural changes helps the physician to avoid fatal diagnostic errors.

The greater curvature is more frequently affected by blastomatous process of mostly diffuse character than was believed in the 1990s. Therefore, discovery of signs of cancer infiltration at this localization must suggest the use of »extreme« technologies: ingestion of greater amounts of contrast medium, maximum permissible inflation of the stomach. These measures give more accurate information on the presence or absence of infiltrative cancer of the greater curvature of the stomach with or without ulceration.

To conclude this section, it is necessary to note that, like cancer of the anterior wall, cancer of the greater curvature has many »latent« aspects which should be considered today by both diagnosticians and clinicians. First and foremost is the considerably greater percentage of endophytic (diffuse) cancers at their early stages, and also the important role of updated means of radiological diagnosis such as ultrasonography, CT, and MRI in their detection.

Cancer of the Anterior Wall

Even today popular opinion holds that cancer of the anterior wall is an extremely rare incidence. In supporting of this point of view, allusion is made to the absence of statistical data on the frequency of new growths at this localization in the great majority of publications. Based on our experience, we do not agree with this opinion. The more so that some other authors have the same view of this problem as ours (T. Hirota et al. 1984; W. Meyer et al. 1987). They indicate the tendency to an increasing proportion of cancers of the anterior wall. D. Brandt et al. (1989) state that the percentage of cancer of the anterior wall in the antral part of the stomach is the same as that of tumors located on the posterior wall in this part of the stomach. Our opinion on this problem coincides with that of researchers who believe that the anterior wall is the site where gastric cancer occurs more frequently than is believed by many authors. But diagnosis of new growths at this localization is difficult because their possibility is underestimated. Cancer of the anterior wall does not show clinically until evacuation dysfunction of the stomach or of the esophagus develops due to severe circular narrowing of the organ. This usually happens in patients with far advanced cancer when it is no longer possible to locate the primary site of the tumor. Screening programs developed in Japan make it possible to significantly improve detection of primary cancers of the anterior wall. This stimulated researchers in other countries to take a new look at the problem [143, 239]. Our research also confirms this standpoint [31, 34, 223, 224].

The special methodological approach to diagnosis of cancer of the anterior wall consists in special projections for this region of the stomach body and its antral part, and in using additional techniques such as »mild and incomplete« compression under fluoroscopy guidance (Fig. 147). The non-standard nature of anterior wall imaging made roentgenologists pay special attention to the examination procedure itself. This involved changes in methodology. Thus, Hisamichi et al. [144] recommended that the patient ingest the first portions of barium sulfate suspension in the prone position, which gives unexpected results. Roentgenological screening conducted by this method revealed a markedly increased incidence of early cancers of the anterior wall of the stomach [142, 143].

▼ **Fig. 147 a.**

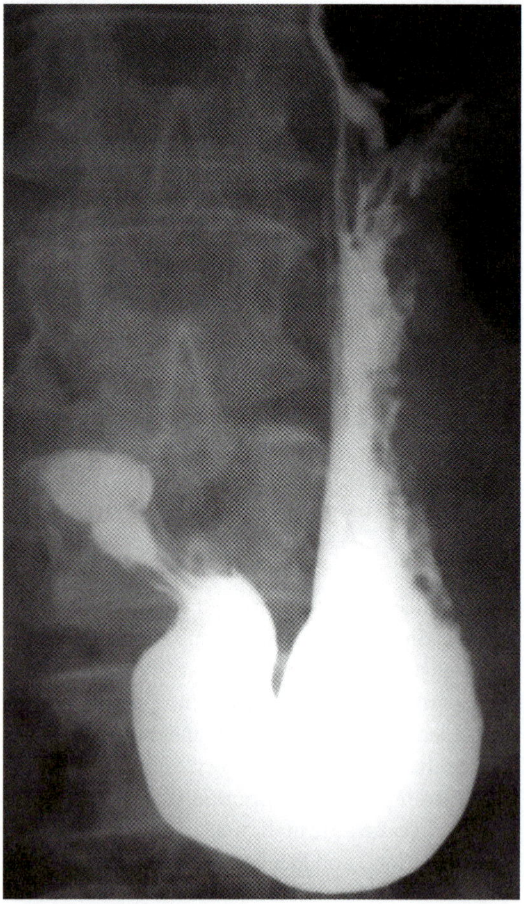

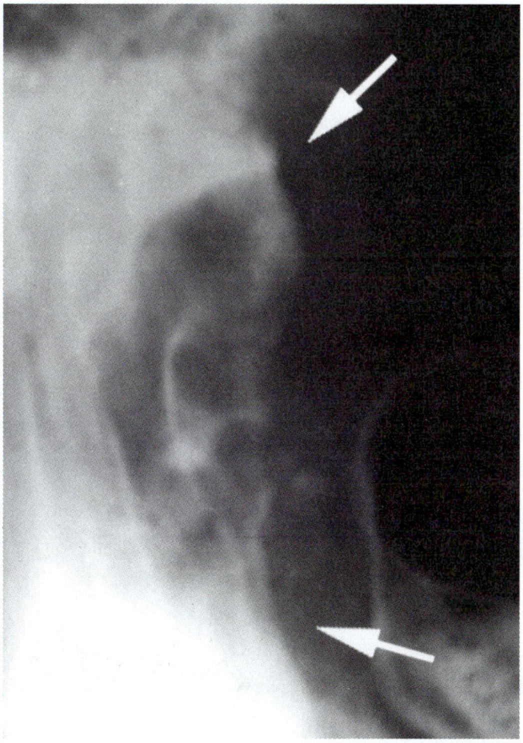

▲ Fig. 147 b.

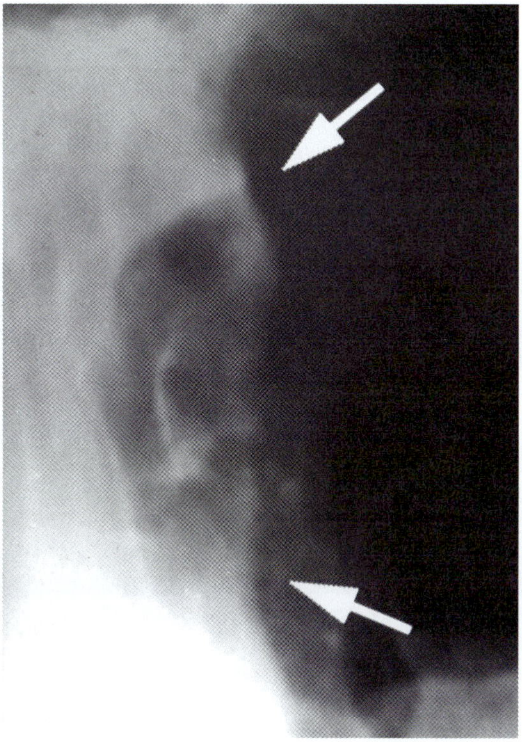

▼ Fig. 147 c.

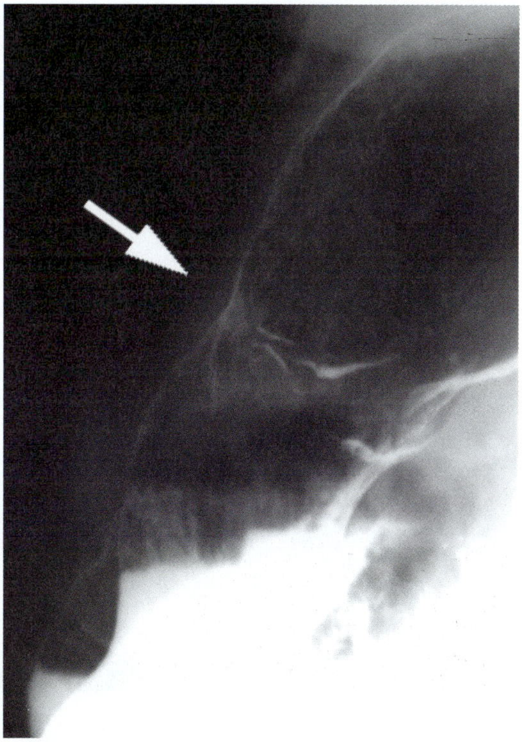

▲ Fig. 147 d.

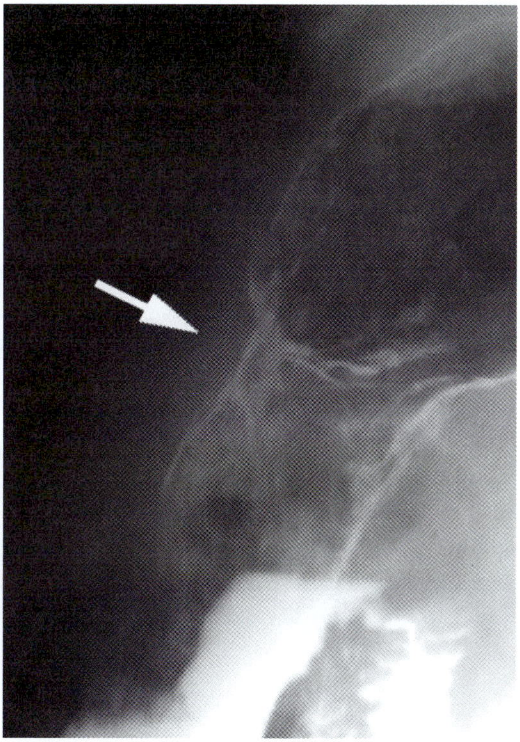

▼ Fig. 147 e.

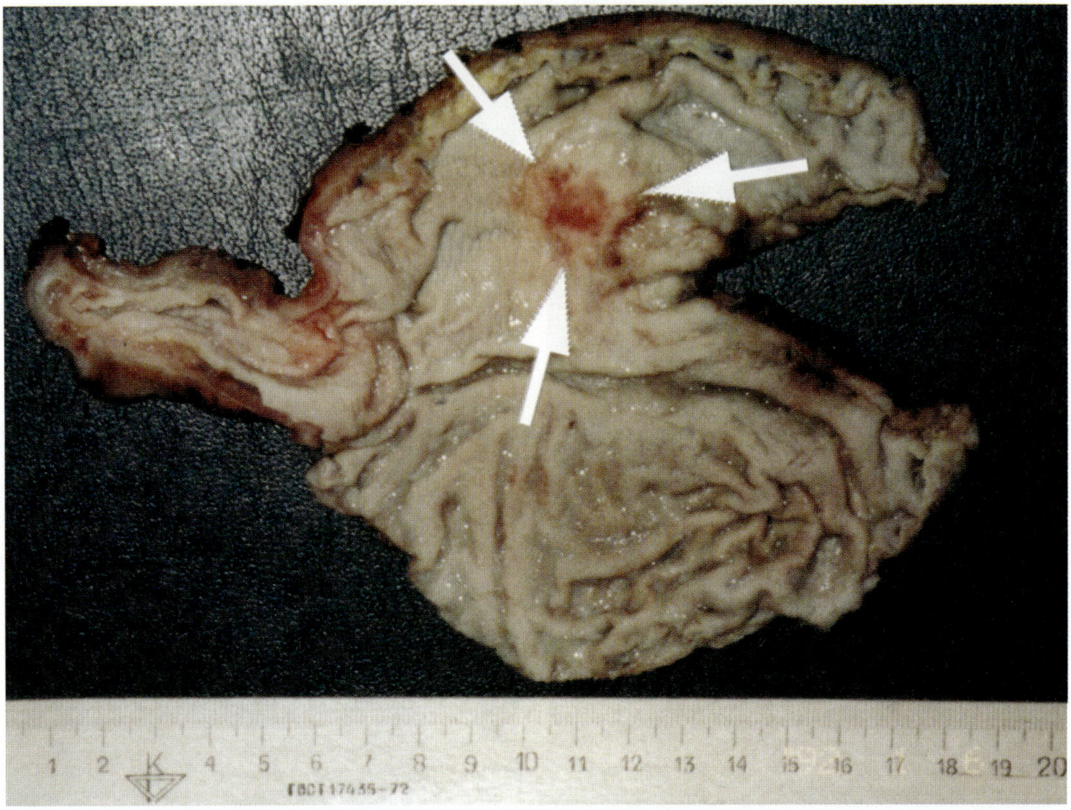

▲ Fig. 147 f.

▼ Fig. 147 g.

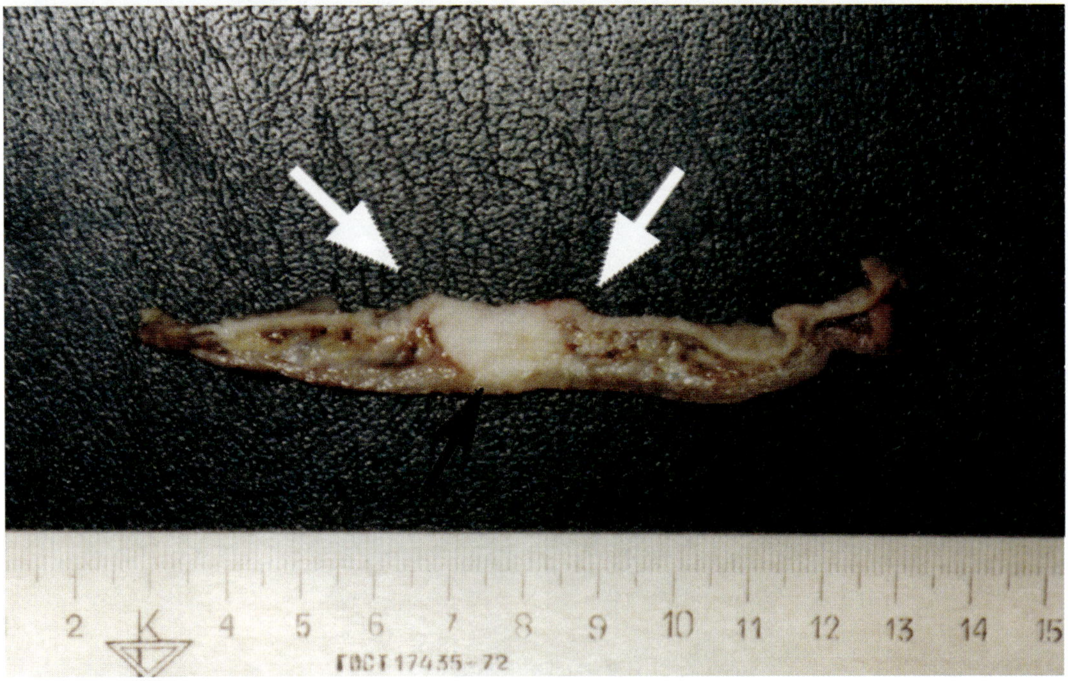

Fig. 147 a–g. Female patient A., age 56. Diagnosis: gastric cancer. **a** Stomach roentgenogram (tight filling, vertical position, anterior projection): organic changes are not detectable. **b, c** Stomach roentgenograms (tight filling, vertical position, left half-oblique projection), dosed compression: slight compression visualizes a depot of contrast medium on the anterior wall of the stomach body in the form of a spider surrounded by a ridge of infiltrated tissue with folds terminating at the periphery (arrows). **d** Stomach roentgenogram (double contrast, vertical position, left anterior oblique projection): the anterior wall of the upper third of the stomach body is thickened due to intramural infiltration (arrow); the folds converge toward the affected site. **e** Stomach roentgenogram (double contrast, vertical position, left lateral projection): with optimal projection, more distinctly visualized is thickening of the anterior wall of the upper third of the stomach body due to intramural infiltration (arrow) and the folds converging toward the involved part. Conclusion: Infiltrative-ulcerous cancer of the anterior wall of the upper third of the stomach body. **f** Macrospecimen of the resected stomach: ulceration with an atypical relief is seen on the anterior wall (arrows). **g** Fragment of the macrospecimen (strip): the stomach wall is thickened due to white intramural infiltration of mostly mucous and submucous coats (white arrows); initial invasion of the muscular coat (black arrow). Histologically, signet-ring cell carcinoma.

The complexity of the skiagram suggested the necessity of searching for optimal approaches to the diagnosis of cancer at this location. Some authors proposed special projections and techniques. The following seem to be the most important:

1. Left anterior oblique projection, more suitable for visualization of the pyloric ring
2. Left lateral projection
3. Posterior straight or left oblique projection in the horizontal position

In our practical work, we usually use the following techniques. Where it is necessary to examine the anterior wall of the antral part, we use tight filling of the stomach with a slightly excessive amount of barium sulfate suspension and turn the patient to the left lateral projection, taking a series of X-ray pictures under compression. The anterior wall of the stomach body is easy to image using one of the standard projections: left lateral projection in the vertical or horizontal position, both with tight filling and double contrast (Fig. 148).

With special emphasis on the diagnosis of cancer with its primary location on the anterior wall, we want to note once again how updated technical facilities can change our concept of the pathology under discussion. Information adequate for the preoperative establishment of diagnosis can be obtained only in cases where the methodology agrees with the technical components of the diagnostic process. As applied to infiltrative cancers located on the anterior wall, we want to discuss some problems we have encountered in our practical experience. We have observed situations in which such tumors spread to more vulnerable anatomical structures, such as the lesser curvature and the greater curvature of the stomach. Minor changes, often called partial changes on the contour, suggested early or minor cancer. But the projections used specifically for visualization of the anterior wall not only removed any doubt of the tumor, but also verified its primary location on the anterior wall. [28, 223].

Using the necessary additional methods, which differ depending on the location of the tumor in the stomach body or its antral part, we obtained quite specific signs of tumor infiltration. These included local thickening of the wall over short distances with converging folds, which produce an indistinct stellar pattern, or certain contraction, and asymmetry of mucosal relief. The signs detectable with double-contrast radiology are supplemented by the traditional signs of uneven contours in the presence of tight filling and disfiguring changes which become apparent with compression of the involved part of the stomach, if the tumor is found in the lower third of the stomach body and its antral part.

By filling the stomach with a slightly greater portion of barium sulfate suspension at the phase of tight filling and applying the minimal possible compression, it is possible to visualize such signs of early cancer of the anterior wall as spiders (under 0.6–0.8 cm) against the background of the relief of the anterior wall of the stomach (▸ Fig. 55). When dosed compression is applied in such situations, it is possible to see at this level a distinct (limited to 1 cm) thickening of the wall with one or two folds terminating at this level.

In other words, tight filling of the stomach with the above mentioned additional meals and dosed compression form a special complex in current radiological diagnosis which can reveal early manifestation of gastric cancer. This becomes feasible if the physician remembers that roentgenogastroenterology can give important results in diagnosis of gastric cancer, and if the radiologist disposes of sufficient knowledge and skills in using the methods and fundamental signs.

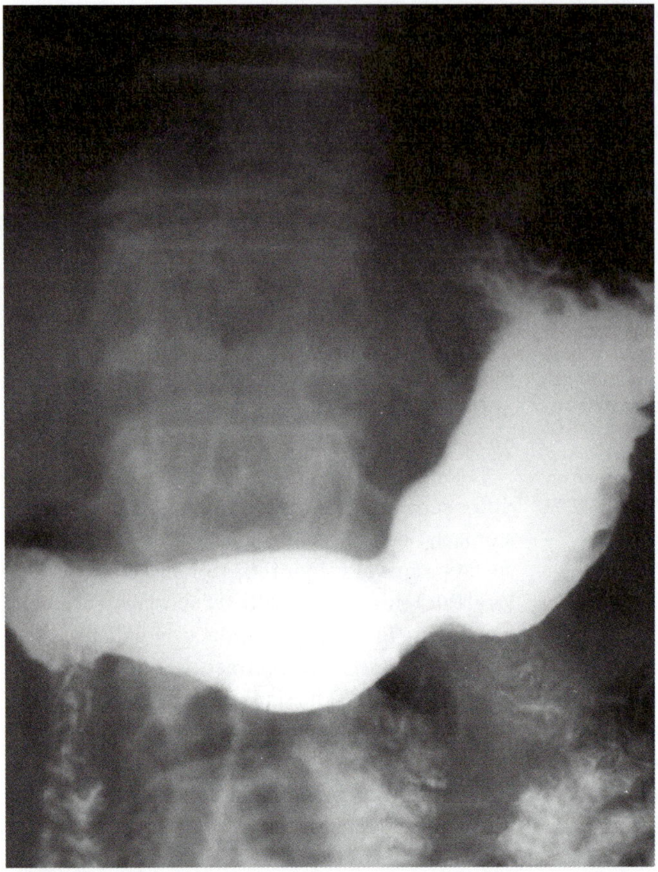

▲ **Fig. 148 a.**

Fig. 148 a, b. Patient D., age 62. Diagnosis: gastric cancer. **a** Stomach roentgenogram (tight filling, vertical position, anterior projection): organic changes are not detectable. **b** Stomach roentgenogram (double contrast, horizontal position, left lateral projection): the anterior wall of the lower third of the stomach body is thickened due to intramural infiltration with folds converging toward it (arrow). Conclusion: Minor infiltrative cancer of the anterior wall of the lower third of the stomach body. The patient was operated. Histologically, adenocarcinoma with the signet-ring cell component.

Fig. 149 a–d. Female patient S., age 56. Diagnosis: gastric cancer. **a** Stomach roentgenogram (tight filling, vertical position, anterior projection): horn-shaped stomach. **b** Stomach roentgenogram (double contrast, horizontal position, anterior projection): no organic changes are found; stomach walls are elastic and of normal thickness. **c** Stomach roentgenogram (double contrast, horizontal position, left lateral projection): anterior wall of upper third of the stomach is thickened (arrow). **d** Stomach roentgenogram (double contrast, vertical position, left lateral projection): anterior wall of upper third of the stomach body is thickened due to intramural infiltration with the folds converging toward it (arrow). Conclusion: Minor infiltrative cancer of the anterior wall of the stomach body. The patient was operated. Histologically, signet-ring cell carcinoma.

▼ **Fig. 148 b.**

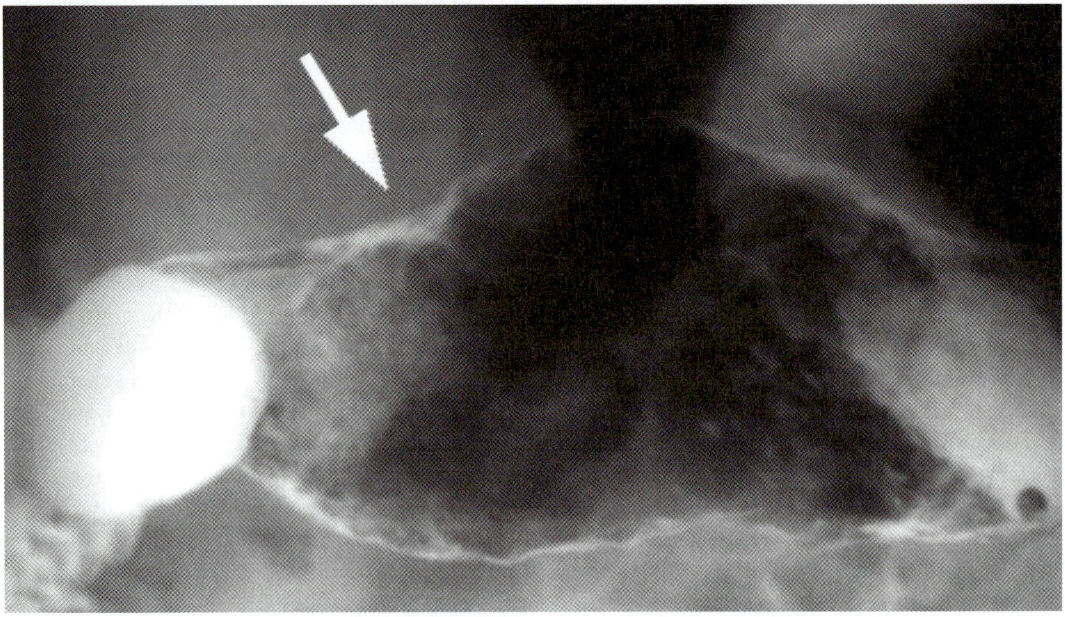

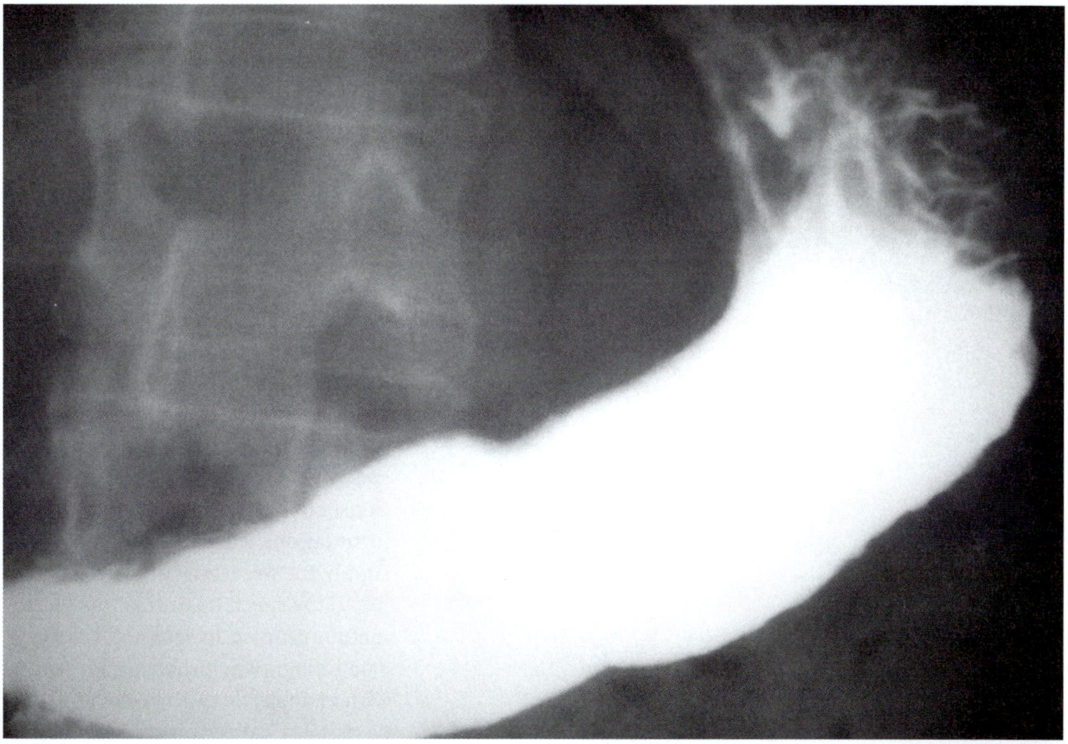

▲ **Fig. 149 a.**

▼ **Fig. 149 b.**

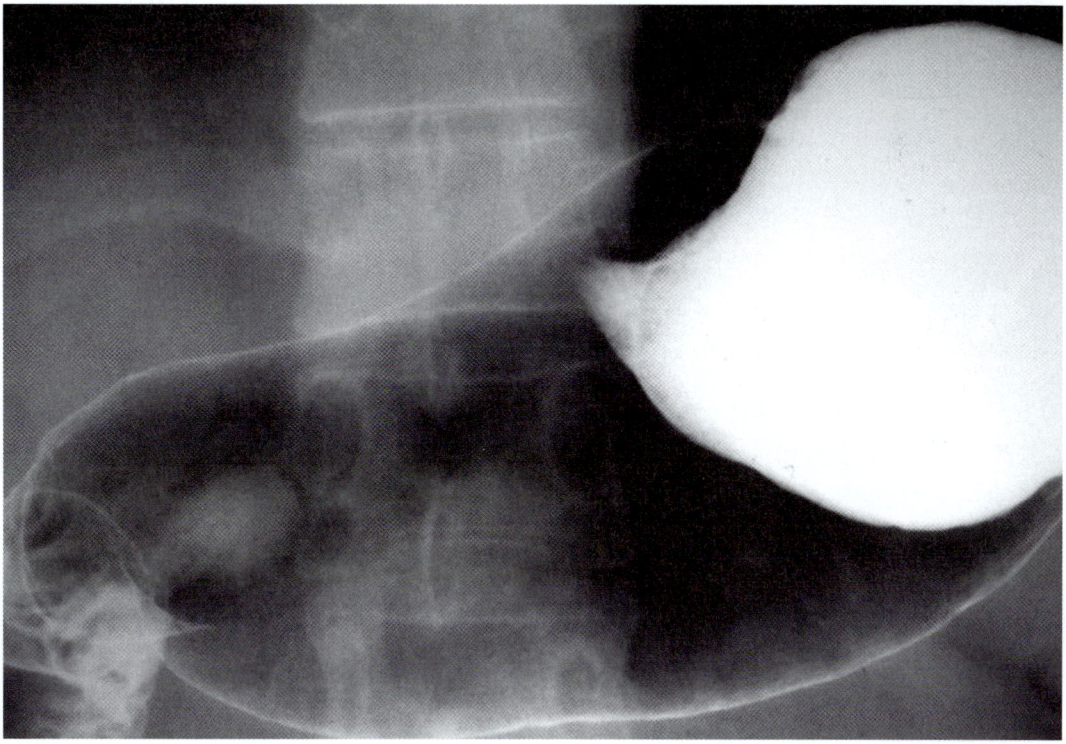

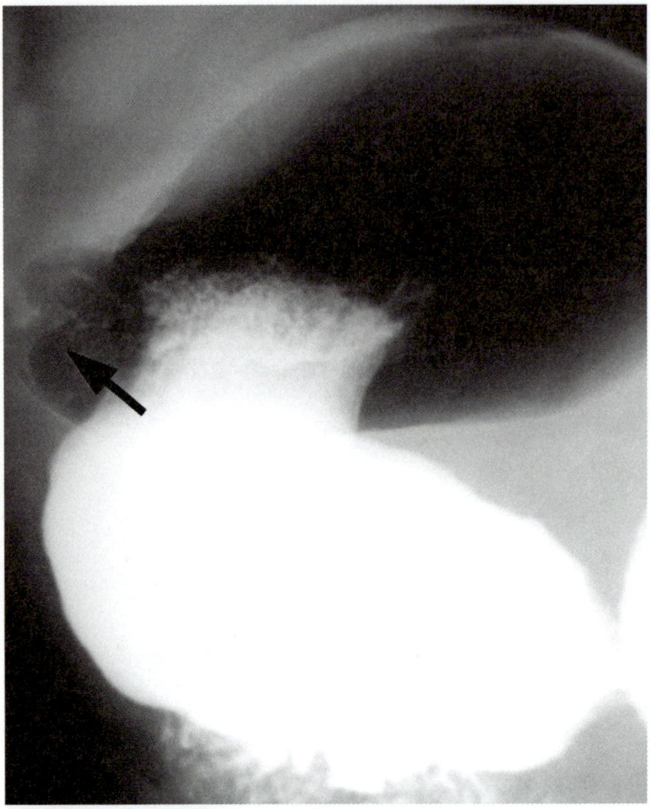

▲ Fig. 149 c.

The additional tools available to radiological diagnosis and the improved methodological approaches to detecting gastric cancer can provide a new assessment of the structure of tumors not only by their localization, but also, in most cases, by the character of spread of the malignant process. The accumulated material shows the necessity of revising the role of radiological examination in the early diagnosis of diffuse cancer. Potentials of radiological diagnosis are important not only to create optimal conditions for taking tissue specimens for histological examinations, but also to solve some problems in situations where endoscopy fails to supply the necessary information owing to the special nature of the blastomatous process. In such cases, complicated diagnostic problems associated with endophytic cancers can be solved by radiological examinations, which visualize signs that can be considered sufficiently objective (Fig. 149).

▼ Fig. 149 d.

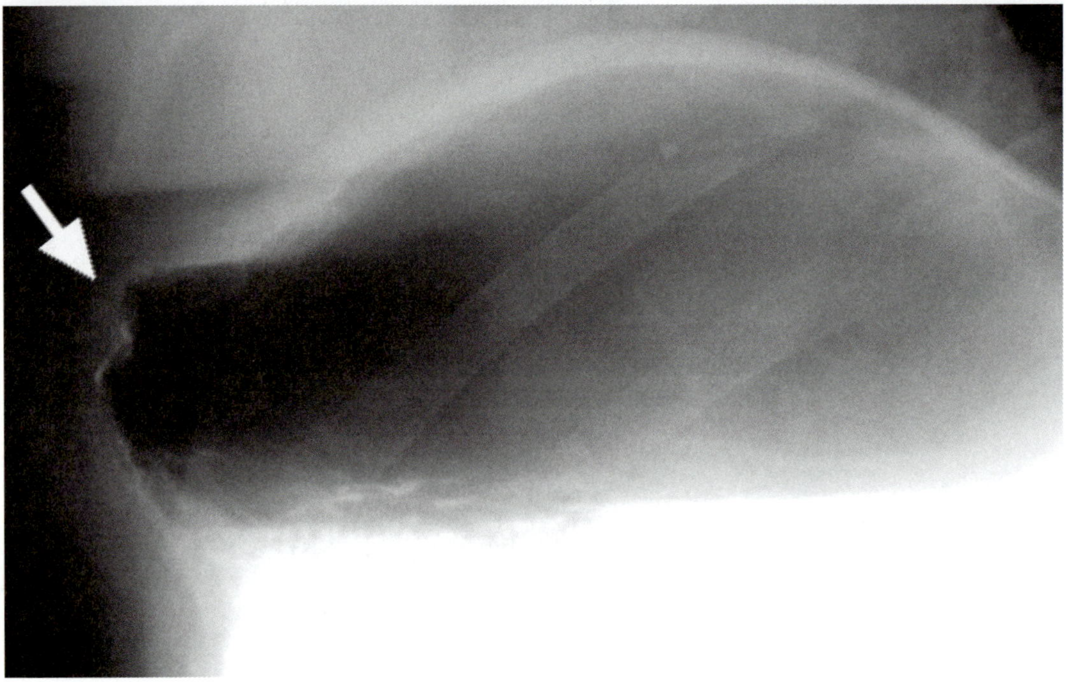

In view of what has been said, the problems of diagnosing cancer in those parts of the stomach that are inaccessible for adequate examination due to their specific anatomical features can be considered in quite a new aspect. While the studies on the anterior wall were started only recently, such anatomical parts of the stomach as the upper and the pyloric parts are discussed in any manual or study worthy of mention. These manuals and studies, however, do not consider the methodological and semiotic »supplements« to radiological examination of the stomach that we have mentioned here, made necessary by the substantial changes that have taken place in the morphogenesis of cancer and regarding its primary localization in various parts of the stomach.

The methods currently used to examine the upper part of the stomach rely on adequate impregnation of its mucous membrane with barium sulfate suspension. This is attainable by tight filling of the stomach and (in view of the specific relief of the mucous membrane) by adequate stretching of the stomach fundus using a gas-producing mixture with double contrast. Adequate selection of a projection for taking X-ray pictures is another important prerequisite to a good examination of the upper part of the stomach (Fig. 125). Although the current standardized method calls for inspection of this region with the patient in several positions, additional techniques must be used in each particular case in the presence of even minimal deviations from the X-ray »standard« [27, 33, 35]. The main projections for examination of the upper part of the stomach are the following:

- Vertical position:
  a. Anterior
  b. Left lateral
- Horizontal plus half-vertical positions:
  a. Left posterior oblique
  b. Left lateral
  c. Left anterior oblique
  d. Right anterior oblique

The most effective positions (as proved by practical experience) are left posterior oblique and left lateral projections with the patient in the horizontal position or half-vertical position, especially when the cardia is examined (Fig. 126).

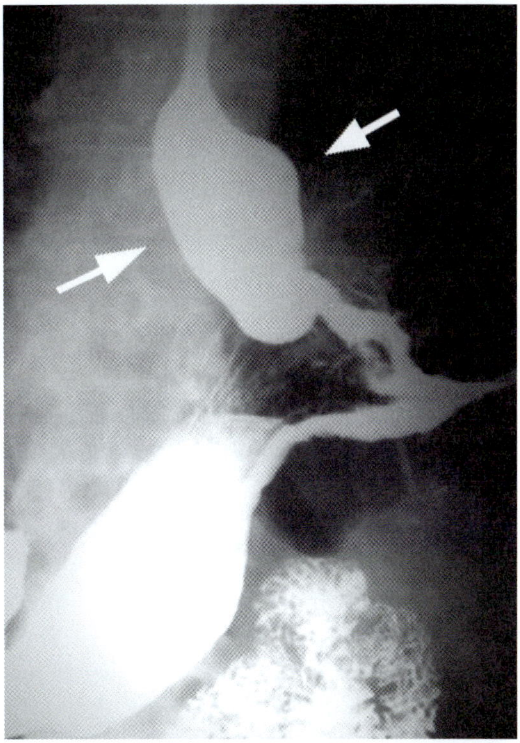

▲ Fig. 125 a.

▼ Fig. 125 b.

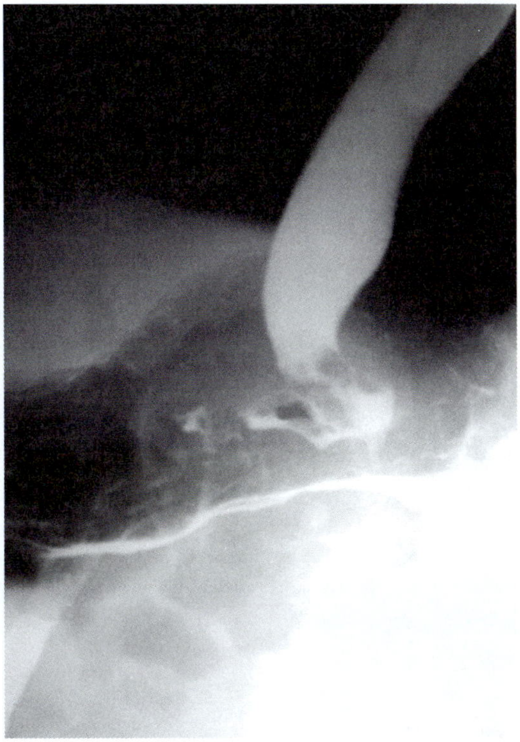

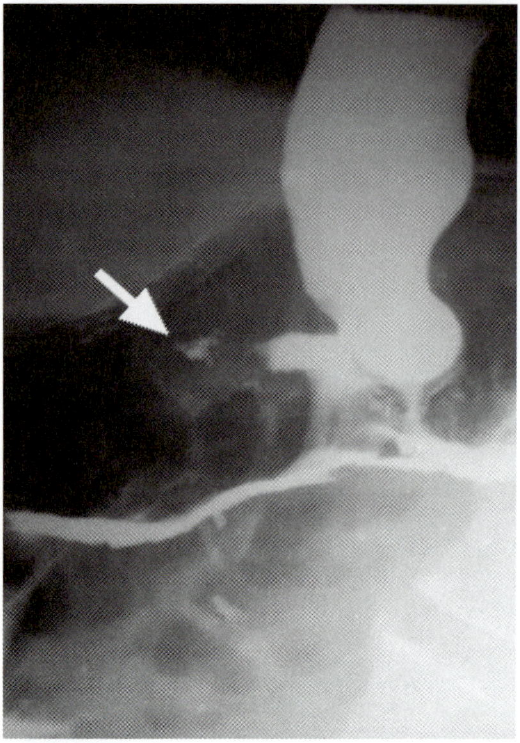

▲ Fig. 125 c.

Fig. 125 a–d. Patient K., age 68. Diagnosis: gastric cancer. According to the patient's estimate, he had been ill for a month, since the day when he first experienced difficult passage of food through the esophagus. A week earlier, epigastric pain developed, for which the patient sought medical aid. Anamnesis revealed the following: for about 8 months the patient had experienced attacks of unmotivated general weakness, occasional discomfort after ingesting solid food, which made him drink water. Later the patient adapted to a special diet and no longer felt discomfort. **a** Stomach roentgenogram (tight filling, vertical position, anterior projection) at the moment of contrast medium passage through the gastroesophageal junction: marked deformation of the upper part of the stomach, the wall of the lesser curvature is thickened, the abdominal segment of the esophagus is strongly disfigured and narrowed in the immediate vicinity of the cardia, its walls are uneven and rigid due to infiltration, suprasthenic dilation of the esophagus over the point of narrowing (arrows) which suggests long-standing difficult patency. **b** Stomach roentgenogram (double contrast, vertical position, left lateral projection) at the moment of contrast medium passage through the gastroesophageal junction: the abdominal segment of the esophagus near the cardia is narrow; atypical relief of the cardioesophageal junction. **c** Stomach roentgenogram (double contrast, vertical position, left lateral projection) at the moment of contrast medium passage through the gastroesophageal junction: uneven narrowing and disfiguring of the abdominal segment of the esophagus,

▼ Fig. 125 d.

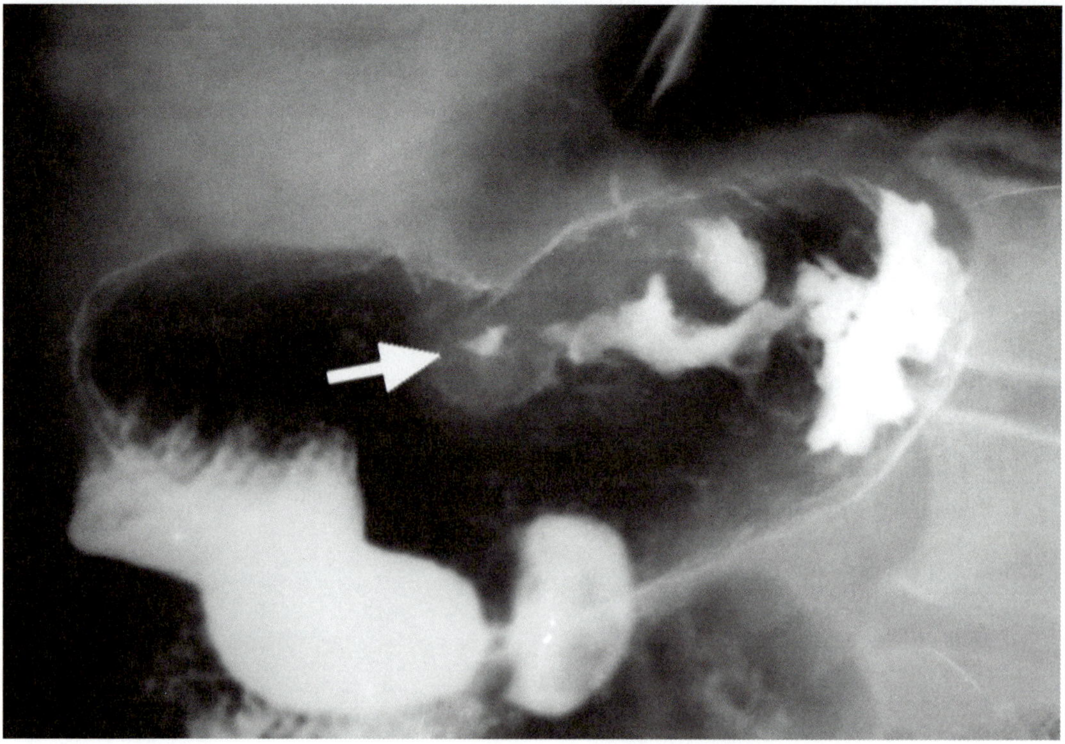

suprasthenic dilatation of the esophagus above the infiltrated part, a depot of contrast medium surrounded by a ridge of infiltration (arrow). **d** Stomach roentgenogram (double contrast, horizontal position, left lateral projection): anterior wall of the upper part is thickened due to intramural infiltration; more distinctly visualized is a depot of contrast medium surrounded by a ridge of infiltration (arrow). Conclusion: Infiltrative-ulcerous cancer of the upper part of the stomach with invasion of the esophagus. The patient was operated. Histologically, signet-ring cell carcinoma.

Fig. 126 a–c. Female patient T., age 68. Diagnosis: gastric cancer. **a** Stomach roentgenogram (tight filling, vertical position, anterior projection) at the moment of contrast medium passage through the gastroesophageal junction: moderately pronounced deformation of the subcardiac part, insignificantly shortened lesser curvature, its contour is uneven, marked deformation of the abdominal segment of the esophagus. **b** Stomach roentgenogram (double contrast, vertical position, left lateral projection) at the moment of contrast medium passage through the gastroesophageal junction: the abdominal segment of the esophagus is unevenly narrowed. **c** Stomach roentgenogram (double contrast, horizontal position, left posterior oblique projection): atypical relief of the cardiac rosette (cardioesophageal junction), the specific radiating pattern is absent. Conclusion: Infiltrative cancer of the upper part of the stomach with invasion of the esophagus. The patient was operated. Histologically, signet-ring cell carcinoma.

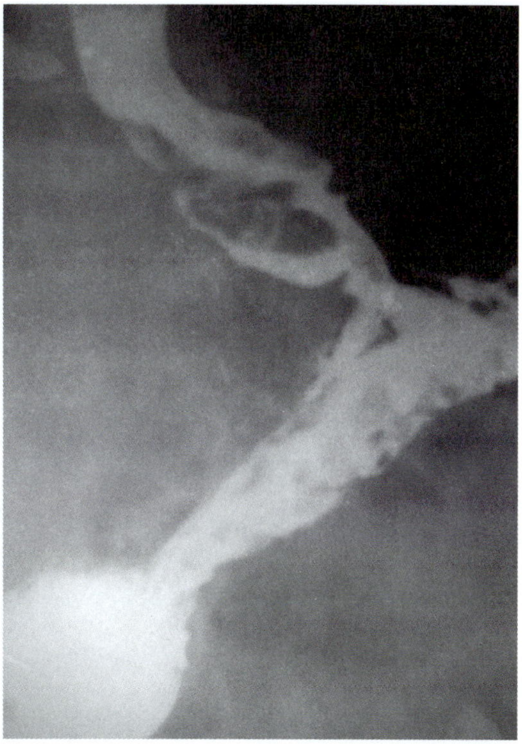

▲ **Fig. 126 a.**

▼ **Fig. 126 b.**

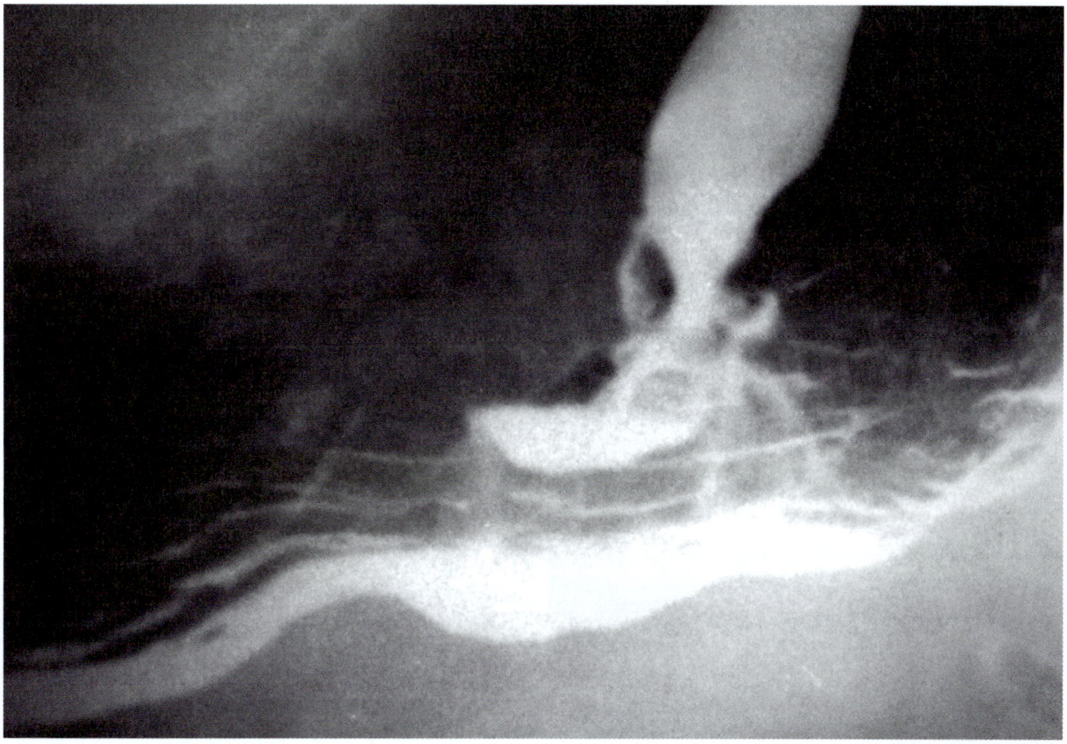

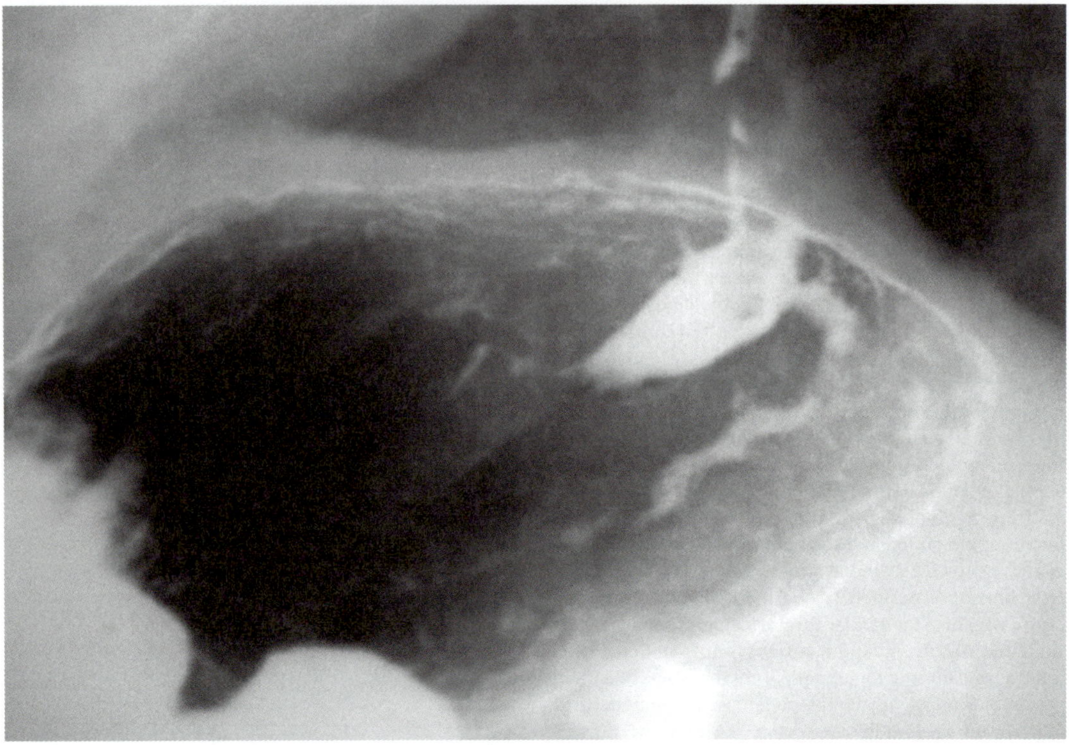

▲ **Fig. 126 c.** ▼ **Fig. 127 a.**

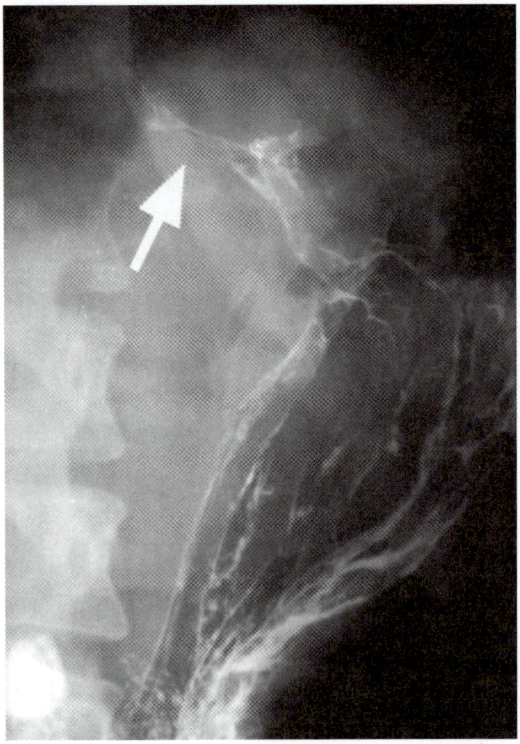

Fig. 127 a–f. Female patient B., age 60. Diagnosis: gastric cancer. **a** Roentgenogram of upper part of the stomach (vertical position, anterior projection): the air bladder is disfigured due intramural infiltration of the upper part of the stomach, the abdominal segment of the esophagus is narrowed unevenly (arrow). **b** Roentgenogram of upper part of the stomach (vertical position, left lateral projection): the walls of the subcardiac and cardiac parts are thickened due to intramural infiltration, light central spot of the ulcer crater (arrows). **c** Roentgenogram of upper part of the stomach (vertical position, left lateral projection) at the moment of contrast medium passage through the gastroesophageal junction: the abdominal segment of the esophagus is narrowed unevenly, its contour is eroded and uneven (arrow), atypical relief of the cardiac cardioesophageal junction. **d** Roentgenogram of upper part of the stomach (double contrast, horizontal position, left lateral projection): a ridge of infiltration with the light center (arrows) is visualized in the projection of the subcardiac part and cardioesophageal junction. Conclusion: Infiltrative-ulcerous cancer of the upper part of the stomach with invasion of the esophagus. **e** Macrospecimen of the resected stomach: tumor tissue of the upper part of the stomach with the ulcer in the center (black arrows). Infiltration spreads onto the esophagus (white arrows). **f** Fragment of the macrospecimen (strip): stomach wall is thickened due to white intramural infiltration (arrows). Histologically, adenocarcinoma with the signet-ring cell component.

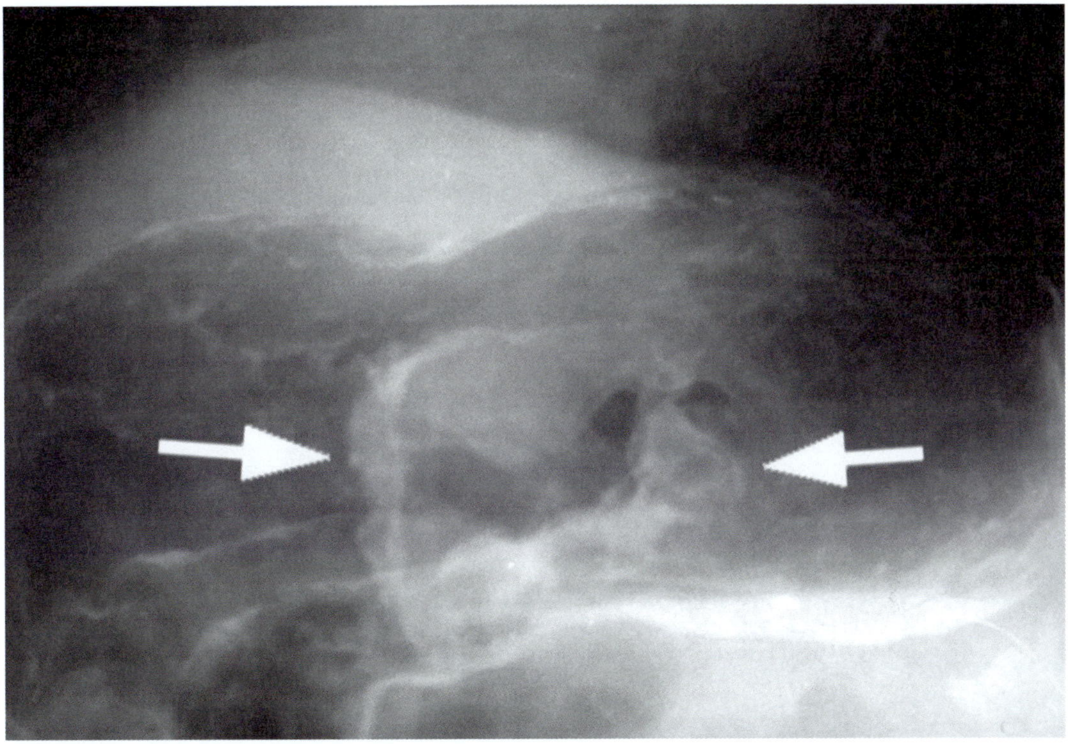

▲ **Fig. 127 b.**

▼ **Fig. 127 c.**

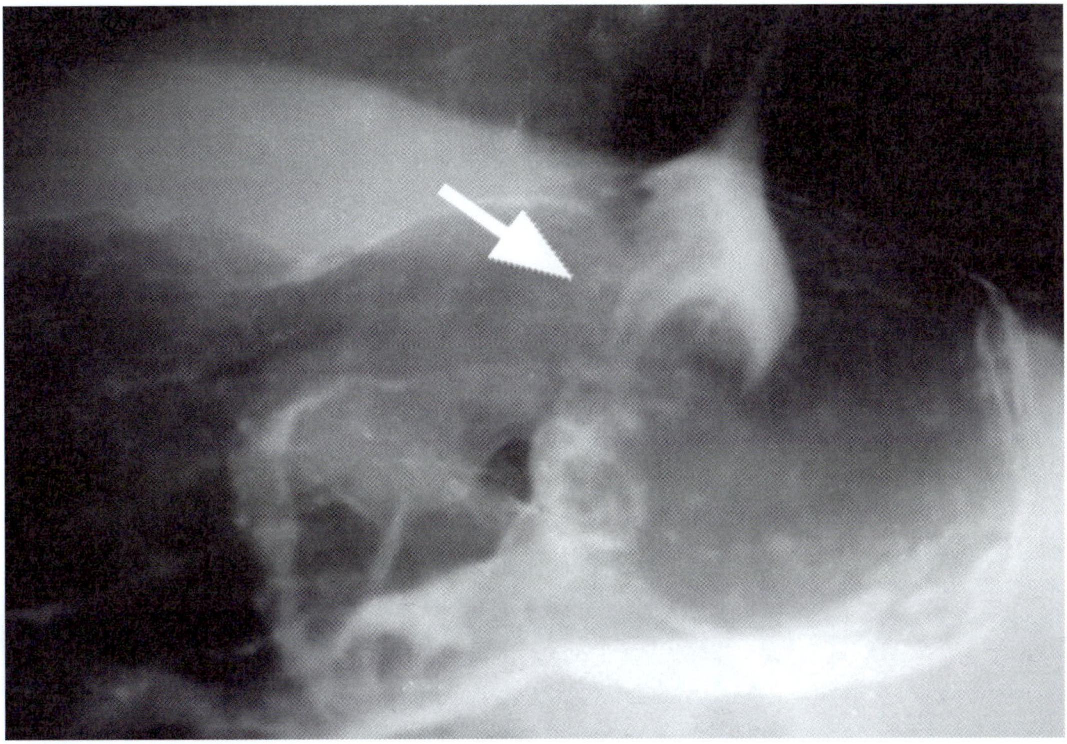

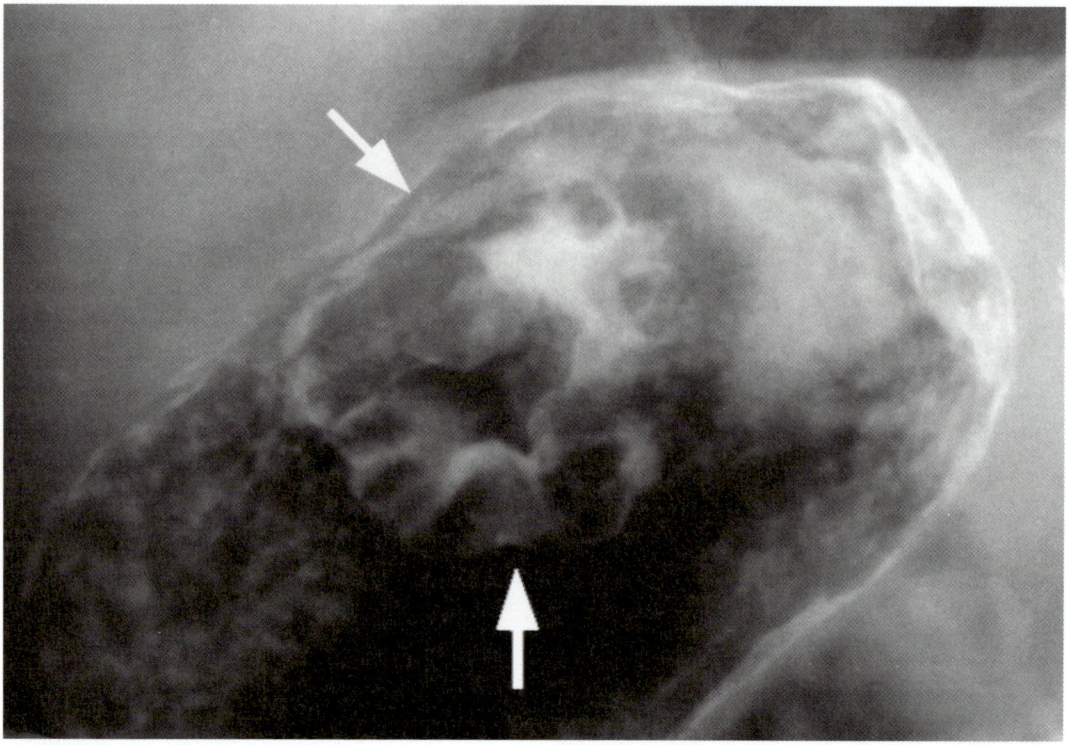

▲ Fig. 127 d.

▼ Fig. 127 e.

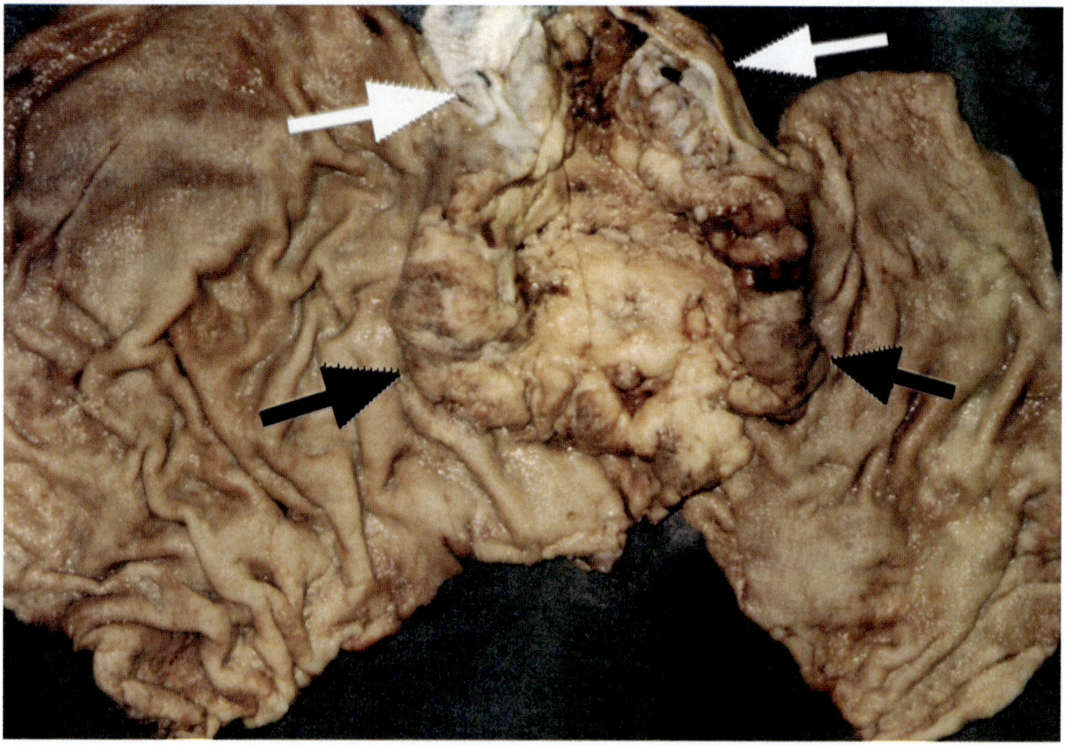

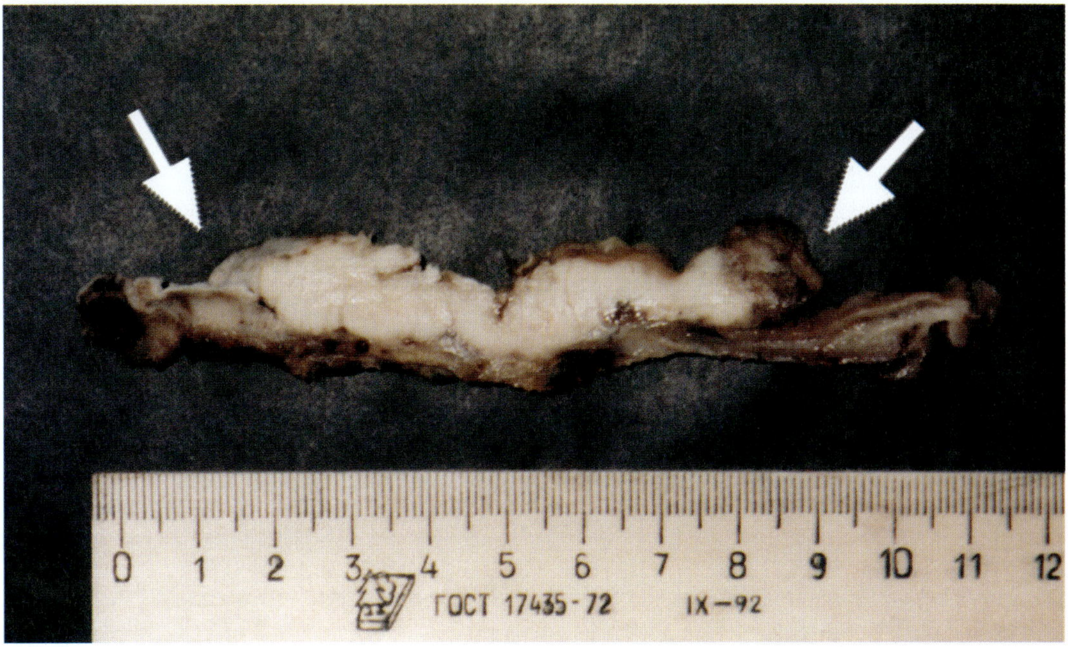

▲ **Fig. 127 f.**

Before discussing radiological semiotics, it is necessary to dwell on some aspects that are characteristic for this localization. Opinion has it that cardioesophageal cancers are different in some aspects from tumors in other parts of the stomach. This pertains mostly to exophytic growth, considerable association with intestinal metaplasia, histological differentiation which is more conspicuous compared with cancers of other localizations in the stomach, etc. Therefore, the sign proposed by Kirklin (1939) is still considered to be the main one in roentgenological diagnosis of proximal gastric cancer. However, according to our observations, diffuse tumors generally prevail in the upper part of the stomach. We observed a predominantly intramural character of tumor propagation in more than 70% of cases of blastomatous affection of the upper part of the stomach. In other cases, we usually observed mixed growth of the tumor (■ Fig. 127).

While appreciating the serious research conducted by many authors, we explain this phenomenon as follows. Keeping in mind the role of submucous infiltrative cancers, we think that the tumor most probably spreads from the underlying parts (the greater curvature in particular). Infiltrative cancer known as linitis plastica, which affects the entire stomach, has long been known. Spread of the tumor in the proximal direction was reported by T. Okamoto et al. (1988), and Levin at al. (1990). They noted that affection of the upper part of the stomach is characteristic more of young patients than of the elderly. At the same time, the problem of diagnosing infiltrative cancer of the upper part of the stomach remains unsolved.

8

Radiological Examination in Screening for Gastric Cancer

Improvement of the early diagnosis of malignant new growths is among the most important problems in the Russian health-care system. Gastric cancer remains one of the leading pathologies in the structure of oncological morbidity and mortality.

Early diagnosis of gastric cancer is important for the long-term results of treatment. Thus, the 5-year postoperative survival of patients in whom cancer is diagnosed in its early stage is 95–100% [168, 251, 268]. But despite the introduction of endoscopy into practical medicine the diagnosis of gastric cancer has not improved. The early diagnosis of gastric cancer patients does not exceed 1–3%, which indicates a very low efficacy of the existing organizational forms of screening. As before, gastric cancer is detected in patients in its third or fourth stage, when the potential of radical surgery is very low (Fig. 150). So-called test laparotomies or forced palliative operations are done in 13–28% of cases [76]. In mass-scale examinations of groups at risk

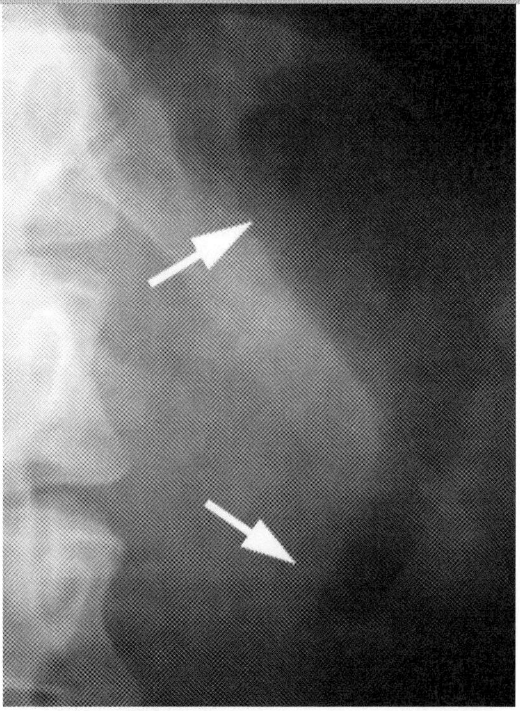

▲ **Fig. 150 a.**

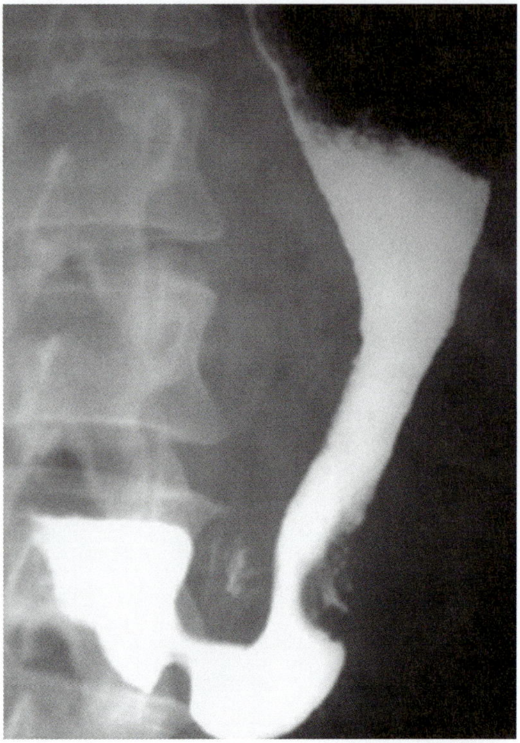

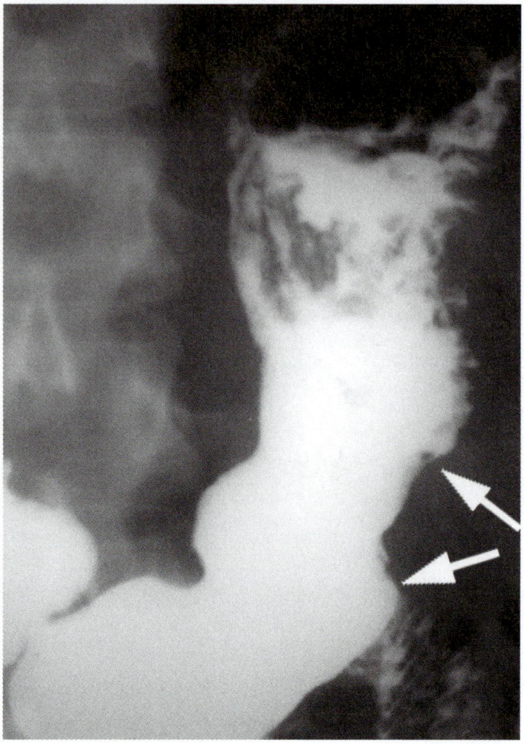

▲ **Fig. 150 b.** ▼ **Fig. 150 c.** ▲ **Fig. 151 a.**

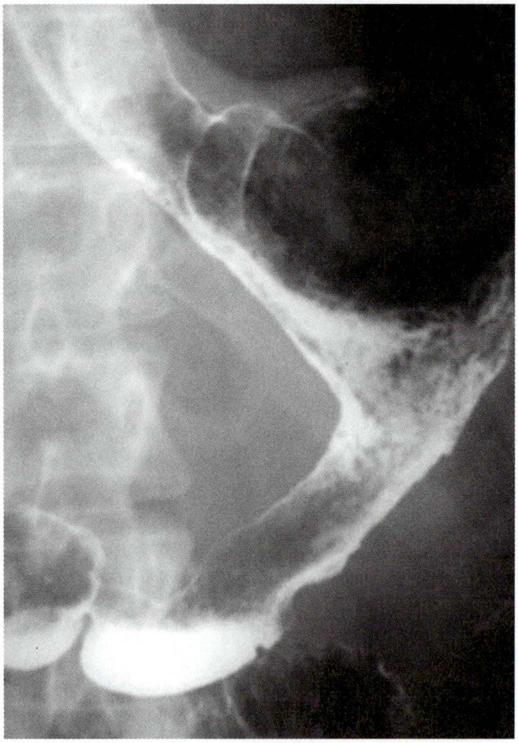

Fig. 150a–c. Patient P., age 60. Diagnosis: gastric cancer. **a** Stomach roentgenogram (vertical position, anterior projection): sign of gas redistribution in the air bubble; the air bubble has the shape of a comma; the stomach walls are thickened (arrows). **b** Stomach roentgenogram (tight filling, vertical position, anterior projection): the capacity of the stomach is diminished; the stomach is disfigured (rigid tube), it contours are uneven. **c** Stomach roentgenogram (double contrast, horizontal position, anterior projection): circular infiltration of the distal part and the body of the stomach, marked rigidity of the walls. Conclusion: Infiltrative cancer of the stomach.

Fig. 151a–d. Patient N., age 52. Diagnosis: gastric cancer. The patient has no complaints. From anamnesis: gastric cancer patient in the family. **a** Stomach roentgenogram (tight filling, vertical position, anterior projection): uneven and eroded contour of the greater curvature in the lower third of the stomach body (arrows). **b** Stomach roentgenogram (double contrast, horizontal position, anterior projection): the walls of the lower third of the stomach body are thickened due to circular infiltration (arrow). Conclusion: Infiltrative cancer of the lower third of the stomach body. **c** Macrospecimen of the resected stomach: the wall is firm, white intramural infiltration is seen (arrow). **d** Fragments of the macrospecimen (strips): the stomach walls are thickened due to intramural infiltration (arrows). Histologically, signet-ring cell carcinoma.

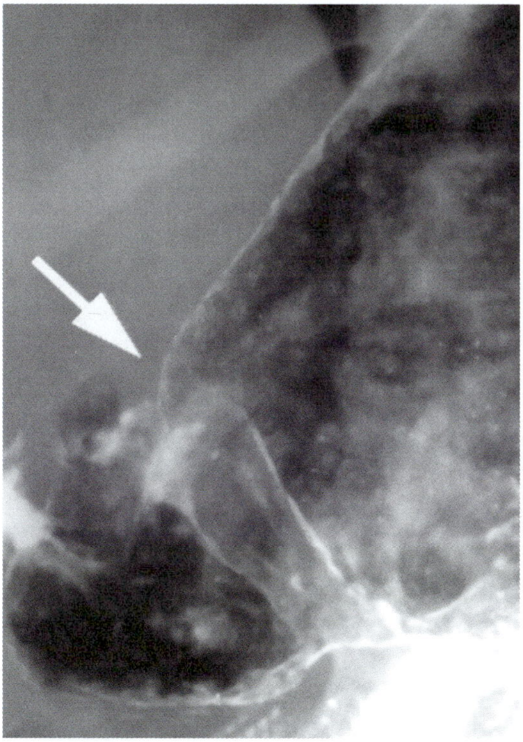

▲ **Fig. 151 b.**

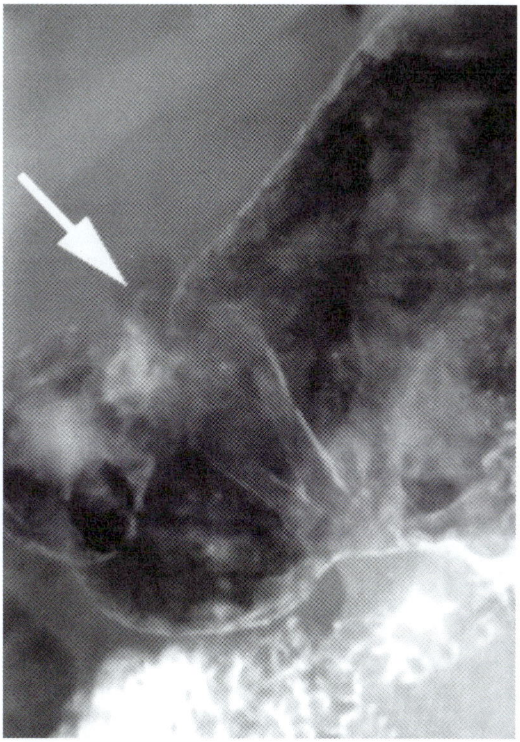

▲ **Fig. 151 b.**

▼ **Fig. 151 c.**

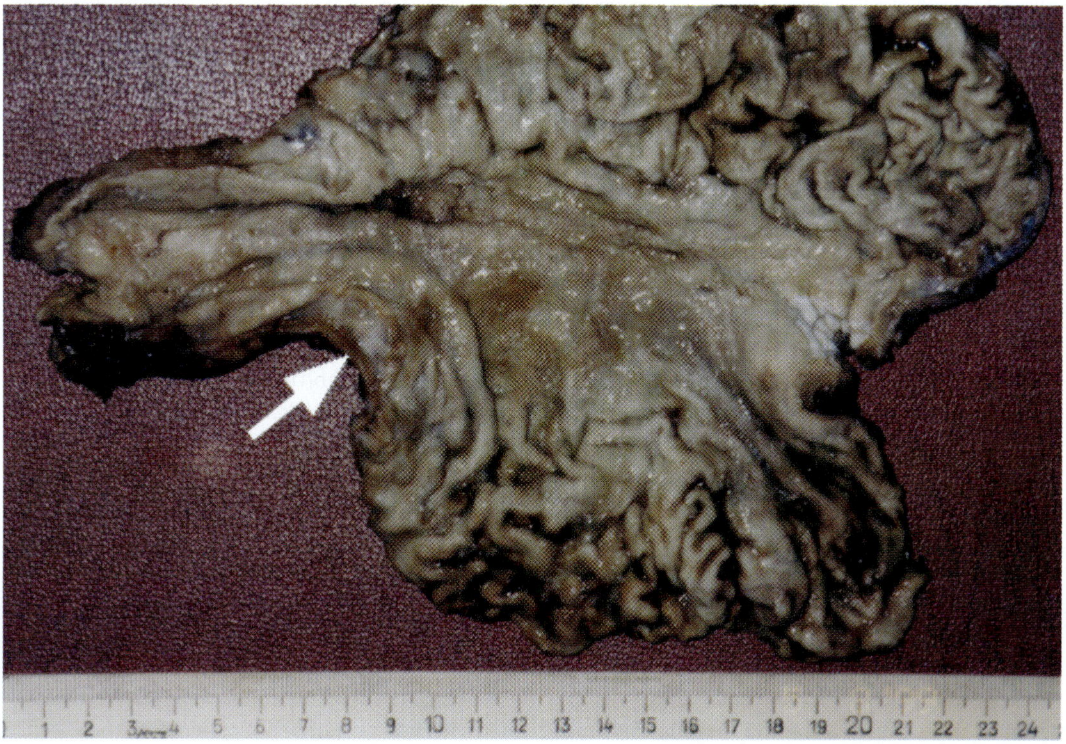

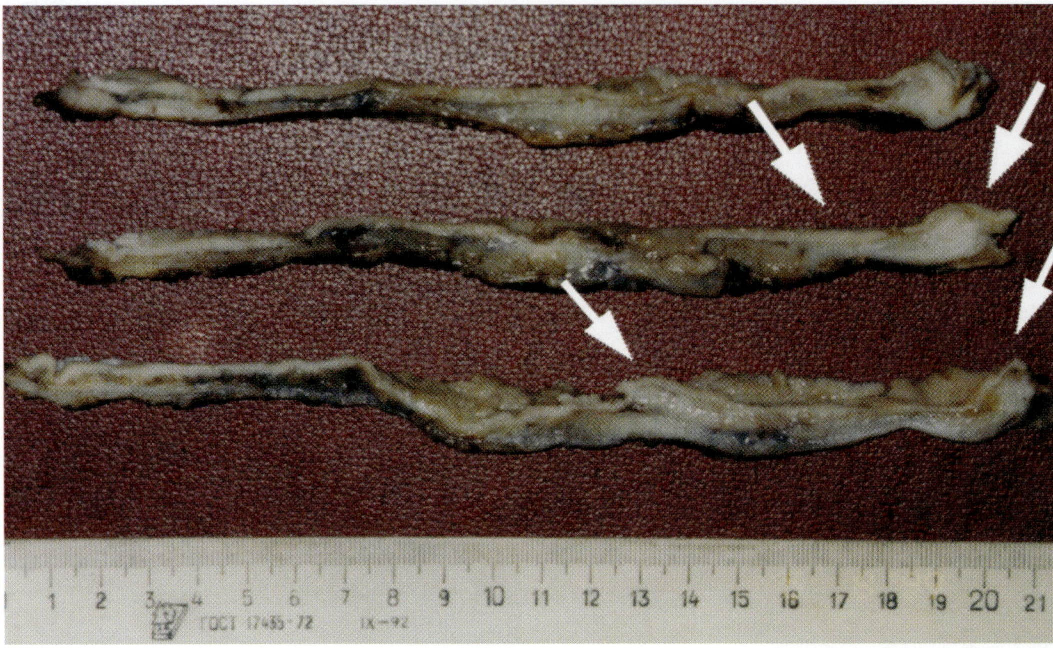

▲ **Fig. 151 d.**

for gastric cancer, the proportion of disease revealed in its initial forms increases to 30–40%, while mass-scale screening of a whole population increases this to 45.7% [143, 223]. This implies that further advances in gastric cancer control depend largely on improvement of the organizational system, based on the principle of active detection of the disease at the stage when, in the absence of clinical symptoms, the patient does not seek medical aid (Fig. 151).

The problem of screening for gastric cancer has long been discussed in the medical literature. The authors allude to the experience of Japan, which developed and introduced to practical use a program for active detection of gastric cancer. The program is oriented at diagnosis of the early forms of gastric cancer and is based on radiological examination with subsequent selective endoscopy. Thus, the 5-year survival is on the whole higher among patients in whom gastric cancer was diagnosed as a result of screening than among patients in whom the disease was diagnosed during a visit to the doctor (86% versus 61%, respectively) [134].

In Russia, the program of selective screening for gastric cancer, based on an initial X-ray examination with subsequent selective endoscopy, was undertaken in the Moscow region (population 5 million) [57, 58, 223]. MONIKI is one of the medical institutions where, in 1980, a special department was equipped with a Toshiba unit for gastrofluorography of the stomach. We have examined more than 36 000 patients. This made it possible to summarize the accumulated experience in selective screening for gastric cancer [52, 56, 57].

An important stage was the formation of groups of persons who were examined by X-ray methods. Most of the subjects selected were patients who did not have any special complaints of gastric dysfunction but were assigned to the risk group for gastric cancer. They were selected by questioning at various clinical departments (hematological, endocrinological, neurological, and others). The following factors were taken into account: familial susceptibility, long-standing nutritional disorders, abuse of alcohol or smoking tobacco, and other risk factors. In addition, we conducted planned outpatient examinations of subjects with chronic diseases of the stomach, mostly chronic gastritis with reduced acidity of the gastric juice, anemic patients, and patients who visited the doctor for the first time because of various forms of gastric discomfort.

Using standard methods, we effectively examined a very large number of patients. In the absence of organic pathologies, X-ray views were taken in the standard projections and subsequently studied (the obligatory component of examination). If changes were detected in the stomach, the number of X-ray views necessary was decided by the radiological diagnostician individually in each particular case.

In evaluating the results, we want to point out the advantages of test examinations, during which the proportion of detected tumors of the stomach extending over a distance 3–4 cm was three times less than during examination of patients with clinical signs of gastric pathology. On the whole, of the 36 000 selectively screened subjects, gastric cancer was diagnosed in 680 patients (1.94%); in 170 of them (25%) the muscular coat was not invaded (■ Fig. 152) [75].

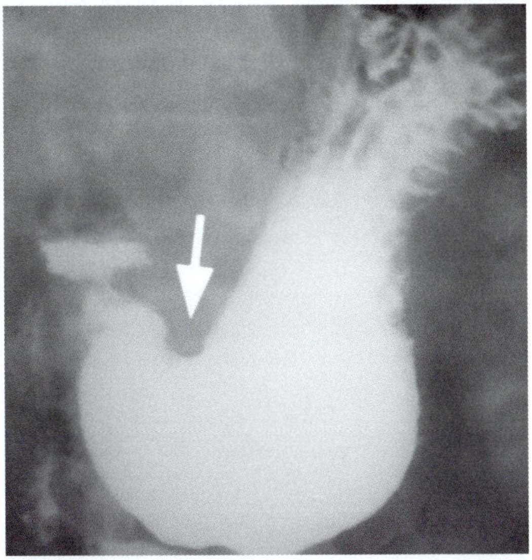

▲ Fig. 152 a. ▼ Fig. 152 b.

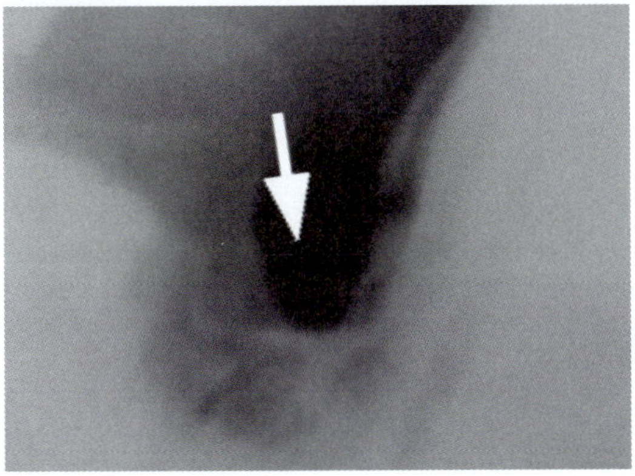

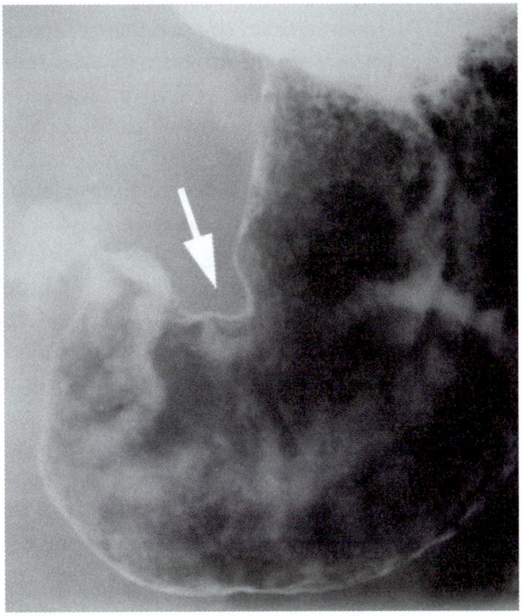

▲ Fig. 152 c. ▼ Fig. 152 d.

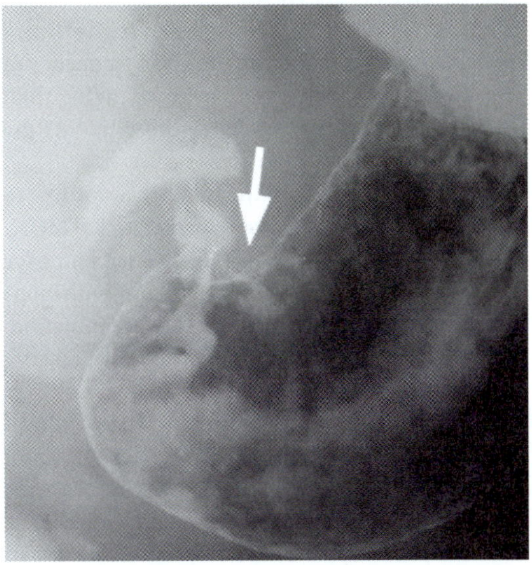

■ **Fig. 152a–d.** Patient Z., age 58. Diagnosis: gastric cancer. **a** Stomach roentgenogram (tight filling, vertical position, anterior projection): uneven contour of the lesser curvature (arrow). **b** Stomach roentgenogram (tight filling, vertical position, left half-oblique projection), dosed compression: more distinctly visualized is uneven contour of the lesser curvature of the antral part (arrow). **c, d** Stomach roentgenograms (double contrast, horizontal position, right anterior oblique projection): the wall of the lesser curvature is thickened and rigid due to intramural infiltration (arrow). Conclusion: Infiltrative cancer of the lesser curvature of the antral part of the stomach.

A comparison of the efficacy of gastric cancer detection by various screening programs shows that screening of risk groups is more effective. As we have already indicated, the frequency of gastric cancer detection in such investigations is 1.94%, much higher than the average in mass-scale screening in Japan (0.12%) or in the countries of Latin America (0.4%). However, in selective screening, only subjects predisposed to tumor disease are examined, and the percentage of cancer patients detected is therefore much higher than during mass-scale outpatient screening. While estimating the frequency of early gastric cancer detection, it is necessary to indicate that selective screening programs are much less effective compared with mass-scale screening of a population. In Japan, for example, early gastric cancer was diagnosed in 57.6% cases of cancer patients, whereas at MONIKI the rate was only 25%. The main objective of any screening program is to reduce mortality and to increase the 5-year survival. Although these parameters are far worse at MONIKI than in Japan, we can still report a sufficiently high efficacy of selective screening, because the 25% frequency of early gastric cancer detection is much higher than the statistical average at specialized hospitals in Russia and in most other countries (5–7%).

X-ray examinations of the stomach according to the complex standard method worked out at MONIKI to evaluate the efficacy of selective screening for gastric cancer included fibergastroscopy with biopsy as the main additional method of examination. Endoscopy was indicated for subjects with any deviation from the X-ray standard, namely, malignant and benign tumors, ulcers, marked hypertrophy of the mucosal folds, including Ménétrier's disease, various deformations of the stomach, etc. Patients who needed a additional examination were directed to the endoscopist. These amounted to 6–7% of the X-ray examined subjects, not exceeding 3–4% in the group of outpatient subjects who had no significant complaints, and 8–9% of patients with marked gastric complaints (◘ Fig. 153) [30, 56, 223].

Since gastrofluoroscopy does not rule out the danger of ionizing radiation for large population groups, equivalent and effective doses were first measured. Tissue doses were determined by the method of thermoluminescent dosimetry on an anthropomorphic phantom, with full modeling of conditions of the method worked out. The overall time of 60 exposures was determined; simultaneously, we determined the duration of exposure to high voltage at all stages of the cycle. The total time of radiation exposure was 33 s. It appeared that during fluoroscopy of the stomach, the equivalent load on the bone marrow, the stomach, the liver, the kidneys, and the spleen is much lower according to our program than with other modifications of X-ray examinations. The effective dose was about 1.43 mSv. Note that the effective dose in traditional fluoroscopy with image enhancement (without spot filming) is 2.2 mSv, and without image enhancement – 4.2 mSv/min; with one X-ray picture taken, the equivalent dose is 1.1 mSv. Thus, screening according to our method significantly reduces the effective dose. Modern digital X-ray units reduce it by 20–30 times, some of them even by 40 times. By using computer technologies to process the findings and doing away with

▼ Fig. 153 a.

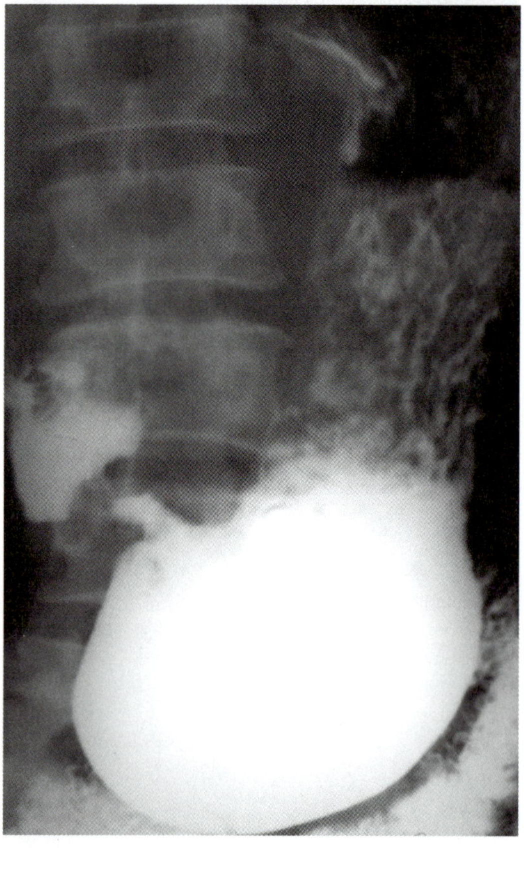

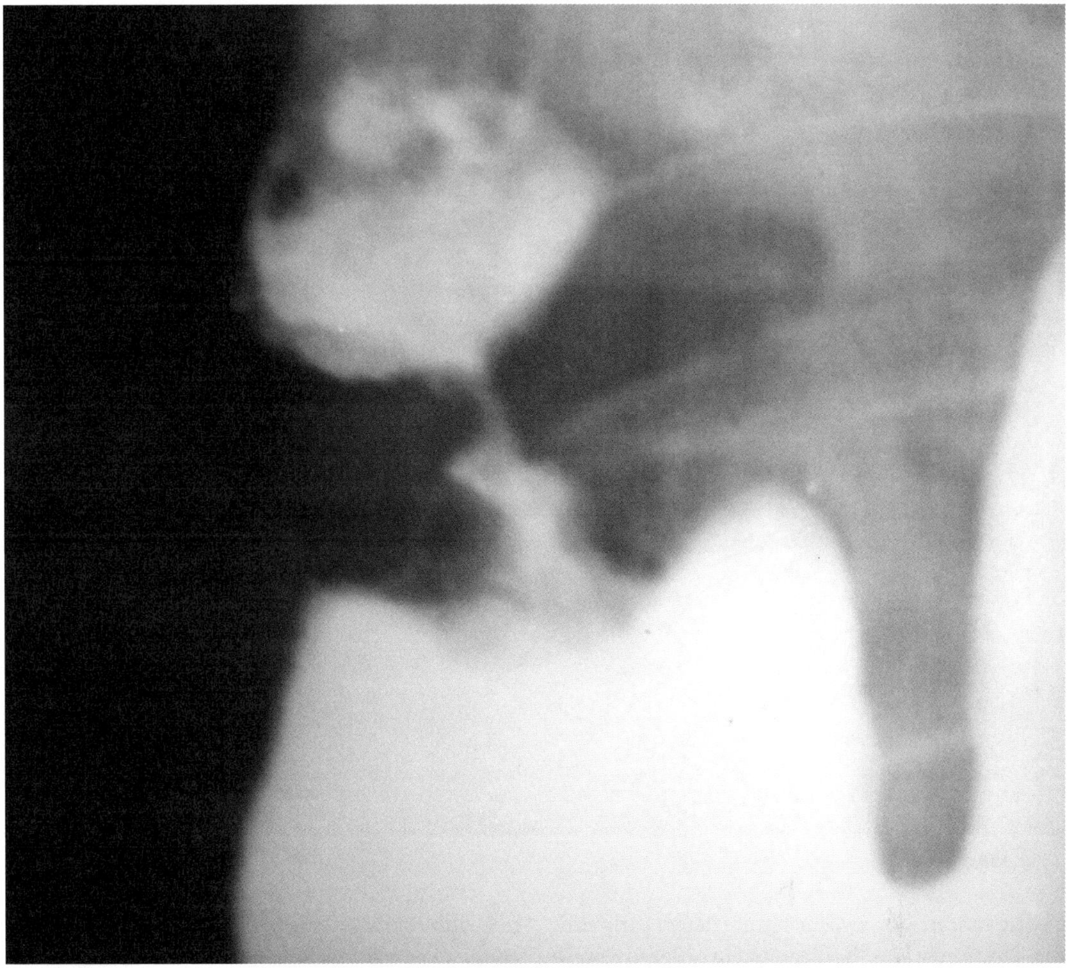

▲ **Fig. 153 b.**

■ **Fig. 153a–c.** Patient L., age 61. Diagnosis: gastric cancer. Complaints of gastric discomfort after meals. Occasional vomiting in the evenings. **a** Stomach roentgenogram (tight filling, vertical position, anterior projection): the sinus and the antral part are ectatic; marked deformation of the pyloric part. **b** Stomach roentgenogram (tight filling, vertical position, anterior projection): the pyloric part is unevenly narrowed due to circular infiltration; the evacuation function of the pylorus is disordered. **c** Stomach roentgenogram (double contrast, horizontal position, anterior projection): the walls of the pyloric part are thickened and rigid, the intramural infiltration spreads to the lesser curvature of the antral part of the stomach (arrows). Conclusion: Infiltrative cancer of the pyloric part of the stomach. Endoscopy reveals marked narrowing of the pyloric part of the stomach. Histological examination of the bioptates taken during endoscopy verified signet-ring cell carcinoma.

film technology, the radiologist will be able to increase the zone of his interest, increase or decrease the contrast of the image, measure the extent of infiltration of the stomach wall, conduct three-dimensional reconstruction, etc. The effective dose in these cases will be so insignificant that the discussion about the danger of ionizing radiation for the patient will be precluded.

China conducted its own screening. Their method was based on determining micro amounts of blood in gastric contents. A patient swallows a test strip, which is then pulled back from the stomach with a thin string within a few minutes. If blood is contained in the stomach in micro quantities, the strip changes color. In other words, this is a qualitative test for the presence of blood in the stomach. The test should by no means be considered specific for

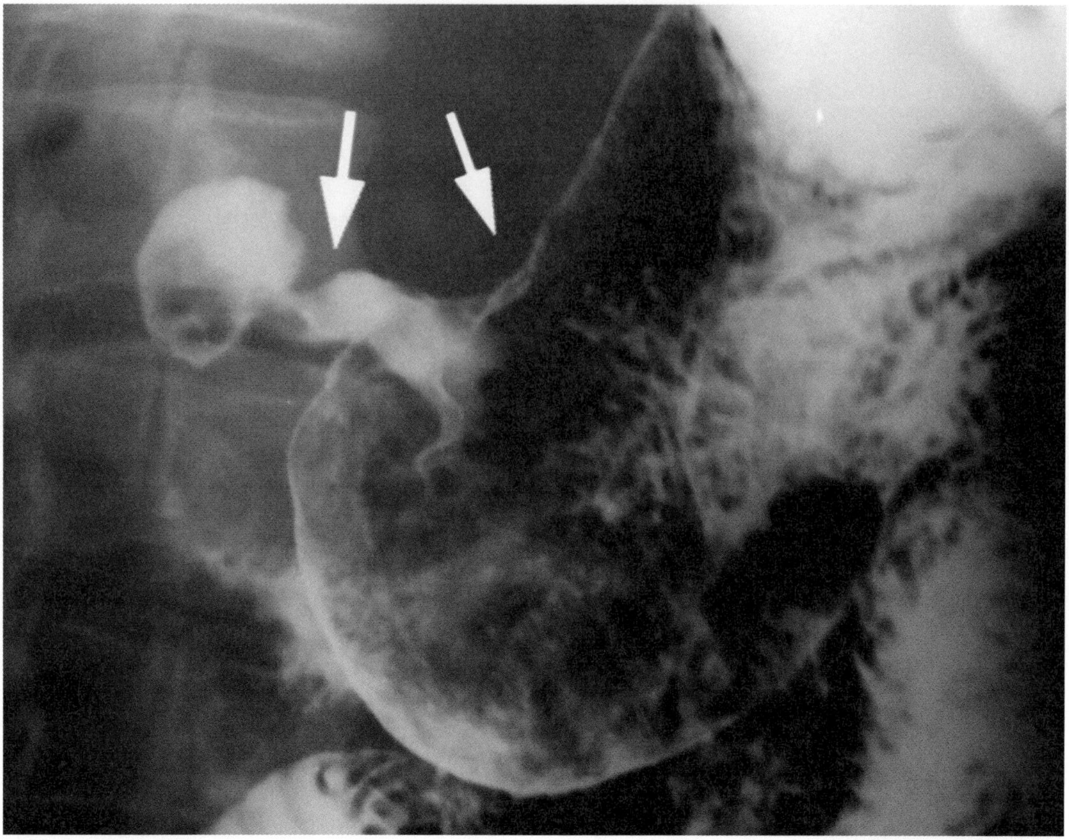

▲ **Fig. 153 c.**

gastric cancer. Moreover, it cannot detect early cancer: The tumor must be ulcerated in order to release blood into the stomach cavity. It therefore follows that this test cannot be used in screening for gastric cancer. Its only indisputable benefit is low cost.

An active search for ways to increase the efficacy of the method with simultaneous reduction of its cost continues. Screening for pre-cancerous conditions is one of them. It has long been known that patients with atrophic gastritis are a risk group for gastric cancer. It has been established that decreased concentration of pepsinogen I and a changed pepsinogen I-to-pepsinogen II ratio closely correlates with atrophy of the gastric mucosa. ELISA data on serum pepsinogen I also indicate its reduced concentration in gastric cancer patients: the lower the differentiation, the lower this level. But the pepsinogen I level is lower in patients with chronic atrophic gastritis than in patients with highly differentiated cancer of the stomach.

In healthy subjects, the pepsinogen I level in the serum is 123.6 ±11.7 ng/ml. In patients with highly differentiated gastric cancer it is 58.2 ±3.5 ng/ml, in those with less differentiated cancer 37.4 ±3.4 ng/ml, and in patients with atrophic gastritis 51.1 ±4.7 ng/ml [25].

It is believed that the sensitivity and specificity of determination of the pepsinogen level for the diagnosis of gastric cancer in the screening program are 84.6% and 73.5%, respectively. This is not bad for an indirect diagnostic method. But it should be remembered that this approach may be informative for the detection of only certain types of gastric cancer, i.e., cancers originating in the presence of atrophic gastritis, namely, distal gastric cancer. Atrophic changes are not an obligatory companion of proximal cancer of the stomach, the incidence of which has increased dramatically in recent years. A similar situation occurs with inclusion of serological markers of antibodies to H. pylori in screening programs, because it is mostly distal cancer of the stomach that is associated with H. pylori infection. It follows that if we use these screening programs, we will miss one third of gastric cancer patients. Such screening by no means meets our requirements. In addition, many problems require verification as regards H. pylori. The problem needs thorough studies.

It can thus be definitely concluded that, in the near future, screening programs based on the traditional X-ray examination with subsequent selective endoscopy will remain one of the most effective ways of increasing the efficacy of gastric cancer detection, especially at its early stages. It should be admitted, however, that mass-scale screening of a population for gastric cancer is an expensive enterprise and can be conducted only with adequate financial support from the government. As for Russia, selective screening may be acknowledged as practicable based on financial considerations, although its efficiency in revealing early forms of gastric cancer is lower. Therefore, it is necessary to be especially careful in selecting subjects into risk groups, and this work should be done by physicians of prophylactic and therapeutic medical institutions.

Of course we do not mean the extensive use of gastrofluorography, which is now outdated. But experience in selective screening, which has been accumulated at MONIKI, suggests its sufficiently high efficiency. In accordance with the concept adopted by the Ministry of Health of the Russian Federation concerning the development of radiological diagnosis up to 2010, this method can become the basis for early diagnosis of gastric cancer.

To conclude the discussion of screening for gastric cancer, it is necessary to emphasize some aspects which, we think, include all major problems connected not only with screening but with the general gastric cancer problem. Unfortunately, some are of the opinion that the study of most problems connected with gastric cancer has already been completed. They refer to the diagnosis of gastric cancer, where the leading role belongs to endoscopy. They also refer to treatment, where the main efforts are directed at further introduction of surgical operations into practical medicine; this can help patients with pronounced forms of cancer. But they almost completely disregard the problem of diagnosing gastric cancer in its initial stages. This discouraging situation will not change as long as this tendency persists, and this is especially discouraging, because gastric cancer makes up 10–12% of all oncological diseases in most regions of the world, Russia included.

Summary

In our monograph we have tried to demonstrate the infeasibility of excluding radiological diagnosis, first and foremost the traditional X-ray examination, from the algorithm for diagnosing gastric cancer. We have produced convincing evidence and explanations for the indispensability of the X-ray, which should be used along with endoscopy.

The current morphological and clinical characteristics of gastric cancer suggest that only the combined use of X-ray and endoscopy can change the discouraging situation with regard to relatively early diagnosis of the disease. Radical change is also very difficult without screening. Selective screening may become a reasonable alternative in countries with limited economic potential, Russia included. It is very important to attach greater importance to outpatient services in the attempt to improve the control of the disease. Diagnosis and treatment might thus be radically facilitated. Therefore, the tendency to minimize outpatient use of X-ray examinations works against improving the diagnosis of gastric cancer. All these aspects are discussed in detail in the monograph.

Although the main purpose of the monograph is to describe the current role of the X-ray examination in the diagnosis of gastric cancer, the book also covers some problems related to the epidemiology and morphology of the disease in order to disprove the existing underestimation of X-ray potential in early diagnosis.

While describing radiological diagnosis, we dwell on its methodological and semeiotic principles, as well as on the special importance of each method. These include the traditional radiological and ultrasonographic methods, computed tomography, and magnetic-resonance imaging. While we value these methods, above all MRI, unlike some other researchers, we rely not only on endoscopy but also on the traditional X-ray, because we believe it greatly increases the objective value of the findings and potentials of each separate method.

A special chapter in the monograph is dedicated to our view of the relationship between endoscopy and X-ray in the diagnosis of gastric cancer. The particular value of the clinical findings, which are included in practically all chapters, is their dependability based on surgical and anatomical evidence.

We realize that it will be very difficult to change existing views on gastric cancer diagnosis, where priority is given to endoscopy alone.

This position is, unfortunately, taken not only by health-care authorities and most clinicians, but also by some leading radiological diagnosticians. All we can do is ask them to read this monograph, which is based on more than 30 years of continuous practical experience. It is our firm conviction that this book can contribute to solving the vitally important problem of diagnosing gastric cancer.

References

Publications in Russian (in English titles in parentheses).

1. Антонович ВБ (1987) Рентгенодиагностика заболеваний пищевода, желудка, кишечника. (**Radiological diagnosis of esophagus, stomach and intestine**). М.: Медицина
2. Араблинский ВМ, Мамонтов АС, Седых СА (1992) Комплексная лучевая диагностика в определении распространенности рака пищевода (**Complex radiological diagnosis in staging cancer of the esophagus**). Вестн. рентгенологии и радиологии. 1:32
3. Араблинский ВМ, Седых СА, Мамонтов АС и др (1991) Роль компьютерной томографии в диагностике регионарных метастазов рака пищевода и проксимального рака желудка (**CT diagnosis of regional metastases of cancer of the esophagus and the proximal part of the stomach**). Сов. медицина 9:26–29
4. Аруин ЛИ, Капуллер ЛЛ, Исаков ВА (1998) Морфологическая диагностика болезней желудка и кишечника (**Morphological diagnosis of gastrointestinal pathologies**). М.: Триада-Х
5. Богер ММ, Мордвинов СА (1988) Ультразвуковая диагностика в гастроэнтерологии. (**Ultrasonographic diagnosis in gastroenterology**). Новосибирск: Наука, p 158
6. Василенко ВХ, Раппопорт СИ, Сальман ММ и др (1989) Опухоли желудка. Клиника и диагностика. (**Stomach tumors: clinical course and diagnosis**). М.
7. Голдобенко ГВ, Канаев СВ, Кныш ВИ и др (1999) Рак желудочно-кишечного тракта-проблемы лучевой терапии (**Gastrointestinal cancers: radiological treatment**). Вопр. онкол. 45:198–201
8. Давыдов МИ, Германов АБ, Лагошный АТ и др (1998) Основные пути улучшения результатов хирургического лечения рака желудка (**Improving results of surgical treatment of gastric cancer**). Вопр. онкол. 44:499–503
9. Давыдов МИ, Лагошный АТ, Стилиди ИО, Тер-Ованесов МД (1996) Пути улучшения результатов хирургического лечения рака проксимального отдела желудка (**Improving**

results of surgical treatment of gastric cancer). Рос. онкол. журн. 1:17–19
10. Давыдов МИ, Тер-Ованесов МД (2000) Современная стратегия хирургического лечения рака желудка (**Strategies in surgery of gastric cancer**). Современная онкология. 2:4–11
11. Ивашкин ВТ, Портной ЛМ (1998) Нужны ли нам государственные стандарты применения лучевой диагностики в гастроэнтерологии? (**Radiological diagnosis standards: Are they necessary?**). Рос. журн. гастроэнтерол., гепатол., колопроктол. 8:27–35
12. Калиновский ВП, Гамаюнова ВБ, Шумаков АР, Хансон КП (2000) Радиоимунологический анализ сывороточного пепсиногена 1 у больных хроническим гастритом и раком желудка (**ELISA of serum pepsinogen 1 in chronic gastritis and gastric cancer**). Вопр. онкол. 46:153–155
13. Кармазановский ГГ Вилявин МЮ, Никитаев НС (1997) Компьютерная томография печени и желчных путей (**Computed tomography of liver and bile ducts**). М.: Паганель-Бук, р 358
14. Кишковский АН (1984) Дифференциальная рентгенодиагностика в гастроэнтерологии (**Differential diagnosis in gastroenterology**). М.: Медицина
15. Кузин МИ, Шкроб ОС, Беличенко ОИ и др (1991) Магнитно-резонансная томография в диагностике некоторых хирургических заболеваний (**Magnetic-resonance tomography in diagnosis of some surgical diseases**). Хирургия 9:107–113
16. Логинов АС (1988) Проблемы современной клинической гастроэнтерологии (**Problems of current clinical gastroenterology**). Хирургия. 12:134–136
17. Лемешко ЗА (1987) Об ультразвуковом исследовании желудка (**Sonographic examination of the stomach**). Клинич. медицина 6:67–71
18. Малиновский НН, Захаров ПИ, Терновой СК, Савчук БД (1987) Сочетанный метод КТ и гастроскопии в диагностике рака желудка (**Computed tomography and gastroscopy in diagnosis of gastric cancer**). Хирургия 11:8–11
19. Мамонтов АС, Бойко АВ, Соколов ВВ и др (1997) Диагностика рака пищевода. Т1-2 N0M0: Пособие для врачей (**Diagnosis of gastric cancer: Manual**). М.
20. Момот НВ, Поляк ЕЗ, Иваницкий СМ и др (1992) Компьютерная томография в диагностике рака желудка и оценке его распространенности (**Computed tomography in diagnosis of gastric cancer and its staging**). Вестн. рентгенологии и радиологии 3:34–39
21. Монахов АС (2001) Раннее выявление опухолевых заболеваний по цитогенетическим критериям, определяемым в лимфоцитах периферической крови (на примере рака желудочно-кишечного тракта у человека) (**Early detection of tumors by cytogenetic criteria in patients with gastrointestinal cancer**). Вопр. онкол. 47:401–407
22. Оота К и др (1982) Гистологическая классификация опухолей пищевода и желудка (**Histological classification of gastric and esophageal tumors**). Международная гистологическая классификация опухолей. № 18. Женева: ВОЗ, р 44
23. Пасечников ВД, Чуков 03 (2002) Эпидемиология рака желудка (**Epidemiology of gastric cancer**). Рос. журн. гастроэнтерол., гепатол., колопроктол. 3:18–26
24. Поддубный БК, Кувшинов ЮП, Кашин СВ и др (2002) Современные эндоскопические методики диагностики и лечения предопухолевой патологии и раннего рака желудка (**Endoscopic diagnosis and treatment of pre-tumor pathology and early gastric cancer**). Рос. журн. гастроэнтерол., гепатол., колопроктол. 3:52–56
25. Портной ЛМ (1979) К вопросу о рентгенологической диагностике «маленького» рака желудка (**X-ray diagnosis of minor gastric cancer**). Вестн. рентгенологии и радиологии. 6:29–35
26. Портной ЛМ (1985) О месте рентгенологии в диагностике рака желудка (**Role of X-ray examination in diagnosis of gastric cancer**). Вестн. рентгенологии и радиологии. 5:75–78
27. Портной ЛМ (1998) Современная лучевая диагностика в выявлении рака верхнего отдела желудка (**Modern radiological diagnosis of cancer of the upper part of the stomach**). Вестн. рентгенологии и радиологии. 5:13–21
28. Портной ЛМ (2001) Современная лучевая диагностика в гастроэнтерологии и гастроэнтероонкологии. (**Modern radiological diagnosis in gastroenterology and gastroenterooncology**). М.: Видар-М, р 218
29. Портной ЛМ, Денисова ЛБ, Сташук ГА и др (2000) Магнитно-резонансная томография в

диагностике рака желудка (по материалам рентгено-МРТ-анатомических сопоставлений) (**Magnetic-resonance tomography in diagnosis of gastric cancer**). Вестн. рентгенологии и радиологии. 5:26–40
30. Портной ЛМ, Дибиров МП (1991) Современные перспективы улучшения выявления рака желудка (Обзор литературы) (**Current prospects for improving diagnosis of gastric cancer**). Вестн. рентгенологии и радиологии. 1:57–60
31. Портной ЛМ, Дибиров МП (1993) Лучевая диагностика эндофитного рака желудка (**Radiological diagnosis of endophytic gastric cancer**). М.: Медицина, p 272
32. Портной ЛМ, Дибиров МП, Лесин ЕБ, Банина ВБ (1992) Рентгенологическая и эндоскопическая диагностика начального рака желудка (**Radiological and endoscopic diagnosis of early gastric cancer**). Рос. мед. журн. 2:16–22
33. Портной ЛМ, Ивашкин ВТ Казанцева ИА и др (2003) Современная лучевая диагностика рака желудка (**Current radiological diagnosis of gastric cancer**). Рос. журн. гастроэнтерол., гепатол., колопроктол. 3:22–43
34. Портной ЛМ, Казанцева ИА (1997) Современный подход к диагностике рака желудка (**New approach to diagnosis of gastric cancer**). Рос. журн. гастроэнтерол., гепатол., колопроктол. 4:16–22
35. Портной ЛМ, Казанцева ИА, Вятчанин ОВ и др (2003) Рак верхнего отдела желудка: современные проблемы его диагностики (**Cancer of the upper part of the stomach and its diagnosis**). Вестн. рентгенологии и радиологии. 1:4–22
36. Портной ЛМ, Казанцева ИА, Гаганов ЛЕ и др (2000) Диагностика эндофитного рака желудка (по материалам сопоставления лучевого и патоморфологического исследования) (**Diagnosis of endophytic gastric cancer**). Рос. онкол. журн. 4:12–25
37. Портной ЛМ, Казанцева ИА, Исаков ВА (1997) Диагностика рака желудка: состояние проблемы, перспективы совершенствования, клинико-морфологические аспекты (**Diagnosis of gastric cancer: problems and prospects for improvement**).Тер. архив. 69:42–48
38. Портной ЛМ, Казанцева ИА, Нефедова ВО, Чекунова ЕВ (1997) Современные возможности лучевой диагностики рака желудка (**Potentials of radiological diagnosis of gastric cancer**). Рос. онкол. журн. 5:7–14
39. Портной ЛМ, Казанцева ИА, Сташук ГА, Гаганов ЛЕ (2002) Современные проблемы и трудности диагностики проксимального рака желудка (**Current problems om diagnosis of distal cancer of the stomach**). Рос. журн. гастроэнтерол., гепатол., колопроктол. 4:31–41
40. Портной ЛМ, Казанцева ИА, Сташук ГА и др (2000) Современная лучевая диагностика рака желудка (сопоставление лучевых и морфологических методов исследования) (**Current radiological diagnosis of gastric cancer**). Вестн. рентгенологии и радиологии. 6:19–29
41. Портной ЛМ, Каушанская ПВ, Зильберт ЗП (1972) К вопросу о возможностях рентгенологического выявления рака большой кривизны желудка (**Potentials of X-ray diagnosis of cancer of the greater curvature**). Вестн. рентгенологии и радиологии. 2:73–81
42. Портной ЛМ, Легостаева ТБ, Трипатхи С (1998) Транс-абдоминальная ультрасонография в диагностике диффузного рака желудка (**Transabdominal sonography in diagnosis of diffuse gastric cancer**). Рос. журн. гастроэнтерол., гепатол., колопроктол. 3:50–55
43. Портной ЛМ, Легостаева ТБ, Яурова НВ, Гаганов ЛЕ (1999) Ультразвуковая диагностика рака желудка (**Sonographic diagnosis of gastric cancer**). Рос. онкол. журн. 4:22–29
44. Портной ЛМ, Марченко ВА, Конина ЕВ, Нефедова ВО (1978) К вопросу о роли пневмогастрографии в дифференциальной диагностике изъязвлений желудка (**Pneumogastrography in differential diagnosis of stomach ulceration**). Вестн. рентгенологии и радиологии. 1:11–19
45. Портной ЛМ, Марченко ВА, Конина ЕВ, Нефедова ВО (1978) Рентгенологическая диагностика язвенной болезни желудка на различных этапах ее лечения (**Radiological diagnosis of peptic ulcer at various stages of its treatment**). Вестн. рентгенологии и радиологии. 6:11–19
46. Портной ЛМ, Марченко ВА, Леонов ВА (1975) Клинико-рентгенологическая характеристика рака желудка у лиц молодого возраста (**Clinical and X-ray symptoms of gastric cancer in the**

young). Вестн. рентгенологии и радиологии. 6:21–28
47. Портной ЛМ, Нефедова ВО, Туровский БМ и др (1980) К вопросу о дифференциальной рентгенодиагностике изъязвлений большой кривизны желудка (**Differential X-ray diagnosis of ulceration of the greater curvature**). Вестн. рентгенологии и радиологии. 5:21–28
48. Портной ЛМ, Нефедова ВО, Чекунова ЕВ (1997) Возможности современной компьютерной томографии в диагностике рака желудка (**Computed tomography in diagnosis of gastric cancer**). Вестн. рентгенологии и радиологии. 3:7–14
49. Портной ЛМ, Романов ГА, Лесин ЕБ, Туровский БМ (1984) Современные возможности клинико-рентгеноэндоскопической диагностики эндофитного рака желудка (**Clinical, X-ray, and endoscopic diagnosis of endophytic gastric cancer**). Вестн. рентгенологии и радиологии. 2:5–11
50. Портной ЛМ, Рослов АЛ (1986) Ультразвуковое сканирование в диагностике заболеваний органов брюшной полости и забрюшинного пространства (Обзор литературы) (**Sonographic scanning in diagnosis of pathologies of the organs of the abdominal and retroperitoneal space**). Вестн. рентгеноогии и радиологии. 5:70–77
51. Портной ЛМ, Рослов АЛ, Дибиров МП (1991) Ультразвуковое исследование в диагностике опухолей желудка (**Sonographic examination in diagnosis of gastric tumors**). Вестн. рентгенологии и радиологии. 6:30–37
52. Портной ЛМ, Симованян КВ, Рослов АЛ (1988) К вопросу о малигнизации язвы желудка (Обзор литературы) (**Malignant transformation of peptic ulcer**). Вестн. рентгенологии и радиологии. 5:65–70
53. Портной ЛМ, Ставицкий РВ, Хасидашвили ИШ и др (1985) Дозиметрическое обоснование массового применения гастрофлюорографии (**Dosimetric substantiation of mass-scale gastrofluorophotography**). Вестн. рентгенологии и радиологии. 4:6–9
54. Портной ЛМ, Сташук ГА, Денисова ЛБ и др (2000) Современные возможности лучевой диагностики рака желудка (традиционное рентгенологическое, ультразвуковое, компьютерно-томографическое и магнитно-резонансно-томографическое исследования) (**Radiological diagnosis of gastric cancer: sonography,computed tomography, and magnetic-resonance tomography**). Мед. визуализация. 2:3–14
55. Портной ЛМ, Суренчик ВИ, Туровский БМ и др (1988) О стандартизации рентгенологического исследования желудка (**Standardization of X-ray examination of the stomach**). Вестн. рентгенологии и радиологии. 2:70–76
56. Портной ЛМ, Туровский БМ (1983) К вопросу о рентгенодиагностике органического стеноза выходного отдела желудка (**Radiological diagnosis of organic stenosis of the pyloric part of the stomach**). Вестн. рентгенологии и радиологии. 3:65–72
57. Портной ЛМ, Туровский БМ, Калужский АА (1983) К вопросу о современной крупнокадровой флюорографии желудка (**Large-frame fluorophotography of the stomach**). Вестн. рентгенологии и радиологии. 5:5–12
58. Портной ЛМ, Туровский БМ, Калужский АА и др (1986) Роль современной флюорографии в выявлении рака желудка при проведении диспансеризации населения (**Fluorophotography in detection of gastric cancer**). Вестн. рентгенологии и радиологии. 1:65–69
59. Портной ЛМ, Туровский БМ, Симовонян КВ, Калужский АА (1984) О месте двойного контрастирования в диагностике рака желудка (**Double-contrast radiology in diagnosis of gastric cancer**). Вестн. рентгенологии и радиологии. 4:27–34
60. Портной ЛМ, Тюрин ИЕ, Юрьев АС (2002) Лучевая диагностика в Российской Федерации: современное состояние и перспективы развития: Метод. пособие (**Radiological diagnosis in Russia**). М., p 98
61. Роман ЛД. Стойко ЮМ, Вербицкий АМ, Карачун АМ (2000) Дифференциальная диагностика хронической язвы и изъязвленного рака желудка (**Differential diagnosis of chronic ulceration of the stomach**). Вопр. онкол. 46:217–220
62. Роттенберг ВИ (1993) Опухоли желудка Патологоанатомическая диагностика опухолей человека: Руководство для врачей: В 2-х т. (**Tumors of the stomach: pathologo-anatomic diagnosis of human tumors**). Под ред. Краевского НА, Смолянникова АВ, Саркисова ДС М.: Медицина, p 543
63. Савельев ВС, Исаков ЮФ, Лопаткин ГА и др (1985) Руководство по клинической

10

эндоскопии (**Manual of clinical endoscopy**). М.: Медицина, p 543

64. Седых СА, Араблинский ВМ, Мамонтов АС (1995) Возможности КТ с денситометрией в уточнении местной распространенности рака пищевода (**Computed tomography with densitometry in verification of local spread of esophageal cancer**). Вестн. рентгенологии и радиологии. 3:43–44
65. Серов ВВ, Аруин ЛИ, Роттенберг ВИ и др (1985) Дисплазия и ранний рак желудка (**Dysplasia and early cancer of the stomach**). Архив патологии 11:6–13
66. Серов ВВ, Золоторевский ВБ, Берестова АА (1990) Ранний рак желудка: морфология, гисто- и морфогенез (**Early gastric cancer: morphology, histo-, and morphogenesis**). Архив патологии 5:70
67. Симонов НН, Гуляев АВ, Правосудов ИВ и др (1998) Приоритетные направления и перспективы в лечении рака желудка (**Trends in and prospects for treatment of gastric cancer**). Вопр. онкол. 44:246–250
68. Соколов ЮН (1975) О некоторых анатомических особенностях области привратника в рентгеновском отображении (**Specific anatomic features of imaging of the pyloric region.** Вестн. рентгенологии и радиологии. 6:5–17
69. Соколов ЮН, Антонович ВБ (1981) Рентгенодиагностика пищеварительного тракта (**X-ray diagnosis of gastric cancer**). М.: Медицина
70. Соколов ЮН, Усова НА, Рохлин ЭА (1975) Диагностика малых (начальных) раков желудка на новом этапе (**Diagnosis of minor gastric cancers**). Вестн. рентгенологии и радиологии. 2:5–18
71. Сташук ГА (2003) Магнитно-резонансное исследование желудка (методика, семиотика) (**Magnetic-resonance examination of the stomach**). Вестн. рентгенологии и радиологии. 2:32–41
72. Федоров СН, Белогубова ЕВ, Гуляев АВ и др(1998) Клонирование амплифицированных нуклеарных последовательностей ДНК члена семьи с высоким риском возникновения рака желудка (**Cloning of nuclear DNA sequences in a family with high risk for gastric cancer**). Вопр. онкол. 44:30–31
73. Фридман ЕГ, Слесарева ЮГ (1988) О роли рентгенологического исследования в выявлении раннего рака желудка (**X-ray examination in diagnosis of gastric cancer**). Сов. медицина 9:86–89
74. Чиссов ВИ, Старинский ВВ, Ковалев БН, Ременник ЛВ (1996) Состояние онкологической помощи населению Российской Федерации (**Oncologic aid to population in Russia**). Рос. онкол. журн. 1:5–12
75. Чиссов ВИ, Старинский ВВ, Ременник ЛВ и др (1997) Основные показатели состояния специализированной онкологической помощи населению России в 1996 г (**Specialized oncological aid to population of Russia in 1996**). М.
76. Шумаков АР, Федоров СН, Калиновский ВП, Хансон КП (1999) Анализ экспрессии генов пепсиногена А при раке желудка (**Pepsinogen A gene expression in gastric cancer**). Вопр. онкол. 45:238–240
77. Яров ВП, Саар ХЭ, Виллано НП (1991) Клиническое значение гистологической классификации рака желудка по Laurent (**Histological classification of gastric cancer after Laurent**). Вопр. онкол. 1:45–48

Publications in other languages

78. Aabakken L (1999) Clinical symptoms, endoscopic findings and histologic features of gastroduodenal non-steroidal anti-inflammatory drugs lesions. Int J Gastroenterol Hepatol 31:19–22
79. Aaron JB, Johnson CD, Stephens DH, et al (2001) Carcinoid tumors of the stomach: a clinical and radiographic study. Am J Radiol 176:947–951
80. Adashek K, Sanger J, Longmire WP (1979) Cancer of the stomach – review of consecutive ten-year intervals. Ann Surg 189:6–10
81. Admassie D (1996) Relative sensitivity of barium swallow examination in the diagnosis of esophageal pathology. East Afr Med J 73:201–203
82. Altshuler JH, Shaka JA (1966) Squamous cell carcinoma of the stomach. Review of the literature and report of a case. Cancer 19:831
83. American Joint Committee on Cancer (1983) Manual for staging of cancer, 2nd edn. Lippincott, Philadelphia, p 67
84. Angelleli G, Brindicci D, Macarini L (1991) La TC nello studio delle lesioni della parete del apparato digerente. Radiol Med 81:83–89

85. Antonioli DA, Goidman H (1982) Changes in the location and type of gastric adenocarcinoma. Cancer 50:775–781
86. Appelman HD (1992) A cohort study of stomach cancer in high-risk American population. Cancer 69:2867–2868
87. Aranha GV, Georgen R (1989) Gastric linitis plastica is not a surgical disease. Surgery 106:758–763
88. Auh YH, Lirn TH, Lee DH, et al (1994) In vitro MR imaging of the resected stomach with a 4,7-T superconducting magnet. Radiology 191:129–134
89. Award JA, Lee EY, Wang TC, et al (1990) Effect of mucosal thickening near gastric carcinoma on the endoscopic diagnosis of malignancy. Dig Dis Sci 35:317–320
90. Baert AL, Poex L, Marchal G, et al (1989) Computed tomography of stomach with water as an oral contrast agent. Technique and preliminary results. J Comput Assist Tomogr 13:633–636
91. Baife DM, Koehier RE, Karstaedt N, et al (1981) Computed tomography of gastric neoplasms. Radiology 140:431–436
92. Balthazar EJ, Siegel SE, Megibow AJ, et al (1995) CT in patients with scirrhous carcinoma of the GI tract: imaging findings and value for tumor detection and staging. Am J Roentgenol 165:839–845
93. Barrett NR (1950) Chronic peptic ulcer of the oesophagus and "oesophagitis". Br J Surg 38:175–182
94. Blaser MI, et al (1997) Helicobacter pylori strains are created equal: Should all be eliminated? Lancet 349:1020–1022
95. Blot WJ, Devesa SS, Kneller RW, Fraumeni JF (1991) Rising incidence of adenocarcinoma of the esophagus and gastric cardia. JAMA 255:1287–1289
96. Borrmann R (1926) Geschwulste des Magens und Duodenum. In: Henke F, Lubarsh 0 (eds) Handbuch der speziellen pathologischen Anatomie und Histologie, vol 4. Springer, Berlin, pp 3–34
97. Boyacioglu S, Dolar E, Acar Y, et al (1993) Ultrasonographic scoring system: an auxiliary to differential diagnosis of pathologies. J Clin Ultrasound 21:97–101
98. Breaux JR, Bringaze W, Chappius C, Coha I (1990) Adenocarcinoma of the stomach: a review of 35 years and 1710 cases. World J Surg 14:480–586
99. Cameron I, Marion R, Billi B, Brendan D (2001) Is Helicobacter pylori infection in childhood a risk factor for gastric cancer? Pediatrics 107:373–380
100. Capella C, Cornaggia M, Usellini L, et al (1984) Neoplastic cells containing lysozyme in gastric carcinomas. Pathology 16:87
101. Capella C, Frigerio B, Cornaggia M, et al (1984) Gastric parietal cell carcinoma – a newly recognized entity: light microscopic and ultrastructural features. Histopathology 8:813
102. Caron de Fromentel C, Soussi (1992)T P53 tumor suppressor gene: a model for investigating human mutagenesis. Genes Chromosome Cancer 4:1
103. Carter KJ, Schaffer HA, Ritchie WP Jr (1984) Early gastric cancer. Ann Surg 199:604
104. Chen MC, Tsang YM, Kung CH, et al (1993) Computed tomography of gastric carcinoma using water as a contrast agent. J Formos Med Assoc 92 [Suppl]:140–145
105. Chia MM, Langman JM, Hecker R, et al (1988) Early gastric cancer: 52 cases of combined experience of two South Australian teaching hospitals. Pathology 20:216
106. Cho JS, Kim JK (1994) Preoperative assessment of gastric carcinoma: value of two-phase dynamic CT with mechanical IV injection of contrast material. Am J Roentgenol 163:68–75
107. Coggon D, Barker DJP, Cole RB, et al (1989) Stomach cancer and food storage. JNCI 81:1178
108. Correa P (1985) Clinical implications of recent developments in gastric cancer pathology and epidemiology. Semin Oncol 12:2
109. Correa P (1992) Human gastric carcinogenesis: a multistep and multifactorial process: First American Cancer Society Award Lecture in Cancer Epidemiology and Prevention. Cancer Res 52:6735–6740
110. Correa P, Cuello C, Duque E (1970) Carcinoma and intestinal metaplasia of the stomach in Columbian migrants. JNCI 44:297
111. Craanen ME, Dekker W, Blok P, et al (1992) Time trends in gastric carcinoma: changing patterns of type and location. Am J Gastroenterol 87:572–579
112. Current Opinion (1998) Helicobacter pylori and gastric cancer. Highlights of an expert round-table workshop held in the UK, spring
113. Day DW (1987) The stomach. In: Morson BC (ed) Alimentary tract, vol 3. Churchill Livingstone, Edinburgh, p 149
114. Dux M, Roeren T, Kuntz C, et al (1997) MRI for staging of gastric carcinoma: first results of ex-

perimental prospective study. J Comput Assist Tomogr 21:66–72
115. Eaton H, Tennekoon GE (1972) Squamous carcinoma of the stomach following corrosive acid burns. Br J Surg 59:382
116. Eckardt VF, Giebler W, Kauzler G, et al (1990) Clinical and morphological characteristics of early gastric cancer. A case-control study. Gastroenterology 98:708–714
117. Elischer J (1911) Fortschr Rontgenstr 18:332
118. Esaki Y, Hirokawa K, Yamashiro M (1987) Multiple gastric cancers in the aged with special reference to intramucosal cancers. Cancer 59:560
119. Evans DMD, Cleary BK (1979) The sites of origin of gastric cancers and ulcers in relation to mucosal junctions and the lesser curvature. Invest Cell Pathol 2:97
120. Fiocca R, Villani L, Tenti P, et al (1987) Characterization of four main cell types in gastric cancer: foveolar, mucopeptic, intestinal columnar and goblet cells. An histopathologic, histochemical and ultrastructural study of „early“ and „advanced“ tumours. Pathol Res Pract 182:308
121. Fiocca R, Villani L, Tenti P, et al (1990) The foveolar cell component of gastric cancer. Hum Pathol 21:83
122. Fishman EK, Urban BA, Hruban RH (1996) CT of the stomach: spectrum of disease. Radiographics 16:298–300
123. Frohling W (1979) Fruherkennung des Magenkarzinom. Therapiewoche 29:1791–1792
124. Fuchs CS, Mayer RJ (1995) Gastric carcinoma. N Engl J Med 333:32–41
125. Fukuya T, Honda H, Kaneko K, et al (1997) Efficacy of helical CT in T-staging of gastric cancer. J Comput Assist Tomogr 21:73–81
126. Fujita S (1978) Biology of early gastric cancer. Pathol Res Pract 163:297
127. Fujita S, Hattori T (1977) Cell proliferation, differentiation and migration in gastric mucosa: a study on the background of carcinogenesis. In: Farber E (ed) Pathophysiology of cancerogenesis in digestive organs. Tokyo, pp 21–36
128. Funaco A, Tsubono Y, Tsuji I, et a (1995)I The evaluation of screening for gastric cancer in Miyagi Prefecture, Japan: a population-based case-control study. Int J Cancer 60:45–48
129. Griffin MR (1998) Epidemiology of nonsteroidal drug-associated gastrointestinal injury. Am J Med 104 [Suppl 3A]:23–29
130. Grin PHR, O'Tool KM, Slonim D, et al (1988) Increasing incidence and excellent survival of patients with early gastric cancer: experience in a US medical center. Am J Med 85:658–661
131. Gutmann RA (1956) Le diagnostic du cancer d'estomac a la periode utile. Paris
132. Gutmann RA (1960) Sur les cancers gastriques imisibles a l'operation. L'Union Med Canada 11:1351–1361
133. Hanazaki K, Sodeyama H, Wikabayashi M, et al (1997) Surgical treatment of gastric cancer detected by mass screening. Hepatogastroenterology 44:1126–1132
134. Hanssen LE, Nyre'n O, Hsing AW, et al (1996) Cancer in patients with gastric or duodenal ulcer disease. N Engl J Med 335:242
135. Harrison JC, Dean PJ, Vander Zwaag R, et al (1991) Adenocarcinoma of the stomach with invasion limited to the muscularis propria. Hum Pathol 22:III
136. Hasegawa S, Semelka RC, Noone TC, et al (1998) Gastric stromal sarcomas: correlation of MR imaging and histopathologic findings in nine patients. Radiology 208:591–595
137. Hassan HA, Sharma VK, Raufman J-P (2001) Changing trends in gastric carcinoma at a university medical center. A twelve-year retrospective analysis. J Clin Gastroenterol 32:37–40
138. Hattori T (1993) DNA ploidy pattern and cell kinetics. In: Nishi M, Ichikawa H, Nakajima T, et al (eds) Gastric cancer. Springer-Verlag, Tokyo, pp 184–195
139. Hattori T, Hosokawa Y, Fukuda M, et al (1984) Analysis of DNA ploidy patterns of gastric carcinomas of Japanese. Cancer 54:1591
140. Herrera-Goepfert R, Reyes E, Hernandes-Avila M, et al (1999) Epshtein-Barr virus-associated gastric carcinoma in Mexico: analysis of 135 consecutive gastrectomies in two hospitals. Mod Pathol12:873–878
141. Hilton DA, West KP (1992) c-erbB-2 oncogene product expression in gastric carcinoma. J Clin Pathol 45:454
142. Hirota T, Ochiai A, Itabashi M, et al (1991) Significance of histological type of gastric carcinoma as a prognostic factor. Stomach Intest 26:1149
143. Hisamichi S, Sugawara N (1983) Mass screening for gastric cancer by X-ray examination. Jpn J Clin Oncol 14:211–223
144. Hisamichi S, Sugawara N, Fukao A (1988) Effectiveness of gastric mass screening in Japan. Cancer Detect Prev 11:323–329

145. Holburt E, Freedman SI (1987) Gastric carcinoma in patients younger than age 36 years. Cancer 60:1395
146. Holscher AH, Bollschweiler E, Siewert JR (1995) Carcinoma of the gastric cardia. Ann Chir Gynaecol 84:185–192
147. Holzknecht G, Jonas S (1908) Die radiologische Diagnostik der intra- und extraventrikuloren Tumoren. Wien
148. IARC Monographs on the Evaluation of the Cancerogenic Risk (1994) Lyon, p 61
149. Ichikura T, Tomimatsu S, Okusa Y, et al (1993) Comparison of the prognostic significance between the number of metastatic lymph nodes and nodal stage based on their location in patients with gastric cancer. J Clin Oncol 11:1894
150. Ihekwaha TN, Solanke T (1984)F Carcinoma of the oesophagus. Br J Surg 71:116–118
151. Imazeki F, Omata M, Nose H, et al (1992) p53 mutations in gastric and esophageal cancer. Gastroenterology 103:892
152. Japanese Gastric Cancer Association (1998) Japanese classification of gastric carcinoma, 13th edn (in Japanese). Kanehara, Tokyo
153. Japanese Society for Esophageal Diseases (1995) Japanese Classification of gastric carcinoma, 1st English edn. Kanehara, Tokyo
154. Japanese Society for Esophageal Diseases (1999) Guidelines for the clinical and pathologic studies on carcinoma of the esophagus (in Japanese with English diagnostic terms), 9th English edn. Kanehara, Tokyo
155. Ji B-T, Chow W-H, Yang G, et al (1996) The influence of cigarette smoking, alcohol, and green tea consumption on the risk of carcinoma of the cardia and distal stomach in Shanghai, China. Cancer 77:2449
156. Karnei H (1984) Study of stroma in scirrhous gastric carcinoma. Nagoya J Med Sci 47:23–34
157. Karnei H, Watanabe T, Terabe K, et al (1984) Study of stroma in scirrhous gastric carcinoma. Nagoya J Med Sci 47:23–34
158. Kang BC, Kirn JH, Kim KW, et al (2000) Value of the dynamic and delayed MR sequence with Gd-DTPA in the T-staging of stomach cancer: correlation with the histopathology. Abdom Imaging 25:14–24
159. Komaki S (1986) Gastric carcinoma. In: Meyers MA (ed) Computed tomography of the gastrointestinal tract. Springer, NY pp 23–54
160. Korenaga D, Saito A, Baba H, et al (1990) Cytophotometrically determined DNA content, mitotic activity, and lymph node metastasis in clinical gastric cancer. Surgery 107:262
161. Kastan MB, Oyekwere O, Sidransky D, et al (1991) Participation of p53 in the cell response to DNA damage. Cancer Res 51:6304
162. Kato I, Tominaga S, Ito Y, et al (1990) A comparative case-control analysis of stomach cancer and atrophic gastritis. Cancer Res 50:6559
163. Kato M, Saji S, Kanematsu M, et al (2000) Detection of lymph-node metastases in patients with gastric carcinoma: comparison of three MR imaging pulse sequences. Abdom Imaging 25:25–29
164. Kelsen D (1982) Treatment of advanced esophageal cancer. Cancer (Philadelphia) 50:2576–2581
165. Kernohan N, Cox L (1996) Regulation of apoptosis by bcl-2 and its related protein: immunohistochemical challenges and therapeutic implications. J Pathol 179:1–3
166. Kirn J-P, Hur YS, Yang H-K (1995) Lymph node metastasis as a significantly prognostic factor in early gastric cancer: analysis of 1,136 early gastric cancers. Ann Surg Oncol 2:308–313
167. Kim JJ, Jung HC, Song IS, et al (1997) Preoperative evaluation of the curative resectability of gastric cancer by abdominal computed tomography and ultrasonography: a prospective comparison study. Korean J Intern Med 12:1–6
168. Kitaoka H, Yoshikawa K, Hirota T, et al (1984) Surgical treatment of early gastric cancer. Jpn J Clin Oncol 14:283
169. Kiwamu O (1997) Gastric cancer screening program in Japan. World Gastroenterol News May:24–25
170. Klauber MR, Lyon (1978)L Gastric cancer in a coal mining region. Cancer 41:2355
171. Kocher HM, Linklater K, Patel S, et al (2001) Epidemiological study of oesophageal and gastric cancer in south-east England. Br J Surg 88:1249–1257
172. Kodama Y, Inokuchi K, Soejima K, et al (1983) Growth patterns and prognosis in early gastric carcinoma. Superficially spreading and penetrating growth types. Cancer 51:320
173. Krajewski S (1995) Immunohistochemical determination of in vivo distribution of Bax? A dominant inhibitor of bcl-2. Am J Pathol 146:20–26
174. Kuerbitz SJ, Plunkett BS, Wash WB, et al (1992) Wild type p53 is a cell cycle checkpoint determinant following irradiation. Proc Natl Acad Sci U S A 89:7491

10

175. Laheij RJ, Strootman H, Verbeek AL, Jansen JB (1999) Mortality trend from cancer of the gastric cardia in the Netherlands 1969–94. Int J Epidemiol 28:391–395
176. Lane DP (1989) Worrying about p53. Curr Biol 2:581
177. Lauwers GY Scott GV, Karpeh MS (1995) Immunohistochemical evidence of bcl-2 protein expression in gastric adenocarcinomas. Cancer 75:2209
178. Laurent PA (1965) The two histologic main types of gastric carcinoma. Acta Pathol Microbiol Scand 64:34
179. Laurent PA, Nevalainen JT (1993) Epidemiology of intestinal and diffuse types of gastric carcinoma: a time-trend study in Finland with comparison between studies from high- and low-risk areas. Cancer 71:2926–2933
180. Lee DH (2000) Two-dimensional and three-dimensional imaging of gastric tumors using spiral CT. Abdom Imaging 25:1–6
181. Levin MS (1995) Role of double-contrast upper gastrointestinal series in the 1990s. Gastroenterol Clin North Am 24:289–308
182. Levin MS, Creteur V, Kressel H, et al (1987) Benign gastric ulcers: diagnosis and follow-up with double-contrast radiography. Radiology 164:9–13
183. Levin MS, Rubesin SE, Herlinger G, et al (1988) Double-contrast upper gastrointestinal examination: technique and interpretation. Radiology 168:593–602
184. Levin MS, Kong V, Rubesin SE, et al (1990) Scirrhous carcinoma of the stomach: radiologic and endoscopic diagnosis. Radiology 175:151–154
185. Lutz H, Petzolt R (1976) Ultrasonic patterns of space-occupying lesions of the stomach and the intestine- Ultrasound Med Biol 2:129–132
186. Maartmann-Moe H, Hartviet F (1990) Underdiagnosis of carcinoma of the stomach and the elderly: a 25-year autopsy study. Eur J Surg Oncol 16:417–422
187. Maetani S, Tobe T, Hirakawa A, et al (1980) Parametric survival analysis of gastric cancer patients. Cancer 46:2709
188. Margulis AR, Brandt DJ (1989) The changing face of gastrointestinal radiology. Semin Roentgenol 24:231–238
189. Maruyama K, Baba Y (1994) Gastric carcinoma. Radiol Clin North Am 32:1233–1252
190. Matsusaka T, KodamaY, Soejima K, et al (1980) Recurrence in early gastric cancer. A pathologic evaluation. Cancer 46:168
191. Matsushita M, Oi H, Murakami T, et al (1994) Extraserosal invasion in advanced gastric cancer: evaluation with MR imaging. Radiology 192:87–91
192. Murayarna H, Imai T, Kikuchi M (1983) Solid carcinomas of the stomach. A combined histochemical, light and electron microscopic study. Cancer 51:1673
193. McCormick D, Hall RA (1992) The complexities of proliferating cell nuclear antigen. Histopathology 21:591–594
194. Miller AB (1978) Asbestos fibre dust and gastrointestinal malignancies, review of literature with regard to a cause/effect relationship. J Chronic Dis 31:23
195. Minami M, Kawauchi N, Niki T, et al (1992) Gastric tumors: radiologic-pathologic correlation and accuracy of CT staging with dynamic CT. Radiology 185:173–178
196. Ming S-C (1986) Classification of gastric carcinoma. In: Filipe MI, Jass JR (eds) Gastric carcinoma. Churchill Livingstone, Edinburgh, p 197
197. Ming S-C (1973) Tumors of the esophagus and stomach. In: Atlas of Tumor Pathology, 2nd edn, Fascicle 7. AFIP, Washington, DC
198. Ming S-C, Goidman H, Freiman DG (1967) Intestinal metaplasia and histogenesis of carcinoma in human stomach. Light and electron microscopic study. Cancer 20:1418
199. Misiewicz JJ, Pounder RE, Venables CW (1988) Diseases of the gut and pancreas. London, 3:385–386
200. Misumi A, Misumi K, Murakami A, et al (1989) Endoscopic diagnosis of minute, small and flat early gastric cancers. Endoscopy 21:159–164
201. Moertel CG, Bargen JA, Soule EH (1957) Multiple gastric cancers. Review of the literature and study of 42 cases. Gastroenterology 32:1095
202. Mod M, Iwashita A, Enjoji M (1986) Adenosquamous carcinoma of the stomach. Cancer 57:333
203. Mori H, Soeda O, Kamano T, et al (1982) Choriocarcinomatous change with immunocytochemically hCG-positive cells in the gastric carcinoma of the males. Virchows Arch A Path Anat 396:141
204. Mori M, Enjoji M, Sugimachi K (1989) Histopathologic features of minute and small human gastric adenocarcinomas. Arch Pathol Lab Med 113:926–931
205. Morson BC, Sobin LH, Grundmann E, et al (1980) Precancerous conditions and epithelial dysplasia in the stomach. J Clin Pathol 33:711

206. Motoyama T, Saito K, Iwafuchi M, et al (1985) Endodermal sinus tumor of the stomach. Acta Pathol Jpn 35:497
207. Murakami T (1972) Pathomorphological diagnosis. Definition and gross classification of early gastric cancer. Early gastric cancer. Gann Monograph on Cancer Research, no 11. University of Tokyo Press, p 53
208. Nakatani H, Sakamoto H, Yoshida T, et al (1990) Isolation of an amplified DNA sequence in stomach cancer. Jpn J Cancer Res 81:707
209. National Cancer Institute (1994) Annual cancer statistic review: 1973–1991. Department of Health and Human Services, Bethesda, Md.
210. Neugut A, Hayek M, Howe G (1996) Epidemiology of gastric cancer. Semin Oncol 23:281–291
211. Nevalainen T, Jarvi OH (1977) Ultrastructure of intestinal and diffuse type gastric carcinoma. J Pathol 122:129
212. Okada M, Kojima S, Murakami M, et al (1983) Human gastric carcinoma: prognosis in relation to macroscopic and microscopic features of the primary tumor. J Natl Cancer Inst 71:275
213. O'Connor PM, Jackman J, Jondle D, et al (1993) Role of p53 tumor suppressor gene in cell cycle arrest and radiosensitivity of Burkitt's lymphoma cell lines. Cancer Res 53:4776
214. Ohguri T, Sato Y, Koizumi W, et al (1993) An immunohistochemical study of c-erbB-2 protein in gastric carcinomas and lymph node metastases: is the c-erbB-2 protein really a prognostic indicator? Int J Cancer 53:75
215. Oi H, Matsushita M, Murakami T, Nakamura H (1997) Dynamic MR imaging for extraserosal invasion of advanced gastric cancer. Abdom Imaging 22:35–40
216. Oohara T, Aono G, Ukawa S, et al (1984) Clinical diagnosis of minute gastric cancer less than 5 mm in diameter. Cancer 53:162–165
217. OPCS Mortality statistics 1974–1985. HMSO, London
218. Orlowska J, Jarosz D, Pachlewski J, Butruk E (1995) Malignant transformation of benign epithelial gastric polyps. Am J Gastroenterol 90:2152–2159
219. Parkin PM (2001) Global cancer statistics in the year 2000. Lancet Oncol 2:533–543
220. Parkin PM, Pisani R, Ferlay J Estimates of the worldwide incidence of twenty-five major cancers in 1990. Int J Cancer 80:827–841
221. Polotsky BE (1992) Some aspects of multiple esophageal and gastric cancer. Semin Surg Oncol 8:46–49
222. Portnoi LM, Dibirov MP (1995) Radiodiagnosis of endophytic gastric cancer. Begell House, NY, Wallingford (UK)
223. Portnoi LM, Kazantseva IA, Isacov VA, Nefedova VO, Gaganov LE (1999) Gastric cancer screening in selected population of Moscow region: retrospective evolution. Eur Radiol 9:701–705
224. Portnoi LM, Denisova LB, Nefedova VO, et al (2000) Accuracy of MRI of diseases of the stomach. European Congress of Radiology, SS1401a: Scientific Programme and Book of Abstracts. Vienna, p 223
225. Portnoi LM, Denisova LB, Nefedova VO, et al (2000) Efficacy of MRI in determining tumor size and local expansion of gastric carcinoma. European Congress of Radiology, SS1401a: Scientific Programme and Book of Abstracts. Vienna, pp 222–223
226. Potente G, Ossi MF, Torriero F, et al (1994) Computed tomography in the preoperative staging of gastric cancer. Radiol Med (Torino) 87:76–81
227. Radi MJ, Fenoglio-Preiser CM, Bartow SA, et al (1986) Gastric carcinoma in the young: a clinicopathological and immunohistochemical study. Am J Gastroenterol 81:747
228. Ruck P, Wehrmann M, Campbell M, et al (1989) Squamous cell carcinoma of the gastric stump. A case report and review of the literature. Am J Surg Pathol 13:317
229. Rodi W (1997) „Neue Morphologie" in der Pancreasdiagnostic – Ultraschall, Computertomografie. Verh Dtsch Ges Pathol 7:231–238
230. Rossi M, Broglia L, Maccioni F, et al (1997) Hydro-CT in patients with gastric cancer: preoperative radiologic staging. Eur Radiol 7:659–664
231. Rybak DJ (1987) Early gastric carcinoma diagnosis in Japan: radiologic, endoscopic, and pathologic alert. Mt Sinai J Med 54:413–416
232. Saitoh H, Okuno Y, Suzuki M, et al (1997) Various manifestations of early and advanced gastric cancer in gastrointestinal series (GIS). Radiat Med 15:259–265
233. Sandier RS, Holland KL (1987) Trends in gastric cancer sex ratio in the United States. Cancer 59:1032
234. Scatarige JC, Di Santis DJ (1989) CT of the stomach and duodenum. Radiol Clin North Am 27:687–706
235. Schlemper RJ, Itabashi M, Kato Y, et al (1998) Differences in the diagnostic criteria used by Japanese and Western pathologists to diagnose colorectal carcinoma. Cancer V. 82:60–69

10

236. Schlemper RJ, Kato Y, Stolte M (2001) Review of classification of gastrointestinal epithelial neoplasia: differences in diagnosis of early carcinomas between Japanese and Western pathologists. J Gastroenterol 36:445–456
237. Schlemper RJ, Riddel RH, Kato Y, et al (2000) The Vienna classification of gastrointestinal neoplasia. Gut 47:251–255
238. Shino Y, Watanabe A, Yamada Y, et al (1995) Clinicopathologic evaluation of immunohistochemical E-cadherin expression in human gastric carcinomas. Cancer 76:2193
239. Shirakade H (1972) Double contrast studies of the stomach. Thieme, Stuttgart
240. Shirakade H, Nishirawa M, Shigeo K (1982) Atlas of X-ray diagnosis of early gastric cancer. Idaku-Shoin, Tokyo, NY
241. Shirakawa T, Fukuda K, Tada S (1996) New method for evaluation of perigastric invasion of gastric cancer by right lateral position CT. Eur Radiol 6:358–361
242. Sohn KM, Lee JM, Lee SY, et al (2000) Comparing MR imaging and CT in staging of gastric carcinoma. Am J Roentgenol 174:1551–1557
243. Solcia E (1996) Intestinal and diffuse gastric cancers arise in a different background of helicobacter pylori gastritis through different gene involvement. Am J Surg Pathol 20 [Suppl 1]:8–22
244. Spigelman AD, Murday V, Phillips RKS (1989) Cancer and Peutz-Jeghers syndrome. Gut 30:1588
245. Stehr PA, Gloninger MF, Kuller LH, et al (1985) Dietary vitamin A deficiency and stomach cancer. Am J Epidemiol 121:65
246. Stemmermann GN, Brown C (1974) A survival study of intestinal and diffuse types of gastric carcinoma. Cancer 33:1190
247. American Joint Committee on Cancer (1992) Stomach. Manual for staging of cancer, 4th edn. Lippincott, Philadelphia, pp 63-67
248. Stout AP (1942) Superficial spreading type of carcinoma of the stomach. Arch Surg 44:651
249. Suehiro S-I, Nagasue N, Abe S-I, et al (1986) Carcinoma of the stomach in atomic bomb survivors. A comparison of clinicopathologic features to the general population. Cancer 57:1894
250. Sussman SK, Halvorsen RA, Illeskas FF, et al (1988) Gastric adenocarcinoma: CT versus surgical staging. Radiology 167:335–340
251. Sue-Ling HM, Martin I, Griffith J, et al (1992) Early gastric cancer: 46 cases in one surgical department. Gut 33:1318-1322
252. Tahara E (1995) Molecular biology of gastric cancer. World J Surg 19:484
253. Takahashi M, Hasegawa R (1986) Enhancing effects of dietary salt on both initiation and promotion stages of rat carcinogenesis. In: Hayashi Y (ed) Diet, nutrition and cancer. Scientific Societies Press, Tokyo, pp 169–182
254. Takahashi M, Kokubo T, Furukawa F, et al (1983) Effect of high salt diet on rat gastric carcinogenesis induced by N-methyl-N'-nitro-N-nitrosoguanidine. Jpn J Cancer Res 74:28
255. Takahashi M, Ota S, Shimada T, et al (1995) Hepatocyte growth factor is the most potent endogenous stimulant of rabbit gastric epithelial cell proliferation and migration in primary culture. J Clin Invest 95:1994
256. Takasu S, Tsuhiya H, Kitamura A, et al (1984) Detection of early gastric cancer by panendoscopy. Jpn J Clin Oncol 14:243–252
257. Takayama T, Shiozaki H, Shibamoto S, et all (1996) Beta-catechin expression in human cancers. Am J Patho 148:39
258. Tatsuta M, Okuda S, Taniguchi H (1981) Endoscopic diagnosis of early gastric cancer in the cardiac portion. Gastric Cancer 53:27
259. Tersmette AC, Offerhaus GJA, Tersmette KWF, et al (1990) Meta-analysis of the risk of gastric stump cancer: detection of high risk patient subsets for stomach cancer after remote partial gastrectomy for benign conditions. Cancer Res 50:6486
260. Thompson WM, Halvorsen RA, Foster WL, et al (1983) Computed tomography for staging esophageal and gastroesophageal cancer: reevaluation. Am J Roentgenol 141:951–958
261. Tsuburaya A, Nogushi Y, Matsumoto A, et al (1994) A preoperative assessment of adjacent organ invasion by stomach carcinoma with high-resolution computed tomography. Surg Today 24:299–304
262. Tsuda K, Hori S, Marakami T, et al (1995) Intramural invasion of gastric cancer: evaluation by CT with water-filling method. J Comput Assist Tomogr 19:941–947
263. Tsukuma H, Mishima T, Oshima A (1983) Prospective study of „early" gastric cancer. Int Cancer 31:421–426
264. Tsukuma H, Oshima A, Naraharab H, Moriic T (2000) Natural history of early gastric cancer: a non-concurrent, long-term, follow-up study. Gut 47:618–621

Printing: Krips bv, Meppel
Binding: Stürtz, Würzburg